AF716751

Medicine at Sea

The History and Practice of Medicine in the Field

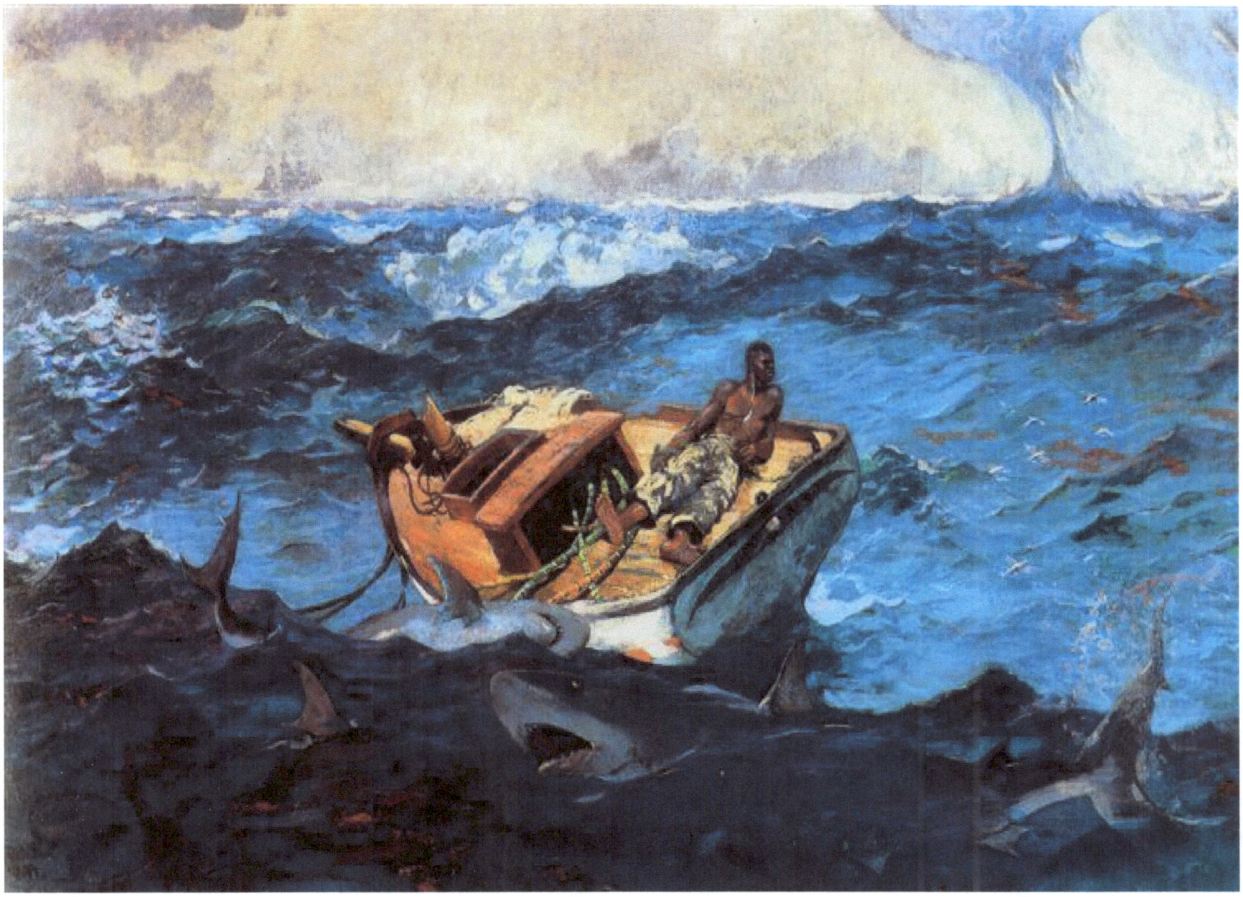

"The Gulf Stream" by Winslow Homer, Metropolitan Museum of Art

"To learn to pray, go to sea" 16th century Portuguese sailor proverb

Dr. Dickie Lynn Hill, USCG Ship's Surgeon

Medicine at Sea

Third Edition, copyright TXu 2-176-416
Paperback: 9798893973488
Hardback: 9798893973495
February 2025

For information or to purchase book contact
Dickie Hill
707-328-4884
dickiehilldo@yahoo.com

Foreword

"There are three sorts of people: those who are alive, those who are dead, and those who are at sea" —Aristotle

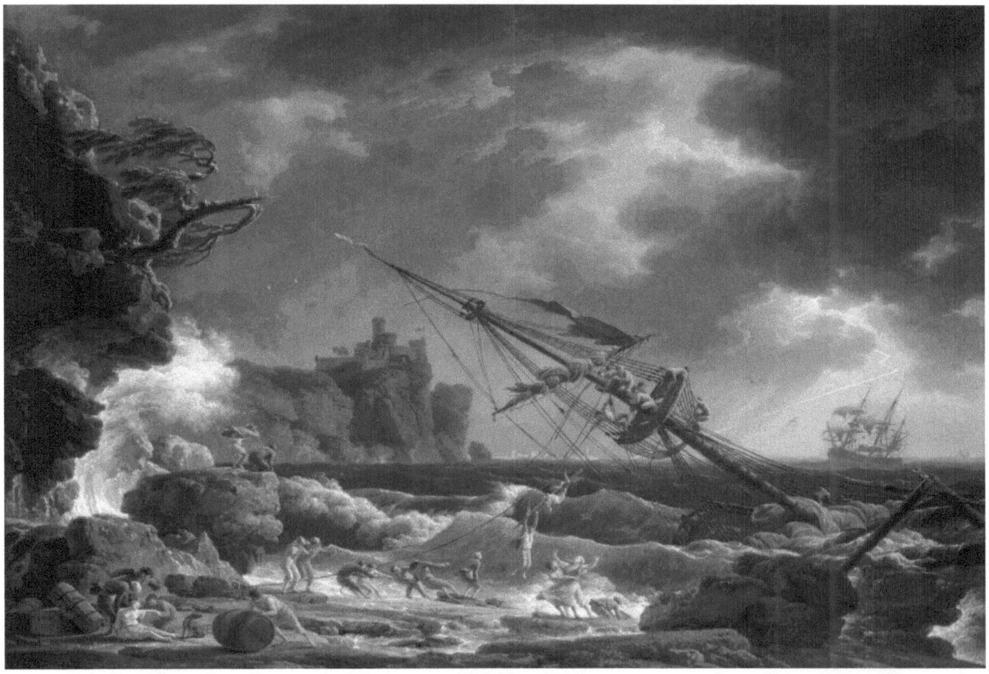

"The Shipwreck" Claude-Joseph Vernet, 1772. Going to sea has been and continues to be risky with storms, pirates, ill-found vessels and navigation mistakes endangering life and limb.

The pages in this text are about the history, science and practice of medicine at sea and in the field. The practical portion is written for those providing medical care in isolated environments of a ship, in the wilderness or after natural disasters where individuals with limited formal medical education may be pressed into duty. Similar circumstances have been common throughout history. Only in the last one century did medical education lasting several years. Before that, most medical care delivered at sea and on land was performed by men and in some cases women, with little to no formal medical education, trained by apprenticeship only. All too often, this medical care was not adequate.

This book started with a series of lectures that began in 1983 while the author began teaching at the California Maritime Academy in the graduate continuing maritime education and to the undergraduate midshipmen. In its earliest form, this text was little more than handouts of lectures in outline form. Sometime later, it came to the author's attention that these notes, with much missing information, had been copied and "bootlegged" onto sea going vessels, primarily in the Alaskan fishing fleets. The author was not displeased that lecture outlines were being used by people outside the classroom, but concerned that notes were incomplete, not well organized and did not represent the full context of the author's lectures. This, more than any other stimulus, brought about the first two editions of "Medicine at Sea".

Today, medical care at sea and in the field may be in the hands of lay officers with little formal medical training (when compared to professionally trained personnel). Very few ships carry physicians, nurses or other medical personnel, yet there are thousands of people at sea every day, some becoming ill or injured. This would be true on land in the event of an earthquake, hurricane or other large natural disaster, when medical centers are overwhelmed. In recent years, many communities have been stripped of their medical assets, at least in California with assets now concentrated in large vulnerable institutions. When the toilets quit flushing, these institutions will be mostly ineffective. It is fortunate that today sea-going personnel and others can prepare themselves with education that allows deployment of quality medical care in the field, provided they have access to a proper modern medicine chest.

It is the responsibility and the right thing, for the vessel's master, no matter the size of the ship, to provide health care. The same could be said for a family, community leaders and those that venture off the grid. Health care can be given competently with tools and skills available to non-physicians because of the innovations in the field of medicine in the last seventy years. Simple laboratory tests on urine are available, making it possible to diagnose diabetes, hepatitis, urinary tract infection, pregnancy, determine hydration, detect kidney stone, and kidney disease. The use of modern safe and effective antibiotics greatly increases the success of treating infections such as appendicitis, pneumonia, wound infections and other serious conditions that were often fatal until recently. More importantly, management of heart attack, trauma, shock and burns can be taught to lay people for emergency use.

For a nonprofessional medical person who might be pressed into service as a medical officer, these are exciting times. With training, outside reading, practice and a proper field medicine chest, one can provide a quality of diagnosis and treatment, never experienced by the great physicians of the past. The author told students at the beginning of each course, that if they travelled back in time to the Second World War, with the knowledge, training and equipment discussed in class, they would be one the premier field medical officers in the world! This text contains the author's own perspective on what this training should involve and the contents of a modern chest's contents. Some liberty has been taken in explaining the basic medical sciences such as physiology, biochemistry, pharmacology and others in the interest of making things flow. For this, the author apologizes to the purist. This book contains examples of stories that differ than what has been promoted as true and the author has tried to justify a different view of history. Current philosophy contends that it takes four years of premed followed by 5-8 years of graduate medical education to function as a medical officer whereas in the past a medical officer could be highly affected with little to no formal training.

The author wanted a book that would be readable, unlike many medical texts that only serve as a reference. This text will hopefully be more than a text to look up topics when medical problems arise but one that is enjoyable to read. There are numerous incidents where medicine in the field played large roles, both positive and negative in human history. In some cases, totally changing history with diseases, organisms and human behavior. Some of these stories are in the following pages. Medicine's foundation sciences of chemistry, microbiology, anatomy and physiology are included to remove some of medicine's mystery. The author's lectures and text used history as a major vehicle of instruction since students seemed to grasp medicine more completely. The author feels strongly that a better understanding of the past is important in the study of any topic, especially medicine. George Santayana's often quoted "Those that cannot remember the past are condemned to repeat it" is true today as it has in the past. Students complained that most textbooks are barren of illustrations. Several voiced that while reading the earlier "Medicine at Sea" editions, if several pages were void of pictures, continued reading was suppressed. Therefore, this text is heavily illustrated, the pictures giving both the reader and author a visual of the written words.

As a live-aboard sailor, former Naval medical officer and maritime medicine educator, the author has been fortunate to encouter people otherwise denied to the general public. Sailors are generally attentive as students and haved enhanced the author's library with thier personal "sea stories". One such encounter was with the captain of the Royal Dutch Shell tanker that refueled the submarine, the USS *Permit* in 1942 that evacuated Douglas MacArthur's staff and family off the island of Corrigador (this contradicts the offical accounts of MacArhur evacuation by tiny wooden PT boats over hundreds of miles of open ocean patrolled by Imperial Japanese warships and aircraft). McArthur was ordered to leave thousands of his stranded troops by direct orders of President Rosevelt. Troops who later endured the Bataan Death March and three years of brutal imprisonment. While the submarine took on fuel, the captain hosted the General and his of family and staff to dinner. Weeks later, the captain was forced to surrender his tanker and crew to Imperial Japan and begin internment in the Philipines. As a ship's comanding officer, the Dutch captain was incarcerated with General Wainwright and other senior officers where he witnessed the fevers and dysentaries of the POW camp that soon overwhelmed the medical officers. Assistants were trained, and after practice, elevated to medical officers as they had been throughout history. When the tanker captain was captured he wieghed 230 lbs, yet MacArthur immediately recognized him after years of harsh captivity at 130 lbs. After thanking him for the dinner and fuel during his escape, ask if he felt fit enough to command a tanker again. The US Navy had more ships than experienced captains and soon the Dutchman was commanding an American ship. Stories from an eyewitness to history's great events are part of the evolution of this book.

Another sea story comes from a former United States Marine enlisted tank commander, who fought and wounded on Okinawa. In the late 1960's, he finished a steel boat in Australia, and with little offshore experience, sailed back to California. The book "Sail East Through the Great Barrier Reef" by Harry Neely was the story of that trip with wife, two young children and a single young Australian for crew. Based on his expereince, Harry begins the book with: "why would anyone go to sea when they could be in jail? There is hot food, a stable bunk, its safer and you meet a higher class of people". This is a similar to Samuel Johnson's description of sailor on an 18th century British warship was the same as being in jail, only more dangerous. After experincing combat in the Pacific, the fear Harry Neely ncountered when his son developed a fever in the middle of the Pacific Ocean was more fightening. He had no medical training, a tiny first aid kit and in the 1960's, no way to obtain help in the middle of the Pacific Ocean. Fortunately, like most fevers, it resolved without treatment. These and other encounters, flavor this text.

It is not the intent of this text to train people to be their "own physician", something even a doctor should not attempt, except if necessary. That does not mean that this text and the course of instruction it represents is not capable. It is meant to be fully functional when other medical care is not available. In talking with former students and hearing about their medical experiences, they believed that the medical care they rendered was the best available at that time. In any case, sound medical knowledge is useful in determining the difference between good and bad medical advice. This book is dedicated to the men and women who go down to the sea in boats. In war and peace, their jobs carry a higher risk of death and injury than any other trade, and the importance of competent medical care is woven through this text. There are many accounts of the injured and ill feeling "a divine relief" when touched by a medical officer. Do not underestimate the power of simple care in the field that begins with calm, confident touch and voice.

"The Art is long, and life is short" described the practice of medicine during the time of Hippocrates when medicine was practiced exclusively in the field. Greek history is an early source of documented field medicine and laid the foundations of medicine practiced today. The following pages contain discussions of diseases, medical officers, personalities affected by medical consequences along with battles and transformations altered by some aspects of medicine. The author believes medicine is a life-long interest and wishes every medical officer good luck and following seas.

"The further backwards you look, the further forward you can see". Winston Churchill

"There is no greater teacher than the past" unknown

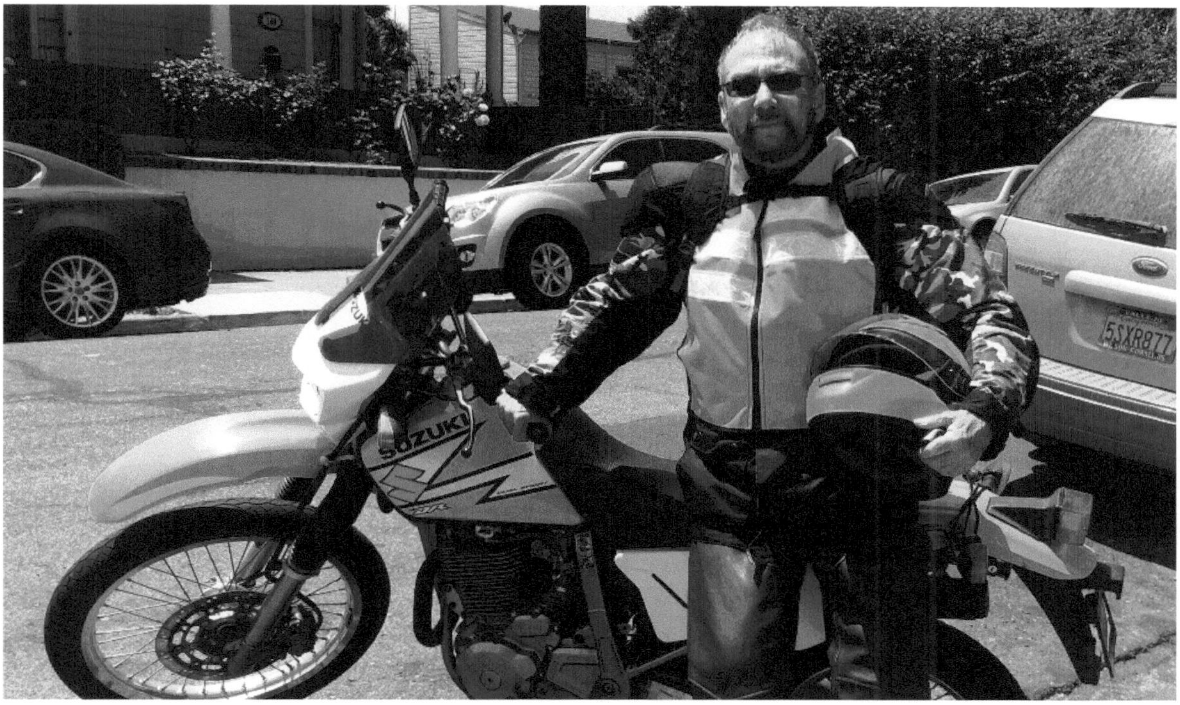

Dr. Dickie L. Hill DO, Osteopathic Physician and Surgeon

Lieutenant Commander, Medical Corps, United States Navy Reserve

United States Coast Guard Licensed Ship Surgeon, Serial Number 7210

Table of Contents

Introduction

Medicine is as old as the human race, as old as the necessity for the removal of disease." Heinrich Haeser-19th century medical historian

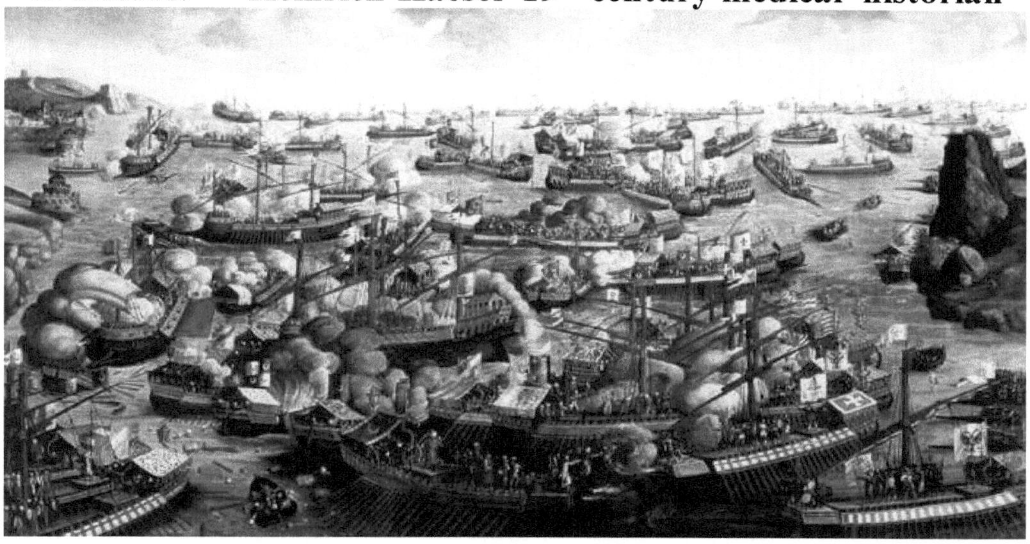

Vasari's painting depicting the Battle of Lepanto off the west coast of Greece on October 5, 1571. In four hours, some 100,000 men and over 400 ships fought one of Western Civilization's great sea struggles. The battle, six years after the Siege of Malta and five years after Suleiman the Magnificence died at the Siege of Szigetvar, blunted Islam's attempts to conquer more of Europe. At Lepanto (near the sites of Salamis, where Greece defeated a larger Persian fleet and Actium, where Augustus defeated Anthony and Cleopatra) the Christian fleet led by twenty-four-year-old Don Juan of Austria, the illegitimate son of Charles V, met the Turkish fleet, rowed by Christian galley slaves. Charles V and his son Don Juan were two of the few effective Hapsburgs in a family that ruled Europe for centuries. Don Juan had the advantage of heavier guns and a new type of warship, the Gallese, fresh from the great Arsenal at Venice. The six Gallese ships were a cross between a Mediterranean galley and a sailing ship of northern Europe. Massive ships of their day delivering withering broadsides with the heaviest guns afloat designed with six guns for forward firing. At the end of the battle, 20-30,000 Muslims were dead and over 15,000 Christian galley slaves were freed. The numbers and the severity of the injuries confronting field surgeons after a battle of this magnitude would be unimaginable by modern medical officers. Thousands with burns, penetrating wounds of sword, spear and the more dangerous, wood splinters. During the battle, a young naval officer, Miguel de Cervantes had his lower left arm shattered and amputated. He likely recovered because of field medical training he learned from his apothecary-surgeon father. On his return to convalescence, his ship was captured by Algerian pirates, and he endured five and one-half long years as a slave in North Africa. As a slave, he learned "patience in the face of adversity" and later wrote one of history's great novels, "The Man of La Mancha", better known for the main character, "Don Quixote". Cervantes died on April 23, 1616, on the same day as Shakespeare. Although well-known writers of their day, they could not have met, as William Shakespeare never travelled beyond his village of Stratford and the city of

London. Shakespeare had no documented formal education and more importantly no access to a reference library. Yet the author of the Shakespeare plays, must have had access to a reference library and experienced firsthand knowledge of the cities where the stories, especially those in Italy were portrayed. Some history taught in high school and college is based on the Shakespeare plays. How could the details about 1600-year-old Roman Empire and other history in Shakespeare's plays be known without a reference library? Edward de Vere did meet Cervantes in Milan, Italy after his imprisonment and unlike Shakespeare had access to several reference Libraries in Europe. In contrast to Shakespeare, Edward de Vere traveled widely and lived in the cities where Shakespeare plays occurred. The overt sexuality and bisexuality implied in many of the Shakespeare plays were out of place in Elizabethan London, a city sexually repressed and backward compared to the courts and cities where Edward de Vere was an honored guest. The real writer of Shakespeare's plays was likely the bisexual, Edward de Vere, 17th Earl of Oxford. Had the Turks won the Siege of Malta and the Battle of Lepanto, much of Europe would have fallen under the repressive curtain of Islam and the world would have never known the Shakespearean plays, regardless of who wrote them.

The author believes modern field medicine began with the Crimean War and America's Civil War with the introduction of anesthesia, injectable morphine and the newly discovered beneficial effects of handwashing and wound cleaning (although it took decades for the medical community to embrace). The First World War introduced blood transfusions for shock, tetanus toxoid reduced wound infections and X-rays allowed abdominal surgery for removal of foreign bodies were major breakthroughs. All came into wide use in the field during and after the conflict. Chest surgery and antibiotics emerged during the Second World War. In Korea, major surgery was moved close to the front with the MASH, mobile army surgical hospital. In Viet Nam, surgery was brought to the firefight with trauma-trained enlisted medical officers using simple tools to save lives at the site of injury. In the recent Middle East wars, field surgery occurred as close as possible to the front. The sooner the care, the better the outcome has been the goal of field medicine. The last one hundred and fifty years of medical advancement, highly encouraged by warfare, has expanded the effectiveness of field medicine. The purpose of the author is to tell the story of medicine in the field using earlier foundations, both the good and the bad. The story, older than recorded history, likely begins with the rise of trade, centralized control and the empathy humans often show for the injured and ill.

Shipping, trade, conflict and field medicine came early in the development of human settlements connected by water. Surplus of foods and other resources, almost all transported by water required vessels, sailors and some form of medical care to be effective. Transport by water continues as the most efficient medium for moving resources, and successful sea transport needs well-built vessels crewed by trained, hopefully healthy crew. Sailors are valuable and keeping them fit for duty is a boon to any shipping enterprise as it would be for armies, explorers and migrations. Although there are scant records of medical care until six thousand years ago, fossil records of repaired fractures and skull trephinations prove that field medicine was in use long before that time. Egyptian ships of four thousand years ago carried trained medical officers and extensive medicine chests; some contents still used today. Early cultivation of wild wheat (emmer) domesticated in the Mesopotamian River valleys led to an explosion of grain production in the plateaus of central Anatolia (modern Turkey) and the coastal flood plains of inland seas entering the Mediterranean, joining slaves and salt as primary early cargo for Western civilizations.

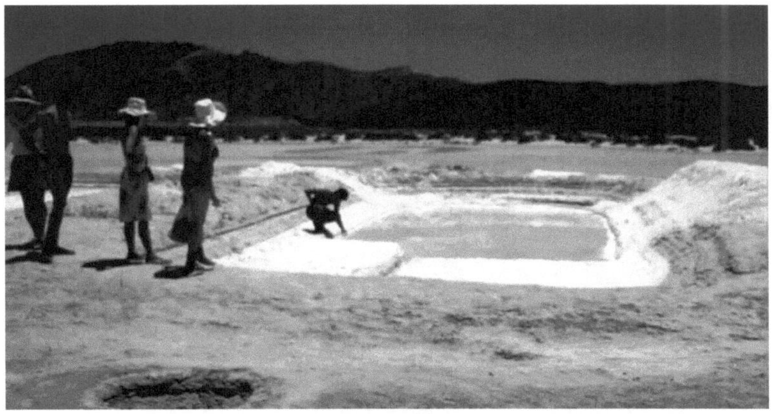

Salt mine on a waterless and unoccupied island in the Sea of Cortez. Controlling salt works, providing slaves to mine salt and ships to transport it were trade pillars of Greek and Roman empires. Rome controlled its empire by controlling all salt works.

Most shipping in the Mediterranean basin was coastal and riverine, however, some trade and travel required long and dangerous sails across open water. Open water sojourns were the "ones at sea" that Aristotle was describing in the opening statement of this text. At the time of Christ, the city of Rome depended on constant resupply of grain, as 90% of inhabitants were fed by the state. When the grain ships, especially those coming from far away Egypt, were delayed by unfavorable winds, riots occurred in a city more densely population than modern Washington, DC. Most of Rome's residents were homeless, often diseased, existing on near starvation diets, totally dependent on food from the state. Rome's leaders knew grain ships were more important to control the rabble than the Pretorian Guard troops.

Urak (Ereck in the Old Testament) was one of the first to grow wheat in excess, as the city state was built on a vast inland freshwater sea (as was Angkor Wat in Cambodia) connected to the Persian Gulf (Arabian Sea) in what is now Iraq. Urak is the source of Western Civilization's earliest record of field medicine and shipping. The city collected goods and people from around the world concentrating power and knowledge. It is likely medical officers gathered here, sharing ideas and skills from world travel. Clay cylinders found here contain medical texts, even a description of medical malpractice. The ruins of this early city contain "Fish Eyes", pearls only found in Ceylon, artifacts from China, ivory from central Africa and trade goods from the western Mediterranean basin. The complex being unearthed at Gobekli Tepe predates Urak by at least six thousand years and are older than any previous ruins demonstrating a much earlier human civilization. Domestication of plants and animals along with metal smelting suddenly appeared in the known world where Gobekli Tepe is located. There are now dozens of sites being discovered in Turkey that even predate Gobekli, proving a previous advanced civilization "jumped started" the current civilization. These structures dated to the end of the last ice age 12,000 years ago and were deliberately buried 8,000 years before the present. Cotton was first domesticated in central Turkey along with the four tools needed to change a raw cotton boll into cloth. Surprisingly, cotton's domestication and the invention of these four tools occurred in distant cultures on other continents, at the same time! Implying widespread knowledge from previous worldwide civilization. Biochemically and medically, cotton is an excellent dressing for wounds as its microscopic structure is ideal for "wicking" fluids from wounds.

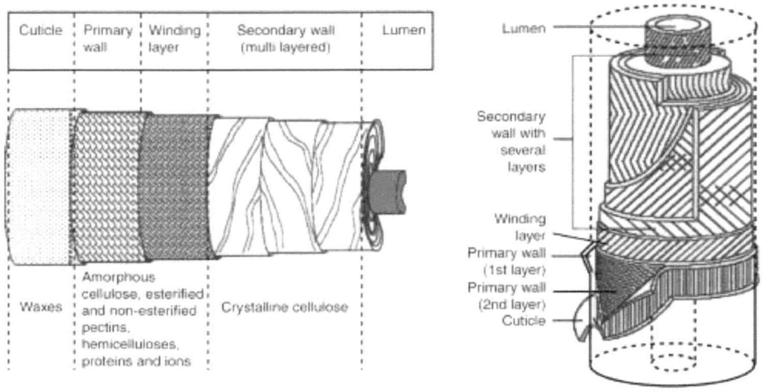

The layers and natural engineering of a cotton fiber appear as if it was designed to function as dressing. National Archives

Improved fishing technology, irrigation, sanitary engineering and field medicine employing surgical procedures and drugs, some still in use, appeared at the same time as cotton production. Medical officers of this early period must have spent most of their professional lives in the field and at sea, as there are no early mentions of hospitals. Hippocrates, Aristotle, Galan, Avicenna, Maimonides and Ambrose Pare are six of the better known of early medical officers. Each spent time at sea, in the field and all experienced combat.

Shipping, trade and field medicine grew with the coming of the Bronze Age, as copper and tin mines were often far apart, necessitating long-distance transport. Some of the earliest known metal works are the bronze smelting ruins of Catal Huyuk in Anatolia (Turkey), which is close to the ruins of Gobekli Tepe. Tin from Britain and Afghanistan connected the early Celtic culture with those of central Asia by shipping, drawing Alexander to the East and Julius Caesar and Rome to the West. The Bronze Age collapsed over a few short decades as iron replaced the more brittle bronze as the metal of trade, because of its supremacy in agriculture, warfare and shipping. Twelve centuries before Christ, "The Sea People" with iron spears and long swords erased cities and cultures in one of history's mysterious disappearances. The 13th and 12th centuries BC were a bad time for early western civilizations, as iron swept the battlefields of larger armies fighting with outdated bronze weapons, climate change, disease, famine and war swept the Mediterranean.

Iron ore, because of its weight and bulk, could not be easily carried on the backs of animals or people, required ships to transport it in bulk. An iron plow tills the soil more deeply with less effort, increasing agriculture output. Iron warfare led to a greater variety of wounds, increasing the need for field surgery. Iron products improved surgical tools and greatly enhanced sea worthiness of ships, as iron nails and fittings strengthened the hull. The science of metallurgy and the ability of ships to gather iron ore from far away sources led to denser, more powerful cultures arising around the shipping ports of the world, increasing infectious diseases while spreading new ones. Most of history's great plagues rode the hulls of ships and changed the world. Port cities suffered massive death rates during history's pandemics. During Black Death, seaports were ravaged due to ship-borne infections while isolated inland villages escaped.

The development of pottery in Japan and China as early as 10,000 B.C. and in southern Europe 5,000 years later, gave a tremendous boost to shipping. Kiln-fired clay amphora pots allowed a wider variety of products (wine, oil, preserved fruits and vegetables) to be shipped to places where these trade goods were not produced. With trade, came travelling medical officers, dispersing the skills and agents of medicine. The first ships surgeons mentioned by name were Machaon and Podalirius, according to Homer's "Iliad" were skilled in extracting embedded weapons, binding wounds and applying soothing dressings. Field surgeons have been a mixed lot through history, in their earliest form, they likely resembled a Shaman-Priest with physical medical skills and knowledge of medicinal plants. The medicine developed slowly and painfully by the Greek and Roman world of the Mediterranean Basin, all but disappeared from Western Europe during the Dark Ages, emerging later during the Renaissance with help from the East. This lack of competent field medicine hindered the rise of sea power among European nations.

Medicine emerged slowly in Medieval Europe after shipping increased. When European Crusaders met the superior medical care of Islam, they were amazed that the Saracens had physicians, surgeons, medical schools, field hospitals and effective medicine chests. Eastern medical officers were much different than the barber-surgeons brought from Europe. The returning Crusaders bought back silk, Far-East spices, physicians with medical and historical manuscripts, pieces of the True Cross, body parts of Saints and the bacteria that caused leprosy. The Crusades stimulated long range shipping and an increased need for medical officers after the Europeans were driven from the Holy Lands. In the centuries following the Crusades, there were plenty of opportunities for newly trained physicians to travel.

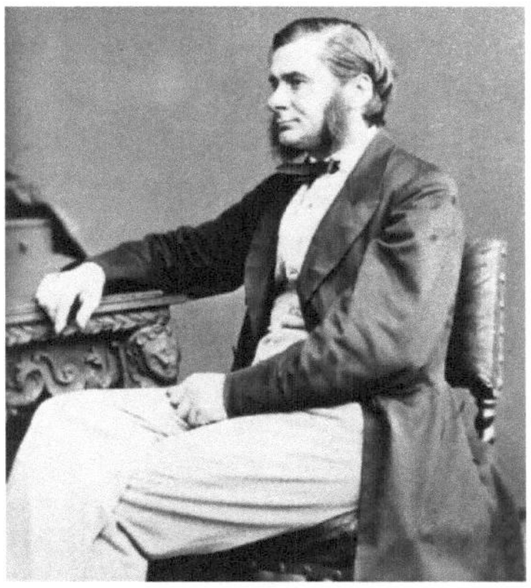

Thomas Henry Huxley (1825-1895), evolutionary biologist and staunch defender of Darwin was an uncommon Ships Surgeon of the mid-19th century, and the HMS Rattlesnake was fortunate to have such a trained medical officer. Many naval medical officers during this period were former common seaman that learned the trade as surgeon's mates, some with questionable training while others were alcoholics and drug addicts. Too many of these apprenticed-trained medical officers were barely literate and unclean, maiming and killing with incompetence. The medicine chest carried by Huxley and those before him bears little resemblance to a modern chest but did carry items still used today such as opium-based drugs, heavy jells of oils (aloe) and in the case of a chest from the Royal Egyptian Navy of the 11th Dynasty (1500 BC), a drug for the relief of abdominal pain obtained from butchered cows. Ox gall has been rediscovered and is now used to dissolve gall stones without surgery. Huxley's offspring include Aldous Huxley, author of "Brave New World"

and Julian Huxley, like his ancestor, an evolutionary biologist and founder of UNICEF. Garrison

Some medical officers went to sea for the romance and challenge, while many had no other opportunities, and there is always a few running away. There were university-trained scholars that became famous scientists and writers such as Thomas Huxley, who after graduating from London University, entered the Royal Navy for adventure. Within a year of graduating, he was the medical officer aboard the HMS Rattlesnake for a five-year circumnavigation of the globe. Upon his return, he published important papers on marine zoology, wrote the "Elementary Biology" and "Comparative Anatomy of Man and the Higher Apes" as well as texts of invertebrate anatomy and general physiology. Among the defenders of Charles Darwin's, he was a respected champion. Unfortunately, too many field medical officers were void of formal education, their training uneven and taught by poor mentors, while some were grossly incompetent like Thomas Huggan, the medical officer on the HMS *Bounty*.

Much travel in the past was on the water, and physicians famous enough to make it into history, spent time at sea. Hippocrates recorded cases aboard ships and on the battlefield. The best-known Roman physician, Galan (129-199 AD) began his medical practice caring for injured gladiators, rising to the rank of Surgeon-General to Emperor Marcus Aurelius (considered Rome's greatest leader), campaigning with him at sea and land for decades. Later in life, Galan recorded everything he had learned about medicine in the field, in dozens of large volumes, most of which lost to history. What little remained served as one of the foundations of Western Medicine. After the fall of Constantinople in 1453, large numbers of Greek, Arab, Armenian and Hebrew physicians bearing medical texts appeared in Europe where manuscripts were translated into Latin. Greek was the first and true language of Western medicine until the Middle Ages when Latin translations of medical writings of Hippocrates, Aristotle, Pliny, Celsius, Dioscorides, and Galan appeared in Europe. Latin became the language of medicine and science for the western world because outside the Catholic clergy in Europe, literacy was rare. Latin, although seldom spoken, had connected the educated of Medieval Europe with a common written form for medicine and science for centuries, trapping them in an archaic language. By the Middle Ages, Latin was no longer spoken, described as a dead language. The bulk of medical and scientific terminology is still largely based in Latin; however, some medical terms had no Latin equivalent, leaving some words in original Greek and Arabic forms.

Just one year ago tonight my love I became your blushing bride
You promised I'd be happy, but no happiness I find
For tonight I am a widow
In the cottage by the sea

-Unknown author-

The sailor in the young widow's lament and tens of thousands of others might have been saved with simple medical care. There have always been competent medical officers, unfortunately few ships carried one until the late 19th century. One of the best medical officers during the Age of Maritime Exploration (17th-19th century) was James Lind, educated in medical college in Scotland is credited with proving that citrus fruit treated and prevented scurvy, that "baking" the clothing and bedding of sailors killed lice and fleas, greatly reducing the risk of typhus. Lind also established the British-Indian medical education system. A system that has trained more physicians than all other world systems combined. Had Lind's treatments been followed since their discovery in mid-18th century, thousands of sailors, soldiers and civilians would have been saved, since scurvy and typhus were still killing into the 20th century.

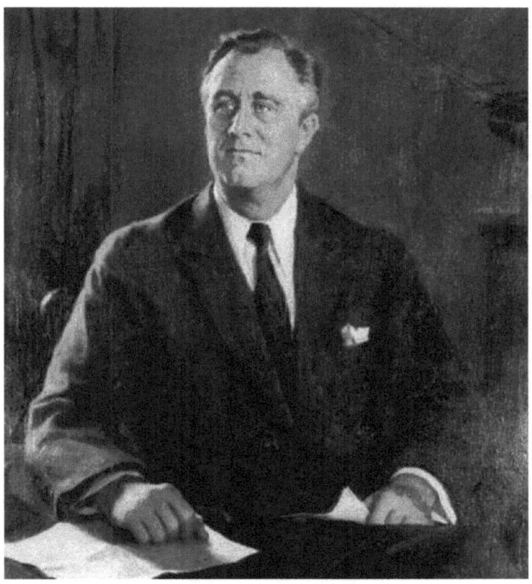

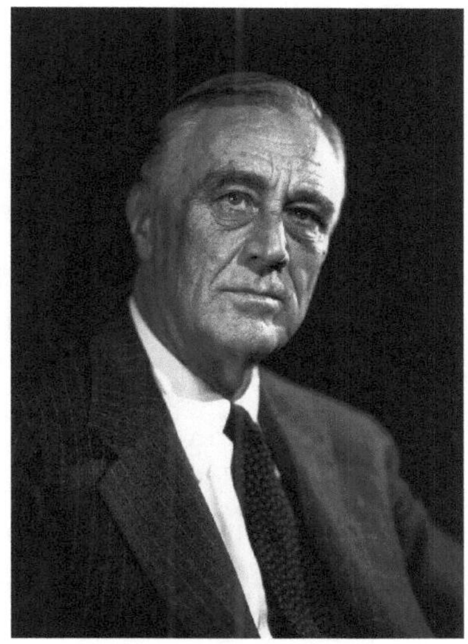

Franklin Delano Roosevelt, 1882-1944, 32nd president of the United Srates and only president to be elected four times. The painting on left in 1934 during his first term and the photo on right in 1944, near the end of his life reveal the ravages of stress, untreated hypertension, tobacco and alcohol abuse. FDR contracted polio, a gastrointestinal virus that invades across the blood brain barrier and attacks the anterior horn cells in the spinal cord at 39 years of age, leaving him paralysed in both legs. At the time of FDR's death in early 1945 from multiple strokes there was no effective treatment of hypertension, even for the president. FDR's blood pressure in his last six months was 240/180 yet he continued to smoke and drink. The author finds it interesting that FDR, Winston Churchill and General Douglas Mac Arthur, three giants of World War II had a common ancestor. Perhaps there is something to "blue bloods". National Archive

As mention earlier, the field medicine discussed in this text begin with the Crimean and Americn Civil War and was steadily advanced with the Great War, World War II, the Korean War, the Viet Nam War and has been expotentially increasing with medical training in the last fifty years which encompassed the years when the author trained and practiced.

The Crimean War 1855-57

The Dawn of modern Field Medicine

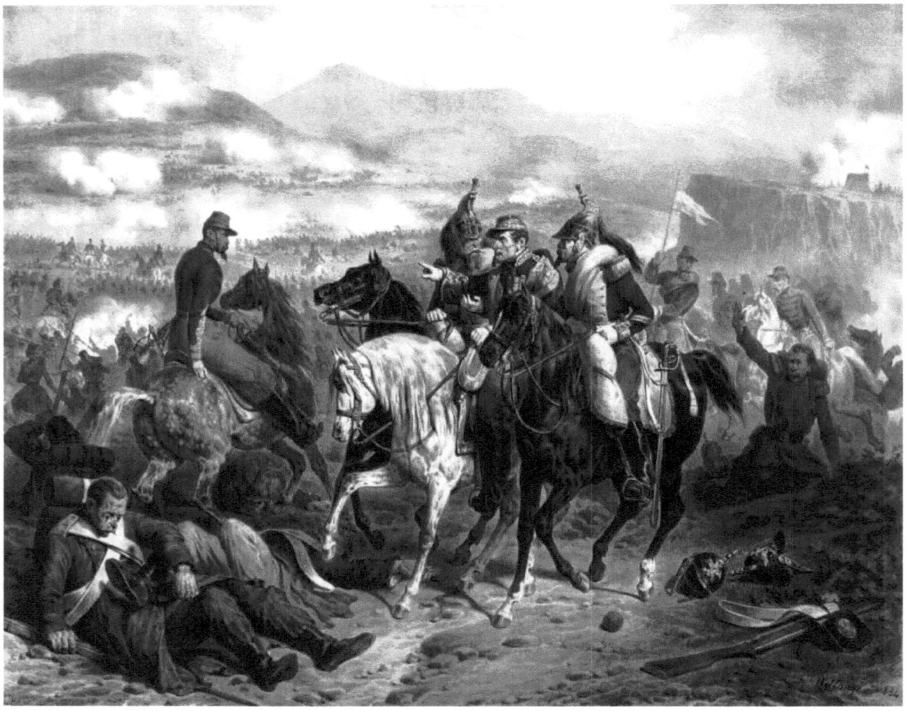

French Commander Marshall Saint-Arnaud who was dying of stomach cancer in great pain, leading troops near the front at the Battle of Alma River. Painting by Belange

The Islamic Middle East in 1833 was an unsettled place, as it is today. A single generation before the Crimean War, Mehmet Ali, the ruler of Egypt, led an army driven by Islamic fervor out of the Nile delta through Syria and encamped at the gates of Constantinople. This "Jihadist Army" was on the verge of taking both the city and perhaps the Ottoman Empire precipitated massive responses from Western Christian powers. France and England sent fleets to the Dardanelles, while Russia landed an army of over 30,000 between Mehmet Ali and the city, saving the Ottoman Empire for almost another century. Twenty years later, Constantinople (Istanbul) was again vulnerable, risking the balance of power in the eastern Mediterranean. This time it was Imperial Russia threatening to capture the city connecting the Black Sea to the Mediterranean. In three previous generations, Russia had defeated Turkey in seven wars, lifting the yoke of Turkish Islam off the Christian populations along the Danube River. By the mid-19th century, Russia was poised to defeat Turkey again, with Constantinople and control of the Straits of the Dardanelles, becoming a maritime power in the Mediterranean Sea. Many in Western Europe feared all this was within Imperial Russia's grasp. France and England would not tolerate Jihadist occupying Constantinople twenty years before, nor would they allow it to be controlled by Russia now. For the first time England and France were allied in one of the few times in history where a major war was fought by a European Alliance on the side of a Moslem power against a fellow Christian Nation. Even though most fighting took place in and around the Crimean Peninsula, it was a world war, with fighting in the Baltic Sea and the western Pacific Ocean as English warships attacked the forts protecting St. Petersburg and Russia's Siberian eastern outposts.

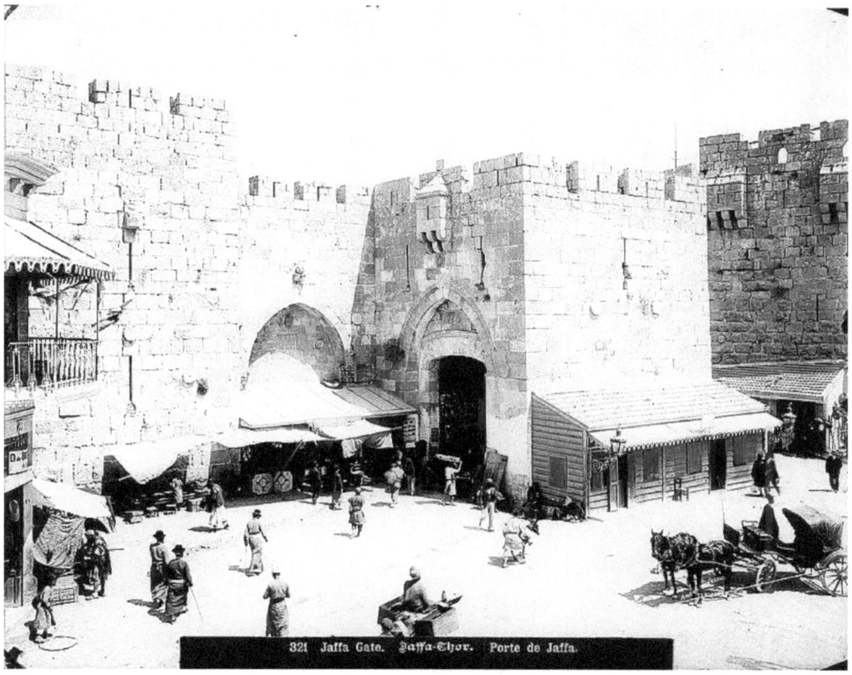

Jaffe Gate embedded in massive walls, of 19th century Jerusalem.
National Library of Congress

The bloody forge of the Crimean War was started by a tiny spark in a city that has spawned and continues to spawn wars, Jerusalem. Random isolated acts of violence between Roman Catholic and Orthodox clergy in the Holy City, i.e., stealing icons, defacing buildings, even physical fights with injuries and a few deaths, had gone on for decades. But one such minor act of violence between Roman Catholicism and Eastern Orthodox led to a world war. Just as most skin wounds are minor self-limiting injuries but when combined with factors of contamination, diabetes and poor wound care, a simple wound can have larger consequences. Just as a small wound can turn deadly, the normally self-limiting religious disturbance 1,432 kilometers from the Crimea brought about a major event, costing the lives of millions while providing a killing ground for the new rifled musket, industrial age artillery, the telegraph and the emergence of modern field medicine.

France, looking for a fight, responded to the disturbance in Jerusalem with threats on behalf of persecuted Catholics. The aged Tsar Nicolas I, who had fought against the French and Napoleon, responded with his own military threats in defense of the Orthodox population. Napoleon III (nephew of the first Napoleon) was anxious to prove his military acumen, reestablishing France as a world military power, as his uncle had done four decades earlier. In addition to promoting a war with Russia, his later military ambitions led him to invade Mexico during the American Civil War, placing Austrian Archduke Maximillian on the throne of Mexico briefly. After the Civil War, some Confederate officers and men joined Maximillian and the French army in a losing war against Mexican nationalists. Cinco de Maya is a celebration of the May 5th, 1862, Mexican victory over French forces at the Battle of Pueblo. During Napoleon III's aggressive reign, Indochina was invaded and unlike Mexico, remained French for almost 100 years. His hubris led to declaring war on Prussia in 1869, in a war where he was captured, Paris occupied, ending the 2nd French Empire, and the creation of Germany. A creation that invaded France twice in the 20th century.

In 1854 France was again trying to be a world power while Imperial Russia was looking for a reason to justify "a holy" war against the Turks, using protection of Orthodox Christians as a pretense. Peter the Great and Catherine the Great's goal of Russia capturing Constantinople and the control of the Straits of the Dardanelles, appeared nearing reality. It was a "perfect storm" of conflicting powerful forces ignited by a tiny act. Just as the single act of the assassination of Austria's Archduke Ferdinand in Sarajevo in the summer of 1914 started the conflagration of the Great War. In medical biochemistry, a single tiny enzyme can instigate a series of chemical reactions resulting in great changes within the cell.

Few wars in human history displayed levels of incompetence on the scale of the Crimean War, especially in field medicine. It was poorly planned, poorly executed and poorly led, resulting in deaths of a million combatants and an unknown number of civilians, most from poorly engineered medical science. Perhaps all this misery did some good, as it gave the world some needed improvements in medicine including field sanitation, field anesthesia, medical engineering, the elevation of nurses to the rank of officers and the evolution of triage. Concepts that emerged and continue today. The Crimean war saw the first extensive use of the rifled musket with the "expanding" Minnie' projectile. The recently developed telegraph, a forerunner of the internet, connected the war to the populations of France and England in real time, creating big problems for the military and the Government's control of information. Uncensored facts from journalists in the field contradicted the fake news from the military, especially when reporting on conditions of medicine in the field.

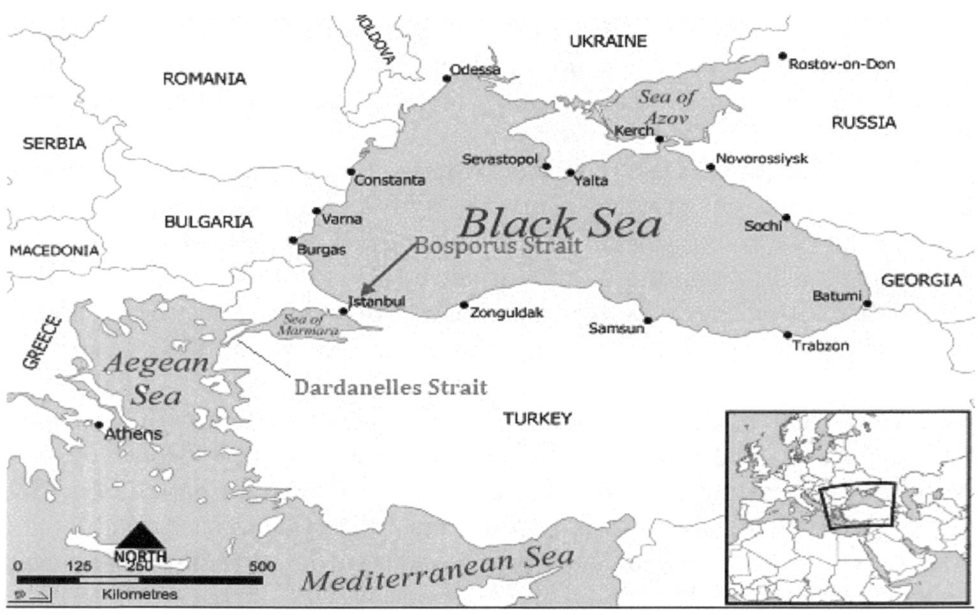

The Black Sea and its major cities note the tiny exit at Istanbul (Constantinople). Wiki-commons

Contradictory information from the war front brought down the British government of Prime Minister Aberdeen, forcing his surrendering the position to one of Queen Victoria's least favorite politicians, Palmerston. Henry John Temple, 3rd Viscount Palmerston, known as "Pam" to the press and common people, served twice during Victoria's reign, dying in office 1865, at the age of 80 during his second term. Palmerston was a rabid Imperialist who planned to use victory in the Crimean War to dismember the Russian Empire, giving the Crimea Peninsula, including the

Christian lands around the Caucasus Mountain regions back to Turkey, transferring Finland to Sweden, the Baltic States to Prussia, Bessarabia to Austria and the establishment of an independent Poland. War aims totally unacceptable to Russia, and none were included with the Treaty of Berlin which ended the war. Even before the Crimean War ended, England under Palmerston, begin fighting the Anglo-Persian War 1856-57 against Russian's ally, Persia. All part England's "Great Game" with Imperial Russia, as there were British agents in Kazakhstan and Russians in Afghanistan. Palmerston is regarded as one of England's great politicians, maintaining the balance of power in Europe while defending British colonies. With his backing, England started the Second Opium War in 1857 while at the same time, reacted ruthlessly in putting down the Indian Sepoy Rebellion of 1857. Palmerston along with the Queen Victoria and the British Royal Navy were keen to break the Union blockade of Confederate ports in 1861 during the American Civil War, especially after the HMS Trent affair. However, the Queens's consort, Prince Albert, although dying of typhus, was instrumental in preventing England and France from starting a war with the Northern States. Albert overruled his wife, the Prime Minister and the Royal Navy clamoring to break the Union naval blockade of Confederate ports, allowing President Lincoln to apologize for Captain Charles Wilkes (perhaps the worst officer in the US Navy history) illegal diplomatic violation. The HMS *Trent* affair almost brought England and France into the American Civil War when Wilkes fired upon and detained an unarmed British warship transporting the Confederate ambassadors to Europe.

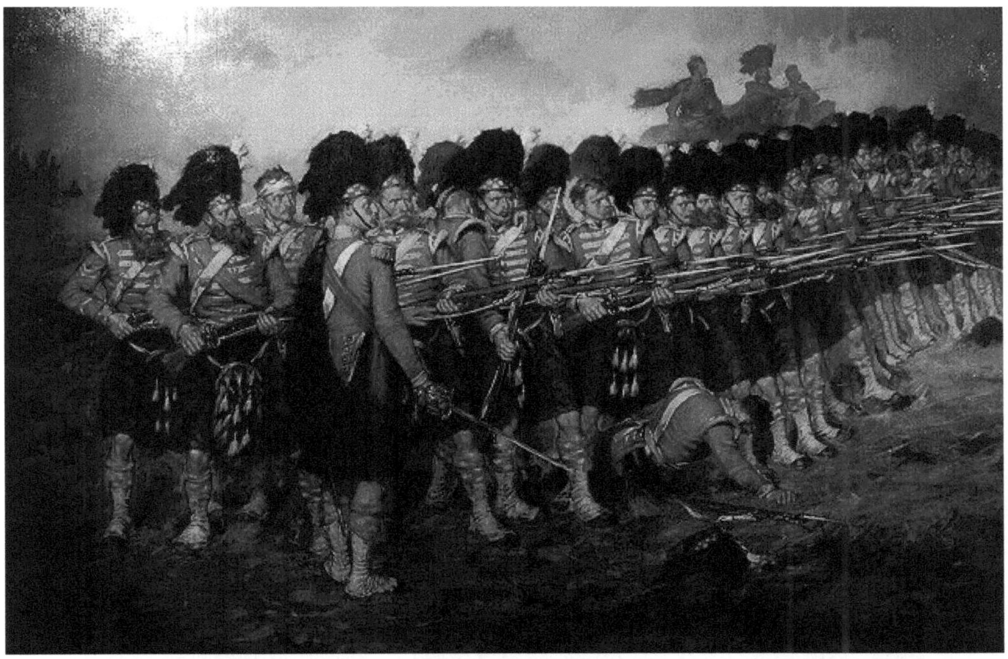

"The Thin Red Line" Robert Gibb's painting of a small British unit holding off Russian cavalry charge, the rifled musket ended most cavalry charges.

The three main field commanders in the Crimea had significant medical problems, and in an environment ripe with fevers and drastic weather extremes, was not a place for older infirmed field commanders. The Allies first stop after Istanbul was Varna, at the mouth of the Danube River, where the army sickened and died in great numbers. Clearly no competent medical officers were consulted since the Danube delta and the surrounding lands were experiencing a massive epidemic of cholera. It was a bad time to have tens of thousands of gastrointestinal tracts adding their fecal discharge to the milieu. After suffering loses of irreplaceable men and materials, for reasons not well known, the armies and navies decided to attack the Imperial Russian Naval Base in the Crimea. Perhaps fleeing cholera?

England sent Lord Raglan, a commander-in-chief who had not seen conflict since losing his right arm at Waterloo, forty years earlier. Raglan was an amazing young combat officer, (like US Grant) leading from the front in a dozen battles and at Badajoz, was the first man through the breach. However, courage alone seldom wins wars, let alone organize and lead an invading army far from home. Upon arriving in the theatre, Lord Raglan, now in his seventh decade was too weak to board the French flagship using his single arm and yet was to command an expeditionary army. The decorated veteran had spent the past four decades occasionally attending Parliament, lecturing at war collages, some hunting and horse riding on his estate. He had no recent combat experience, had never commanded a large body of men, was frail, partially crippled, and seemed a poor choice for command of an army far from home. Generally, going to sea and to war is not for the aged and fragile. Field Marshall, FitzRoy James Henry Somerset, Baron Raglan would have never passed a fit for duty exam by a competent medical officer. England later sent Redvers Buller as commanding officer in Boer War and John French as commander of the British Expeditionary Force in World War I, both poor choices.

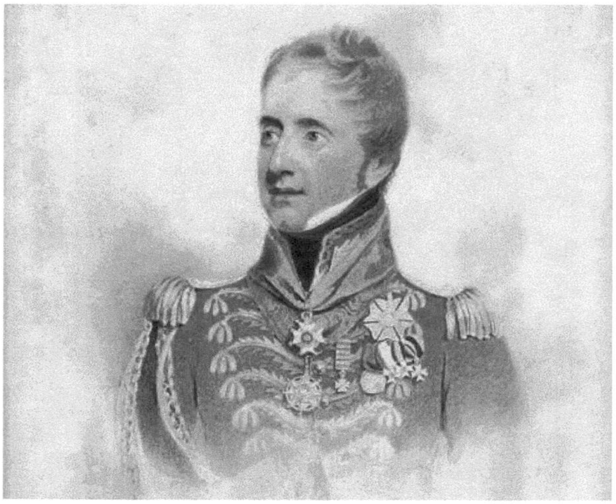

A young Lord Raglan, before his wounds and multiple fevers. By the time of his death in the Crimea, his chronic medical problems added to infectious disease, had left him a thin, bald weakened old man. Medically unfit to command. Painting by William Haines

France sent Saint Arnaud, who like the Ulysses S. Grant had problems in peacetime after brilliant careers as young combat officers. Fighting under Napoleon, Arnaud acquired combat experience and like General Grant, excelled at war. Arnaud prospered in the years of peace, unlike Grant who failed at peaceful endeavors. As a civilian, Arnaud became a popular theatre actor and owned a chain of pawn shops in Paris. Due to unscrupulous business activity and scandals with married women, he joined the French Foreign Legion and fled to Algeria. Once back in the arms of combat, Arnaud excelled, becoming an early advocate of the new rifled musket firing the Minnie' ball. The increased range and firepower of a rifled barrel allowed him to develop new tactics in quelling desert tribes. In some cases, bringing formally rebel tribes into the French armies of North Africa.

The revolutions that swept Europe in 1848 ended the 2nd French Republic, overthrown by a military coup led by Napoleon III and the army. Arnaud's brigade played a major role in the creation of the 2nd French Empire proclaimed by Napoleon's nephew, and the former stage actor's popularity among the people of Paris threatened Napoleon III's leadership. Fearing Arnaud's growing support among civilians and the army, Napoleon III made him a Major General and sent him back to Algeria and then even further away as commander of The Army of the East in Turkey's support against Russia. After brief successes, especially storming the Alma River, he died of stomach cancer and was replaced by the less forceful, Pelissier. Early in the war, the British command was furious that leadership of the war would be shared with Arnaud, a former "actor" of less than noble birth with a scandalous history. The entire general staff of the British Army were high-born aristocrats, their numbers peppered with family members. Lord Raglan had five nephews serving as ADC's. Imagine the old dying patriarch, sitting in his headquarters surrounded by his young family members.

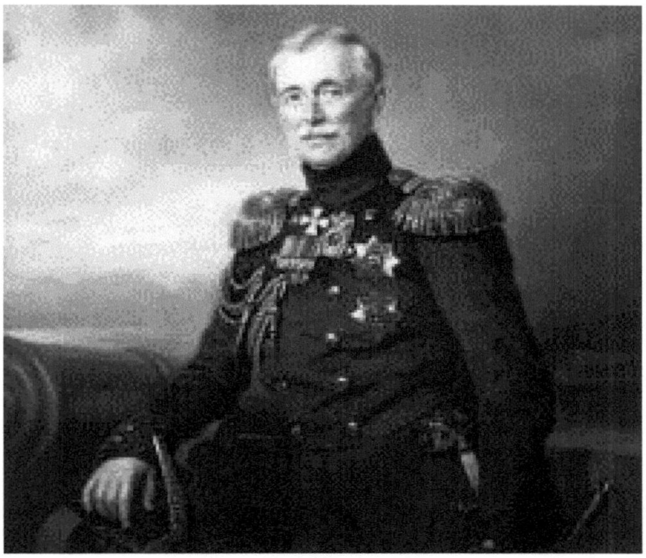

Admiral Menshikov by Franz Kruger, Hermitage Museum

The third Christian leader was the aristocratic Russian admiral, Alexander Sergeyevich Menshikov, the senior Imperial officer in the Crimea when war started. He too, was in his mid-sixty's and had serious medical problems resulting from a wounding in previous combat. He was unfit to command a navy, let alone an army. As a junior officer, he had fought with Tsar Nicolas I against Napoleon and later endured traumatic castration via cannonball during the Siege of Varna in the Turkish War 1828-29. He was brave, yet a poor administrator, stalling the combat ability of the Russian Navy before the war and later proved to be an even worse field commander of the Russian army in the Crimea. At the Battle of the Alma River, most historians believe even an inept commander would have been victorious, however, Menshikov was so flagrantly incompetent, the Russians defending the high ground with more troops and more cannon, retreated from a strong position. The Russian army fleeing into Sevastopol with little order, left the city wide open to the enemy. By not following the Russian army into Sevastopol, a long twelve-month siege over a Russian winter resulted. The city would have fallen easily, if the British, after supporting the French assault, had followed on the heels of Russians.

Most World History texts about the Crimean War were from the British perspective, implying the British Army and Royal Navy were the primary combatants. This is hardly true, as the French under Arnaud were much better fed, better equipped and better led. The French landed with engineers for sanitation and built wood housing, deployed a medical department and commissary for food and clothing. On the other hand, British soldiers seldom had tents, food, medical care, or safe drinking water, let alone housing. The largest set battle of the war was at the Alma where the French competently led by Arnaud, fought bravely, stormed and breached the Russian line with the English in support.

In most cases, medical care and sanitation were even more primitive in the Russian army than the allies. While fighting the Turks in the Hungarian Campaign of 1848, the Russians suffered 708 killed, while 57,000 were admitted to field hospitals with fevers. Even during peacetime, 65% of the massive Russian army was too ill for duty, primarily from cholera due to poor medical engineering. The Russian Army at the Siege of Sevastopol was fortunate to have a powerful medical asset in the person of Nikolai Pirogov, a peace-time professor of surgery at the Academy of Military Medicine in St. Petersburg. He was the first surgeon to use the general anesthetic ether in the field, not just for amputations but also to calm the injured when arriving at the hospital, preventing collapse (shock) associated with severe pain and despair. Anesthesia aided his triage of the injured and is considered one of his great achievements in field medicine. Under anesthesia, Pirogov was able to post a survival rate of 65% for amputation of upper extremity compared to barely 10% for the English surgeons. John Hall, a senior British surgeon in the Crimea, did not believe in anesthesia but "the smart of the knife" as a powerful stimulant in preventing collapse. "Better to hear the man bawl lustily than to sink silently into the grave".

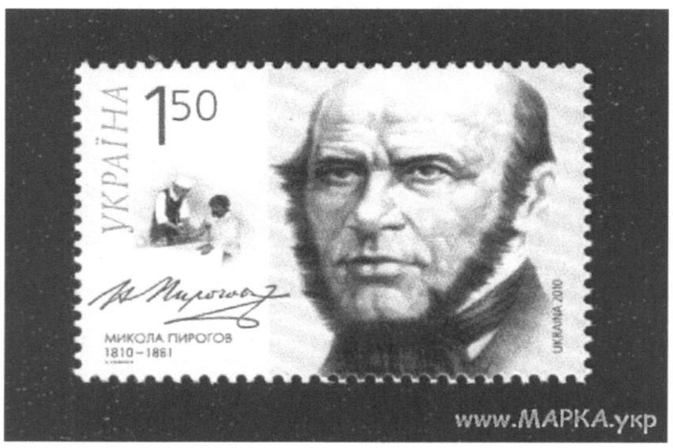

Soviet era stamp honoring Dr. Pirogov

Pirogov argued successfully that having women care for wounded improved morale, whereas the British medical department was adamantly against females among the troops. Grand Duchess Elana Pavlona, Tzar Alexander's sister-in-law was the Russian "Florence Nightingale", carried nurses, food, medicines, and supplies 1,000 kilometers over rough roads to the fight. Aside from the high-born Pavlona and England's Nightingale, the war created 18-year-old Daria Mikhailova, who sold all her meager processions after her sailor father was killed to purchase horse, cart, dressings and food to care for the wounded. She became known as "the heroine of Sevastopol", symbolizing the patriotic spirit of the Russian female. By the battle's end, Daria and others were living through a new type of industrial warfare as thousands of artillery rounds fell on the city every day.

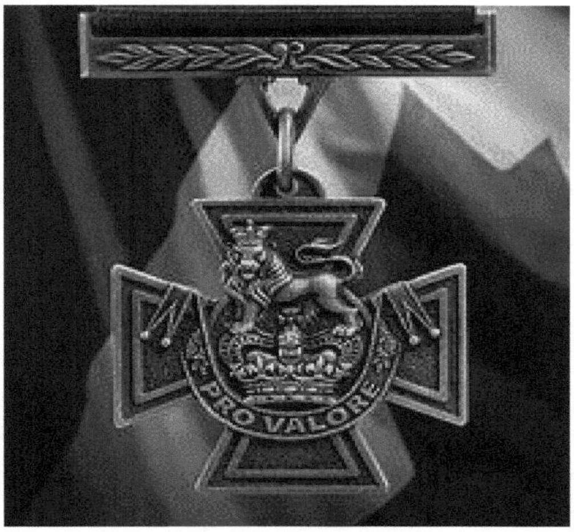

The Crimean War brought about creation of the Victoria Cross, the highest award for bravery in Great Britain, equivalent to the United States Medal of Honor. It was a new medal, created to reward bravery in all classes of soldiers, not just officers. The original crosses were made from melted Russian cannons captured at Sevastopol. Queen Victoria and the English, for the first time saw their ordinary soldiers as more than drunken thugs (since one third were poor Irish), wanting to see instead, Christian saintly martyrs. British War Museum

After the one-year siege, October 1854 to September 1855, the Russians quietly abandoned the now destroyed city. Russia lost 450,000 men in the Crimean War with 250,000 in and around Sevastopol, yet the siege was later celebrated as a victory of Russian bravery and resistance. For those that do not believe history repeats itself, Sevastopol was again besieged by Nazi Germany in 1941-42. During the siege, over 20,000 tons of bombs fell in June alone. Russia lost over 300,000 souls in the 20th century siege, creating another story of heroism of Russia in the Crimea and further justification of Russia reclaiming the Crimea in the 21st century.

The war made no economic sense. By the middle of the 19th century, Western Europe, especially England and France needed the Russian forest products of the Black Sea for timber and pitch for their navies as well as grain shipped from Russia's breadbasket, the Ukraine. Russia was also a major export market for manufactured goods of these two nations. A war in this area between these nations would greatly impede this trade. The Russian army was huge, the largest in Europe, however it was spread over several thousand miles of border. In 1854 Russia had only 650 miles of railroads (England and France had tens of thousands of miles by this time) and very poor roads making the movement of troops slow and fraught with losses. In the age of enlightenment, literacy rates were rising throughout Europe, however the Russian army was barely 0.2% literate, making written orders seldom readable even for officers in the field. Leo Tolstoy fought at Sevastopol and used his experiences of combat in writing the novel "War and Peace" about the War of 1812. For hundreds of years, large numbers of these illiterate troops had protected the Christians under Ottoman Turkish rule, believing in Russia's obligation to the Slavic people of the Balkans. In 1914, when Austria threatened the Slaves in Serbia that Russia had been protecting from Islam, Imperial Russia went to war. Before the Crimean War, the British press was anti-Russian and pro-Turkey, describing the Russian bear as a form of vicious tyranny over the poor defenseless Turks. An example of journalism promoting only one view. Early in the war, when the Turks overran Christian areas of Armenia and Georgia, they raped, murdered and took slaves. Some of these

Christians ended up being sold in the slave markets of Constantinople in full view of the French and English diplomats, soldiers and press! News ignored by reporters and editor's intent on encouraging the war.

There were American and other foreign army observers, including future commander of the Union Army, George McClellan who witnessed the lack of supply and training in the combatants, especially of the British Army. This may explain why McClellan's Army of the Potomac was the best trained, equipped and supplied army in history. Raglan in overall command of British soldiers was blamed for the infamous "Charge of the Light Brigade" among other disasters. As the war grew grimmer and criticism greater, fighting both the Russians and the British press, he lost hair, weight, patience and the day after he declared "there is no cholera in my camp" to the press, he died of cholera. To send an ancient warrior halfway around the world leading an army attacking the Russians on their own ground, should have been opposed by competent medical officers. Some 2 million soldiers, French, British and Turks fought against Imperial Russia, mostly in the Crimea, where 25% became causalities. The poor medical care led directly to the demand for better field medicine, led in part by Florence Nightingale who emerged into history during the Crimean War.

Medical care in the field owes much to Florence Nightingale. The world is a better place because she was the right person at the right time in the right place, the Crimean Peninsula, mid-19th century. She was a highly unusual female, coming to prominence during a highly usual war. Unusual in that the Christian nations of France, England and Sardinia were fighting as allies with the Moslem nation of Turkey against Christian Imperial Russia. Ms Nightingale was attractive, processed a quick intellect, well-rooted confidence and descended from ancestors who were staunch abolitionists that helped outlaw slavery in the British Empire. She was fortunate in Victorian England at a time when women were generally not educated, to have a father that believed his three daughters deserved the first-class education usually reserved for boys. He taught them Greek, Latin, Italian, mathematics, literature and writing. Ms Nightingale was raised in Greece, Italy and later England, travelling as an adult through Europe and Egypt. Her experiences in Egypt led her to write "Letters from Egypt: A Journey on the Nile, 1849-1850", about a spiritual revelation in the ancient temple at Thebes. The author also experienced a metaphysical sensation while visiting the temple of Thebes as a medical student.

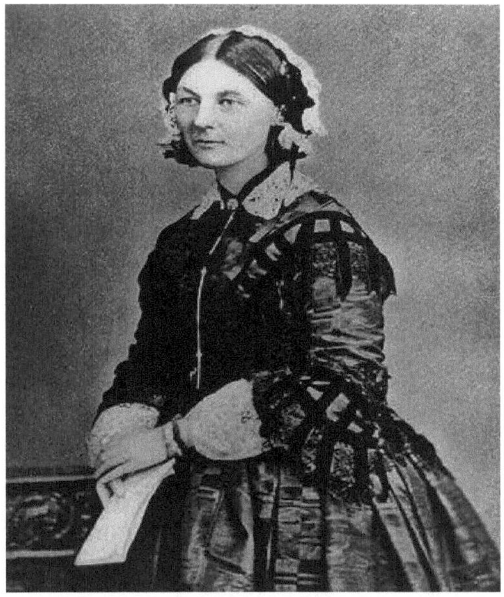

Florence Nightingale, 1860. British War Museum

Ms. Nightingale wrote over 200 medical related books and papers, written in simple plain English and founded the pillar concepts of civilian medical sanitation. Concepts are important today for people enjoying safe water and sewage disposal. Ms. Nightingale is largely responsible for elevating nurses to the level of officers (as Caesar had done for field medics). Before Ms. Nightingale, most nursing was done by "camp followers", women with husbands in the army, widows and unmarried with children, following in the wake of armies. Camp followers were certain to contain courtesans, giving the group a tainted place in history. Nightingale and other Europeans (especially Mary Clarke in the British Indian Public Health system) and later Americans (Clara Barton), who like Florence, had family name, education, stubbornness, relationships with politicians, and celebrities gave them the ability to attract respect in a male dominated system.

In the beginning, the British Army did not want her help, placing restrictions, delays and denials in her path to the war. However, the press, with the invention of telegraph, sent home the problems of the war, especially the dearth of medical care. The truth combined with her political connections allowed her to "bully" herself to Turkey. When Ms. Nightingale finally got to Istanbul, hundreds of miles from the actual fighting, she and her team found conditions "horrific" in the huge barracks turned into hospital at Scutari. Her regular correspondence with her close friend and supporter, Sidney Herbert, who became Secretary of War during the Crimean War, allowed her to continue to the front where the medical conditions were worse. The wounded were not even being fed, dressing changes were barely attempted, and men were dying needlessly. Shortly after her care commenced at the Scutari hospital where hundreds of wounded were languishing, the death rate fell from 42% to 2%. No wonder the Army did not want her around! Remember, "Truth is the first victim of war".

There are feminists today that feel Florence Nightingale has been given too much credit for success done by other women. They believe she was not a strong voice for the women's rights, especially voting, in mid-19th century England where women were being imprisoned for suffrage, and therefore her accomplishments have been devalued. The very competent Great War author, Lyn

McDonald defends both her reputation and her work as changing forever, the positive role that nurses play in war. This author agrees with Ms. McDonald.

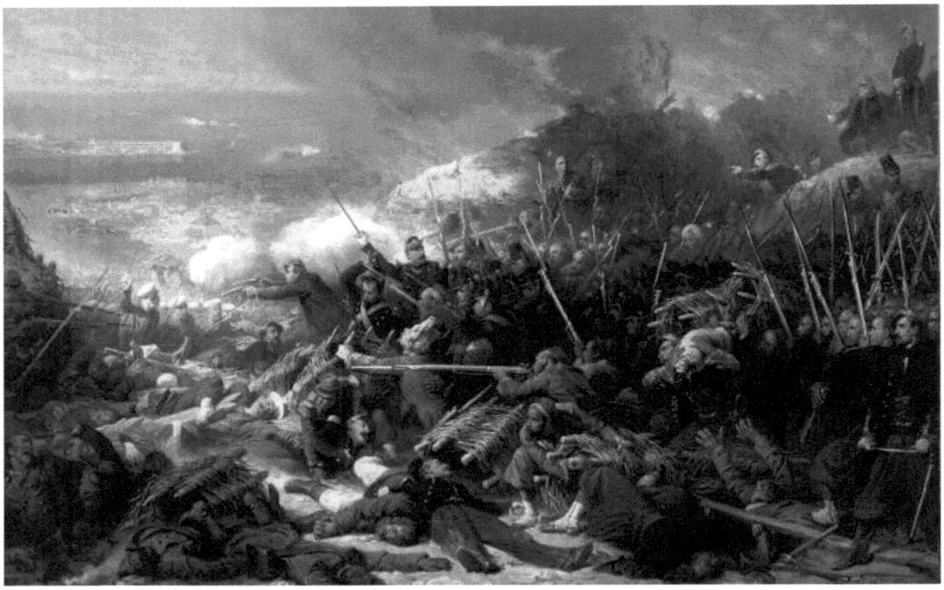

The French Zouaves assault the Malakoff Redan in the Siege of Sevastopol during the war on the Crimean Peninsula created large numbers of extremity injuries. William Simpson

Amputations were the mainstay of surgery in combat medicine and even with competent surgeons were often the only option when extremities mangled by high velocity projectiles, leaving scattered bones and bullet fragments. In the field it was really the only choice, especially with hundreds of injuries. Interestingly, bullet wounds to joints made it easier to save the extremity in high velocity wounds as opposed to the long bones since the joint absorbed the impact, sparing the splintering of bone. Fortunately, management of extremity injuries is now less gruesome; however, amputations are still common in warfare and civilian trauma (think of an earthquake).

In extremity wounds, first control bleeding with direct pressure, and later after the victim has been stabilized, pack with firm dressings or close with sutures. Infection control is paramount and there is no replacement for thorough wound cleaning, proper wound dressing and antibiotics. Thoroughly washed wounds have a much lower incidence of infection. A large syringe is useful in gently pushing water through the wound and into pockets and cavities. Antibiotic (deodorant) soaps are useful in the lavage, iodine solution (Betadine) has years of use in disinfecting wounds. Silver sulfonamide (Silvadene) is effective as a local antibiotic covering the wound with thin layer and then covered by the placement of non-stick dressing (Adaptic, Telfa, etc.) which is then covered with soft absorbent layers of cotton (4x4 gauze) held in place by gentle compression around the wound. The dressing should be kept clean and dry, changed daily, more often if dressing becomes soiled or wet. The biochemistry of cotton makes it an asset in wounds, as the shape of individual cotton fibers acts as a straw, drawing fluid, reducing stagnation and infection. The wound should be inspected every day for signs of spreading redness, swelling, tenderness and heat. Red streaks leading from the wound back towards the central body is a poor sign, especially with a fever. Controlling bleeding, cleaning and dressing the wound in the beginning, is always superior to treating a later infection. It is easier to prevent infection than to treat a wound that has become infected.

Tetanus immunizations are effective and strongly recommended by the author every 10 years, reduced to 5 years with dirty wounds. Tetanus has a long ugly history in wounds. For centuries, battles left men writhing in pain with the slow painful death of tetanus. In over 40 years of medicine, the author saw a single case of tetanus (lockjaw) as a young medical student in the mid 1970's. The victim was an elderly widow living alone on a farm near Ada, Oklahoma. One of her cows stepped on her foot breaking the skin and fracturing several underlying bones while spreading fresh manure into the wound. She cleaned the wound placed some type of homemade dressing and soldiered on. When brought to the hospital her wound was beginning to heal, however she had tetanus, which is more of a poisoning than infection. The tetanus bacteria produce a powerful toxic chemical resulting in extreme muscle tetany (Latin for painful shortening of muscles). Anyone who has ever had a leg cramp can appreciate pain levels when all your muscles are cramping! The poor lady was bowed with only the back of head and her heels touching the bed. She was in severe pain and unable to swallow her saliva, slowly drowning even with near-constant suctioning through her clenched jaws. Not a pretty picture. Every battle in human history left tetanus causalities, men crying in pain, begging for a quick death. Tetanus toxoid, similar enough to the real toxin prevents tetanus and became in widespread use during the Great War.

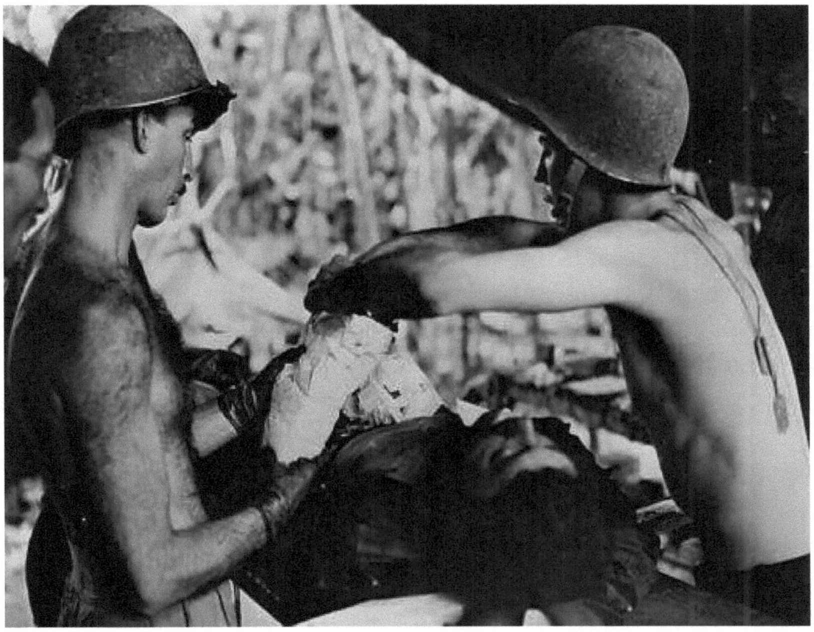

New Guinea, World War II, Field Medical Officer George Marks performing surgery in the field. Except for antibiotics, anesthetics, anesthesia, X-ray and better training, little has changed for medical officers in combat almost 100 years after the Crimean war. Medical officers wearing helmets indicate this field surgery is close to the front. National Archives

Shock

French word "to strike against"

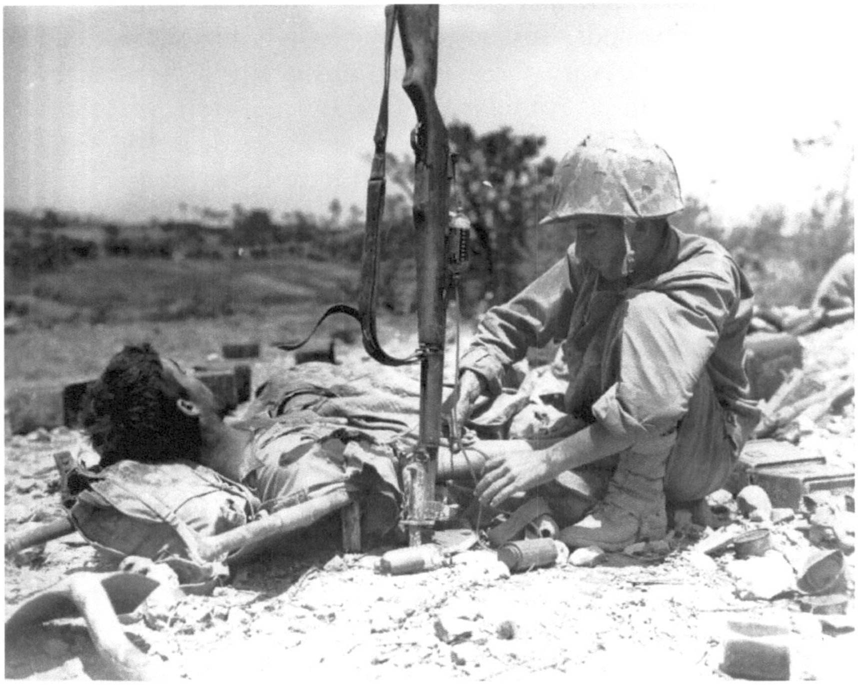

Okinawa May 1945 saw widespread use of plasma in the field for shock. Dr. Charles Drew developed a form of dried blood that, when mixed with water, was injected directly into circulation. For the first time in known history, shock could be treated by replacing circulating fluids in the field. Morphine for pain and plasma for shock saved many lives. The eighty-two-day battle for Okinawa consumed 250,000 lives, was the largest battle in the Pacific War and the only battle where both commanding generals were killed in action. 82, 000 American causalities portended the enormous costs the invasion of Japan would require. The "butcher bill" of Okinawa helped make the decision to drop atomic bombs on Japan's home islands instead of landing troops. National Archives

Shock occurs when there is inadequate circulating fluid, the elixir required to maintain life. Although shock is life-threatening, it can be treated in the field in many cases unlike in the past. After securing airways, breathing and circulation in the injured, continue to monitor for signs of inadequate circulating fluid. Signs include altered level of consciousness (confusion, poor response to stimulation, unconsciousness), low blood pressure, pale cool skin, rapid weak pulse, increased breathing rate, sweating, thirst and in severe cases, coma. In its infancy, shock may slowly, almost silently remove fluid from circulation. Detecting the subtle beginnings of shock requires more than passively waiting for the above symptoms to appear. To enhance survival, it is paramount that shocks can be identified early and treated aggressively, especially in isolated environments. Diagnosis of shock in its early form is possible with repeated careful physical examination. Check the pulse every few minutes, recording rate and strength. Measure blood pressure with the victim lying flat on the back (supine) and repeated in a sitting position. This "tilting" can indirectly reveal the cardiovascular system's response to the stress of pumping blood uphill to the brain. A fall in blood pressure and an increased yet weakened pulse with this maneuver are signs that a person has inadequate circulating fluid. A positive "tilt test" should prompt aggressive treatment of shock. Many have died in the past and continue to perish from treatable shock.

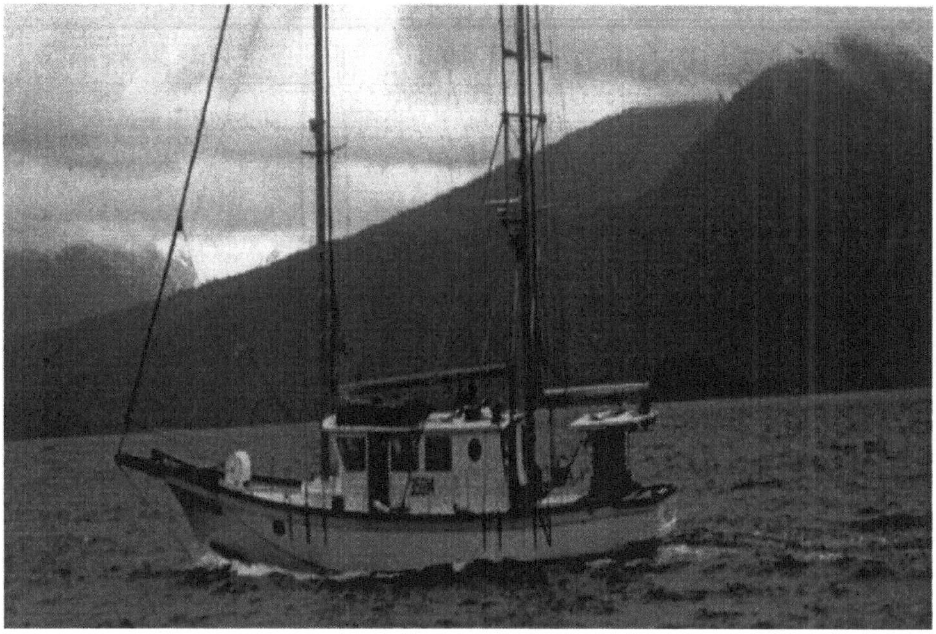

The US Public Health Service rates the maritime industry as the most dangerous profession for death and maiming, with the fishing industry leading the way. Even the small fishing vessel above, deep within the inland passage of Alaska, should carry a modem medicine chest and be trained in medical emergencies at sea. There is no way to predict what might happen in this isolated environment and if possible, this vessel should be as prepared to deal with medical problems as would a larger ship. Photo by author

For adequate blood flow, there must be a pumping heart, sufficient pressure in the arteries and enough fluid available to deliver oxygen and carry away carbon dioxide. Shock ensues when there is loss of blood flow within the arteries and smaller arterioles, interrupting the orderly flow of blood. When this happens, the brain and other central organs and tissues are deprived of the means to function properly and more importantly, to survive. Cells can live for a short time using non-oxygen dependent pathways, but this cellular struggle produces more toxic waste. Waste that can damage and even kill when shock is not prevented or reversed quickly.

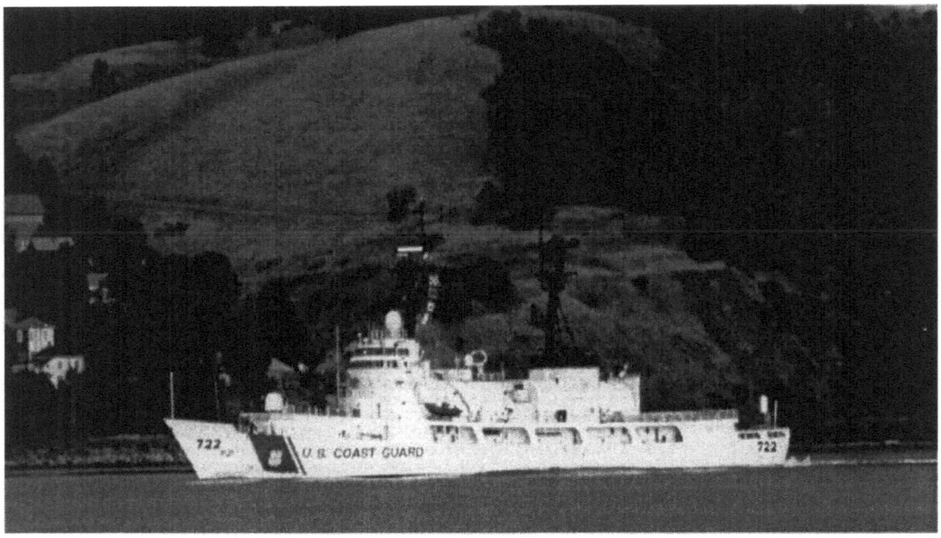

The cutter above in the California Delta is one of the largest operated by the United States Coast Guard and although it contains an extensive medicine chest to deal with most medical emergencies, it unlikely carries a physician. The medical officer on this vessel is likely a senior enlisted, well trained in field medicine. Photos by author

Recognition and Treatment of Shock

The initial management of suspected shock includes simple measures of confident touch, warming and reassuring, loosening any tight clothing at the waist and throat (even a T-shirt may constrict at the neck) and elevating the feet to encourage the flow of blood back to the central organs. After assuring that airway, breathing and circulation are adequate, a series of blood pressures are recorded during the **Tilt test**. The tilt test begins with a blood pressure reading obtained with the patient lying down, the brain the same level as the heart. The patient's head is then raised to 45 degrees, if unconscious, the head is elevated above the heart by gently placing something soft under the victim's back. Blood pressure is taken every few minutes, watching for a drop of either the top or bottom number of the blood pressure. If either number decreases by 10 mm of Mercury, it is a positive tilt test and treat the person immediately with placing feet above the head, loosening clothing, boots and cover with blanket.

The tilt test is a dynamic stress maneuver, measuring both heart function and amount of circulating fluid. A properly done tilt test may detect a dropping blood pressure before the other signs of shock appear. It is possible for blood pressure to fall, and pulse to weaken after trauma with the injured complaining of few symptoms. Yet they should be monitored closely, as it may portend a deeper injury even in the asymptomatic. In fractures, burns, penetrating injuries and other forms of trauma, a tilt test should be part of the initial exam and repeated every few minutes until the threat of shock has passed. Indications of reduced danger include an alert patient who is taking fluids, producing urine and hopeful.

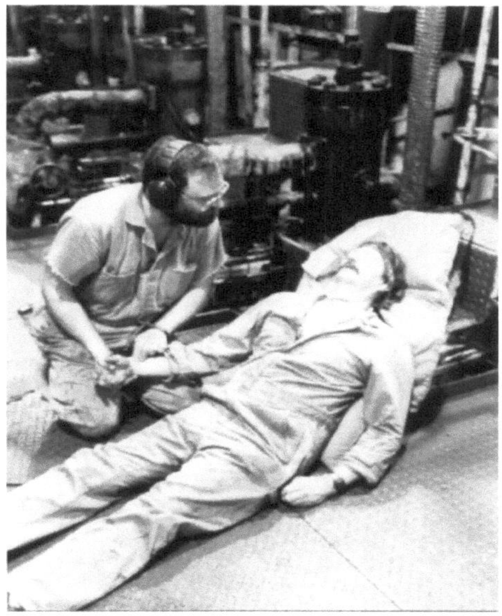

Stimulation in noisy engine room where stethoscope replaced with fingers in tilt test.

MAST pants have come into use in the USA by emergency personnel managing shock in the field but have fallen in use by military. However, they may have value in the field, as application is not difficult, and have been helpful at maintaining adequate circulating fluid. These suits contain many air bladders that are inflated first at the feet and continuing upward in progressively larger bladders over the thighs and the pelvic area. Filing the bladders flushes blood from the lower body back into the central area where it can be circulated to the brain and kidneys. At the same time, MAST pants act as an effective tourniquet in reducing blood flow into the lower body and may be useful in splinting lower body fractures. The author has no firsthand experience in their use.

Intravenous fluids can only augment circulating blood, rarely replace it completely. Even at high flows, IVs deliver less fluid than drinking a large glass of water. To get fluid into circulation quickly, give electrolyte drinks by mouth. Even small sips are frequently taken are better than dripping fluids through a tiny needle precariously anchored in a vein. If victim is alert and can drink, offer electrolyte-rich fluid, found in commercially available powder form, or mix 1 teaspoon of sugar and ½ teaspoon of salt in 500cc/1 pint of water. If available, add a small amount of citrus juice. Alcohol, although a stimulant, may play a detrimental role in early shock and has been responsible for many deaths over the years at sea and battlefields. Inserting IVs may be helpful, but the gut is the preferred site for fluid replacement. Some form of powdered electrolyte preparation should be part of every medicine chest. Fluids can be effective given rectally with placing lubricated hollow tube deep into rectum and giving electrolyte fluid when victim unable to take oral fluids and an IV is not practical. The author's wife and daughter while on a backpacking trip saved the life of a diabetic experiencing an episode of volume-depleted shock in the wilderness with electrolyte fluids given rectally with a camelback water bottle and tube.

Triage

From old French to "cull" or sort out

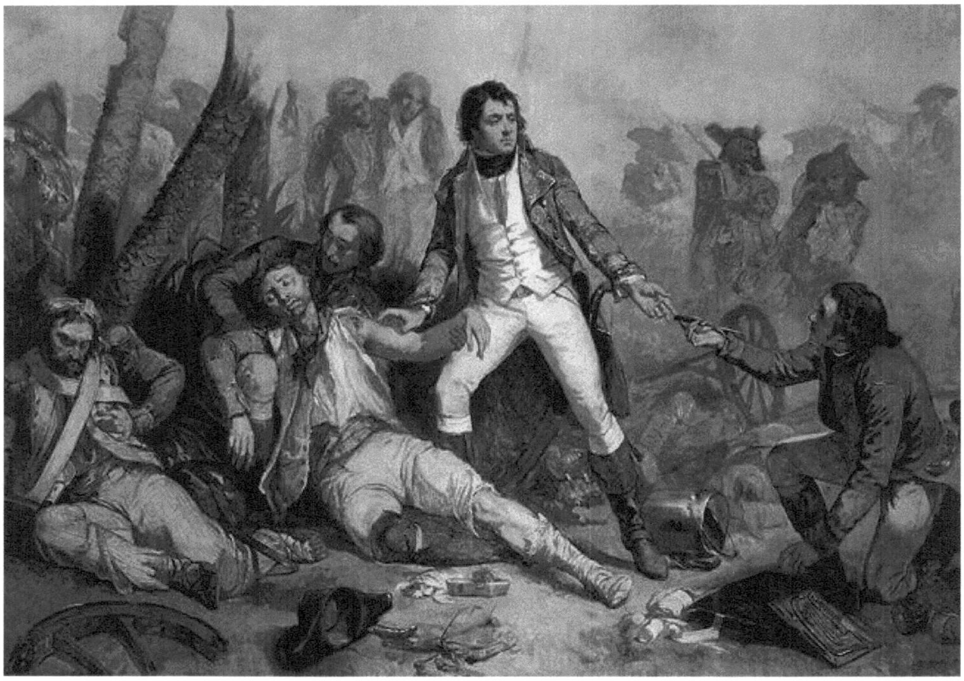

"Field Surgery" by Charles-Louis Muller depicting Napoleon's chief field surgeon, Dominque Larrey and the concept of triage. National Museum of Paris

Deciding in multiple casualties, which receive initial and how much care, requires planning. Often personnel and resources are limited, requiring efficient distribution. Saving limb and life requires careful systematic examination and prompt evaluation in multiple injuries. Triage in combat is the opposite of triage in a civilian ER. During battle, field medical officers were sorted wounded on basis of severity of injures as one would, after multiple causalities in a civilian hospital. However, during a battle the most lightly wounded are treated first, as they can quickly be returned for combat duty. The more severely injured are placed at the end of care, as they require more time and resources. The reverse would occur in a civilian mass causality scenario where the most serious would be first attended. Battles have been won when medical officers quickly treated and returned large numbers of wounded to duty. Medical officers traditionally were unarmed and boldly displayed their medical intentions, however in combat scenarios, American medical officers display neither rank nor profession as medical officer are high asset targets. The author during naval medical training was encouraged to qualify with small arms to defend wounded and staff. A few classmates refused to take up arms for ethical beliefs while in uniform.

Causes of Shock

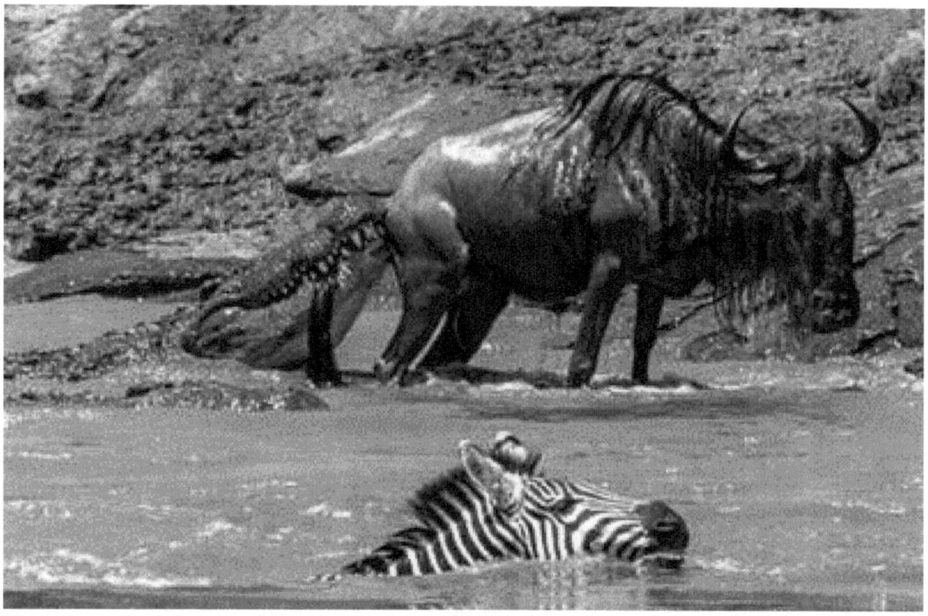

The "wildebeest syndrome" is a non-medical term coined by the San Francisco 49er football coach, Bill Walsh when his team appeared to lay down and die, after the Minnesota Vikings scored three quick touchdowns. On the Serengeti, animals such as the wildebeest, sometimes lay down and die from non-fatal wounds when confronted with being "eaten alive" and the only escape is death. There must be "a kill switch" animals can deploy to commit suicide. When engaged, it is the author's belief that fluid is released from circulation and enters the "third space" within the body resulting in shock. This kill switch is why some people after falling overboard and pulled from the water quickly, are dead, while others can last for hours in the water. Thus, the wildebeest syndrome is unique to each person. Photographed in the Mara River, Kenya where migrating herbivores must run the gauntlet of the carnivore crocodile-infested water crossings. Tumblr

There are many events and conditions that can trigger the phenomenon of shock. And shock is a phenomenon, not a disease, but a complicated body-wide event. It is different in every case and unique in every victim. Many causes of shock are treatable in the field, while some are hopeless even in the hands of a surgical unit. With skill, equipment and medications, heart attack, bleeding, head trauma, pneumothorax, infection, envenomation (direct injection of an alien foreign substance into circulation), anaphylaxis, extreme pain or terror, diabetes, heat and cold injuries can be managed. Heart attack is the most common cause of shock in the United States and in the field (excluding combat). The only effective management of heart attack in the field is effective CPR, fluids and cardiovascular drugs until the heart has returned to normal function and there is adequate circulating fluid.

Blood loss is a common cause of shock in trauma. This loss can be external when a blood vessel's wall has been opened to the outside world with visible evidence of bleeding. Blood loss can be internal, when it occurs within an organ or a body cavity, invisible to direct exam. External bleeding is managed with direct pressure over the bleeding site or just proximal (between the wound and the heart) to it. Direct pressure is best applied with a clean dressing firmly held in place. Tourniquets offer limited use in bleeding, since they constrict not only the violated vessel but all others in the area, leading to tissue damage and perhaps tissue death. If the tourniquet is employed, loosen for ten minutes every hour and blood pressure cuffs make excellent tourniquets. There are instances where shock can occur in non-lethal injuries. In these cases, severe pain, fear and panic can lead to hypovolemic shock without apparent blood loss. Circulating fluid is lost as it leaves circulation and enters "the third space", the space outside the cardiovascular system and outside the cell.

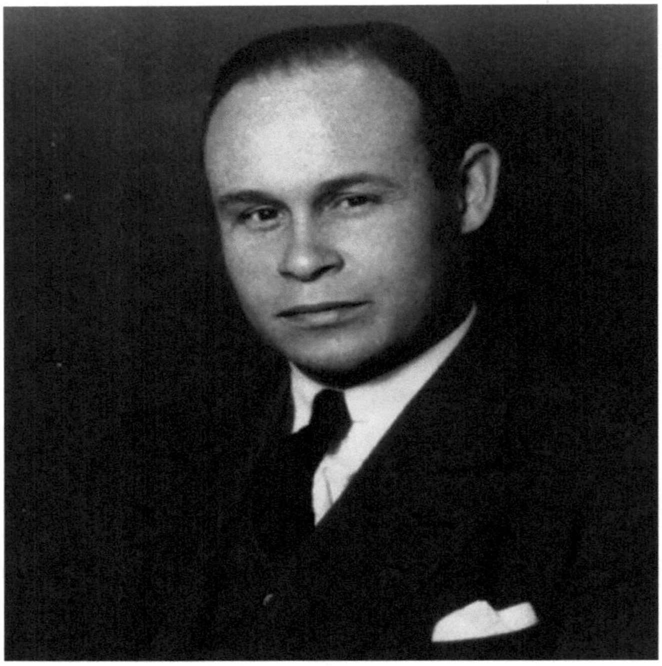

Charles Drew MD, African American physician and researcher who indirectly saved lives of thousands of Allied soldiers in World War II and later with his development of dried plasma. Dr. Drew is one of history's greatest life savers. His preserved plasma, the liquid portion of blood, primarily albumin, was developed in 1938 just in time for the Second World War. Dr. Drew promoted plasma for its longer storage and proved it was just as effective as whole blood to manage volume depleted shock when carefully dried and later reconstituted into fluid plasma. His medical contributions became controversial when he refused to separate blood and plasma based on race. Charles Drew was an outstanding student and athlete at Amherst, and later graduated second in his medical school class at McGill University in Toronto. He was the first African American to get post-doctorate degree from Columbia and the first African American to become an examiner for the American Board of Surgery. During the war, he argued successfully against separating Negro from Caucasian blood, proving that human blood is "colorless". After the war, he became disillusioned with the Red Cross when they returned to separating blood based on race. He was killed in an auto accident while attending a conference in Tuskegee, Mississippi, the site where the Federal government experimented on African American inmates with syphilis. At only 45, he was a great loss. The descendants of the lives he saved could be reading this book. His plasma is on the list of essential medications by the World Health Organization. National Library of Medicine

Internal bleeding is difficult to diagnose and probably impossible to treat without surgery. It should be suspected when the signs of shock appear following trauma with no apparent bleeding sites. Abdominal trauma can result in bleeding from the blood-rich liver and spleen while fractures to large bones such as the hip, thigh, and pelvis are known to produce excessive internal bleeding. Most people would recognize many of the obvious signs of shock, such as pale cool skin, low blood pressure, rapid weak pulse, unconsciousness, dilated pupils, rapid shallow breathing, and sometimes the bluish tint of cyanosis to the skin. All are late signs.

In treatable shock, diagnosis should not wait for the late signs of inadequate circulating fluid since treatment in the field is best effective when employed early. If too much time passes with little or no circulation, the body may suffer serious damage even when the injured survives the initial event. With the advent of highly skilled ambulance crews, more shock victims were successfully resuscitated in the field, and transferred to the hospital after shock had been reversed. However, they sometimes survived shock, only to experience a delayed death caused by damage to lungs, kidneys and other organs by the cell's own toxic wastes. This damage occurs when circulation is restored and toxins produced during shock, primarily in the stagnant muscle tissue, are flushed into the blood. They are then carried to the unprotected lungs and kidneys, where these natural poisons destroy tissue. Destruction prevented by early and aggressive treatment of shock. Management of shock in the field has been a recent development. During the First World War, shock victims were given a cigarette, since nicotine appeared to increase pulse, improve skin color and alertness while alcohol in low doses delivered similar responses. Both could exert a detrimental effect in shock and should be avoided in these modern times.

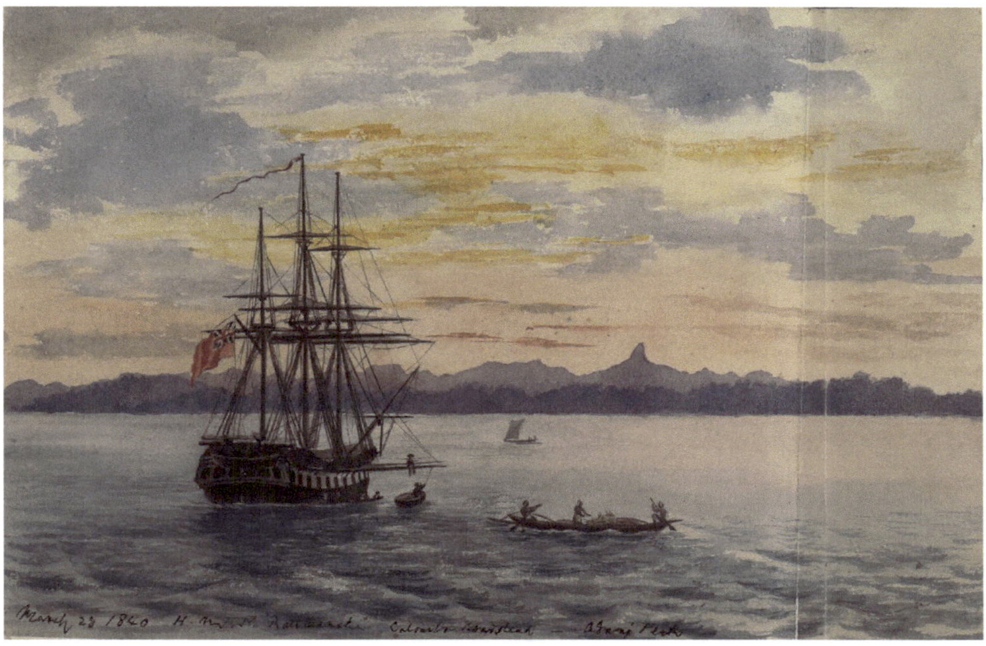

The HMS Rattlesnake (Thomas Huxley's ship), painted by Edward Cree, a mid-eighteenth-century Ships Surgeon. Dr. Cree served in the Royal Navy throughout the Far East, surviving fevers, wounds and typhoons. A typical tour of duty in the Far East theatre for a surgeon and other Royal Navy officers was ten years with only a minority surviving to see merry ole England again. During his years at sea, Cree completed and published over 1500

paintings and drawings with a written journal. In his years in the Far-East, he must have seen many sailors and Marines die of shock from injuries, fever, heat stroke and cholera as he helplessly stood by their death bed. Cholera was and continues to be a major cause of shock, as fluids pour from the rectum. Cholera could kill a healthy person in a single day and quickly spread through ship, camp, army and city.

As previously written and in the author's lectures, some concepts are important enough to repeat such as the initial management of shock: including simple measures of warming and reassuring the person, loosening any tight clothing at the waist and throat (even a T-shirt may constrict at the neck), removing boots and elevating the feet to encourage the flow of blood back to the central organs. After assuring airway, breathing and circulation are adequate, a series of blood pressures are recorded using the Tilt Test. Once again, the tilt test begins with a blood pressure reading obtained with the patient lying down, the brain the same level as the heart. The patient is then raised to 45 degrees, if unconscious, the head is elevated above the heart by gently placing something soft under the victim's back. Blood pressure is taken repeatedly, watching for a drop of either the top or bottom number of the blood pressure. If either number decreases by 10 mm of Mercury, it is a positive tilt test. The tilt test by stressing the cardiovascular system (heart and circulating fluid) may reveal a dropping blood pressure before the other signs of shock. A positive tilt test may be present in an injured person who is alert and complaining of few symptoms yet is in early stage of shock. In fractures, burns, deep penetrating injuries, and other forms of trauma, a tilt test should be part of the initial exam and repeated until the threat of shock has passed.

Anaphylactic Shock

Anaphylactic shock is a sudden allergic reaction caused by invasion of the deep body through circulation by foreign agent (usually a protein). Although possibly fatal, it is the most treatable form of shock, triggered by an insect or animal bite, food ingestion (shellfish) or with some organic chemicals (pesticides). Shock in these cases is due to microscopic "leaking" fluid from circulation into other spaces (third space) on a massive scale. This reaction occurs primarily when mast cells disintegrate, releasing stored histamine and heparin. Mast cells are a type of lymphocyte found in great numbers throughout the body, with especially large concentrations in the respiratory tract. As a result of mast cell's degranulation, fluid leaves circulation, becoming free fluid (examples are "runny nose", watery eyes in allergies). This release, usually a nuisance, can potentially be a fatal event when huge amounts of mast cells degranulate and enough fluid is "siphoned" from circulating fluid to produce shock. An example of the immune system's inappropriate response to what appears a minor injury. What benefit is for a seventy-kilogram human to be killed by a bee weighing a few milligrams? Anaphylaxis occurs when the victim's blood meets a substance the body's defenses have been "sensitized" to by previous contact. In its most severe form produces the sudden, relentless extreme reaction of anaphylaxis (a Greek word meaning adverse protection).

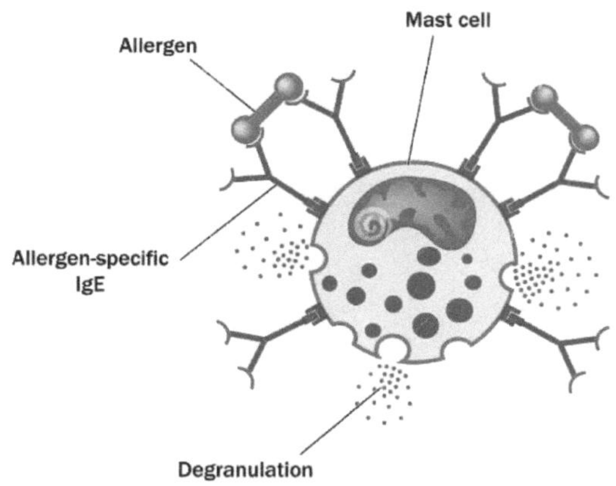

Illustration of mast cell dissolving and releasing heparin/histamine. NIH

An early sign of anaphylaxis appears in the skin as raised red welts (hives) emerging suddenly at one site and then spreading over the body. Breathing may become difficult as the throat tightens as mucus membranes lining the respiratory tract become swollen with fluid that has "leaked" from tiny blood vessels (capillaries). This swelling causes respiratory distress, as increased air is forced into a narrowed respiratory tract stricken by histamine-induced fluids flooding the air compartments. As the rate and force of breathing increases through constricted airways, whistling noises, or wheezing (rhonchi) will be heard with a stethoscope or with unaided ear. Similar reactions are occurring in the gut and elsewhere, where high concentration of mast cells release large amounts of histamine and heparin into circulating blood. The command of such a life-threatening maneuver is an example of the possible danger the immune system may represent to its host. The source of this command, and its reason for existence, is not understood since it serves no useful purpose for survival. A powerful defense requires a powerful offense, one that must be destructive to be effective. The human cell and the body deploy a defense system like “a two-edged sword”. Meaning it can harm as well as defend. The human immune system is probably the most complex in nature and one of the most powerful. Power that can turn on its host.

In anaphylactic shock, the goal of treatment is to prevent or slow the release of histamine while supporting blood pressure and relieving respiratory distress. Antihistamines and epinephrine (adrenalin) may do both. In the intact mast cell, histamine is coupled to heparin, a potent natural blood thinner. On a microscopic level, these two substances cause the thin capillary walls to "weep" fluid from circulation into the spaces between cells. The first space is fluid within the cells (where most of the fluid resides within the body), the second space is circulating fluid and the third space is fluid within the body, not in the first two spaces. On a grand scale, anaphylaxis may siphon enough fluid away from circulation to deny the heart its ability to maintain blood pressure. Treatment, in an event likely to trigger anaphylaxis in a sensitized person (such as one allergic to bee sting), should begin immediately with an antihistamine capsule such as diphenhydramine (Benadryl) 25-50mg. As a rule, the more quickly symptoms develop after envenomation or ingestion, the more serious the reaction.

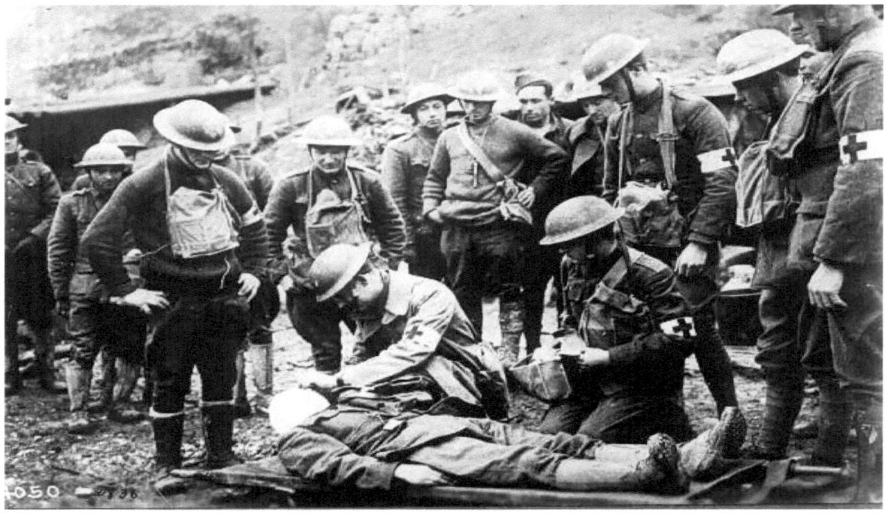

American wounded, Western Front where anaphylactic shock was of little concern as was diabetes induced shock. Clearly a staged photo, as few injured received this much attention. In his memoirs "A Surgeon in Khaki", the author, Dr. A. A. Martin, described being the single surgeon for an entire New Zealand regiment (over 1000 men). The regimental aid station sometimes little more than a standing wall or clump of trees, where he only had enough time and materials to dress wounds and splint fractures. Due to necessity, his apprenticed-trained assistants became medical officers under Martin's supervision. They practiced close to the front where Dr. Martin and much of his staff were killed in action late in the Great War, after serving three years at the front and surviving the earlier Boer War. Medical officers are high value assets and at the same time, expendable. The Great War is only war where more died of battlefield injuries than disease. This was not due to improved field medicine but due to sending masses of men into machine gun and artillery fire over open ground. National Archives

In severe cases of anaphylaxis, an injection (0.3-0.5 cc) or several injections of adrenalin or (epinephrine 1:10,000) must be given, as well as injectable Benadryl (diphenhydramine) 50 mgs. Injected diphenhydramine is more effective than when swallowed. Epinephrine (adrenalin) will work in seconds if injected under the tongue, within minutes if injected shallowly under the skin anywhere on the body. If wheezing is heard in the lungs or sudden shortness of breath develops, an injection of both epinephrine and diphenhydramine is indicated. Adrenalin acts more quickly and forcibly than Benadryl, producing brief side effects of rapid pulse, elevated blood pressure and nervousness. Because of this, epinephrine should be used cautiously in a person who may have heart disease, since it could increase the risk of heart attack. However, in a falling blood pressure, epinephrine is the only drug that will support blood pressure directly. Diphenhydramine, on the other hand, will maintain a longer effect in slowing down histamine release, while causing no adverse effects on the heart. Diphenhydramine (Benadryl) capsule or other oral antihistamines are used in less severe cases of suspected allergic reactions. Every first aid kit should include a separate small "bee sting kit" with a small syringe pre-filled with 1.0 cc of adrenalin and 1.0 cc (50 mg) of Benadryl (diphenhydramine) in both injection and oral form.

Diabetes Mellitus

Greek/Latin for sweet urine

Poorly controlled diabetes may result in shock if glucose is too low or too high. If a diabetic has taken too much insulin or injected the normal amount but has been unable to eat, insulin overdose may result in severe hypoglycemia (low blood sugar), a life-threatening shock. It may be preceded by seizure activity and must be treated immediately with intravenous sugar to prevent brain damage. In emergency rooms, dextrose or glucagon injection is given initially in seizures and shock, if no working diagnosis has been established. If an IV site cannot be accessed quickly, inject the sugar solution directly under the tongue, as this area is filled with large veins. There is little risk from administration of glucose in the field and medicine chests should include some form of glucose, dextrose, fructose or glucagon in a pre-loaded syringe for quick use. Insulin is dangerous in the field without the ability to monitor blood sugar and therefore has little if any value in a field medicine chest. Hyperglycemia (high blood sugar) occurs with too little insulin. It can be the result of illness or stress in a diabetic, elevating glucose with symptoms of fatigue, abdominal pain and thirst. All are signs of high blood sugar, and if glucose climbs into the hundreds, a diabetic coma may occur. Hyperglycemia is managed with high volume fluids. On the other hand, Hypoglycemia (low blood sugar) results from too much insulin or too little food, resulting in hunger, weakness, confusion, seizures, insulin shock.

The goal in management of shock in most cases, especially trauma, is fluid replacement. And the best mechanism to get fluid into circulation is through the gut. Diluted electrolyte solutions are far superior to drinking water as plain water is slow to be absorbed and lacks chemicals cells need. Outside of diabetic shock, low circulating fluid, **hypovolemic shock** is the target to resolve. There are countless stories after battles of the wounded pleading for water and in some early cases, drinking water may prevent the evolution of hypovolemic shock. For the medical officer, fluid replacement is the gold standard and the ability to perform this task is at the heart of shock management. After simple measures and evaluation with blood pressure, fluid replacement is the next step. Intravenous fluid is not the best option, but in trauma, it may be the only choice, and the medical officer should the trained in opening and maintaining a vein. If this fails and the injured is unable to take fluids orally, they can be given rectally with minimal expertise as an enema. Fluid replacement came into wide use during the Second World War and has remained a core skill in the management of hypovolemic shock in the field.

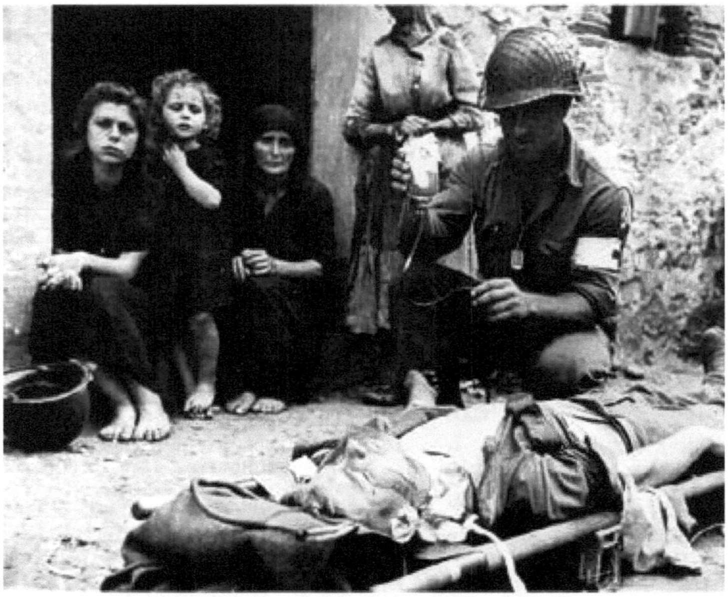

ADMINISTERING PLASMA TO WOUNDED MAN *at 7th Infantry aid station, Sant'Agata*

Giving plasma, a reconstituted blood, was a huge addition to field medicine. Whole fresh blood had been used for decades in hospitals for replacing blood loss in trauma. However, to get whole fresh blood into the field, is much more difficult. The above-enlisted medical officer has the training to catharize a vein and give intravenous preserved dried blood which has been reconstituted with water. Plasma is safe, simple to deploy and highly effective in replacing fluids lost in trauma. A perfect field medicine tool! People in villages of Sicily like those in the photo have witnessed many armies and generations of wounded on their volcanic island. It was in Sicily where the quote "don't kill the messenger" emerges from history. In the 5th century BC, Athens suffered a horrendous defeat at Syracuse, losing an entire navy and army. Almost every family in Athens was affected and the news so bad, the first three messengers were put to death to hide the defeat from public. National Archives

Fluid replacement is the most effective treatment in most causes of shock, even if unknown. There is no substitute for fluid replacement in management of low blood pressure or other signs of shock, and the earlier the better. Modern electrolyte fluid given orally or rectally (if no intravenous accessible) should be given until urine produced, alertness returns, and other treatment rendered as needed. Infections, especially hemorrhagic fevers can cause septic shock which without early aggressive antibiotics and fluids are fatal. Infection can cause a type of hemophilia when clotting factors are consumed within blood vessels, causing bleeding inside and the outside body with ensuing shock. Uncontrolled bleeding is the hallmark of hemophilia. In the field, bleeding with hemophilia is likely beyond management. Hemophilia is inherited and rare, but it has a place in this book.

Defective DNA, an armored train, and a man of God

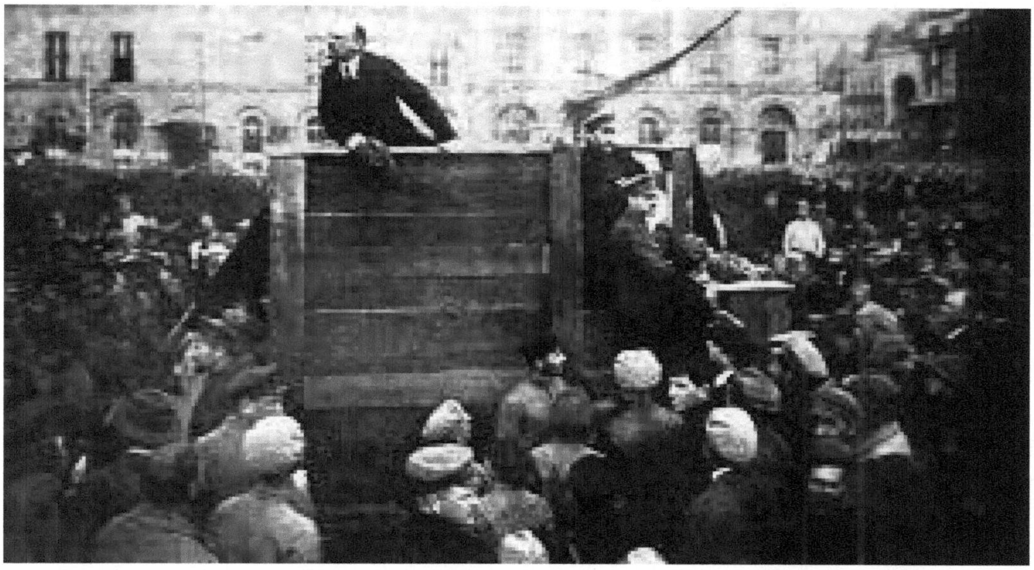

"Without Rasputin, there would have been no Lenin" historian Robert Massey. Without Hemophilia, there would have been no Rasputin. National Archives

Diseases, especially infections, have been major players in human history. The Plague of Athens of 430 BC ended the Peloponnesian War, swept order from the Mediterranean, and created the greatness of Alexander the Great. The Plague of Justinian in the 6th century AD gravely wounded the first great Christian nation ruled from Constantinople, leaving a void in the Mediterranean world quickly filled by Islam. In 632 AD, two years after uniting Arabia, Muhamad died and the religion he created swarmed out of the Arabian Peninsula, conquering Persia in 637, Jerusalem 638, Mosul 641, Alexandra and in Egypt 642, Kabul 642, North Africa, Spain, Cyprus, Sicily and much of Central Asia by 722. They were turned back in western France in 732 at the Battle of Tours, likely saving Christian Europe. Without the Plague of Justinian, Islam might have remained in the Arabian deserts. Black Death during the mid and late 14th century ravaged Europe, directly leading to the Renaissance. All three of these devastating plagues were preceded by large volcanic eruptions in Indonesia and comet strikes resulting in climate changes. In the early 20th century, influenza killed seventy million people and ended the First World War. These infections killed tens of millions, yet a single disease in a single person was just as powerful in changing history.

Hemophilia and Rasputin, a juxtaposition of a rare normally mild inherited medical condition genetically acquired from Queen Victoria and a peasant monk from Siberia, created a perfect storm of weak leadership, pathological motherhood, military defeats, famine, alcoholism and a strong dose of evil that changed the world in the early 20th century. Changes as powerful as any pandemic in history, one that continues to affect the world. Hemophilia is a Greek for blood loving, that was later defined as excessive bleeding after trauma or surgery. Alexis, the fifth child of Nicolas II and Alexandra and only son, thus the heir to the Russian throne, had unfortunately inherited the gene for hemophilia from his German mother, one of Victoria's favorite granddaughters. Alexis' father, Tsar Nicolas II was first cousin to his wife's uncle, King George V, a close geneti c coupling (inbreeding) resulting in a disaster for Russia and for the world. Another ruling European family, the Hapsburgs by 1914 had endured five hundred years of inbreeding, resulting in no competent leadership since the 16th century with Charles V of Spain and his illegitimate son, Don Juan of

Austria. Alexis inherited a particularly malignant form of hemophilia, one that caused large painful bleeds into joints, sometimes with only slight trauma.

During severe episodes, screams of pain from the young prince were heard throughout the palace, agonizing for his parents. There was no treatment for the type of hemophilia suffered by Alexis until late in the 20th century and poor child and his parents' endured years of suffering helplessly. Imperial Russia's humiliation by Japan in the war of 1904-5 (a war Germany's Kaiser William encouraged his cousin Nicolas II to wage), the near revolution of 1907, poor harvests in 1910-11 and reliance on foreign investments battered the leadership of Nicolas II, already a weak leader at best. "The wrong man at the wrong time" Robert Massey describes the tragedy of Nicolas II. 1914 found Europe at peace with no major European wars since Napoleon's defeat at Waterloo. Yet many nations were heavily armed and poised for war when a single incident in the Balkans set off a chain of events, like a chain of chemical reactions within the cell, swept through Europe as quickly as had Black Death. In 1914 the Tsar of Russia controlled Europe's largest army, but a country so primitive, it could not transport, supply nor lead Russia's huge masses of men, animals and materials. The French army knew Russia's aid was critical if war came with Germany and had been pouring large loans and massive engineering into building railroads in western Russia to move the enormous Russian army to the German border. By August 1914, it was almost too late.

The Russia soldier was brave but poorly led and poorly supplied, many sent into battle against the professional German army without food, medical care and in some cases without rifles! Vast number of dead, wounded and abandoned led to great distress at home. The war started with fanfare and enthusiasm that soon turned to despair and anger. A nation and a cell deprived of nourishment and exposed to toxic agents is ripe for failure.

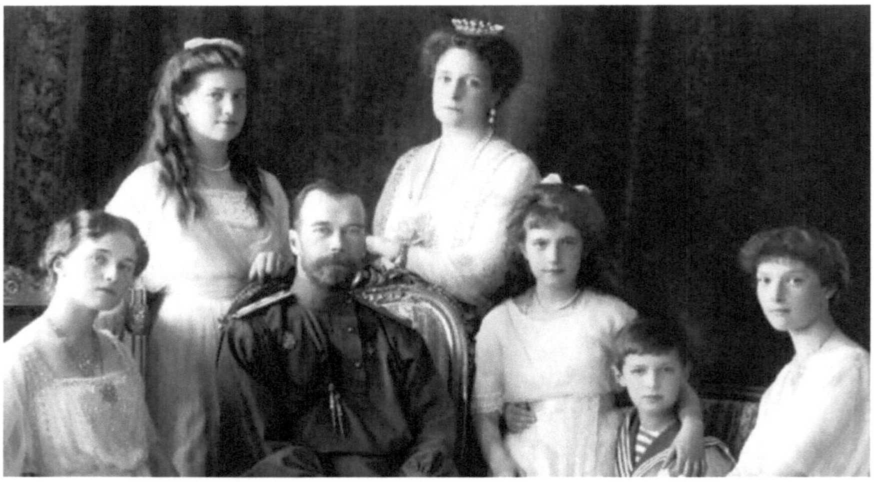

The last Romanov family in happier days. The Tsar and Empress were so invested with the medical condition of their son, they ignored the sickness of their country. They paid for their sins with a brutal slaying of themselves, their five children and the pitiless socialist subjugation of their people. All due to a microscopic misalignment of DNA. The wrong man at the wrong time combined with the wrong disease at the wrong time.
National Archives

Circulating fluid contains twenty factors necessary for blood to clot. One of these is Factor IX, an enzyme necessary in a long line of other chemical reactions, all required in preventing bleeding from wounds. The genes of Queen Victoria contained a DNA defective code for the manufacture of Factor IX and its absence prevents blood from clotting. The cascade of reactions required for these twenty factors to clot blood is too complicated for the author and the reader. This inherited defect is now called Christmas Disease, named for the family where it was diagnosed. There are acquired conditions of bleeding disorders associated with infection and some are serious. Disseminated intravascular coagulation (DIC) occurs in severe infections when the clotting factors are consumed within circulation, leading to widespread internal bleeding and death. COVID-19 in its lethal forms, causes DIC as does other hemorrhagic viral infections such as Ebola, Yellow Fever, Lassa Fever, Rift Valley Fever (the author received an immunization for Rift Valley Fever while in Egypt), malaria and some tick-borne hemorrhagic infections. Just malignant cells, whose innocence has been changed into a force of evil, overcomes normal cells and if strong enough, overcomes the body. Malignant people can overcome a nation. This happened the Russia during the Great War.

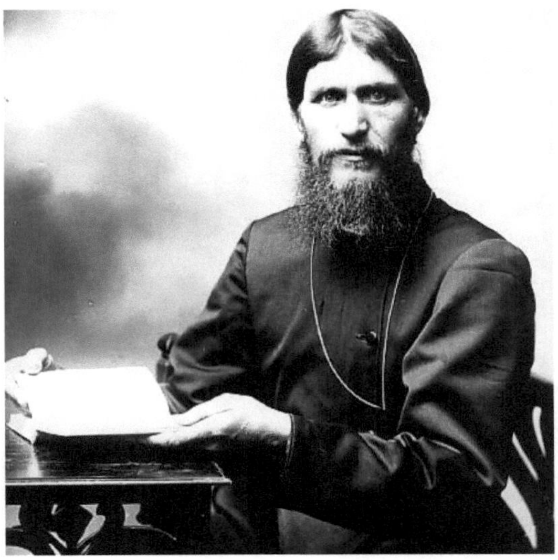

Photo by Kal Bulla 1910, Rasputin looks almost normal in this image.

At no time in history has a single genetic defect wrought such misery on the world. Because there is no parallel in history for a Rasputin and a disease in a single person resulting in so much human tragedy. Empress Alexandra was deeply religious combined with a form of malignant motherhood spending hours in prayer every day for her son's survival. She genuinely believed the monk was sent by God to save her son and his future throne. Rasputin was a powerful person and deployed a force strong enough to penetrate and control the Tsarist government of Russia during the Great War. He was unwashed, had blackened his teeth, barely literate, large, powerful, sexually promiscuous and an alcoholic. Many nights he laid drunk in St Petersburg brothels, yet wives of aristocrats and officers were frequent visitors to his flat. The Empress went against the pleading of her family and government officials demanding Rasputin be expelled from the capital. The Tsar, too weak to confront his German wife, fled from the turmoil and taking personal command of his armies in the field far from the capital. Command that further degraded his army's effectiveness. The Empress was openly called "that German woman" with few allies in St. Petersburg. By 1917,

Rasputin was discharging and appointing ministers at will, further degrading leadership in the eyes of the people. He was finally lured to a meeting where young ladies were promised where he was poisoned by a royal physician, shot, and bludgeoned royal family members. In a government reeling from losses on the battlefield, Rasputin's corruption of leadership and the German injection of Lenin in an armored train filled with gold and revolutionaries, finished off three hundred years of Romanov rule. Germany helped in dismantlement of the government of Imperial Russia, replacing it with three years of civil war and the removal of Russian armies from the First World War. The Soviet Russia that emerged played the major role in defeating Germany in the Second World War.

Blood Pressure

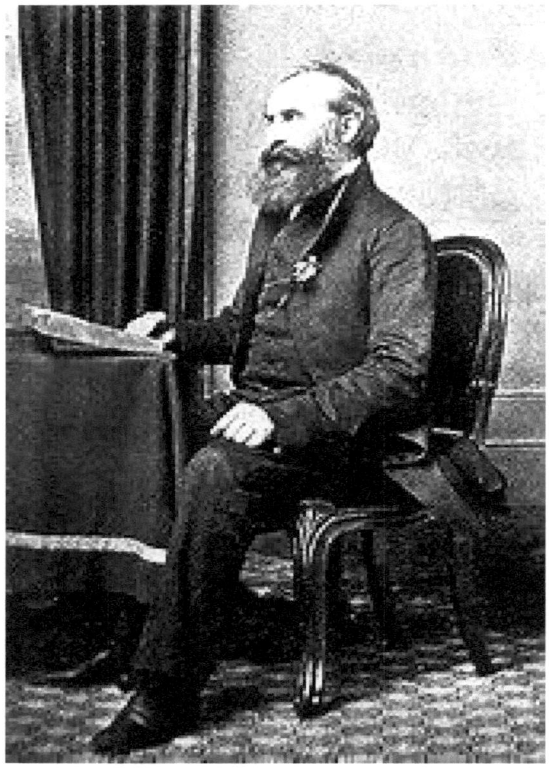

Thomas Hodgkin (1798-1866) one of the world's first pathologists is credited for describing the cancer of the lymphatic system that bears his name and wrote extensively on heart disease. Although he did not measure blood pressure (blood pressures have only been routinely measured since the 1940s), he documented pulse changes in amplitude over the different arteries and in different conditions later verified by the blood pressure cuff and meter. In shock and severe heart disease, blood pressures fall, while in the normal heart, pain and excitement, pressures increase. Careful blood pressure measurement is an important part of most examinations. Garrison

Pressure within the artery can be measured by a simple machine employing a bladder connected to a pressure gauge, that when inflated, compresses, and then completely collapses the walls of the underlying artery. When pressure within the cuff is higher than the pressure generated by contraction of the left side of the heart, the artery underneath the cuff is closed, ceasing blood flow beyond the cuff. The slow release of pressure within the cuff will eventually allow blood flow to "squirt" under the cuff, creating sounds of turbulence which can be detected with a stethoscope listening over the slowly opening artery. The pressure within the bladder when the first heart sound heard is noted on a dial in millimeters of Hg (mercury). The pressure reading on the dial when the first heart sound is heard reflects the pressure in the left side of heart, the pump pressure or systolic pressure. Although it is usually obtained with both a blood pressure cuff and stethoscope, it can be measured with the cuff only. While monitoring the pulse at the wrist, note the pressure in the cuff when pulse is once again felt. This may be necessary in the field, since it must be relatively quiet for one to hear sounds of turbulent blood flow created within the compressed artery by a blood pressure cuff. The author strongly recommends a mechanical blood pressure cuff in the field as the electronic devices are poor tourniquets, are fragile and require batteries.

Blood pressure is recorded in two numbers when the stethoscope is used, the top number is the pressure generated by the heart's forceful contraction (systole). The bottom number represents line pressure within the artery when the heart is at rest (diastole). It is against this lower pressure that the heart must open its valves to discharge each stroke of blood. Elevated diastolic pressure (hypertension) increases work on a heart as it must overcome higher pressures with each beat. A heart beats around 120,000 times each day and when this number is multiplied over months and years, it becomes apparent why hypertension will "wear-out" a heart. Untreated hypertension reduces the life span of heart muscle while increases the risk of stroke, as higher pressures are driven through the brain's small arteries.

Blood pressure often changes as we age. In most Americans, the systolic pressure increases as arteries become stiff and congested, requiring increased pressure to drive blood through narrowing small arterioles. As older vessels become constricted with cholesterol, iron and other debris, they weaken, becoming more likely to leak or rupture at higher pressures. In cultures with little salt and less meat, blood pressure lowers with aging. This would make more sense in protecting the aging human from strokes and heart attacks. The diet of most Americans is not complimentary to aging safely, otherwise it would contain less processed food and more fiber.

Measuring blood pressure in the arm, begins with finding the pulse in the crease of the elbow (brachial artery). This large artery lies close to the skin's surface at the inboard part (medial) of this crease. The pulse should be felt with the index and middle finger pressed firmly into the skin (do not use the thumb, since it has a pulse of its own). Pulse can be taken at this site by counting beats for 15 seconds and multiply by 4, giving beats per minute. Over the site where the pulse is strongest, the stethoscope is placed, with the blood pressure cuff secured above it. Next, locate the pulse at the wrist on the thumb side, the radial artery. Inflate the cuff while feeling the radial pulse, when it disappears the pressure in the cuff has overcome the pressure within the artery. Inflate the cuff 20-30 mm of Hg above this number and slowly deflate the bladder. It is not always necessary to feel for pulse to know how high to inflate the cuff; most people will simply inflate to 140-160 mm Hg and slowly release. As the cuff is slowly deflated, at some point blood will "squirt" under the cuff, freeing itself from the constricted artery and creating a sound. Imagine a flowing silent stream, that when a rock or other object is placed to interfere with the flow, will create turbulence. Turbulence creates noise and the constricting cuff does just that. By creating constriction of flow, the cuff generates the sounds heard through the stethoscope and these man-made sounds are measured on the pressure gauge.

The first clear sound represents the systolic pressure. This number can also be obtained by recording the pressure when the pulse of the radial artery at the wrist returns. Therefore, when a stethoscope is not practical (as in a noisy engine room or during a storm), the systolic pressure can be obtained. The diastolic pressure is the pressure where the last sound is heard as the cuff continues to deflate. This last audible sound is sometimes difficult to hear and cannot be measured without a stethoscope in a quiet setting. Normal pressure is 120/80 for men and varies from that number to 90/60 for women. It is lower in most women, because of the female hormone, estrogen. Blood pressure is highest in morning and any numbers of 140/100 or higher should be evaluated for treatment.

If repeated blood pressure readings are taken, be sure to completely deflate the cuff each time. If the cuff remains inflated for any length of time, it will be uncomfortable and by pooling blood within the arm, will falsely elevate the pressures. The most accurate measures are obtained when the arm, cuff and artery area are at the same level as the heart. In the event of severe bleeding, the blood pressure cuff is an excellent tourniquet, allowing a wide soft constrictor of blood flow. To control bleeding, place the cuff above the bleeding site and inflate just enough to stop. Deflate cuff every 15 minutes unless deflation results in continued blood loss.

Napoleon Bonaparte

General, Emperor and Medical Officer

The chaos of the French Revolution and subsequent invasions by the surrounding monarchies led to the rise of a little-known artillery officer from Corsica. This author believes it takes a stretch of the imagination, to believe Napoleon a Frenchman, as Corsica had not been a part of France until seven years before his birth. He and his family spoke Italian at home and belonged to a minor aristocratic family. In Corsica, families were more like the clans of the Scottish highlanders than French aristocrats. French was not Napoleon's first language, and his French was so bad, it encouraged disparaging remarks behind his back. Later Napoleon with his bad French, conquered most of Europe, toppled kings, princes and queens, rearranged regimes, dissolved borders, creating new nations, imposed the metric system to the continent and pushed medical frontiers, all while destroying large tracts of Europe. Napoleon had little use for the Roman Catholic Church, especially the Inquisition, reducing the power of the Church in the Catholic countries he conquered. He was responsible for combining over two hundred tiny states and cities in central Europe into a handful of departments, making it much easier for Otto Bismarck to create modern Germany later in the 19th century. A creation that invaded France three times in the next seventy years, twice successfully.

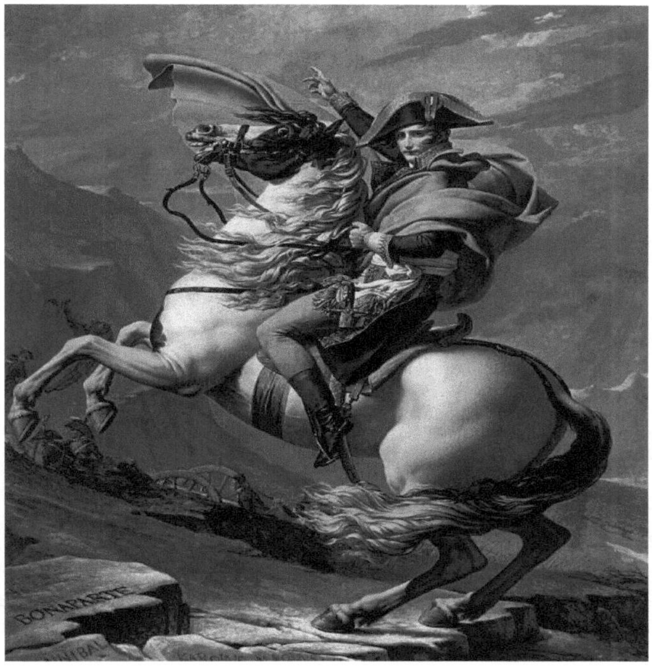

Jacques-Louis David's overstatement of Napoleon crossing the Alps during a break in the weather in the spring of 1800, surprising and defeating the Austrians. He used the Saint Bernard Pass and had no elephants. Hannibal crossed these Alps 2000 years before with elephants with similar results, surprising and defeating Rome at Cannae, where 50,000 Romans fell.

Napoleon believed he was blessed by something greater than himself, as his luck saved him many times early in his reign. In 1792, paperwork detailing his treason as rebel leader in Corsica was lost during the chaos of The Reign of Terror described by Charles Dickens in "Tale of two Cities". Documentation of Napoleon's actions in Corsica's attempt at independence from Revolutionary France would have resulted in his appointment with Dr. Guillotine's invention. In 1793, Napoleon received a spike wound through his thigh while leading from the front, and unlike most similar wounds, did not become infected or lead to an amputation and possibly death. He rose quickly through the fog of wars France was fighting, winning battles, and surrounding himself with a cadre of combat, engineering, and medical officers. By the end of the 18th century, he attained command of all French armies and in a surprise amphibious attack, occupied Malta (evicting the Knights of Malta) without firing a shot, obtained a naval base and a large amount of plunder.

After evading Nelson's British fleet in the Mediterranean, he landed in Egypt and at "The Battle of the Pyramids" destroyed the Mameluke army deploying his five divisions using a new technique of "hollow" squares of infantry with cannons on the corners. This tactic surprised and defeated repeated charges by the legendary Mameluke cavalry. With engineers, artists and historians he gathered and shipped back many ancient artifacts, which remain in French museums today. Much to the chagrin of Egypt. Admiral Nelson and the British were outraged at Napoleon's successful thrust into the Eastern Mediterranean threatening England's power. One artist that joined the French army and rendered many paintings of Napoleon's victories was Louis-Francois Lejeune. As a combat engineer, he carried paint and brushes into battle, becoming an important witness to Napoleon's campaigns.

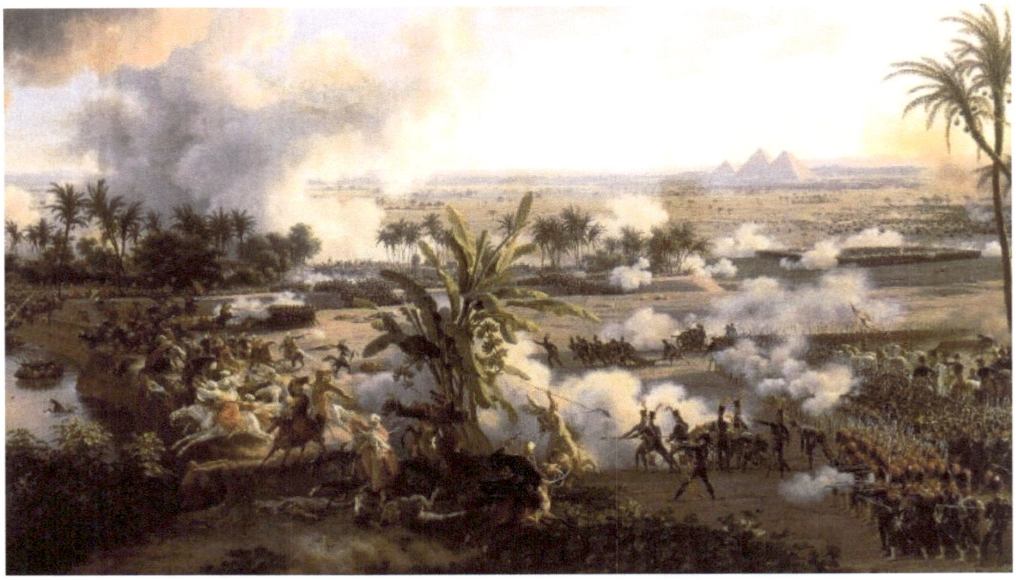

Battle of the Pyramids July 21, 1798, by Louis-Francois Lejeune

The surprising achievements of occupying Malta and Egypt were followed by a British surprise, when Horatio Nelson attacked and destroyed the French fleet anchored in Aboukir Bay, essentially stranding Napoleon and his army. After conquering the Nile Delta and with no navy to evacuate the French army, he attacked north into Syria. In attacking Acre, Napoleon placed his headquarters on the same high ground where Richard the Lionhearted had directed his attack six centuries earlier. In the withdrawal from Syria, the lack of supplies, fevers and thirst drove him back to Egypt. In this retreat (the first of many), Napoleon made a grim request of his medical officers. Captured French soldiers had been cruelly tortured thus far by the Turks, and Napoleon did not want the wounded he was leaving behind to suffer, medical officers under orders deliberately dispensed high doses of opium to end lives silently and pleasantly. A violation of the Hippocratic Oath, yet a humanitarian violation.

Without a navy to resupply him, he knew the French army in Egypt was doomed. So in 1799 he abandoned his army, returned to France, barely escaping capture by the British Navy for a second time due to unexpected favorable winds. Arriving in Paris without thousands of fathers, husbands and sons Napoleon left behind, his continued power was doubtful in Revolutionary France. At this time, he took a desperate gamble, leading the reserve army over the Alps, during a break in spring storms, meeting the Austrians at Marengo. This move, like the German attack through the Ardennes in 1940, was so unexpected, it achieved total victory.

At Marengo, after crossing the Alps, he won the great battle primarily by accident when a rapidly flooding river saved him after overconfidently dividing his army. The fighting was desperate by his outnumbered infantry, firing volley after volley into lines of men fifty to sixty yards apart for over an hour, barely holding until the troops stopped by the river, returned. Napoleon's infantry under his direct supervision at the front and in range of Austrian muskets, had his soldiers urinate on their muskets to prevent gunpowder from igniting when poured down heated barrels. A victory snatched from the "jaws of defeat" further enhanced a supernatural belief in himself.

In early December 1805 at Austerlitz, Napoleon achieved an even more unlikely victory when he abandoned the high ground, turned an army 90 degrees attacking the flank and rear of two larger armies, hailed as "the greatest feat of arms" up to that time. This was the high mark of Napoleon. After the battle he crowned himself Emperor of France, controlling most of Europe and creating many enemies.

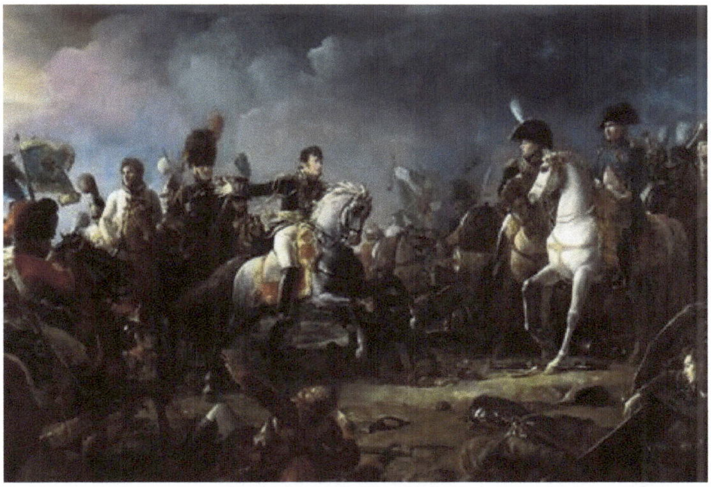

Austerlitz is considered Napoleon's greatest victory, defeating the Emperors of Austria and Russia. Patton's Third Army executed a similar maneuver, turning 90 degrees at the Battle of the Bulge, 1944, again hailed a major feat of arms. Francis Gerard painting

Napoleon's luck begins to change with the invasion of Spain and the slave revolt in Haiti. The microbiology of Haiti inflicted heavy costs on his invincibility. France never subdued Spain but did finally secure Haiti's sugar supply at an extremely high price as sugar was major source of income for Napoleon's wars and empire. During the revolt, the French lost two dozen generals, twenty thousand soldiers and estimated three hundred and fifty thousand civilians including most of the French colonists. The war became brutal beyond imagination as a tiny mosquito and the yellow fever it carried ravaged the French Army, killing many more than did the rebels. Napoleon realized if he could barely hold on to half an island, France could not control the Louisiana Territory against the rapidly growing United States. The Louisiana Purchase that Napoleon sold to Jefferson's government in 1803 was not his to sell. England, Hapsburg Spain and Bourbon France did not recognize the sale until after the United States won the battle of New Orleans in 1815. In addition to needing the money to subdue Spain by selling the confiscated Territory of Louisiana to the United States, he wrote clairvoyantly "I have just given to England a maritime rival". Sugar had become an important part of most lives in early 19th century Europe, and Napoleon's "Continental System" whereby all trade on the continent passed through his hands made French sugar much expensive than sugar in the homes of the English and the people they traded. Russia preferred the cheaper British sugar and other things, openly trading with England in violation of the deal Nicolas I made after his defeat Austerlitz to buy only from France. Napoleon invaded Russia over trade and a personal "slight" by Nicolas I, punishing him by invading, just as Alexander the Great invaded Bactria to punish the murderer of the defeated King of Persia, Darius and the United States invaded Afghanistan to punish the perturbators of September 11, 2001. All three invasions ended badly.

Much of Napoleon's military success was based on logistics; organized field medicine, concentrated use of artillery, commissary to feed both men and horses, clothing the army (six pairs of shoes for each infantryman) and good luck. France had a healthier and therefore more effective army because of his inspired innovative advances in field medicine. He wrote over three hundred papers on field medicine, laying foundations for modern military field medical care. Safe drinking fluids and field sanitation were primary medical pillars in Napoleonic warfare. Soldiers were restricted from drinking from streams or wells and instead were furnished wine diluted with secured water from mobile horse-drawn tankers twice daily. Flogging could result from violating this rule, as Napoleon knew men could quickly sicken and die in large numbers with fevers and dysentery (cholera) from consuming contaminated water. He surmised some agent was in local water that could destroy the army, agents Pasteur discovered generations later. Napoleon spent freely on research into "potable" food such a dried soup, sealing meat in wine bottles and pickled vegetables. He knew preserved meats and vegetables along with safe drinking water were needed in maintaining and deploying an army. Three decades later the English invented canned meats and vegetables, however, the lead used to seal can, negated any advantage of the preserved food. It was lead poisoning that doomed The Franklin Expedition searching for a passage to China over the frozen North America continent in the 1840's. Among other things, the expedition was an experiment of the British Admiralty in long-range sea travel nutrition. This experiment of preserved foods for exploration failed.

Heat Injuries

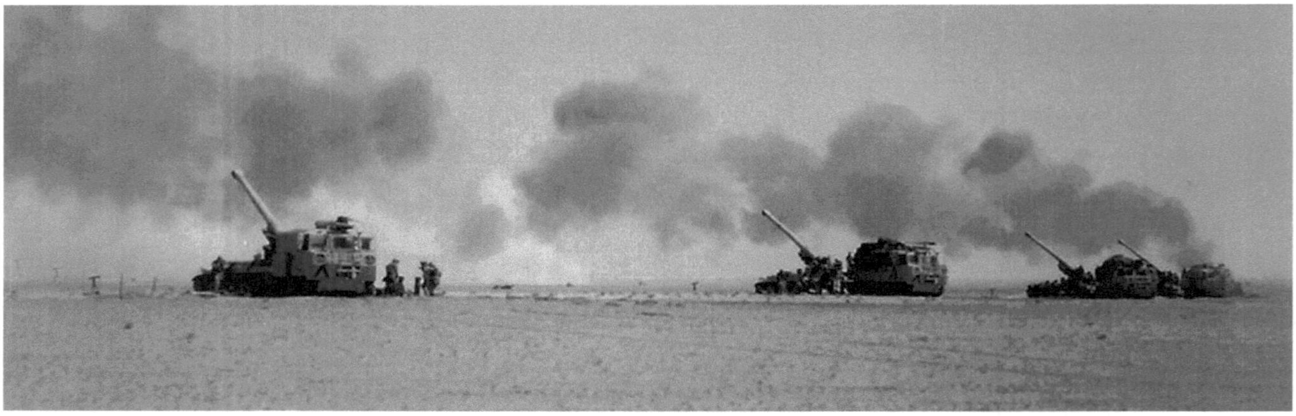

8-inch howitzers from Arkansas in the Mideast desert. Heat injuries accounted for most causalities in the first Mideast invasion 1991 as well as the 1973 Arb-Israeli War. National Archives

Heat injuries have several names, heat stroke, heat exhaustion and heat prostration. They are essentially the same with different levels of severity. All heat injuries begin with inadequate fluid intake which prevents discharging the heat produced in the body's trillions of metabolically active cells. In heat injury, the body temperature rises, and its prevention and treatment consist of fluid replacement and if temperature approaches 104 degrees, immediate cooling! Give fluids until urine is produced while cooling the entire body with cold water with towels or emersion. Heat injuries are believed to be preventable with adequate fluid intake and in the Israeli and American army, losing troops to heat injury are grounds to be relieved of command.

Drinking water safety is one of the most important tools of war as dehydration is a medical condition that has repeatedly played major roles in history. At the Siege of Malta, the defenders had adequate drinking water while the invading Turks did not. The British conquered much of the world by the accidental medical microbiology of boiling water before consumption, to make tea. Drinking tea greatly reduced the incidence of dysentery and was paramount to the British sailor and soldier. During the Battle of Stalingrad, Russian snipers targeted German watercarriers, knowing that thirst would drive German soldiers to drink from contaminated water pools, leading to dysentery. On the 2nd day of Gettysburg, General Longstreet knowing his men had been marching all day in the humid summer heat ordered filled canteens to be given to his troops before attacking the high ground. Unfortunately for the Confederacy, this order was not executed. Had the dry and thirsty Confederate troops attacking Little Round Top been given drinking water before assaulting uphill on a hot Pennsylvania July day, they probably would have carried the Union position and flanked the entire Federal army. Longstreet's infantry under Generals Hood and McLaws arrived parched, overheated and less effective. Dehydration reduces mental and physical capabilities and the brigades under General Hood attacked Little Round Top uphill in a dehydrated state certainly blunted their attack. Drinking water in adequate amounts has won battles. While the lack of safe drinking water has lost them.

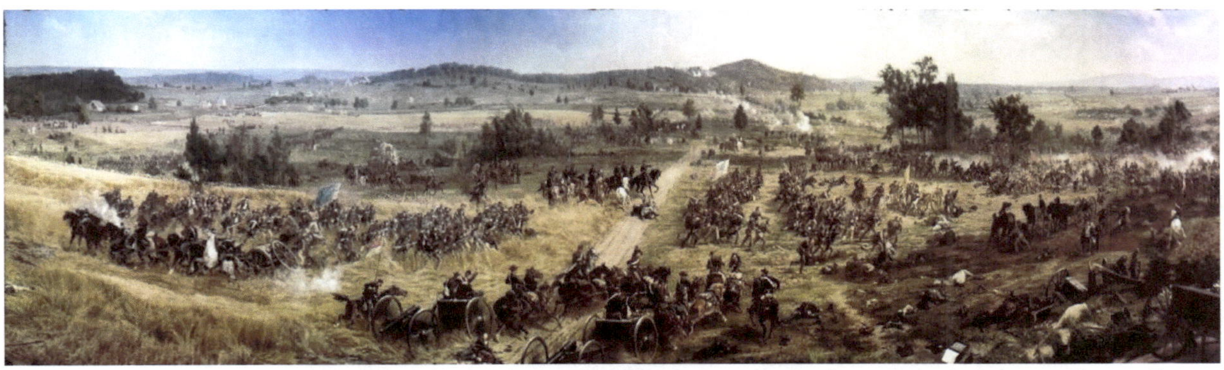

James Longstreet said the fighting his corps preformed on the second day at Gettysburg "was the finest three hours of fighting by any troops on any battlefield in history". Had they been better hydrated, they likely could have turned the Union right flank and won the battle of Gettysburg. In the background of this portion of the Panorama by Paul Philippoteaux shows the high ground Longstreet's two divisions attacked the much larger two Union Corps on a hot Pennsylvania July day.

As impressive as Longstreet's troops fight at Gettysburg, the Confederate soldiers attacking the fortified position at Franklin, Tennessee November 1864 could make a strong case to be included in that class of fighting. At Franklin, Confederate General John Bell Hood sent some 20,000 infantrymen across an open mile-long field into the teeth of an equal number of Union troops backed by thirty-eight three-inch guns. The carnage was worse than the 3rd Day of Gettysburg and the medical care rendered was just as inadequate. Both the Union and Southern armies had endured forced marching to come to battle leaving medical resources well to the rear resulting in medical carnage.

Some historians believe the Confederate attack at Franklin was Hood's punishment for his army's reluctance to attack fortified positions and supposed betrayal of orders. The night before the battle, an entire Union army, almost 25,000 men, hundreds of horses, wagons and cannons "crept" by Hood's sleeping soldiers on a turnpike that was supposed to be sealed. Confederate camps were only a few hundred yards from the road and "the Wizard in the Saddle", Nathan Bedford Forrest with his cavalry were tasked with watching John Schofield's Union army. The next morning when Hood and his officers, including Forrest, saw the turnpike strewn with discarded Union packs, broken wagons and other gear, it was not hard to image the rage in John Bell Hood, a general known for his temper. One officer reported he was "as mad as a rattlesnake", anger likely enhanced by morphine withdrawal. Arriving before Franklin in a late fall afternoon with the sun due to set soon, Hood sent his army in a suicidal assault which failed and wrecked his army. Hood survived unlike most of his senior officers as six of his generals were killed outright, six survived with major wounds and one captured, all leading from the front within the first hour of battle. The day before all this happened, General Hood had fallen from his horse and painfully injured his amputated leg stump, requiring increase doses of morphia for his chronic pain. After the injury, he retreated from his troops to headquarters in a comfortable large estate where he recovered under the influence of opiates while the Union army in a long line stole around his sleeping troops. Just as the medical condition of dehydration played a pivotal role at Gettysburg, the pharmacology of opium played a major role in the failed assault at Franklin, Tennessee.

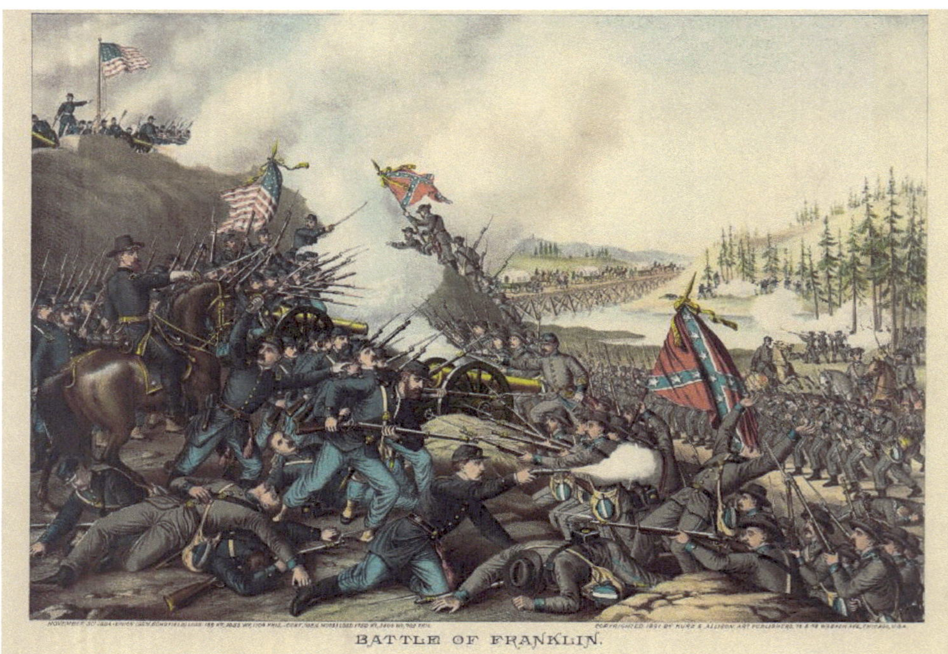

John Bell Hood's catastrophic defeat at Franklin Tennessee, Kurz and Allison 1891

There have been persistent rumors that Hood's behavior at Franklin was affected by the pharmacology of chronic morphia use. After losing 20,000 Confederate troops around Atlanta with frontal attacks, he had assured his officers he would not attack again unless he chose the ground and would avoid frontal attacks. For reasons unknown to history, he abandoned these promises at Franklin. Did the alkaloid purine opium play a role in the order to attack at sunset?

General Hood used opium in the form of laudanum, a tincture of opium dissolved in brandy as well as injected morphine via his medical officer. He lost the use of an arm at Gettysburg and later had a leg amputated at Chickamauga, both painful wounds and chronic pain of his amputated stump were documented. Several field surgeons treated him, the most consistent was Dr. John Darby whose medical records indicate Hood being addicted to opiates. After the Civil War, Dr. Darby with extensive use of laudanum and injectable morphine in the field, immigrated to Europe and found employment in the Franco-Prussian War. A conflict that added 20,000 morphine addicts to the thousands created in the American Civil War. The tiny Franklin community of 750 people had to deal with 10,000 casualties as both armies moved on. Every building, home, church, barn and shed become hospitals with forty-four active hospitals in Franklin the year after war ended. Just prior to the American Civil War, morphine had been extracted from raw opium and the hypodermic hollow metal needle was invented. The miracle drug Sydenham praised in the 17th century became a menace in 19th warfare and continues today in the form of fentanyl.

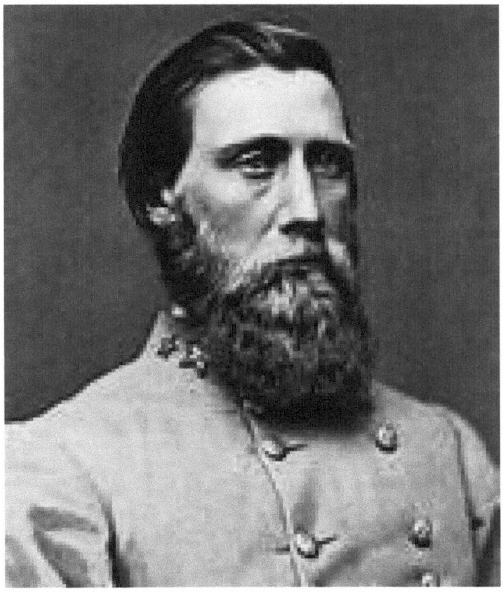

John Bell Hood, West Point class of 1853, fought Indians in the West, was a cavalry instructor at West Point and left parts of his body on several Civil War battlefields. Before the battle of Franklin, Hood was rumored to be having an affair with the same married woman whose husband assassinated Confederate general Van Dorn over similar behavior of his unfaithful wife. Hood was a risk taker and a warrior-general with little imagination in battlefield tactics in the last year of the war, brutality driving his men against superior numbers occupying fortified positions As the Union armies of William Tecumseh Sherman closed on Atlanta in the summer of 1864, the Confederate President Jefferson Davis removed General Joseph Johnston and replaced him with General Hood, considered the worst military decision of the American Civil War by either side. Hood died in 1879 during another Yellow Fever outbreak in New Orleans. National Archives

Introduction to Emergency Medicine

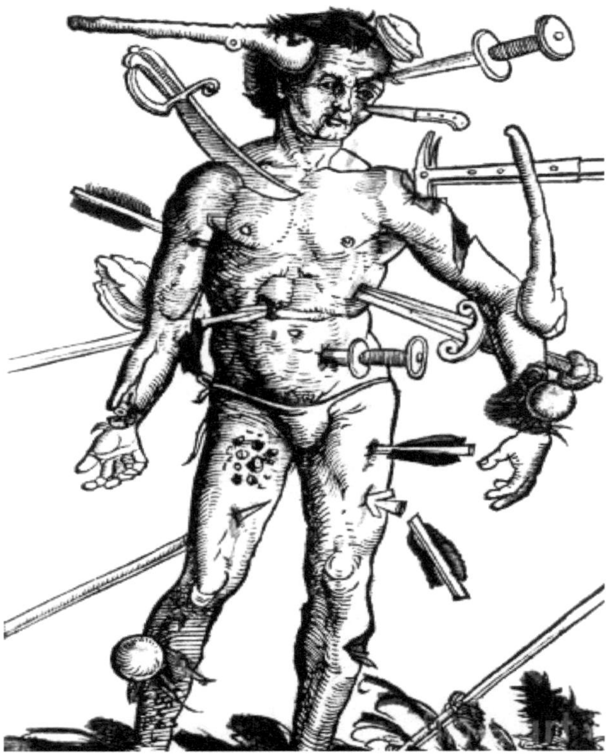

"Wound man" an early 16th century image found in several texts on field surgery

True medical emergencies are fortunately rare. Even in large hospitals, medical emergencies represent a tiny fraction of patients seen in the emergency departments. However, there are no emergency rooms at sea, in the wilderness nor would there be after a large natural disaster. A ship at sea with a medical emergency is a truly unique situation, since not only is a sea-going vessel isolated, is also a moving platform. Whether at sea or on land, people should be prepared to manage medical emergencies with the resources on hand. Unfortunately, some injuries and medical problems are too severe to be managed in the field, even if aided by radio or telephone. As important as the communication link may be for the injured or ill, take care of the victim first, before turning to outside help. Airway, Breathing and Circulation must be established and maintained, bleeding controlled, life-saving drugs given if indicated, early shock ruled-out and treated before turning to the radio. Initial treatment in most medical emergencies is a simple, easy to remember, step-by-step evolution. Review CPR, the Heimlich maneuver, first aid procedures and the use of emergency drugs. Train others in basic field medicine; it is proven to save lives. The goal in most medical emergencies is the recognition, prevention and treatment of shock, whatever the cause. The most important concepts in field emergency medicine, concern reversing shock. Ultimately, humans and other complex organisms die from some form of shock, as blood flow ceases to maintain life. In humans, shock can be prevented and reversed in many cases by simple measures, saving lives formerly lost. These measures include stopping blood loss with direct pressure or tourniquets, gently elevating the legs of trauma victims, thus increasing blood flow to the brain and kidneys, loosening clothing at the neck and waist, giving oral fluids, reassuring in a calm voice and covering the victim with a blanket or coat. Aspirin in the suspected heart attack along with nitroglycerin and heart drugs may prevent heart damage and shock in heart attack. First Aid, CPR and the use of emergency drugs should be part of every lay medical officer's memory. CPR and the Heimlich Maneuver should be taught and reviewed periodically, as they are simple to teach and deploy. In the words of Willie Dixon, a former student of the author, "Remember, the life you save, could be your own".

Shock Revisited

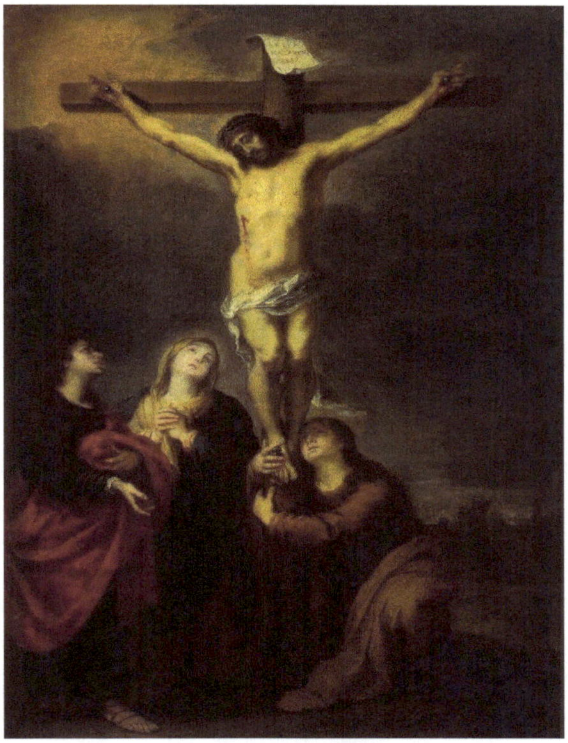

The crucifixion of Christ, by Bartolome Esteban Murillo. This form of death is central to Western Civilization's Christian culture. The cause of death in crucifixion was usually hypovolemic shock.

Most crucifixion deaths are caused by the loss of circulating fluid, as it pools in chest and abdominal cavities. This happens because the chest wall muscles and ribs, which normally act like a bellows, are unable to help the heart in moving blood. The large chest and shoulder muscles suspended from the cross are unsupported and ineffective, the outstretched arms reducing chest wall function. Crucify translates into English as "to make fast to a cross for punishment". Cicero called it "a most cruel and disgusting punishment". Crucifixion was used as an act of terror by armies and governments, making it a public display of a humiliating, gruesome, slow and painful death. Death could take hours to days, sometimes hastened by breaking legs, crushing the chest cavity or in the story of Christ, when a spear thrust to the chest cavity, released a large amount of blood and fluid from the wound. Since Christ died on a Jewish holiday and could not be buried immediately, his body was placed in cool cave and not in the ground. Two generations after Christ's crucifixion over 20,000 Jewish men were crucified in long lines by a Roman army under Titus during the Jewish uprising in AD 69-70. At this time, the Second Temple in Jerusalem was destroyed, the first Temple of Solomon, built to house the "Ark of the Covenant" was destroyed by Nebuchadnezzar in 587 BC when Judea fought on the losing side. Surprisingly, the Ark in the 6th century BC was apparently already missing and not carried into captivity. Searching for the Ark and the Holy Grail have spawned many stories.

Every cell in the body depends upon a constant flow of fluid bringing, oxygen and nutrients, while carrying away waste products and carbon dioxide. This constant flow depends upon a pumping heart and adequate circulating fluid. Interruption of this flow leads to stagnation and ultimately cell death. The single most important thing to prevent loss of limb and life is to keep the adequate flow of fluids moving through the body. Imagine each cell as a separate sea, continually being flushed by larger oceans of fluids, moving with strong and gentle currents passing by and through the cell. The pulse, blood pressure and skin color are reflections of this flow. These are useful signs in the diagnosis and treatment of shock.

The body has internal safeguards to manage shock, releasing chemicals such as adrenalin and cortisol from adrenal glands. Adrenaline (epinephrine) is a powerful rapid-acting chemical that can maintain blood pressure temporarily in the face of injury (the fight-or-flight mechanism). Cortisol has longer-acting similar effects. Both hormones released during stressful events are chemicals designed to help the pumping mechanisms of the heart and increasing pressure in arteries. Cortisol-like steroids are often helpful when injected in shock.

Shock begins when there is loss of pressure within the arteries and smaller arterioles, interrupting the orderly flow of blood. In the brain and central organs deprived of blood flow, only brief periods of interruption are tolerated for survival. Inadequate circulating fluid has cost many lives in combat and other trauma that could have been saved by simple skills in identifying and treating shock. These skills have been discovered and lost and rediscovered and lost again over the centuries. Staunching blood flow, lying the injured down with the feet elevated, reassurance, pain relief and fluids are time-proven measures in reversing shock. Simple measures have changed the tides of battles when leaders were lost needlessly. Some struck by non-fatal wounds, causing superficial bleeding, that could have been easily controlled with direct pressure, tourniquet and elevation. An absence of a medical officer and basic first aid likely changed history early in the American Civil War on the banks of the Tennessee River.

Battle of Shiloh or Pittsburg Landing

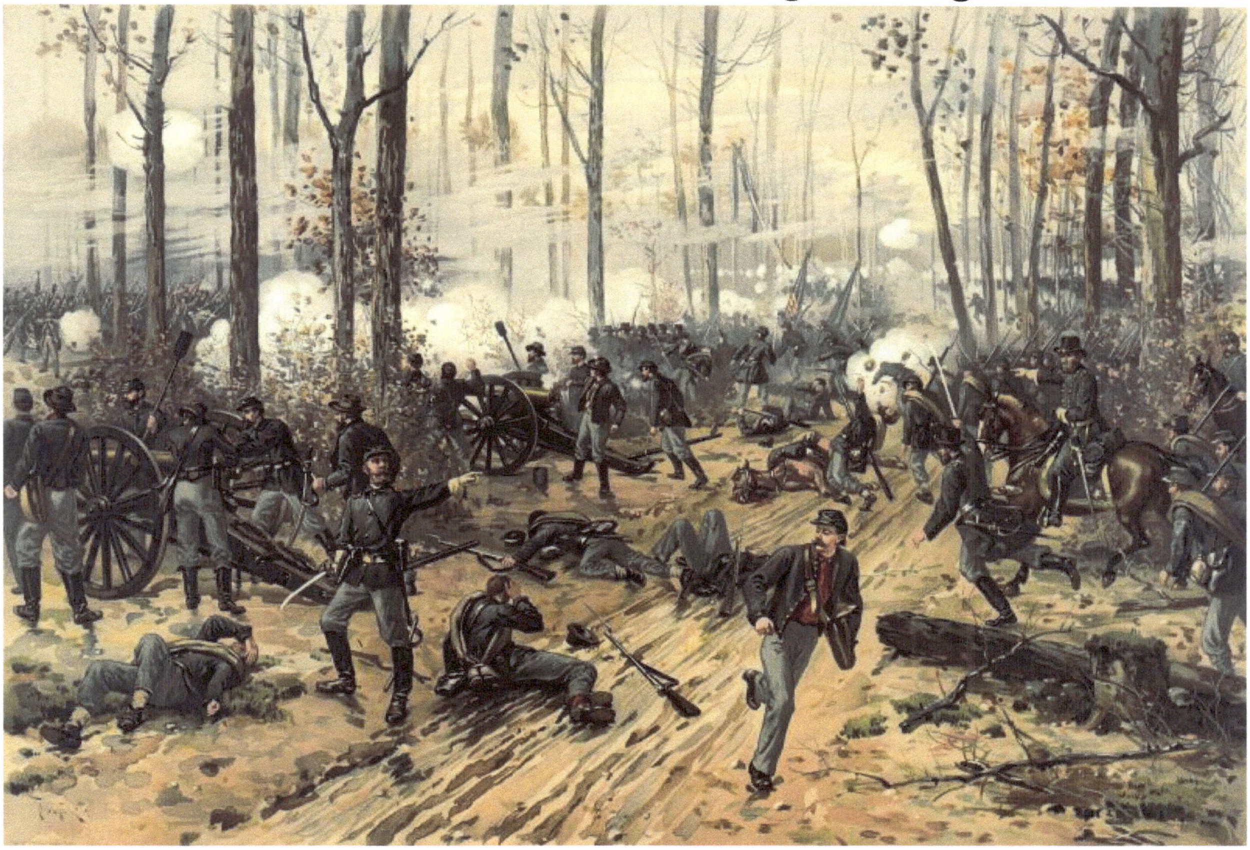

The most lethal site on the battlefield of Shiloh was in the center of the Union line, a sunken road, lined with cannons firing grapeshot and protected by determined infantry who refused to retreat. Painted by Thure Thulstrup, Library of Congress

A preventable lethal wound that should have been non-fatal occurred on April 6, 1862, in the second year of the Civil War when two large opposing armies met on the south bank of the Tennessee River. At a crucial moment in the battle, a superficial wound flowed unimpeded until the injured collapsed, fell from his horse, and died from shock. At the Battle of Shiloh, Albert Sidney Johnson, the Confederacy's most senior and most experienced field commander was maneuvering his army around the exposed flank of the Union Army. Just as his troops were beginning to turn the Union flank, a bullet struck his lower leg (likely a random discharge from a Confederate rifle). Shortly before his wounding, Johnson sternly ordered his personal medical officer to dismount and attend wounded Union soldiers. Southern chivalry and the lack of simple field medicine was a fatal mistake for General Johnson, and some believe, for the Confederacy! In H H Cunningham's book "Doctors in Gray", 1958 LSU Press, Baton Rouge, a footnote contains comments by General Johnson's son that his father's death would have been prevented if he had not insisted his personal physician leave his side and care for enemy wounded. "They are no longer the enemy" were tragically spoken by Johnson soon before his wounding. After Shiloh, "the South never smiled" has been echoed by historians on both sides. For two years following the battle, every structure for miles around the battlefield, homes, barns, chicken coops and sheds were converted into hospitals as it was on the other Civil War battlefields.

Just as the Confederate forces were poised on the left Union flank, a single bullet from a single rifle changed the course of the battle and probably the course of American History. The bullet passed through the lower leg of Confederate general Albert Sydney Johnson severing his perineal artery, filling his boot with blood. Refusing aid and without a medical officer, he stayed erect in the saddle directing the battle at its most crucial moments, without even a simple tourniquet or any attempt to stop the bleeding. When his orderly pointed out the bleeding wound, General Johnson's last words, "its only flesh wound" were spoken just before he fell from his horse. Had he been given simple field medicine and continued to command his army from the ground with legs elevated and tourniquet placed, it is highly probable the Union forces under Ulysses S. Grant and William Tecumseh Sherman would have been trapped, with a river at their back. Here they would have been destroyed or forced to surrender.

Grant was not present on the battlefield when Johnson attacked. He was miles up the Tennessee River on a steamship when he heard the cannon fire, a cup of coffee pressed to his lips. His army had been camped for three days with a river at its back in enemy territory and swampy land on each flank, isolating parts of his forces. No scouting parties had been sent to probe the Confederate forces in Corinth, Mississippi, only twenty miles away and no defensive fortifications built. Grant's army was spread over wide area with poor communicating roads connecting one third of his forces. On the morning of April 6, 1862, an army of over 40,000 well-armed and well-led Confederate infantry overran five Union divisional headquarters, capturing hundreds and sending thousands in panic to the riverbank. "It was a close thing" Wellington said about his victory at Waterloo and the same could be said about the Union victory at Shiloh.

After General Johnson's death, his 2nd in command, General Pierre Gustave Toutant-Beauregard assumed control over the battle, and "leading from the rear" sent arriving troops into the center of the Union line in piecemeal attacks. Beauregard's simple command as pieces of his army went by him were ordered "go to the sound of guns". This maneuver compressed Confederate strength against Grant's strongest position while both flanks remained open. Following the battle, Beauregard and his nearly successful army retreated into Corinth, Mississippi, where his army was ravaged by cholera.

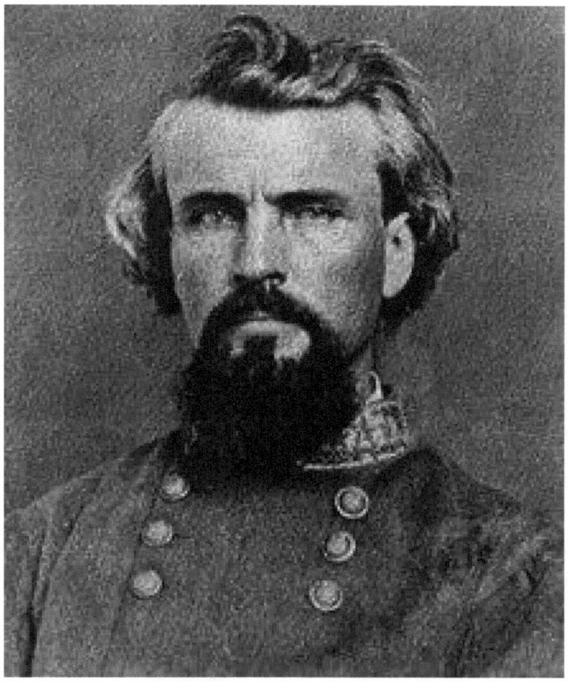

Nathan Bedford Forrest. "The Wizard in the Saddle" played a role in the story at Shiloh. As a child, typhus struck his family, killing several of his 12 siblings and his father. He survived this deadly infection and grew into a large man for his day at 6'2" and almost 200 lbs. Later in life he grew fat, developed diabetes and likely died of a heart attack. His great grandson attended West Point and was the first American general killed in the Second World War. Smithsonian

Nathan Bedford Forest added to his story during the retreat from Shiloh when he attacked a large force of advancing Yankees under Sherman and found himself surrounded by blue infantry. Forest turned, plucked a small Union soldier into the saddle behind him as a human shield and rode to safety. This was the first of many encounters with William Tecumseh Sherman. Before the war he was a slave-trader, Mississippi gambler, plantation owner, known as a killer in duels and street fights, was barely literate with no military training. By the war's end, Forest was considered one of the war's preeminent cavalry commanders and the man Sherman considered his most dangerous and elusive adversary. After the war Forest was a founder and leader of the KKK and a fictional ancestor of Forest Gump.

Except for a single bullet and the absence of a field medical officer, it could have been a very bad day for the Union, and the names of Grant and Sherman remembered not for winning the Civil War, but for grossly incompetent leadership, rivalling any in American History. Even with the loss of General Johnson's flank attack, Grant barely survived the day. Union reinforcements crossed the Tennessee River late on April 6th and the following day pushed the rebels back. Grant was temporarily removed from command due his near-defeat and later with Sherman's help, became commanding general of all Union forces and President. Grant unfairly blamed the near defeat on General Lew Wallace, who later stopped the Confederate army of Jubal Early at the gates of Washington and after living in the Holy Lands as a U S diplomat to the Ottoman Empire, General Wallace wrote "Ben Hur", one of the author's favorite novels.

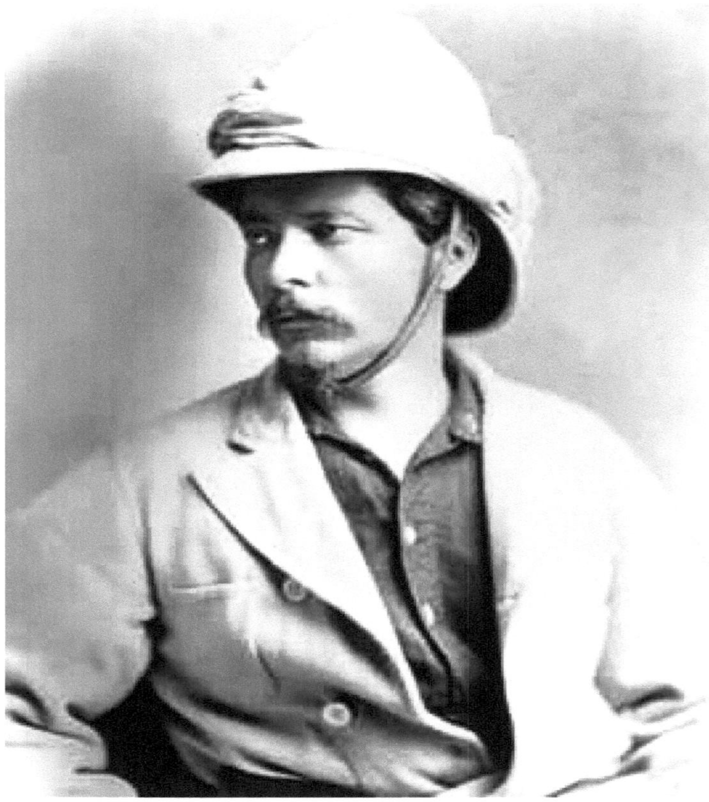

Henry Morton Stanley (not the name he was born with) 1841-1904, one of history's really bad people, first appears in history at Shiloh. His cruelties and enslavements are well documented in "Ghosts of Leopold" by Adan Hochschild.

At Shiloh, Henry Stanley is an eighteen-year-old Confederate private who recently arrived from England. After the war he became an African explorer, newspaper reporter, the first white man to see Dr. Livingstone in several years ("Dr. Livingstone I presume") and King Leopold II of Belgium primary superintendent for the rape, murder and subjugation of the Congo. The Belgium Congo was enormously rich, producing great personal wealth for Leopold because the Congo did not belong to Belgium, it as the King's personal property. Gold, rubber and ivory came out of the Congo while primarily guns and bullets were shipped in. Henry Stanley, as the administrator, ruthlessly forced natives to collect resources, holding their families as hostage. Stanley would shoot natives that refused his orders and replace them in the villages he travelled through by forceful kidnapping. By his own hands he probably killed more Africans than any single person in history.

Treatment of a Suspected Heart Attack

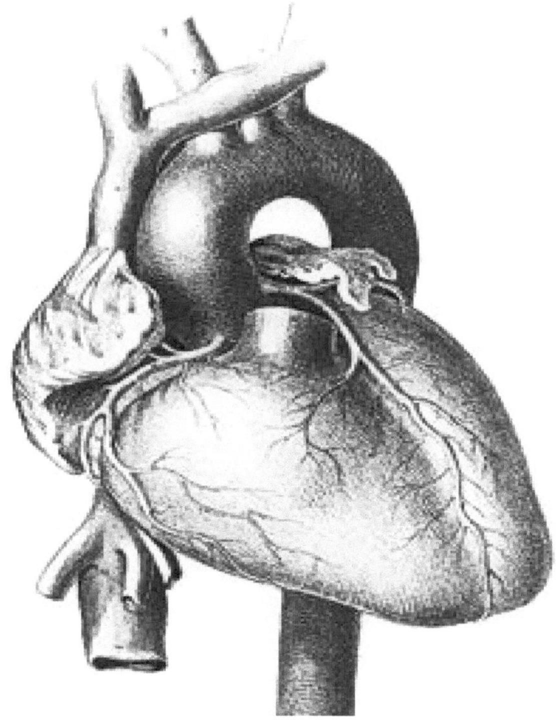

Note the small spidery coronary arteries, spreading over the heart muscle. All blood flow to the constantly working heart muscle is channeled primarily through only three narrow arteries, the right and left coronary arteries and the left anterior branch of the left coronary artery. Angelica Mager

In the field, it may be impossible to discern if chest pain (angina) is truly life-threatening but if there is any doubt, protect the heart! In the hospital there are diagnostic resources aiding the medical officer not available in the field. In the field, one has the patient's story and simple tools of stethoscope and blood pressure cuff. During the author's training forty years ago, there was little else available in the ER and often chest x-ray, EKG and blood work produced scant insight in the evaluation of chest pain. The author remembers a night during internship, when a retired US Navy steward come into the ER, Naval Hospital San Diego, mid-40s, mildly overweight and complaining of chest pain. We did the above studies, determined his physical exam was unremarkable and he left with a presumptive diagnosis of "heartburn" with a prescription for antacids. He returned three hours later DOA (dead on arrival) from a heart attack. Separating "the good, the bad and the ugly" in chest pain is difficult in the field, therefore protecting the heart in chest pain is paramount.

Emergency departments now have blood tests that detect cardiac enzymes released by injured heart muscle, radiographic studies which identify restricted coronary arteries and medical officers with skills to place catheters and stents to open arteries within the heart. Tools not available in the field, where diagnosis relies heavily on the patient's story and the physical exam. Treatment in the field of suspected angina is limited to a few medications; however, these drugs save lives! The important medical history includes what activities brought on chest pain and what relieved it. Any history of similar chest pain and if so, how it was resolved. Chest pain brought on by exertion and relieved by rest is highly suspicious, as physical activity increases workload on the heart, requiring increased coronary blood flow and oxygen. The mismatch between oxygen needs and supply increase heart distress, resulting in chest discomfort. Angina is caused by the heart's need for extra blood flow, a need not being met. Rest reduces demand and often resolves the chest pain. Only a minority of documented heart attacks present with the classic complaints of chest pain radiating into the left shoulder, shortness of breath, sweating and a sense of impending doom. Even vague chest discomfort in a person with risk factors, i.e., male, over 50, history of hypertension, elevated lipids, smoking, increased central body fat and chest discomfort appearing during exertion, increase the risk of angina and heart attack. The higher the blockage in the coronary artery, the greater the damage. Only two coronary arteries supply the entire heart muscle, the right and left coronary. The most common site of blockage is the left anterior descending branch, sometimes called "the widow-maker".

Angina is usually short-lived, seldom lasting more than ten to twenty minutes (chest pain lasting hours is seldom angina). Anginal pain is usually relieved with rest, oxygen, nitroglycerin and reassurance. Pain alone will increase workload on the heart and opiates have a long history of effective use in chest pain, giving euphoria, a sense of wellbeing in addition to pain relief. Angina is a symptom of a possible heart attack and is reversible and treatable with competent care. A heart attack is something different, it is muscle death caused by blockage of blood flow (infarction=dead meat). A heart attack is not reversible but may be softened by protecting the remaining undamaged heart. The location and size of the infarction determines severity. Immediate treatment of suspected heart attack may reduce severity and save a life. Management of chest pain is to prevent or reduce heart muscle death. In chest pain suggestive of angina, protect the heart, save heart muscle, and perhaps save a life. Protection without risk requires a step-by-step approach.

The goal in suspected heart attack is protection with little risk. The following steps provide maximum protection with safe and effective treatments. These medications are safe when used properly while giving the heart an increased chance of survival. Hydration is important, giving fluids may stabilize blood pressure and reduce stagnation. However, if signs of fluid accumulation, ie, swelling in ankles, hearing crackling in lungs, are signs of heart failure requiring fluid management and salt restriction.

Step-by-Step treatment in suspected Angina

Step 1-give aspirin under tongue, crush do not swallow, put patient at rest, loosen clothing, reassure, note skin color, alertness, give oxygen and nitroglycerin if available.

Step 2-take pulse and blood pressure; if these numbers are normal or elevated, give beta blocking heart drug. Listening to heart and lungs, a heart murmur and/or fluid sounds in lungs are signs of reduced heart function.

Step 3- monitor pulse and blood pressure, skin color, alertness, if blood pressure elevated add angiotensin blocker.

Step 4-if chest pain continues, give opiate injection if available.
Continue monitoring, give aspirin and heart drugs every day until care is passed from field to hospital. Regular use of aspirin may prevent heart attack along with lifestyle changes. Reduce salt intake, i.e. no added salt! Stool softeners reduce constipation as "straining" at bowel movements reduces blood flow to heart.

Does Size Matter?

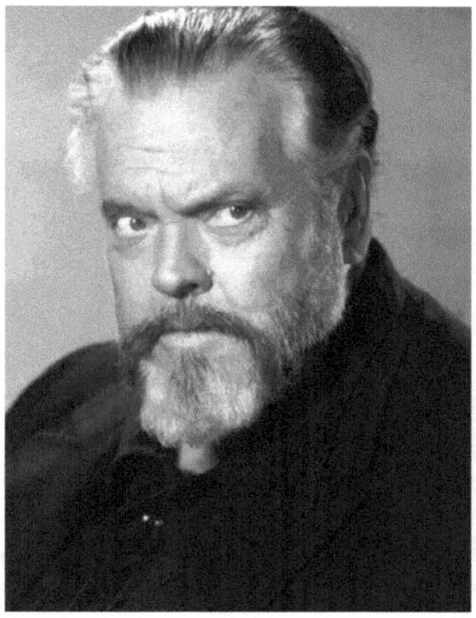
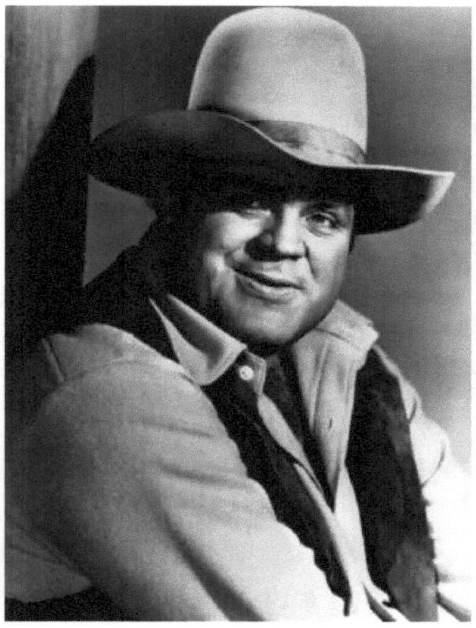
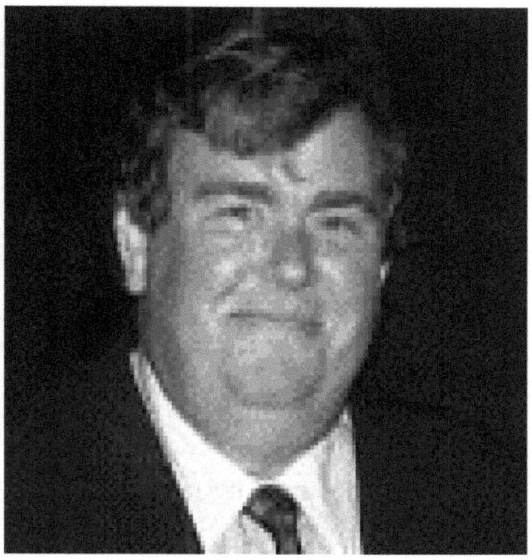

Three famous large men who all died suddenly of heart attacks, Orson Wells, Dan Blocker and John Candy. Large body size increase risk of sudden death.

Robert E Lee and Heart Disease

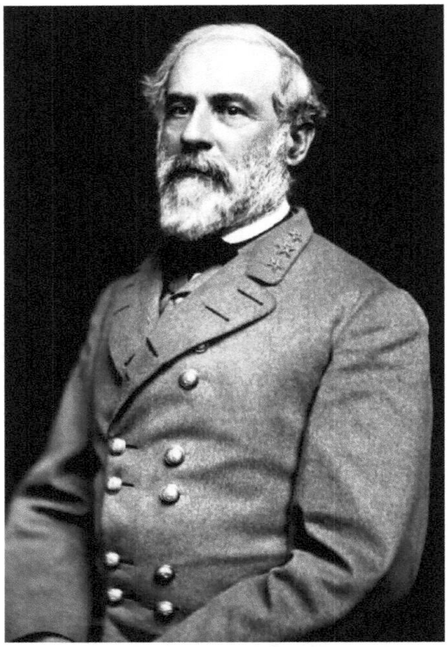

Mid-summer, 1862, Robert E Lee, who had refused command of the Union Army before the war, was given command of the Confederate army defending Richmond after Joseph Johnston wounded. Dividing his forces and exposing aggressive military behavior that would become his trademark, instead of defending Richmond, Lee attacked McClelland, driving the Union army away from the Confederate capitol, back down the peninsula. On July 1, 1862, McClelland's Army of the Potomac turned to fight, choosing a position carefully on the high ground of Malvern Hill. Lee threw his army fruitlessly against an elevated ridge bristling with three-inch guns and rifled muskets experiencing large losses for little return. On September 17, 1862, Lee and McClelland clashed again along the banks, ridges and fields around Antietam Creek. Lee had divided his command into five separate pieces to begin the invasion of Maryland and along the way, a lost copy of his orders was found by the enemy. Had Lee faced almost any other Union general besides McClelland at Antietam, his army should have been destroyed and the war probably ended. As great a reputation as Lee enjoys among Americans, European military schools' analysis of the American Civil War primarily study Grant and Sherman. Lee's worst defeat, Gettysburg, is believed by the author to have been adversely affected by heart disease. National Archives

Lee had a family history of heart disease and by the summer of 1863 his heart was in its sixth decade of service. Three years of war, his loss of many comrades, especially field commanders, fell heavily on Lee, stressful even for a young man. Few of his commanders at Gettysburg were over thirty years old, replacing older, more experienced fallen officers. There are hints his staff officers noted a change in General Lee's health following the battle of Chancellorsville, May 1, 1863. Considered his greatest victory, however Lee was far from pleased, and after the battle, a rare rage took him. If it was indeed a victory, Chancellorsville would cost Lee one-third of his army, over fifty percent of his field commanders and Thomas (Stonewall) Jackson. At Chancellorsville, Lee's army under Stonewall Jackson fell on a Union flank of unprepared soldiers where most threw down weapons surrendering or fleeing to the rear. As the Union commander,

General Joseph Hooker was attempting to stem the retreat, he was knocked unconscious off his horse. After regaining his feet, Hooker was as confused as much of his army and retreated in confusion. Following the battle, knowing what he had lost and the escape of the Union Army, Lee lost his temper, taking his staff and commanders by surprise, as it was extremely rare for him to show anger. Lee knew that two more victories like Chancellorsville, his Army of Northern Virginia would cease to exist. Outbursts of anger are known to precipitate heart attack in an older heart. Lee's victory and loses at Chancellorsville echoed Napoleon's victory and loses at the battle of Borodino in his invasion of Russia.

As the summer of 1863 deepened, Lee planned to invade the North a second time, entering Pennsylvania to force the Union Army to meet him in open combat. The South had so much confidence in Robert E Lee's battlefield prowess, the government in Richmond had prepared a letter for Washington's surrender as soon as the Army of the Potomac was lured into open combat and destroyed. As planning continued through May and June, his staff noted he became easily fatigued, requesting more rest, and to close associates, complained of intermittent sensations of "heaviness". A myocardial infarction resulting in reduced heart function would account for his fatigue and chest heaviness. The movie "Gettysburg" portrays Lee as intermittently tired and relying too much on God's will as does the novel, "The Killer Angels" the movie is based on. Had Lee suffered a heart attack in early May, after the Battle of Chancellorsville, during his anger outburst? In early July 1863 was the largest battle fought on the American continent influenced by a leader weakened by a recent heart attack? The author believes that Lee did indeed suffer a heart attack in early May 1863, and how much this affected his judgement and battle tactics at Gettysburg, is only speculation, but would account for decisions historians have criticized.

In late June, once again Lee divides his invading army, this time into three separate corps (the two leading corps under new commanders) and enters eastern Pennsylvania. His orders are ambiguous, especially to Major General JEB Stuart who rode off with Lee's best cavalry in a different direction. After the Battle of Chancellorsville, Lee told his officers that Hooker lost the battle because he sent away his cavalry. At Gettysburg, Lee made the same mistake. General Stuart left Lee with only two undersized brigades of militia cavalry, forces Lee, like other professional soldiers, seldom respected. On Tuesday, June 30, the leading elements of AP Hill's corps were ordered into Gettysburg to acquire a supposed large store of boots. There were no boots in Gettysburg, no boot manufacturing, no warehouses filled with boots. Part of Lee's army had passed through Gettysburg two days earlier and continued towards Harrisburg. The lack of cavalry to dispel the rumor there were no boots for the following troops was a mistake that precipitated the battle before Lee had concentrated his forces. Cavalry patrols passing back and forth among Lee's divided command would have prevented this lack of intelligence; however, Lee had no effective cavalry. And yet, he was sending large numbers of infantry through enemy territory with no cavalry screen. Strange tactics for a veteran field commander. Lee was "blindly" luring the Union Army towards him, where in open battle, he would destroy it and the win the war. Lee's army was smaller with fewer cannons and little chance of resupply compared to the Union Army of the Potomac, fighting on its own soil, supplied by railroads. It was paramount that Lee makes fewer mistakes and choose the ground to fight on. Neither happened, as this was not the time to have a commanding general compromised with unstable heart disease.

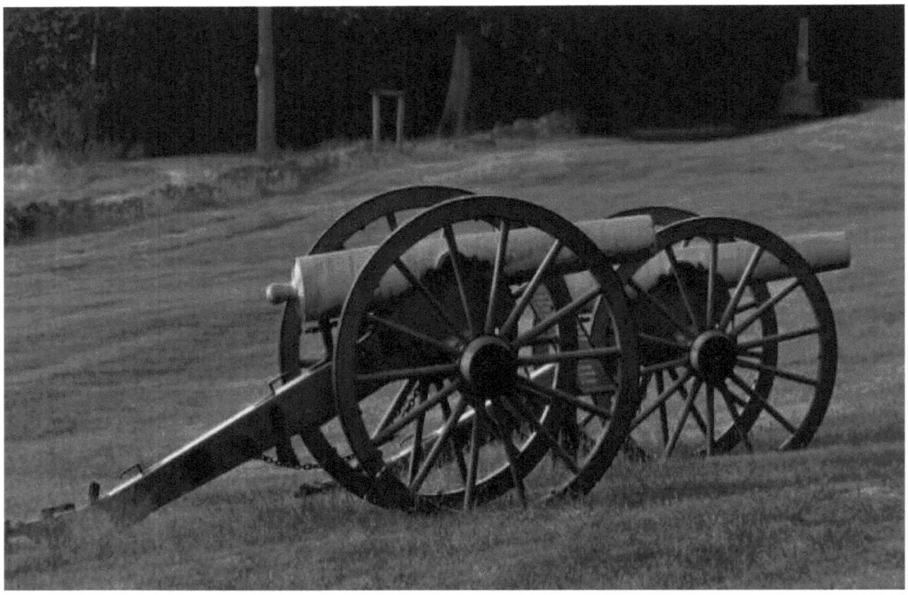

The author and his young son walked the Gettysburg battlefield on a winter sunrise. The air was cold, the cannons were colder. Whether with imagination or not, both felt a powerful sense of awe at what took place here. "Debris of Battle" is a book about the medical carnage at Gettysburg and book "The Madman and the Professor" is a true story about a brilliant Union medical officer that went insane after the battle because of the carnage. There were 350 Union medical officers present during the battle, 13 were seriously injured and 1 was killed in action.

Lee had more troops during the first day and part of the second day; however, the Confederate Army of Northern Virginia was separated into three corps travelling on different narrow roads, spaced miles apart and came to the battlefield in pieces. When Lee arrived at Gettysburg on July 1, the battle was already raging, though he had ordered no attack until his army was concentrated. The myth of boots in Gettysburg had lured a piece of his army into a battle Lee did not control. Wednesday, July 1, Union General Buford with just two brigades (2,500 men) of Union cavalry and six three-inch guns, was tasked with blocking 12,000 men of A P Hill's corps to the west and another 12,000 men of Ewell's corps coming from the north.

With Lee far to the rear issuing vague commands to his generals, the Confederate attacks were poorly coordinated. Instead of waiting for more men, local commanders deployed small contingents of men against the Union cavalry's rear-loading rifles which fire 6-8 shots per minute verse Confederate infantry's muzzle-loading rifles firing 2-3 shots per minute. Because the attacking Confederates lacked strong leadership at the point of attack, Buford's well-led dismounted cavalry held off ten times their number. A healthy and alert commanding general would have been closer to the front, more aggressive and attacked with concentrated force. On the first day of battle, Lee realized the key to the battle was the high hill north of Gettysburg and giving the most fateful orders of the three-day battle Lee sent his aid with the message, "Have General Ewell take that high ground, if practicable". These were not the orders of a competent field commander at the most important moment in the battle. A more vigorous general would have personally led or forced his troops to achieve such an important objective. Certainly Napoleon, Hannibal, Patton and others would not have been that equivocal. Two corps of Union infantry

(20,000) arrived just as Buford's men were about to be flanked. This time the infantry saved the cavalry. At the day's end, even though defeated and forced to withdraw, the Army of the Potomac had retreated to the high ground. As the sun set on July 1, 1863, the veteran Confederate army, with Lee in command and knowing his tendency to attack, was looking up at the untaken high ground, and knew the coming battle would be costly.

Gettysburg, a small town where ten east-west and north-south roads intersected was a part of America that had seen little war. That changed in early July 1863. There are places in Europe, especially Verdun, that have served as battlefields for centuries because of topography and location. The topography around Gettysburg was a natural battlefield with ridges of high ground, open fields for fire, well served by roads and deep woods to hide troop movements. A perfect place for battle, provided the high ground can be defended. The town itself was of little strategic value, however the ground rising north and east of Gettysburg were the keys to the battlefield. The Army of Northern Virginia controlled eight of the ten roads, but the remaining two allowed the Union to reinforce. By the battle's end, artillery pieces and rifled firearms assembled at Gettysburg were the most thus far in human history. In three days of fighting, one third of the combatants were dead, wounded or captured. Even with this violent carnage, fever killed more soldiers at Gettysburg than combat. Lee had brought his medical department with him while the arriving Union army had purposely and tragically left the field surgery units in the rear. Priority on the roads leading to Gettysburg was for combat infantry, cannons, ammunition, drinking water, not field medicine wagons.

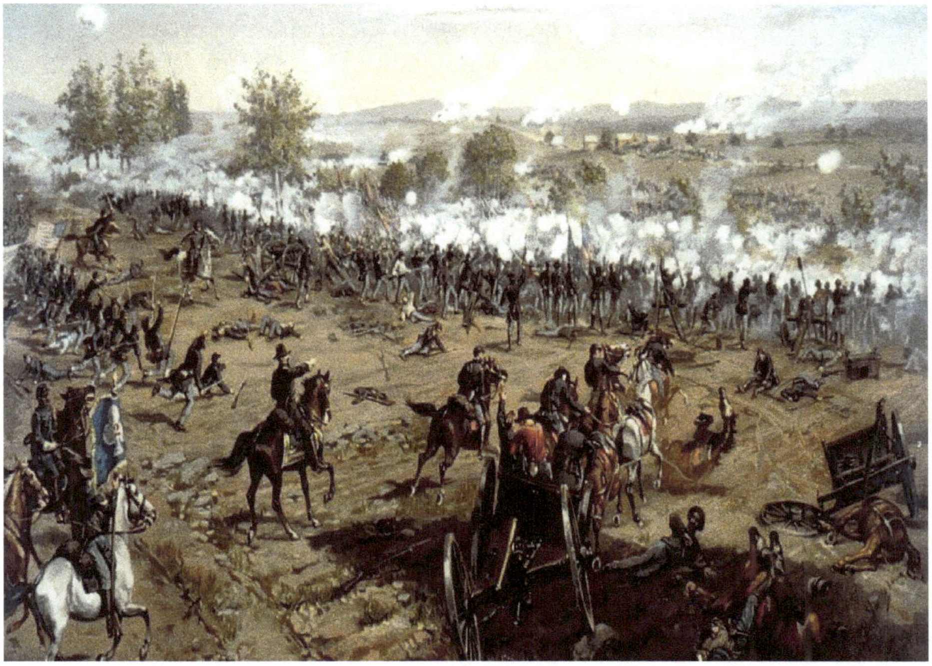

A segment of the large panoramic painting by the French artist, Paul Philippoteau depicting "Pickett's Charge", Lee's last desperate attempt to snatch victory from defeat. Pickett did not lead the attack and only commanded one of three divisions; however, his name has labelled the final charge on the third day. Pickett's Charge is likely the best known in American history, However, Hood's Confederate charge at Franklin, Tennessee was larger, bloodier and even more poorly conceived.

Lee insisted upon attacking the enemy who held the high ground for two days, even though he was unsure of the ground and the numbers he faced. Lee knew he was ill and perhaps dying. Gettysburg was to be the last battle because he believed it could be his last battle and was risking the destruction of the army if his judgement was wrong. To attack the enemy occupying fortified high ground, an enemy with more men and more cannons, were decisions probably made under the shadow of a disabled heart. The entire Gettysburg Campaign occurred in the weeks after Lee's possible heart attack and the first weeks after a heart attack are critical for repairing the heart muscle and rerouting circulation. As the heart begins the process of remodeling, there will be reduced cardiac function, resulting in easy fatigue, less stamina, and reduced mental capacity. In the aftermath of myocardial infarction, rest with a high protein and low salt diet is imperative. In addition to the stress of planning an invasion, the Commanding General of the Army of Northern Virginia insisted on eating the same food as his troops. Lee only had a small serving of meat twice each week and on other days ate greens cooked in saltwater. This sodium load would further aggravate a damaged heart by increasing body fluid. Lee's planning of the invasion, his early management of the battle and the decisions to attack uphill over unknown ground, were likely influenced by an injured heart struggling to heal. After the war Robert E Lee became president of Washington University in Lexington, Virginia where he died of a heart attack in 1870. Hundreds of the combatants, from generals to privates have written their experiences and opinions about the Gettysburg battle, however Lee wrote almost nothing but an after-action report six months later. In January 1864, Lee wrote that he was marching on Harrisburg, the capital of Pennsylvania. This is both not credible and militarily impossible. Some historians had labelled Lee's assertion of attacking Harrisburg as untrue to cover the debacle at Gettysburg. Threatening to cross the two-mile-wide deep Susquehanna River and attack Harrisburg would not have fooled even the worst Union generals. The interval following a heart attack likely not only affected Lee's actions but also his memory of the reasons for the actions.

When the author entered medical training, the belief that nitroglycerin could dilate diseased thickened and stiff coronary arteries was dispelled, working instead by dilating large storage veins and reducing blood return to the heart, thus reducing workload. Recent studies have shown that nitroglycerin does dilate even diseased coronary arteries at the microscopic level. There is a substance, endothelial relaxation factor (EDRF) that when combined with a metabolite of nitroglycerin, nitric oxide, stimulates the coronary blood vessels do dilate. This relaxation factor is normally released by the cells lining coronary arteries and is released in larger amounts during injury. Survivors of heart attacks may release larger amounts of EDRF, especially when nitroglycerin is used in angina. Smoking reduces EDRF, causing vessel constriction in the heart and elsewhere. There are no beneficial effects on the human cardiac physiology from nicotine, only deleterious ones. In addition to heart disease, nicotine damages blood vessels in the brain, increasing risks of strokes. It greatly increases the risks of cancer of the lungs, head and neck, pancreas, colon and even skin.

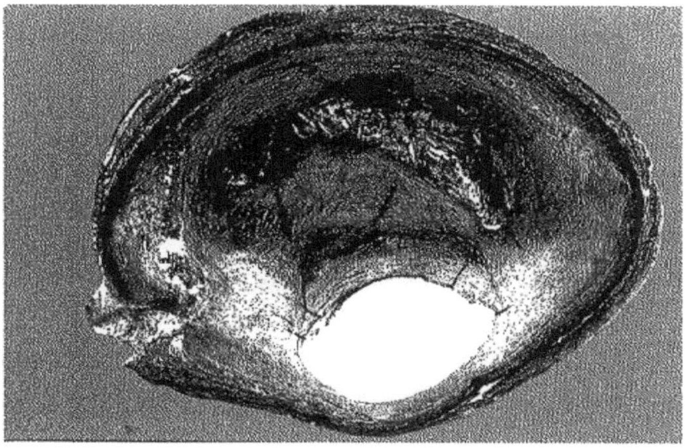

Even though this coronary artery is almost completely obstructed, symptoms of coronary disease may not be noted until exertion. NIH

The obstruction within the pictured coronary artery is a complex mixture of fats (cholesterol), iron, white blood cells, tissue debris and scar tissue. It forms over years, blocking 50-90% of the artery's interior and may remain silent unless the person engages in stressful exercises, pain, anger or fear. It can suddenly be occluded by a blood clot, a blockage sometimes dissolved by "clot busting" agents in the Emergency Department. The "gold standard" test for heart vessel disease include heart catheterization, which measures the actual opening of the coronary arteries. A less invasive test for heart disease is a stress test which is an ECG while exercising. The best predictors of heart disease may be family history and the HDL cholesterol, the higher the better. Levels over 60 mg/dl likely indicate a lower risk of heart disease and HDL levels can be elevated with aerobic exercise and diet. Research is attempting to develop drugs that can lower total cholesterol while elevating the HDL. Alcohol, especially good red wine (life is too short to drink bad red wine) elevates HDL levels in some people.

It is the new blood clot, forming within the constricted walls of the coronary artery, that creates sudden blockage of blood flow. This clot can form within a few seconds under certain conditions or over years in others. There are incidences where blood is more likely to form clots, called "hypercoagulative states" and can lead to the sudden acute heart attack and sudden death. Smoking, low fluid intake in hot weather, elevated platelet count, oral contraceptives, large fatty meals and periods of decreased blood flow can lead to clot formation within heart vessels and other vessels quickly. Some cardiologists believe a single large fatty meal can precipitate a heart attack. An important factor in platelet stickiness is adrenalin. Adrenalin or epinephrine is a normal human hormone that promotes blood clotting, a useful thing in a bleeding wound, but possibly fatal in a heart with constricted coronary arteries. Due to the simple effectiveness of aspirin in dissolving clots, it has become an important drug in the initial treatment of heart attack. In the field, aspirin may be as effective as the later use of the intravenous "clot busting" drugs. Streptokinase, urokinase and others are powerful enzymes, whose use is currently limited to hospitals and are hardly practical in the field. Aspirin must be chewed or crushed and placed under the tongue, where it can be absorbed quickly and make its way to the blocked artery. If swallowed it may not reach circulation fast enough. Adrenalin release in angina and heart attack carries a double threat, increasing workload on struggling heart by increasing oxygen demand and making platelets "sticky", increasing risk of blood clot. For these reasons, adrenalin-blocking beta blockers save lives when used in suspected heart attacks.

Following a suspected heart attack or the development of angina, it is recommended to inhibit future clot formation. A baby aspirin which is only 81 mgs (one-fourth of an adult aspirin) is enough to inhibit platelet stickiness and not enough to promote excessive bleeding from a wound. The author takes half of the 325 mg aspirin every 3-4 days as aspirin poisons every platelet that emerges from the bone marrow for its life, when aspirin is present. If oxygen is available, give at high flows in the beginning, using a mask at 8-10 liters per minute, especially if the victim appears in discomfort. This can be reduced to 2-3 liters per minute by nasal cannula (nose prongs) once the person is more comfortable. Even though oxygen over 21% can be toxic if used for long periods of time, it should be used continuously until the victim is transferred to a physician's care. If this is impractical, continue low flow oxygen until patient is back to normal activities without distress. Beta blockers play an important role in preventing heart attacks, as does blood pressure control.

Examination of the Heart

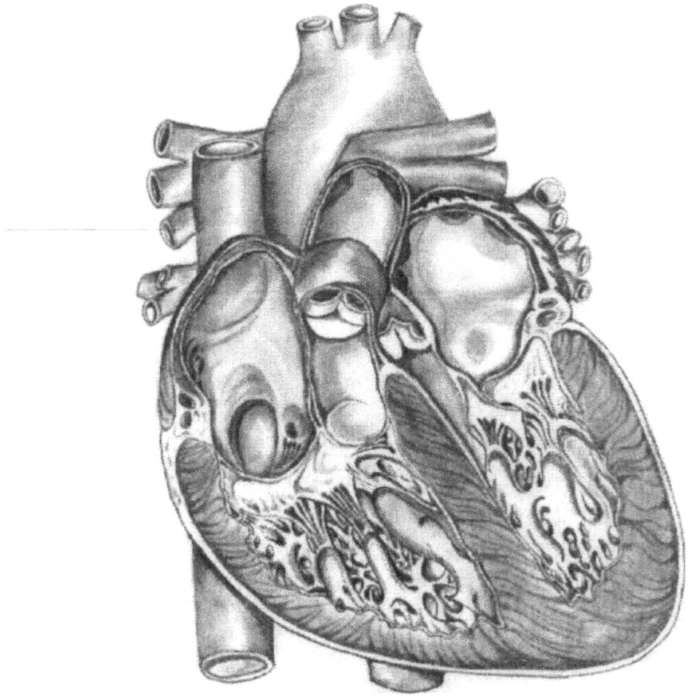

The human heart is a complex mixture of muscle, connective tissue and specialized nerves. Under normal conditions it should last for 100 years beating over 100,000 times each day of a life. The right side of the heart receives blood from the body and pumps it through the lungs where it exchanges carbon dioxide for oxygen. After it returns to the left side of the heart, it is pumped throughout the body. In the adult, 5 liters of blood passes through both sides of the heart each minute at rest. This amount greatly increases with exercise or when the heart is exposed to adrenalin, increasing heart rate and the force of each contraction. If the heart is required to pump against higher pressures for long periods of time, the left side of the heart becomes over-stretched and less effective as a pump, leading to congestive heart failure. Drawing by Angelica Mager

The heart is a fist-sized muscular pump found deep in the chest. Surrounded by bone, fat and tough connecting tissue gives it excellent protection while making it difficult to examine directly. The ancients wrote long papers on examination of pulses, indirectly examining the heart by measuring the strength and regularity of the pulses and listening to the heart sounds with ears on chest. The stethoscope, introduced in the 19th century and slowly accepted, is the mainstay of heart exam augmented by X-ray in the early 20th century, followed by ultrasound, CAT scans (invented by an electrical music research company founded by The Beatles), MRI, radioactive markers and intra-cardiac diagnostics. In the field, only hands, eyes and ears are available to examine the heart, but these are often enough. The "laying on of hands" is the oldest form of physical exam and while seemingly replaced today by technology, it is still the gold standard in field medicine. The heart is deep within the body but being a mechanical organ, it broadcasts its activity through its connecting blood vessels and through the chest wall. This activity can be observed through sight, touch and sound.

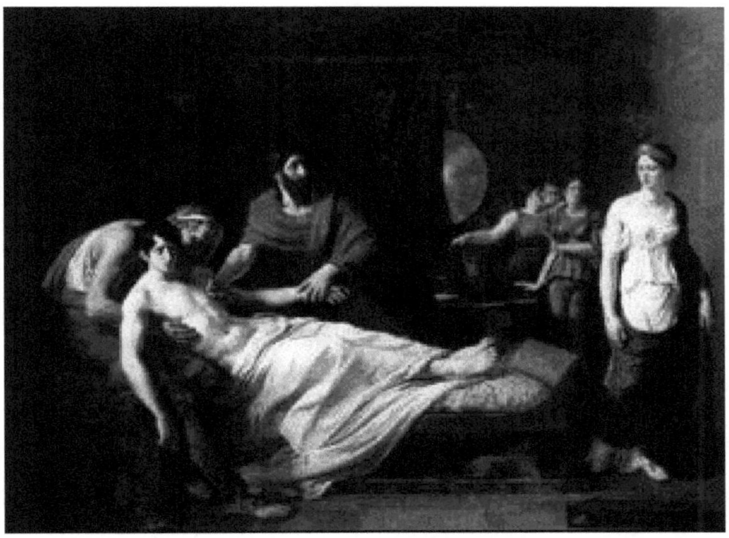

The Greek physician, Erasistratus, measuring pulse with one hand while the other hand lies lightly on chest wall feeling the heart contractions. Jacques-Louis David

From the days of Hippocrates until the early 20th century, examination of the heart was done by feeling the pulse, laying hand upon chest and watching for pulsations in the large neck veins (jugular). These are still useful in the field when combined with stethoscope and blood pressure monitor. The pulse can be appreciated at several sites, the most common are the mid arm in the crease of the elbow (brachial artery), the radial at thumb side of wrist, lower anterior neck (carotid), groin (femoral), behind knee (popliteal) and just behind the lateral ankle bone (posterior tibialis).

Normally the heart rate is measured by locating the pulse and with light pressure of the index and middle fingertip pads, gently press down. Count the pulse for one minute and that equates the heart beats per minute. Most medical officers count for thirty seconds and multiply by two or for fifteen seconds and multiply by four. Normal heart rates vary widely depending on health, age and sex of patient. Certain medical problems will be reflected in the heart rate. Normal heart rate is somewhere around 72 beats per minute; however, this number can range from 50 to 90 and considered normal for that person.

Normal heart rate is regular, beating at nearly exact intervals. Irregular heartbeats can be regularly irregular or irregularly irregular. A regular irregular heart rate is when every 3rd or 4th heartbeat is missing and after the delay is followed by a stronger pulse. This is common, generally not dangerous and caused by an electrical heart block. For many people, this is normal and causes no symptoms. However, an irregular heartbeat emerging after an episode of chest pain is significant and is a physical finding of heart damage. An irregularly irregular heart rate is likely atrial fibrillation, a common condition, and most walk around without treatment. However, atrial fibrillation increases the risk of strokes (cerebrovascular accidents, CVAs) and patients are often given blood thinners to reduce stroke risk. In reducing incidence of strokes, blood thinners increase the risk of bleeding in trauma. For over 100 years, a plant poison, digitalis was the mainstay of atrial fibrillation management, however its use has declined steadily, while a rodent poison, Coumadin is still used in atrial fibrillation, artificial valves and people with previous strokes to prevent blood clots. Neither has use in the field. Beta blockers are safe, if needed in the field for irregularly irregular heartbeat, especially if the heart rate becomes irregular after an episode of chest pain and blood pressure is normal or elevated.

Pulse is normally regular and strong, increasing with exercise and excitement. Weak "thready" pulses may indicate the reduced heart pumping in shock or heart failure. Irregular pulse can be normal in some people, but its development during and after chest pain may indicate problems with the heart's electrical system. A slow steady strong pulse usually indicates good physical conditioning as an athletic heart pump strong and slower. On the other hand, a fast (greater than 90 pulse) at rest often indicates poor conditioning. Pulses less than 50 can be dangerous unless the person is a conditioned athlete. Low pulses are particularly worrisome after a possible heart attack, indicating damage to electrical activity. Beta-blockers drugs often used around suspected heart attack can lower pulse but usually not below 50. Low pulse rate is a contraindication for beta blockers.

Blood pressure readings reflect the strength of heart contractions and the pressure within the artery. High blood pressure is expected in pain and anxiety since the body releases adrenalin, elevating blood pressure by stimulating the heart and contracting blood vessels. Low blood pressure is expected in shock, as there is reduced blood volume to fill arteries. A single blood pressure reading is not adequate to evaluate heart function. Repeated blood pressures are part of a thorough exam of the heart, measured while lying and sitting. Low blood pressure in a suspected heart attack is a poor sign since an elevated pressure would be expected if the undamaged heart.

Listening to heart sounds requires some experience and a quiet setting. These sounds have been heard over thousands of years, first with the ear pressed against the bare chest, followed by a hollow tube, the stethoscope and ultrasound. Although we know much about heart sounds, the actual cause of the heart sounds remains a mystery. They may be the sounds of the heart valves opening, closing or simply the blood being pushed quickly through the constricted spaces of the heart. Under normal conditions the heart sounds consist of a first, S1 and a second S2 sound. The first happens when the heart contracts (systole) and is usually the louder of the two sounds. S2 (diastole) follows quickly after S1 and the two together create sounds described as "lub-dub", "lub-dub", "lub-dub", etc. A heart murmur is a variation of heart sounds. Instead of a crisp "lub-dub" one hears a slurred sound or a low-pitched rumble. Many people have an innocent murmur during the first heart sound; a systolic murmur heard during the ejection phase of the heart's contraction.

More worrisome murmur is one heard during diastole, and all diastolic murmurs are considered pathological and not innocent. The development of a murmur during and after chest pain in a person with no previous history of a murmur likely indicates a heart attack. Dead tissue is now causing new turbulence within the heart. Some murmurs are so turbulent, they can be felt through the chest wall and are called thrills. Finding a thrill in examination of the heart in the field is always significant, some would say exciting. More on the thrill later.

The power of a single field medical officer

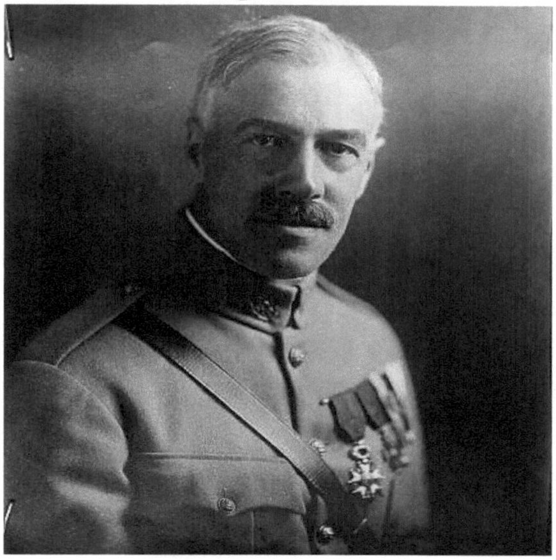

Major Paul Armand-Delille, MC. The Great War in 1915 and 1916 saw offensive failures at Gallipoli and the Somme, both better known than the disaster at Salonika. On the same ground of ancient battles in and around Greece, a single medical officer saved thousands of lives, perhaps an entire French army. National Library of Congress

The French have a rich history of good field medical officers and Armand-Delille was made of that fabric. It was in Gaul, present day France, during the century before Christ's birth that Julius Caesar elevated field medics to the rank of officers. Ambrose Pare, a French field-trained medical officer during the 16th century became the Surgeon General to three French kings and wrote the definitive texts on field medicine during the 1500's in his native French language. However, he was refused admittance to the College of Paris Physicians because he could not read nor write Latin. Pare was the son of a carpenter which was useful to him in field orthopedics, and he was blessed with a wealth of common sense. A famous Pare' quote, "I dressed his wounds and God healed him". So valuable was his reputation, he was smuggled through Spain's Charles V's besieging army into the fortress of Danvilliers to increase morale as he cared for wounded. His presence helped lift the siege. The power of a single medical officer. Pare lived a long and productive life, dying peacefully in bed at 80. He begins a long line of respected French medical officers that continued into the 20th century. Napoleon established high standards for field medicine as experience taught him the value of skilled field medical officers. Dr. Delille, a Great War hero is better known for his accidental release of myxomatous virus used in Australia on his French countryside estate and all but wiping out the wild and domestic rabbit populations in Europe.

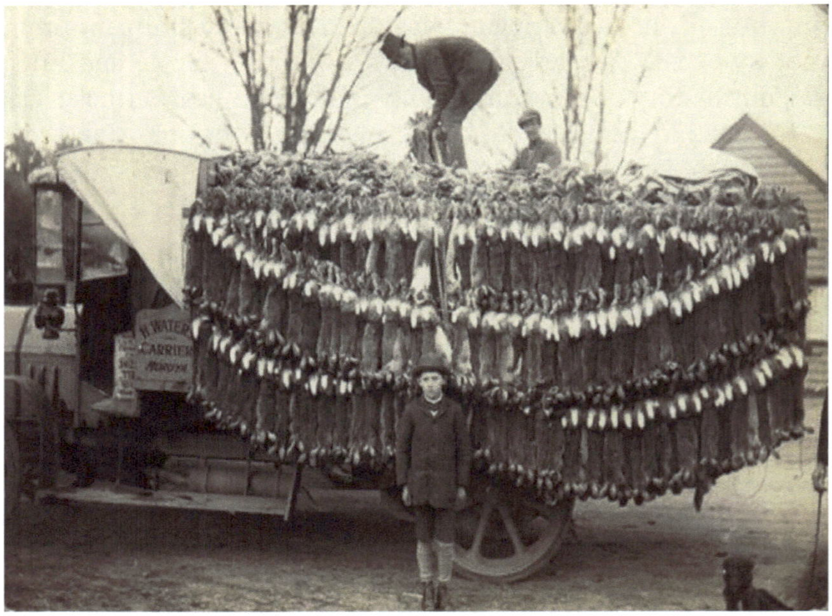

After rabbits were introduced to Australia, they wreaked an environmental disaster, and only controlled by a biological weapon, the deadly myxomatous virus. Museum of Australia

The myxomatous virus was deliberately introduced into Australia for the eradication of a rabbit infestation that was causing massive ecological destruction. In Dr. Delille's retirement and overestimating his knowledge of microbiology, he released myxomatous on his well-fenced estate to kill a rabbit overpopulation, and within weeks they were dead. However, some must have escaped, and his release almost destroyed both domestic and wild rabbit populations throughout Europe. Due to his gross act of environmental malpractice, his heroic role in saving a French army is little known.

Like Alexander Fleming, Delille served as a field medical officer during the Great War, witnessing the ravages of infectious disease. After World War I, both became self-trained bacteriologists and pathologists because of their wartime experiences. Fleming, who discovered penicillin, won a Noble Prize and is better known. Delille was serving in the French army along with British allies when he landed near Salonika, Macedonia in 1916. This force was to invade Austria and Germany through the Balkans. Churchill always believed the Balkans to be the "soft underbelly of the Central Europe". However, Salonika was a poor choice for medical reasons alone as the surrounding areas were among the most notorious in Europe for fevers. It was even worse after ten years of civil war in the Balkans, leaving the area denuded of infrastructure, no safe drinking water, no sewage disposal, no roads to transport supplies, a war-ravaged landscape. It was probably the most medically disadvantageous site on that coast. Cleary competent field medical officers were not consulted.

French medical and engineering officers arrived late, (the British landed with little of each) after most of the invasion force had already become feverish with hundreds dying. Under Major Delille's leadership, standing water was drained, brush removed, and the area sprayed with petroleum products. He brought in huge amounts of quinine, proving for the first time its effectiveness in large numbers of troops. His removal of the mosquito breeding grounds combined with the widespread use of quinine saved the French army clinging to the coast. Salonika or Thessaloniki was founded in 315 BC and became the second largest city in the Byzantine Empire. The early Christian church here received a letter from Paul and is believed to be the first written book of the New Testament. Because of location and importance, it has served as a battlefield in many wars. When the Allies landed, the area had been in conflict for several years in the Balkan Wars and cholera was already established along with malaria. By 1916, it looked like a desert.

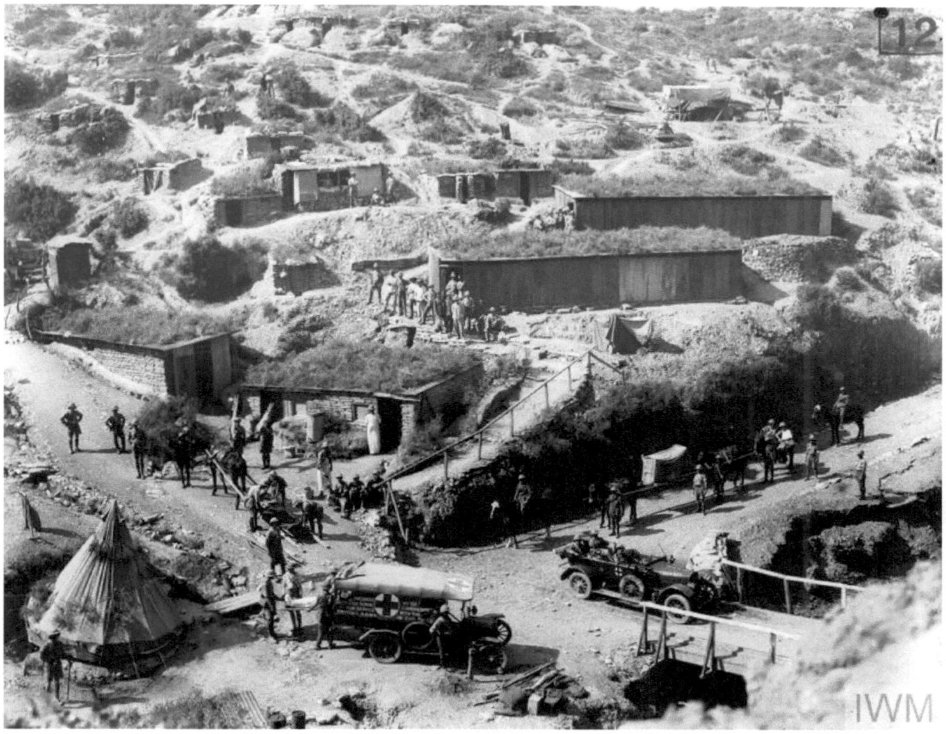

Salonika bunkers resemble the Gallipoli battlefield, Imperial War Museum

Trauma-tpauqa

Greek word for wound

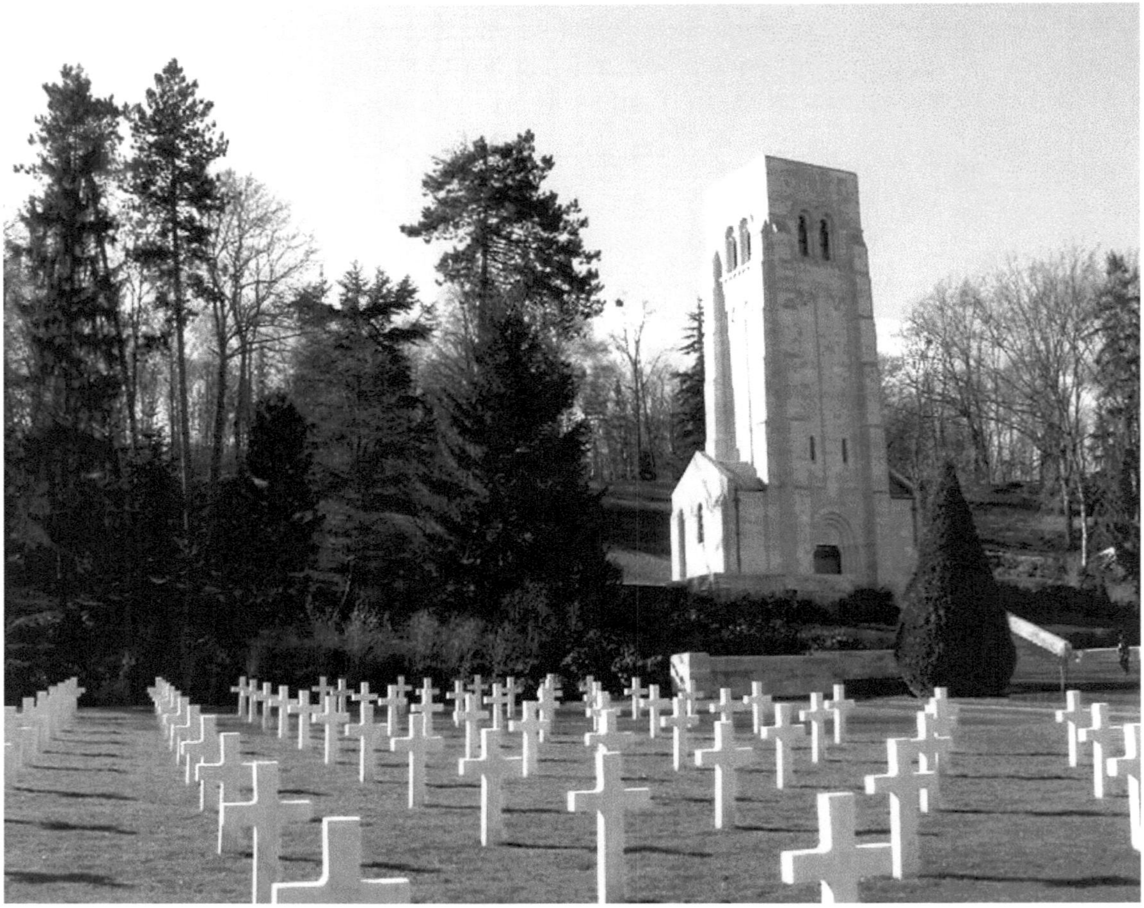

Belleau Woods, June 6, 1918, the United States Marine Corps attacked the fortified high ground rising above the graves, losing thirty-one officers and 1,036 men, more causalities in a single day than in the previous one hundred and forty years of the USMC history. It took several attacks and another 10,000 casualties to finally carry Belleau Woods. Even though the German term "Devil Dogs" was not used for the first time here, the ferocity and enthusiasm exhibited by the Marine attack forever became a nickname the Marines proudly accepted. Marine losses were huge for the small corps, although they pale when compared to the 250,000 French troops lost in the first three weeks of the Great War in 1914. Photo by author

Prior to this battle, the Marines were deliberately kept out of combat while only allowed to managed hospitals and aid stations as the US Army high command did not want the Marine Corps in the fighting. Although eager to fight and following orders, the Marines and their commander, General Smedley Butler, cleaned and organized the medical units previously overwhelmed with arriving American transports filled with sick, dying and dead. With no prior medical expertise, Butler and the USMC did an outstanding job of stabilizing and improving the hospital system of the American Expeditionary Forces. Even before combat in Europe, the United States Marine

Corps was saving American lives while increasing fitness of the forces. Finally obtaining orders from President Woodrow Wilson, who had previously been reluctant to allow Marines and Black troops to participate in combat, the Army deliberately gave the Marine Corps a tough nut to crack, the high ground of Belleau Woods for their first attack. Like the third day at Gettysburg, Marine officers and men, most experiencing combat the first time, looked up at a rocky escarpment defended by a determined enemy with entrenched guns and open field of fire in their front. The Marine high command planning the attack knew it would be costly and the high ground had little chance to be carried by a single advance. They also believed the attack had to be made for the Marine Corps to survive as a fighting force. They commenced the attack over open ground without artillery preparation in waves of unprotected infantry. Something the French and British had discontinued after losing hundreds of thousands of men in frontal attacks. Chest trauma was common on the above battlefield and the field medical officers were awash in it for days below Belleau Woods.

Chest Trauma

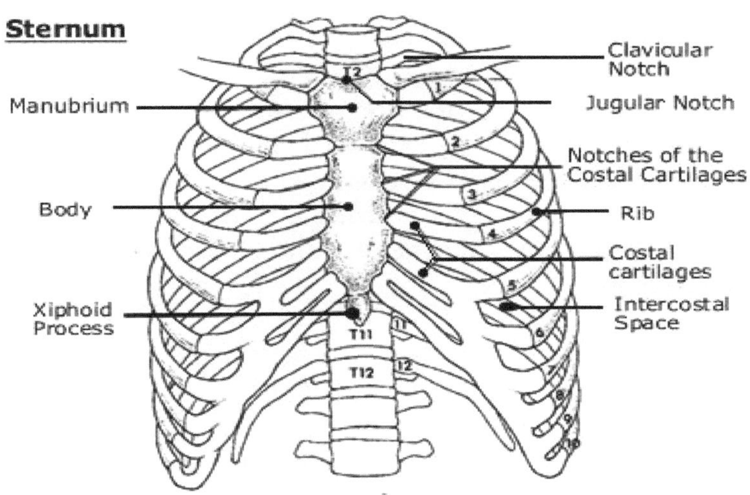

The chest has a well-protected cage of bone, anchored to the strong bones of the pelvis, and supported posteriorly by the thick vertebrae of the spine. The back of the chest is especially well-protected with the ribs at their thickest and the solid bone vertebrae bordered on each side by the shoulder blades. To add extra protection to their backs, sailors and officers braided their long hair or wigs and before battle, coated the braid with a thick coating of tar. When this hardened, it might turn the blade of a saber or soften the blow of a belaying pin. From this practice came the nickname, "tars" for sailors. Tarring hair in the past accounts for the detachable uniform flap worn on the upper back of American enlisted sailors to this day. National Library of Medicine

Chest injuries account for a significant number of deaths in trauma because the chest offers a large target for injurious agents, while harboring two of the most vital organs, the lungs and heart. Fortunately, many former life-threatening injuries can be managed in the field, providing the rescuer has the right tools and appropriate knowledge. Dangerous injuries to the chest lead to shortness of breath (**dyspnea**), moderate to severe pain, falling blood pressure, and a bluish tint (**cyanosis**) to the lips and skin from decreased oxygen.

Deformity of the chest wall is a sign of significant injury, and usually indicates multiple fractured ribs. The lungs, being the largest chest organ are the most likely injured organ in serious rib fractures. In the field, evaluation of chest injuries requires the examiner to use eyes, hands and a stethoscope if possible. The loss or diminishment of breath sounds over the injured side may indicate damage to the underlying lung. The heart is rarely injured because it is encased with a thick tough covering of fat and sinew, lying under the broad protective breastbone (sternum). A serious heart injury would likely lead to decreasing blood pressure and weakening pulse. Life-threatening chest injuries must be identified early and treated aggressively. A stethoscope and blood pressure cuff are useful to diagnose life-threatening chest injuries, while a large bore needle with catheter and a determined attitude are needed for treatment.

Pneumothorax

Greek word for air in chest

Two serious injuries to the chest are the open and closed pneumothorax. These wounds occur when air escapes the lungs, entering the chest cavity or the outside world. Open pneumothorax is easy to identify due to its classic and age-old description as a "sucking chest wound". These wounds are wet and noisy, as air moves through an opening in the chest wall. Initial care consists of covering the wound with a clean dressing, secured on only three sides with tape. This way, the dressing will act like an external one-way valve, allowing air that is drawn in through the mouth to escape through the chest wall. If air cannot escape and becomes trapped between the lung and chest wall, it will create a lethal pressure chamber, the closed pneumothorax. Antibiotics are indicated in all open chest wounds.

Under normal conditions, the lungs are held open within the chest wall by a space (pleural cavity) containing a small amount of negative pressure. Establishment of this pressure is important for survival of a newborn infant and is created in the first minutes to hours of life. This negative pressure is formed when the previously solid and now elastic lungs expand with each breath, becoming air-filled as they are in adults. With each breath, the newborn's lungs expand, stretching elastic tissue which retracts slightly, creating a small amount of negative pressure. The tiny lungs of a newborn repeated attempts to recoil back to their previous smaller size produce enough negative pressure within several hours of life outside the womb to allow the lungs to stay fully expanded. This expansion is life-long, unless the space and negative pressure around each lung is violated, allowing the negative pressure to escape. Air in the chest outside the lung will lead to partial or complete lung collapse.

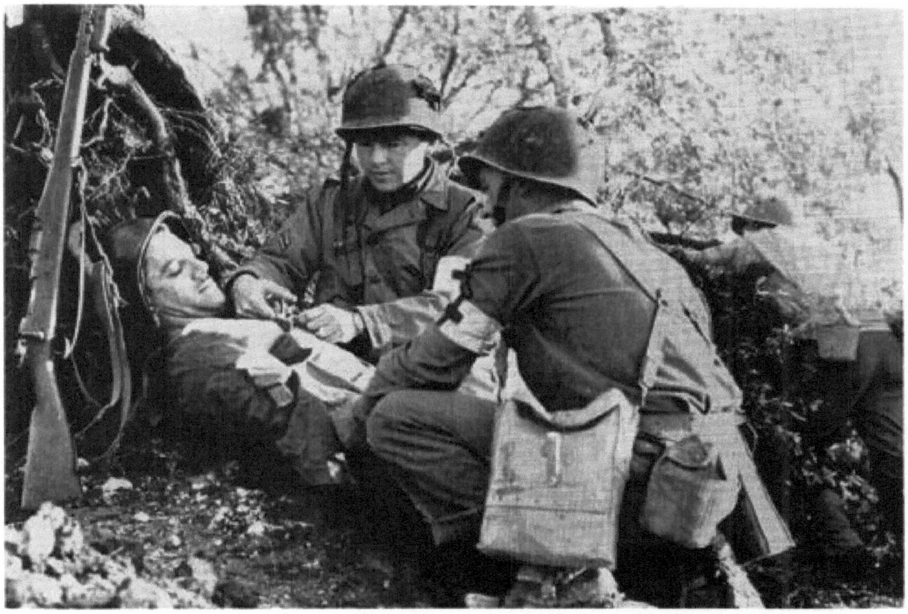

FIGURE 18.—Emergency packing of sucking chest wound by medical corpsmen.

Probably a staged Second World War photo, as the rifle is a World War I 1903 Springfield with an attached bayonet used in training. Soldiers quickly discovered the bayonet reduced accuracy and the rifle was a better club than a spear. In a serious chest wound, head should be no higher than the heart and legs elevated. The opposite is pictured in the above training image.

Open pneumothorax, although serious is generally no longer life-threatening, since infection can now be controlled with antibiotics and infection was the primary killer. Lungs were frequently punctured when the chest cavity penetrated by blades and projectiles. The presence of blood appearing in the mouth with coughing after a chest injury, signaled a lung injury that although not quickly fatal, almost always led to death. On the other hand, the closed or **tension pneumothorax** is life-threatening, necessitating early detection and aggressive treatment. Treatment of tension pneumothorax requires conversion of a closed internal high-pressure wound to an open low-pressure wound, allowing for free passage of air from the high pressure building within the chest to the outside. A tension pneumothorax can result from blunt trauma that may fracture ribs, driving razor sharp bone into lung tissue. Falls impacting the chest or compressive blows can suddenly compress the rib cage rupturing a lung as it would a balloon. The author while on his first clinical rotation, covering an emergency room in a small Oklahoma hospital examined a young man injured in a local rodeo. Hours before, he had been kicked in the chest by a bull he was attempting to ride. He reported slowly increasing shortness of breath and chest wall pain. On exam there was diminished breath sounds over the right chest wall with a dark ecchymosis (bruise) and marked tenderness. On the chest Xray, the right lung was compressed and replaced by a dark air-filled chest cavity. Because the injured was alert with normal blood pressure, oxygen saturation and appeared stable, he was transferred to a larger institution for chest tube insertion, saving the student medical officer from performing a surgical intervention he only knew about in theory.

Tension Pneumothorax-Closed pneumothorax

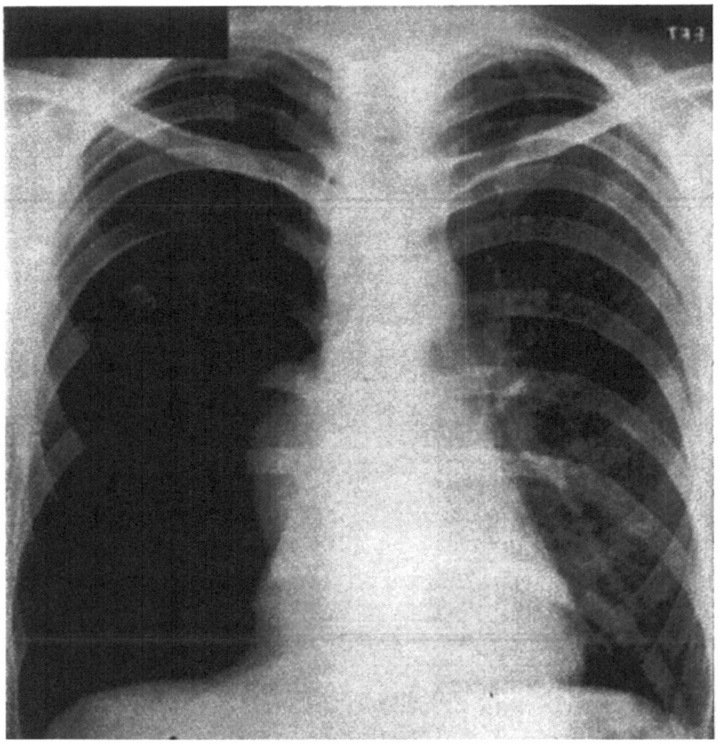

This X-ray depicts a right pneumothorax. The collapsed lung is the white smooth bulge on the right middle chest pushed against the upper heart shadow surrounded by the blackness of no lung tissue. This is an open pneumothorax with no compression nor shift of the heart. Note the blackness of the air-filled right lung space compared to the lung-filled less black left chest. In a tension pneumothorax, the heart would be shifted away from the pressure into the left chest. Film from files

In a closed or tension pneumothorax, not only is the negative pressure around the lung lost, but it is replaced by a deadly increasing positive pressure. With each breath some air leaves the punctured lung, entering and expanding the space between the chest wall and the lung. As breathing continues, the lung becomes increasingly compressed by the rising pressure within the pleural space, which begins to suffocate the heart. The lung may completely collapse, leaving behind a taut, deformed chest wall, overfilled high-pressure chamber, and void of breath sounds as it strangles the heart. It is the heart's struggles to expand and contract that causes the sense of severe breathlessness in tension pneumothorax. Patients surviving the ordeal have described a sensation of impending death and severe respiratory distress. Imagine the perniciousness of having one's breath "knocked out" during an athletic injury and unable to regain it. Treatment is immediate chest decompression, providing an exit for the air and pressure trapped within the thorax. This procedure should only be used in life-threatening situations when other measures have failed, and the victim is in danger of dying.

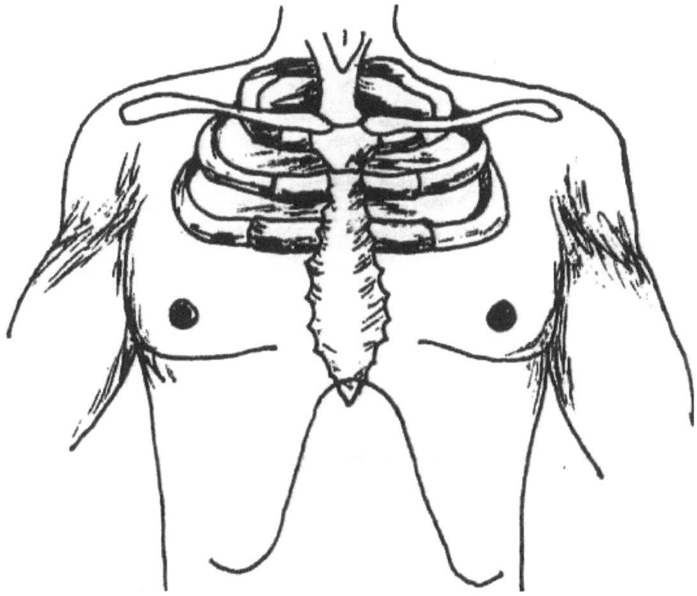

To decompress a tension pneumothorax, a large 3-4 inch long IV catheter (14-15 gauge) is placed through the chest wall over the top of the second rib just inside the nipple line. After a rush of air exits the overfilled lung space, remove the metal needle leaving the soft plastic catheter in place and tape it securely to the chest wall. If a Heimlich valve is not available, it can be made with the fingertip removed from a rubber exam glove. Cut off a finger from the glove and make a slit in the tip of the glove about one inch long and tape the base of the glove's finger to the anchored catheter. This will allow air to pass out of the chest through the glove's slit. Drawing by Julie White

In tension pneumothorax, an air bridge must be established and maintained to release the positive pressure within the chest to the outside air, like clearing ears when diving. The top of the rib is preferred since most vessels and nerves lie on the underside of the ribs. The needle is slowly inserted into the chest until a rush of air (decompression) is achieved

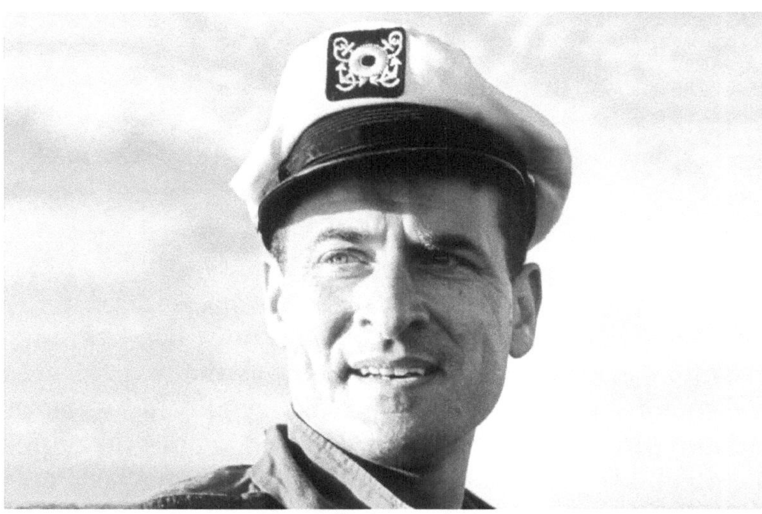

Henry Heimlich, a US Naval medical officer stationed in the middle of the Gobi Desert during World War II at an allied weather station and went on to be one of the most

consequential physicians of the 20th century. The author was fortunate enough to meet him while on the same speaking program. Dr. Heimlich is another example of the power of a single medical officer. National Archives

The successful deployment of this life-saving one-way valve developed by Dr. Henry Heimlich, and implemented in the field by the American corpsman in the Vietnam War, who employed the needle and valve technique saving lives that would have been previously lost. Due to these field medical officers' courage and cleverness, lives were spared during that conflict and are still being saved. Over the centuries, generations of sailors and marines experienced chest punctures by sword, lance or projectile. The gurgling sound of an open chest wound or the appearance of frothy blood at the mouth were death tolls for the injured and dying that littered the aftermath of battle. Hopefully, death came quickly by shock, but many endured the slow death or infection of the even slower one of starvation on a battlefield or vessel abandoned by both victors and losers. A Roman soldier delivered just such a wound to Christ to hurry his death of crucifixion and spare more pain.

Note: Smedley Butler spent 34 years in the Corps, collecting two Medals of Honor and 14 other medals for distinguish service becoming the most decorated Marine who later accused Prescott Bush, the father and grandfather of two American presidents of plotting to overthrow FDR.

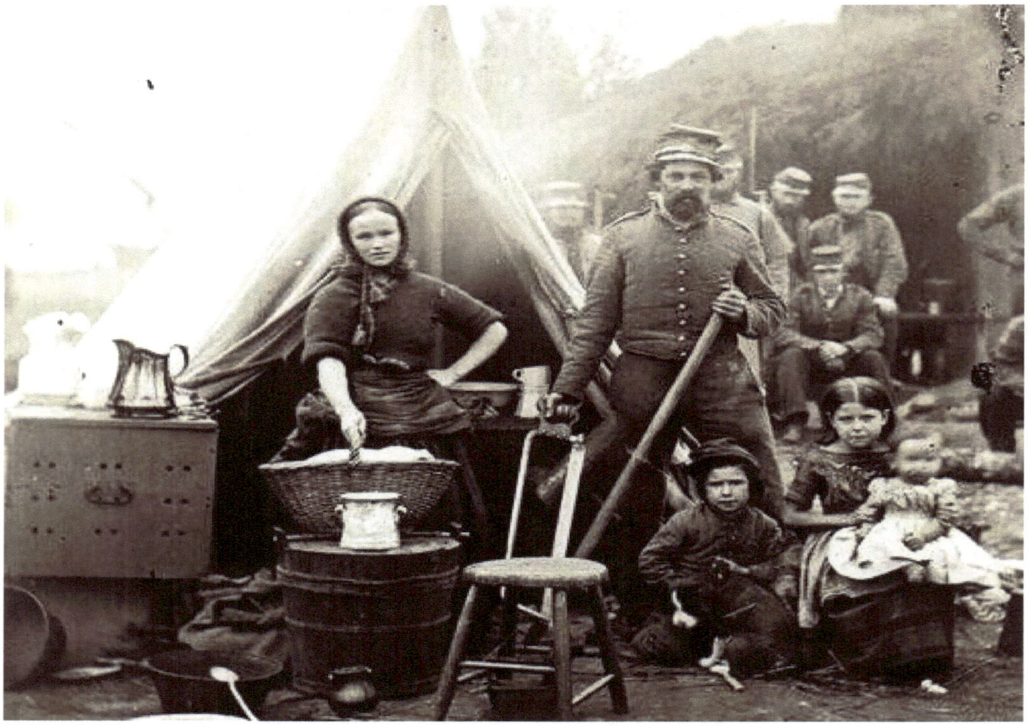

"Camp followers" during Civil War. Every army and most large sailing warships carried women and children, who were part of medical history as they experience the same diseases and often the same wounds. One of the roles in history played by camp followers, those women, children, old and disabled soldiers that followed armies throughout history, was to provide medical care and sometimes mercifully kill the more severely wounded after battles. They travelled with armies and navies as primitive nurses, wives, prostitutes and laundry women, raising children, sometimes fighting, suffering and dying in the same ways

as the men they supported. They collected weapons, dispatched the wounded and were part of the vast amount of unreported history. National Archives

Rib Fracture

Rib fracture generally causes moderate to severe chest pain localized to one area. The appearance of a dark bruise and a popping sensation over the injury site strongly suggest a fracture. The pain is aggravated by deep breathing, coughing and lying on the affected area. **Do not tape the ribs or otherwise reduce chest wall motion** even though it will mildly reduce discomfort. "Strapping the chest wall" has been the standard treatment over the years and while reducing pain, it may lead to more serious complications such as pneumonia. One of the author's attending physicians in the ER would go "ballistic" if an injured sailor came in with a tapped chest for rib fracture. He would call the treating medical officer and strongly question their continued existence as a medical officer. Pain relief with opiates combined with anti-inflammatory pain drugs may be helpful in controlling the discomfort of rib fractures and will allow the victim to breathe more deeply and tolerate coughing in less discomfort. Keep in mind that opiates used for several days will lead to constipation and rib fractures will need perhaps weeks of pain relief. Often an injection of local anesthesia (lidocaine) into the injured area will give temporary relief. The author fractured four ribs in a motorcycle accident while finishing this text and after five weeks was still in significant discomfort but with pain relief was able to deep breath and occasionally cough while firmly holding a pillow against chest. The goal in rib fracture is to prevent pneumonia.

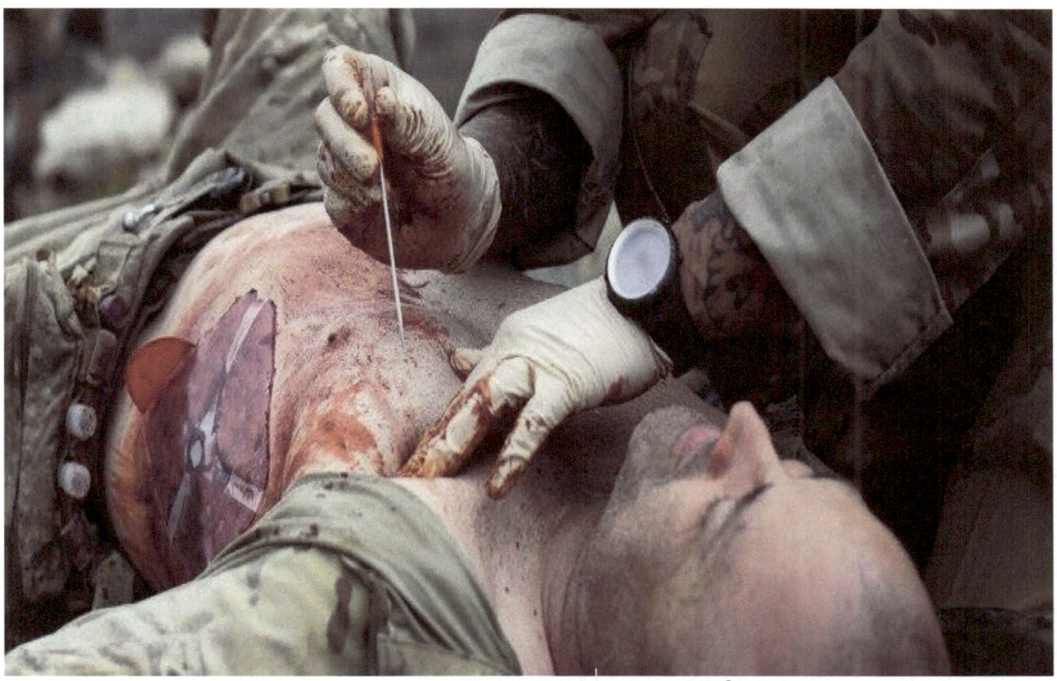

The medical officers' fingers have located the top of the 2nd rib and is preparing to insert the chest tube and decompress a tension pneumothorax. US Army

Head Trauma

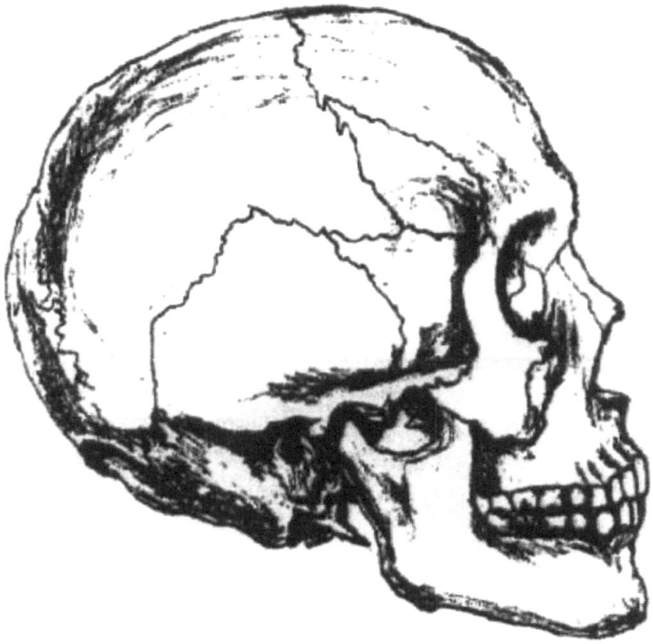

The brain is housed in a rugged, flexible closed box in the adult, composed of bone and layers of connective tissue, each capable of experiencing its own type of injury. Damage to the brain is obvious when the victim is unconscious, or if there is evidence of skull penetration alter trauma. It is important to remember that severe head injury can occur without loss of consciousness (LOC), and signs of severe injury may be subtle, requiring hours or even days to manifest. Therefore, repeat neurological checks on the victim frequently, and do not give pain medicine (especially aspirin or opiates). Checking the neurological system consists of watching for the level of alertness and the pupil size. Aspirin can increase· intracranial bleeding and opiates either oral or injected, can mask the signs of deteriorating brain damage. Signs of change in mental status and pupil size can be "muddled" by opiates. Drawing by Julie White

The Scalp

The scalp is composed of three layers; skin, which in the more fortunate is covered by hair, a fatty layer where the blood vessels reside and the galea, thin scalp muscles and a scant but strong continuous sheet of tendon-like tissue adhering the entire scalp to the bones of the skull. Bleeding into the space between this tissue and the skull forms sub-galeal hematoma, the "knots" that may arise after head injuries. "Scalping" injuries occur when this space is violated, and the skin is lifted from the skull causing much bleeding. It was the Spanish who introduced scalping as a form of torture and trophy taking to the American Indians. Scalping is quick work with a sharp knife since the galea allows the scalp to be separated easily from the skull.

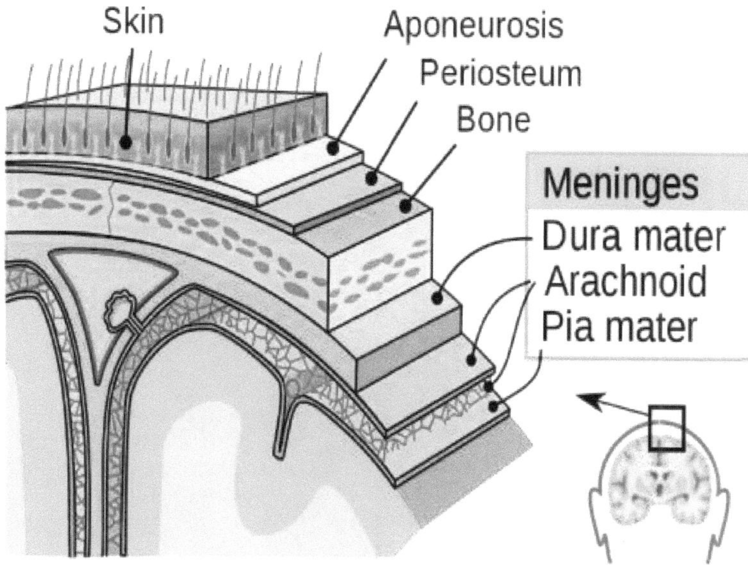

The many layers between the scalp and the brain, NLM

All three layers of the scalp move as one unit allowing for the wrinkling movements of facial expressions and the looseness of the scalp on the skull. The skin is thin in the scalp, but heavily laden with glands that secrete oils and sweat. The layer just under the skin is a thick densely "felted" bed (multiple sheets of fibers matted into a compact single layer) of fat and connective tissue, providing a surprising amount padded protection. Of known animals, the woodpecker has the strongest protection from head trauma due to its unique skull design. A design studied by football and motorcycle helmet manufacturers. The fibers surrounding the skull are oriented in different directions forming a network, like a heavy felt shirt, in which nerves and blood vessels are loosely held. Because of this, when arteries in the scalp are severed, bleeding is more severe and difficult to control, since the severed ends cannot contract, as they do elsewhere in the skin. Bleeding from superficial scalp lacerations can lead to shock if not controlled with direct pressure. In some cases, prolonged pressure will not stop bleeding, requiring the placement of hemostats, staples or sutures to bring bleeding to an end.

Skull

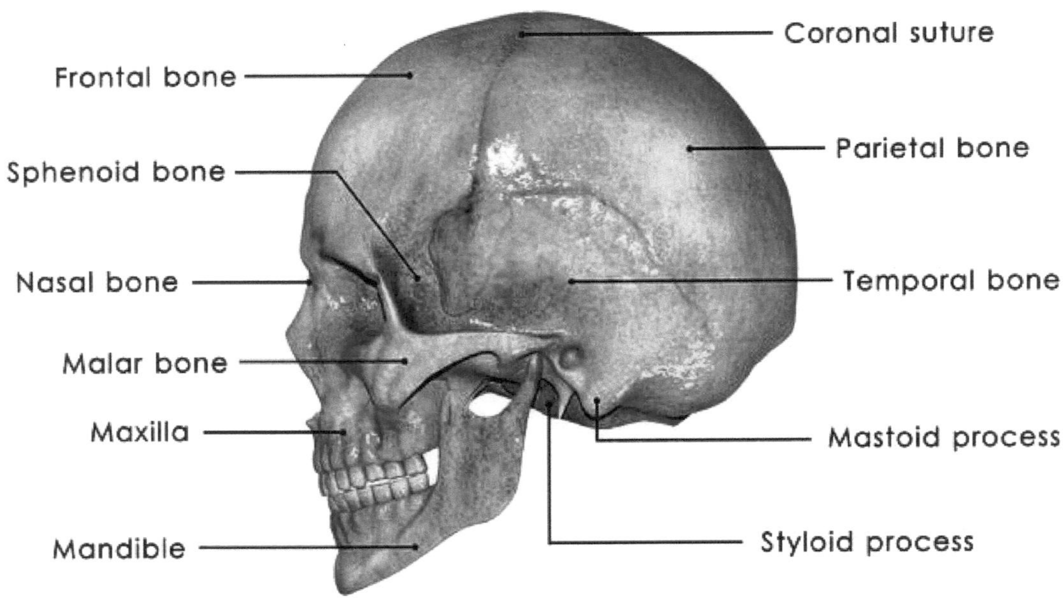

Major bones of the human skull. NLM

The skeleton of the head is composed of flat curved plates of bones, connected by interlocking tiny seams (sutures), appearing like the gill slits of fish. At birth, the larger sutures are open rendering a flexible skull to withstand the head trauma encountered during labor and delivery. The head functions as a “battery ram” forcing open the birth canal with sutures closing slowly during the first months of life. Once closed, the brain is tightly held within its bony vault with only one opening for escape in the event of raising pressure, the foramen magnum (Latin for large hole), an exit at the bottom of the skull from which the spinal cord, blood vessels, and nerves enter and exit the confines of the cranial vault. The human skull is both flexible and durable, light as plastic, strong as alloy steel. Owing to this, the skull can absorb significant blows with little apparent damage. Force can be transmitted to less durable tissue of the brain, resulting in microscopic bleeding and in more severe cases, significant swelling. Swelling and pressure, if continues to increase, can damage fragile brain tissue. Keep in mind that the skull is extremely hard when compared to the brain which it encases, tissue that has the consistency of firm Jell-0. With forces such as those encountered with sudden de-acceleration of the skull, as in a fall or motor vehicle accident, the soft brain is "flung around" within the hard confines of the skull, possibly leading to multiple injury sites and wide-spread swelling. A blow to the head with a belaying pin, ball bat, boom, etc., for an instant, deform the flexible skull inward into the softer brain tissue. The brain can be suddenly and forcefully pushed into the skull opposite the force, producing not just one, but two injury sites. The initial injury site is called the coup and injury to the opposite side of the brain, the contrecoup. Blows to the back of the head are more likely to cause the person to "see stars" since it is the site where the visual center resides.

Meninges

Just underneath the skull and enveloping both the brain and the exiting spinal cord, are layers of protective and nourishing membranes, the meninges. Within the meninges, there are major arteries and multiple, small lake-like venous pools. In head trauma, these can rupture causing a subdural hematoma, which can form slowly over time. Any abnormal change in mental status occurring even days or weeks after head trauma could be a delayed sign of bleeding into or around the brain causing increased pressure. These are more common in alcoholics who fall while drunk and the elderly who awake with no memory of a head trauma. They later report to a medical facility with symptoms of confusion, weakness on one side or coma. Infection of the meninges (meningitis) is serious and can result from penetrating trauma to the skull, carrying skin organisms into the sterile central nervous system. In open head injuries (fractures) infections should be expected and therefore prevented by antibiotics. High fever, neck stiffness, headache and pain on moving the neck are symptoms of meningitis requiring the use of both oral and injectable antibiotics.

The Brain

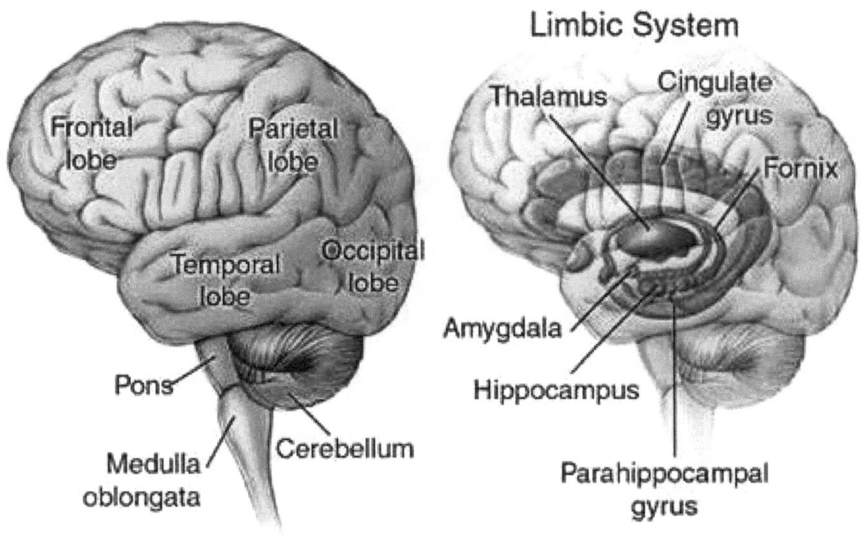

Simplified illustration of the brain, much of its function is still unknown. NIH

There are many ways to describe the deeply textured shape of the brain. Imagine two boxing gloves side-by-side with the thumbs forward and down. These would be the two hemispheres of the higher brain or cerebrum, the site of speech, memory, intelligence, some muscle control, emotions and other yet to be discovered functions. The functions of most of the cerebrum tissue remain unknown. The "hardware" of the brain has been well studied with many sites and structures understood. It is the "software" of the brain that contains most of the secrets of how information is processed and partially stored through a complex chain of electrical-chemical events. We likely have memories of birth and even fetal events, but these memories are difficult for a mature brain to retrieve because it takes several years for the child's central nervous system to develop the software necessary to retrieve memories.

Deep within the brain are lakes and pools of cerebral spinal fluid (CSF), called ventricles. When excessive fluid forms in these subterranean cave-like lagoons in the developing fetus, the skull enlarges (hydrocephaly). Occasionally, trauma will interrupt the normal communication between these pools, blocking the fluid movement from the ventricles to the spinal cord where it exits. Blockage with injury or tumor increases intracranial pressure causing unremitting headaches, nausea, vomiting and pupil dilation. Deeper to the ventricular pools lies the limbic system, the most primitive parts of the central nervous system. Sexuality resides here as does much of the personality. In the microbiology section later in text, the author discusses the role bacteria in the colon affect personality. Mind-altering drugs such as alcohol, marijuana, LSD and most antidepressants exert their effects primarily in the limbic system. On the underside lies the brain stem and sitting atop the spinal cord resides the pons. Here are the vital centers that maintain breathing, regulate heart rate, blood pressure, temperature and muscle tone. In the aft section of the brain is the ball-shaped cerebellum, a site of coordination control. Without the cerebellum, all the motions of the body would be jerky and spastic. Breathing irregularities, elevated blood pressure or fever are possible signs of injury to these deep centers, and when accompanied by coma and muscle rigidity, are the grim announcements of severe brain damage.

Brain Injury

The hallmark of brain injury is alteration of consciousness or decreased alertness. Mental status is monitored by repeated neurological checks of the victim's nervous system including observing the patient's responses or lack of responses to questions, physical stimulation and eye examination. The academics divide unconsciousness into seven levels. Each level measured by the amount of stimulation needed to cause a response. Victims who are not responding to spoken words may withdraw from painful stimulation such as pinching or gently pricking the skin over back of hand with a needle. The less responsive (especially to pain) the deeper the coma.

It is important after head injuries to establish the level of alertness since subsequent examination is compared to the initial mental status. Questions to be asked are time of day, place and date help determine the victim's orientation to place and time. Orientation times four is a medical term for the victim’s ability to know time, date, place and person. Mental status can be further evaluated with simple questions concerning memory and imagination, functions located in more injury-sensitive areas within the brain. Asking about current news events indicates recent memory, information lost early in a worsening head injury. A more sensitive test of mental status requires combination of memory, imagination and insight. Asking "why does a rolling stone gather no moss" or "why should people who live in glass houses not throw rocks" require abstract thought, establishing high levels of brain function. If the patient can move all four extremities in a smooth and appropriate manner, answer thoughtful questions appropriately and focus the eyes; the brain, spinal cord and major nerves are undamaged. Repeated head injuries lead to CTE, chronic traumatic encephalopathy, a common disease in boxers, football players and other activity where the head receives repeated blows.

Increased Intracranial Pressure

Diminishing alertness is likely due to increasing pressure within the head. Therefore, it is important to keep the person awake after a head injury, allowing access to their level of alertness. Death after head injury is caused by increasing intracranial pressure whether from direct bleeding or the swelling associated with concussion. Remember, the brain is encased in a rigid structure and any increase in the size of one part of the brain will come at the expense of another compartment. There is some room for swelling within the cranial vault since fluid in the ventricles can be reduced as blood flow to the brain. The danger begins when all possible cerebral spinal fluids have been removed and blood flow reduced to its lowest level. If the pressure continues to rise, the brain is pushed through its only exit, the foramen magnum. Long before this happens, the pressure will be high enough to effectively shut off the blood flow the brain needs. The brain has a higher demand for oxygen and blood than any other tissue and will not tolerate rise in pressure before brain death occurs. As little as a teaspoon of excess fluid in the closed brain injury could be fatal. There is a diagnostic advantage to the pressure attempts to force (herniate) the brain through the foramen magnum. The nerves that connect the eye to the visual center in the back of the brain lie along the foramen magnum and are compressed early in pressure increases. This leads to an enlarging pupil on the side of an injury and points to the injured side. A dilating pupil is diagnostic for increased intracranial pressure, its sudden appearance or bilateral in head injury is a poor sign.

Narcotics such as morphine and other opiates will cause pupil constriction, blurring this important clinical sign as well as reduce alertness, the two diagnostics findings in the field. These drugs have no place in the management of head injuries or the headache they may cause. Aspirin, since it can increase bleeding, also has no role.

Concussion

Almost all head injuries, even mild ones may result in some swelling. Concussion implies no significant disruption to brain architecture since it usually is a reversible injury. The presence of a headache for several hours after a head injury is suggestive of concussion. Nausea and vomiting are evidence of increased intracranial pressure and are more significant than headache alone. Severe vomiting or seizures may be signs of rapidly developing pressure. The author has seen this with breast cancer that has metastasized to the brain, elevating pressure suddenly, causing intractable nausea and emesis. This is caused when an enlarging tumor increases pressure. Far more common than severe concussion is the post-concussion syndrome. Persistent headache, irritability, easy fatigue, poor concentration and dizziness, lasting a few days to 6-8 weeks is not uncommon after head injuries. Usually managed with rest and mild pain medicines such as Tylenol while avoiding codeine or aspirin.

Management of Life-Threatening Head Injury

In the severe concussion with closed head trauma (no apparent breach of the skull), treatment is reducing intracranial pressure. For thousands of years, this emergency was managed in the field by converting a closed head injury to an open one by trephination of the skull, one of mankind's oldest surgical skills. Trephination was also used for releasing demons, (not unlike the lobotomies of the 1940s and 50s for mental illness), treating headaches, blindness and a wide variety of disorders in addition to head trauma. In modern surgery, burr holes are drilled through the skull by neurosurgeons with surgical precision. In the past it was performed by a field medic spinning a sharp pointed drill, a trephine, back and forth with gentle yet firm skilled hands.

There are methods of reducing intracranial pressure short of field surgery. These involve injecting medications directly into a vein to pull swelling from the brain. Diuretics are drugs that draw fluids from the brain and convert it to urine. A form of concentrated sugar, mannitol, "sponges" fluid out of the brain, lowering pressure and must be injected intravenously (under tongue if no IV available. Another is a powerful short-acting steroid such as Solu-Cortef (125 mg) or dexamethasone (4-10 mg) delivered every two to six hours by injection. Steroids decrease intracranial swelling by reducing the body's inflammatory response at the injury site. Mannitol and steroids can and should be used together and may be enhanced with another urine-forming agent, Lasix a diuretic. These medications to be effective are given through a vein where an IV line has been established. These medications are found on football fields where they save lives. Over-ventilating the patient with some type of breathing apparatus (bag and mask) will lower the amount of carbon dioxide reaching the brain, which also decreases blood flow to the brain and therefore lower pressure.

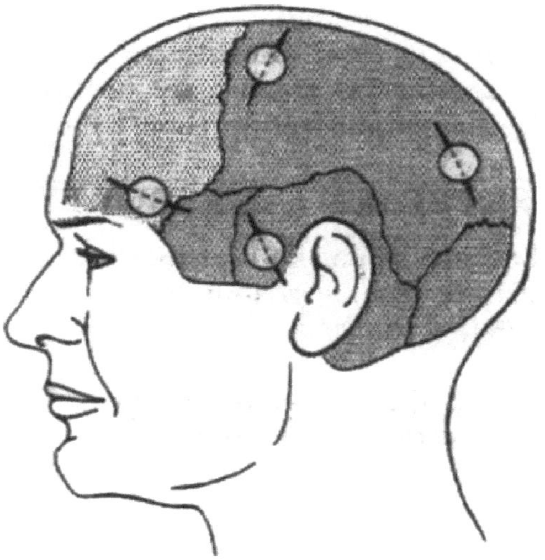

This drawing is from the text "Emergency War Surgery" which has been printed in all languages of nations with armies and navies. It states that indications for burr hole placement include increasing restlessness and headache, dilating pupil on the same side of injury with paralysis of the extremities on the opposite side. As in the illustration, generally, more than one hole is necessary to relieve pressure.

In cases where conservative measures fail to prevent further deterioration of the patient, more drastic measures should be considered. This is the surgical conversion of a life-threatening closed head injury into a less serious open head injury. This procedure should not be considered, let alone attempted, unless circumstances are grim and the person's life "hangs in the balance". An attempt to obtain medical advice via the radio is recommended before attempting trephination in the field! The author's father-in-law in his first and only year of general practice in rural Montana, used a hand brace and bit after a mining accident, performing a successful surgical procedure he only knew in theory. And a classmate in Undersea Medicine School used a battery-powered drill aboard a nuclear submarine to perform successful trephinations. It is not a rare event in the field.

The side for trephination is the side of the dilated pupil. The temporal bone above and on each side of the ear is the most likely site for surgery. This area has been the choice for centuries, since bone here is thin and underlying brain tissue is less easily injured with trephination. Palpate for any small pulses that represent arteries within the scalp that should be avoided. At the chosen site, a 1/2" incision with a knife is made to expose the bone and the skin spread apart. Using extreme care, a hand or powered drill with ¼ inch bit with a stop at 1/4 inch of length is introduced to the bone. After each 1/4 inch of travel, move the stop farther up until the bone of the skull is penetrated. Several holes may be needed to release pressure. Do not expect a sudden burst of pressure release as the swelling and pressure reduce slowly. As pressure reduces, the patient's mental status and pupil size should begin to return to normal. Give antibiotics once the skull has been opened to prevent infection in and around the brain.

Open Head Injury

In the event of a skull fracture, the primary concern is not of increasing intracranial pressure, but infection as an open skull fracture breaches the blood brain barrier. The central nervous system (CNS) is a sterile place where there is little early response to invasion by bacteria. A life-threatening infection such as meningitis or encephalitis can develop quickly when bacteria from the skin or upper respiratory tract breach the brain's protective covering without trauma. The signs of skull fracture are often hidden without use of X-ray or CT scans. If the skull bone is depressed in one area, there can be a "step-off" sensation as fingers probe along the edge of the injury site. Other classic signs of skull fracture are bluish discoloration behind the eardrum and around eyes (Battle's sign) or a clear fluid draining from nose. If an open fracture is suspected after head trauma, antibiotic therapy should begin.

Seizures

Epilepsy Greek word epilepsies meaning seizure

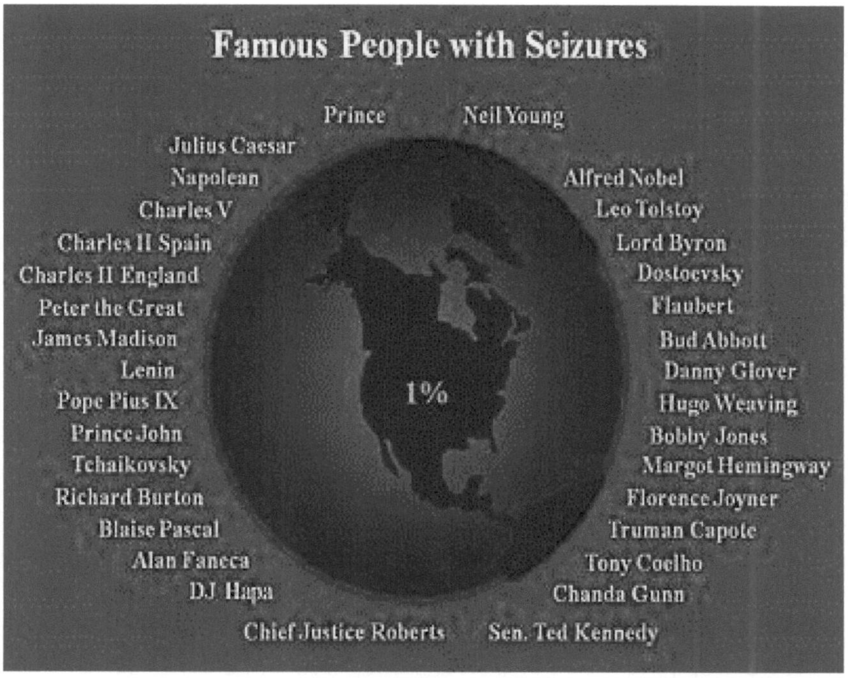

Seizures are common and usually self-limiting, however in alcohol withdrawal and after head injuries, seizures are a poor sign. Based on the above list, seizure disorders do not

prevent productive lives. Nomadic cultures viewed people with seizures as holy, receiving special information during the event. NLM

Seizures take many forms and are loosely defined as a lapse in mentation often accompanied by uncontrolled and sometimes violent contractions of muscles. From petite mal (little seizure) to grand mal (big seizure), seizure activity is usually brief. Exceptions to this include seizures associated with alcohol withdrawal, head trauma, brain tumors and infections. There is generally no memory of the time occupied by seizure episodes. Prolonged grand mal type seizure activity requires lots of energy and oxygen in the brain and muscles, which is difficult to maintain for more than a few minutes, especially if the airway is temporarily closed. This energy release is often followed by a coma-like state as the central nervous system recovers. Grand mal seizures occur when the arms, legs and head react convulsively and uncontrollably lasting seconds to minutes. It is no longer recommended to place a fixed airway into the person's mouth, since it may result in damage to teeth or injury to rescuer fingers. Do not attempt to restrain the victim unless they are in danger of rolling into harm. If the tongue is swallowed or the airway becomes otherwise compromised, the brain's supply of oxygen will be interrupted, bringing the seizure to an end. Most seizures are self-limiting, requiring no treatment other than observation to prevent the person from harm. On the other hand, a dropping blood sugar (hypoglycemia) can cause a seizure, that if not treated with intravenous glucose, dextrose or glucagon, is fatal. Therefore, treatment of seizures of unknown cause should begin with an injection of dextrose IV or injected under the tongue. Some diabetics carry a glucagon kit where 1mg is injected subcutaneously, just under skin. Even though these injections will be of no value in most cases of seizures, it will cause no harm and maybe lifesaving.

Diabetic seizures occur in people who have either taken too much insulin or have fasted while using insulin. Rapid delivery of intravenous glucose or dextrose produces a dramatic response within seconds or minutes of the injection. Seizures caused by low blood sugar are more easily treated than those caused by head trauma, (even days, weeks, or months past the accident), infections such as meningitis, drugs, alcohol either as an overdose or withdrawal, increased intracranial, tumor or when a blood vessel bursts or suddenly clots in the brain (stroke). For seizures lasting more than a few minutes or keep reoccurring, management in the field is limited. Other than giving intravenous glucose, the next drug of choice in controlling seizures is diazepam (Valium) which is effective in dampening the central nervous system's output. In alcohol withdrawal, the development of agitation and visual hallucinations are early signs of DTs (delirium tremors). Delirium tremors are a dangerous entity with an almost 40% death rate even in hospital! During the author's internship, DTs were not rare in a large naval hospital and sometimes treated with IV 80% ethyl alcohol (Ever clear) to prevent withdrawal from becoming fatal. If diazepam is used early, it may prevent possible later seizure activity. The preferred route for administration of diazepam is intravenous. During a seizure or just after, oral pills would be unsafe as the patient could choke. Unfortunately, starting an IV during a seizure could be impossible, leaving intramuscular injection (IM) the only avenue for the drug. This choice of drug administration is unpredictable in how much and how quickly the drug reaches the brain. However, it may be the only way to give diazepam and may be required if the seizure is to be controlled. Even if diazepam does not eliminate the seizure completely, it should reduce its violence. The recommended dose is 10 mg initially, followed by 2-5 mg two hours until desired effects begin to be seen.

In preventing or controlling delirium tremors, 5-10 mg of diazepam can be given every 6-12 hours orally. It is important to control the agitation or nervousness that precedes the tremors since this condition carries a high mortality. If alcohol withdrawal is suspected and the person cannot be removed to a medical facility, it may be necessary to give alcohol to stop the withdrawal process. During the author's internship there were coherent and pleasant patients, yet during withdrawals would have a complete personality change becoming belligerent and combative, pulling out IV lines, hitting and in some cases biting personnel. This was often accompanied by hallucinations, especially seeing snakes and spiders before seizure-like activity commenced. It was paramount to prevent the delirium tremors in its early stages. The author was surprised how a pleasant patient could turn into a monster like the "Dr. Jekyll and Mr. Hyde" character in Robert Louis Stephenson's novel. Alcoholism has a terrible legacy; its biochemistry has changed history.

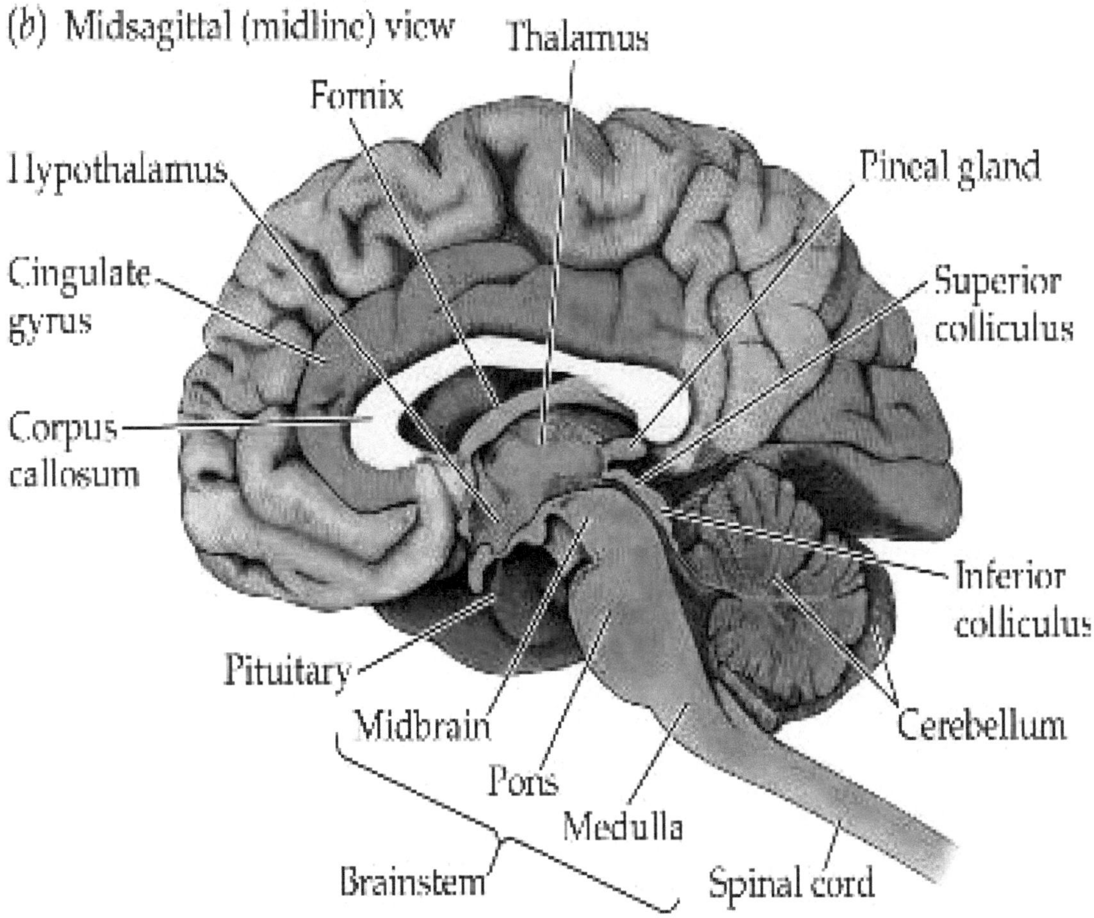

This is a greatly simplified illustration of the major brain structures. More is unknown than known about the brain, especially at the cellular level. In seizures, the normal synchronicity of the brain becomes temporarily non-synchronous. After rest, brain function returns to normal. National Institute of Health

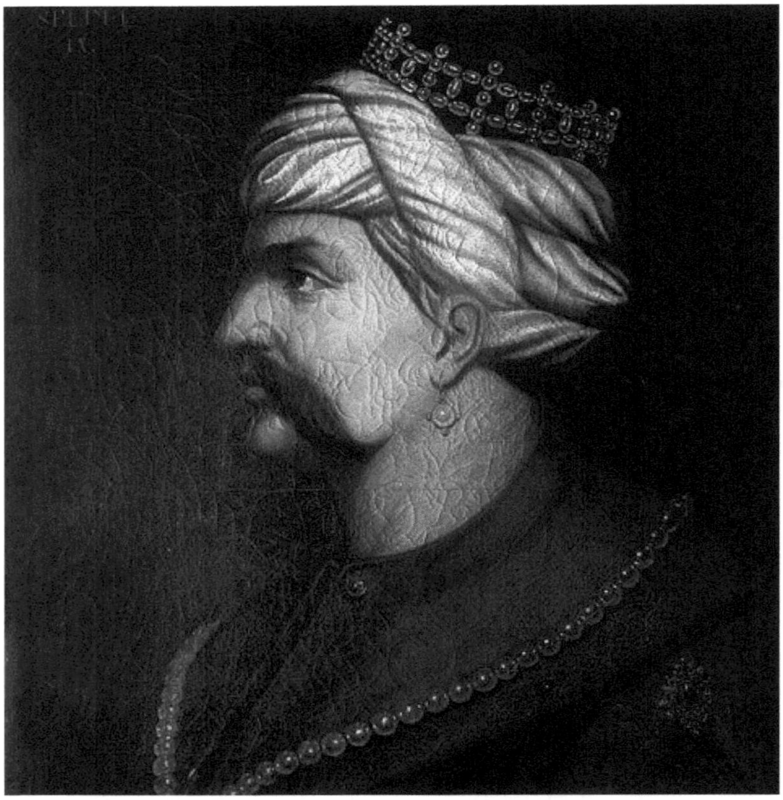

Selim II (1524-1574), the son of Suleiman the Magnificent, was also known as Selim the Drunkard, and is credited with losing much of his father's conquest and beginning a long downfall of the Ottoman Empire. In a large part due to the toxic effects his alcohol consumption. His father was the longest ruling Ottoman Sultan and considered its greatest. His mother, Roxalena (Hurrem Sultana) was one of the great females of the 16th century Islamic world, began life as a Christian in the Ukraine when captured by Islamic Tartars, brought to Istanbul and sold in the slave markets for Suleiman's Harem. She was such a remarkable female, rose to be the Sultan's favorite concubine and later his wife, becoming second in command of his empire. Along with Isabel of Spain, these were two of the most powerful women in the world. Even though alcohol prohibited except for medical use in the Koran, so partial was Selim to Cypriot wine, that he invaded Cyprus to assure his supply. This invasion directly led to the Sea battle of Lepanto, where his father's Turkish Navy was destroyed and the subsequent loss of Greece, Serbia and Bulgaria. Many of his decisions were affected by the corrosive effects of ethyl alcohol on his brain cells. It is hard to underestimate the results of the Battle of Lepanto on the history of Europe as over 70% of the oared-driven galleys in the Mediterranean fought along with 140,000 men and 600 ships (estimates per Roger Crowley, an expert on the battle). There were many players in the battle. In addition to the author of "Don Quixote", Cervantes, there was the English pirate, Thomas Stukeley, an illegitimate son of Henry VIII and a female flamingo dancer, Maria la Bailadora, who distinguished herself during the battle. According to Crowley, it was not until the Battle of Loos in 1915, a battle would have a higher rate of slaughter. Biochemistry of fungi-fermented sugar played a major role in this turning point in history. British Museum

Drowning

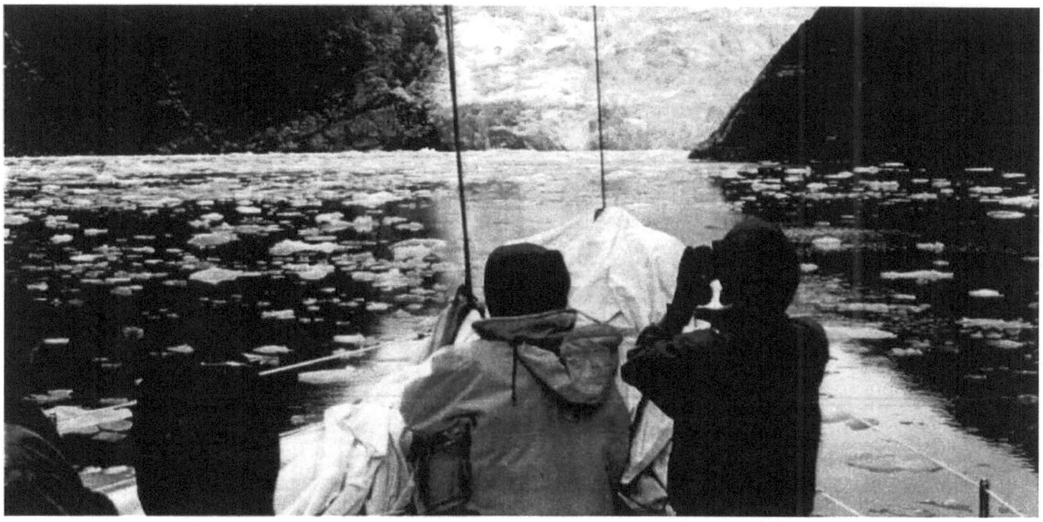

This ice-filled fiord in southeast Alaska is very deep and very cold. Immersion in this water without a survival suit could be fatal within minutes. If someone goes overboard, immediate retrieval and rapid warming is indicated. Remove wet clothing, cover with heated blankets, give warm electrolyte fluid and continue to monitor the victim for hours, as there could be delayed problems with cold water immersion. Photo by author

Immersion in water is always a risk in the maritime environment. In the past, few sailors could swim, nor was there any reason to learn, since falling overboard was almost universally fatal and swimming only prolonged the inevitable. Historically, sailing vessels travelled downwind and could not easily be slowed, stopped or turned around to pick up a man overboard. Thor Heyerdahl in his voyage on "Kon-Tiki" described the absolute eventuality of drowning if a crew member fell overboard, since their vessel with its square sail could only sail in one direction. Modern vessels, although able to stop and turn, would be unable to pick up a man overboard quickly under many conditions, meaning that victims must remain active in their rescue, since minutes and perhaps hours may be spent in the water. Drowning may occur quickly or be delayed, depending upon sea conditions, the health of the victim, the presence or absence of panic, water temperature and the insulation and flotation gear worn by the victim.

In some drowning cases, the patient can receive the best medical care at the stage and later in an intensive care unit, and not survive. Delayed death due to injuries of the internal organs in near drowning victims may not be evident at the time of rescue. It is important to carefully monitor victims that survive the immersion incident for several days, since serious complications of near drowning can begin with mild shortness of breath in the beginning stages and progress to death. Oxygen, fluids and possibly steroids are the only components of a medicine chest that would be useful in management of near drowning while at sea. Before using steroids, attempt to speak to a physician.

Drowning is not simply death from suffocation in water immersion as there are several different possible mechanisms of death in drowning, a death for some that is reversible. In the United States it is the second most common cause of death in children. Near drowning is common in swimming pools, where victims are quickly pulled from the water and given CPR. Unfortunately, some later die from the delayed effects of lung injury sustained while the person was in shock. Chemicals in the water and water temperature play a role in damage to the lung tissue as can infectious materials in the inhaled water (especially swimming pools). Delayed shock is manifested by respiratory distress, increasing shortness of breath, labored breathing and cyanosis (blue skin).

The most common causes of death in drowning are the lack of oxygen to the brain (hypoxia) and cardiac arrest. The later occurs in immersion syndrome, where sudden death results in frigid water when the nervous system reacts with heart-stopping violence. Why this happens is not clearly understood, since people can swim safely in near freezing waters under voluntary or controlled situations. People can fall out of a boat in the San Francisco Bay in 50-degree water and be dead within a few minutes, while others can break the ice in wintertime Chicago and swim without ill effects. Death likely due to uncontrolled fear or terror, over-riding the orderly way the central nervous system maintains blood pressure. Loss of this system's control may lead to an interruption of blood flow to vital organs for only a brief time, cascading a series of events that may terminate life. Panic is the catalyst that allows the internal shock mechanism to trigger a self-destruct response in immersion syndrome. Another possible mechanism of death is suffocation or asphyxia, depriving the brain of oxygen even with the heart still beating. In the drowning victim, this can occur when water enters the lungs through the airway, the so-called wet drowning. In dry drowning, (especially in fresh water) the upper airway develops sudden, severe spasm, closing the lungs to both fluid and air.

Treatment of Immersion Victims

In near or delayed drowning, the lining of the tiny air sacs within the lung become injured. This injury occurs even when CPR is successful in revival of shock, the victim appearing well for several hours or even one or two days. The development of shortness of breath, first with exertion, later at rest, are early signs. The development of fever, blue tint to skin (cyanosis) and chest retraction of labored breathing are signs of worsening conditions. CPR should begin as soon as possible with mouth-to-mouth breathing beginning while the victim is still in the water. By holding the victim's back to your chest with the rescuer's arms embracing the victim, one can sometimes begin CPR. It is unlikely that water will be expelled before the victim can breathe or cough on their own, but the Heimlich maneuver may be useful in expelling fluid from the lungs. The Heimlich maneuver along with mouth-to-mouth, can and begin with the victim still in the water.

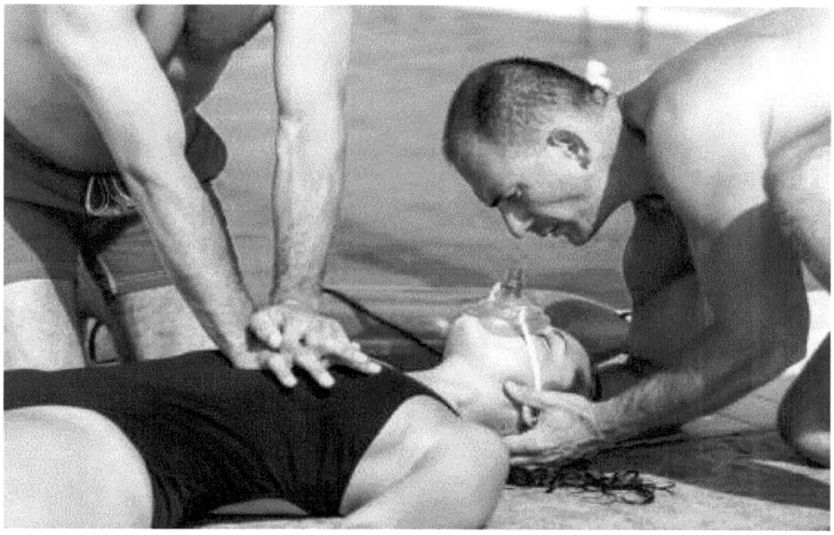

In the life-less drowning victim, 2-person CPR is best. US Public Health

Oxygen should be added to CPR as soon as it is available and used afterwards. It is helpful, since the lung's injury causes increased resistance to oxygen crossing into the blood. An IV is started as soon as possible to ensure a route to administer medications. Sodium bicarbonate given IV, may reduce acid levels formed in the blood during the period of no oxygen. Using steroids such as Prednisone or solu-cortef is somewhat controversial but has been shown to reduce intracranial pressure (ICP) and inhibit damaging inflammatory response within the injured lung. Therefore, in addition to watching for respiratory distress, near drowning victims should be monitored for signs of brain injury. Signs that include headache, confusion, nausea and vomiting. Other medications that are used when intracranial pressure (ICP) is suspected include diuretics such as Mannitol or Dextran. Antibiotics should be started if the water is dirty or if the victim may have breathed vomitus into the lungs. The development of fever in a post-drowning victim requires the use of antibiotics.

Cold Water Immersion

Added to the threat of drowning in cold water is the cold itself. Cold injury (Hypothermia) occurs when the body's central core begins to cool as more heat is lost than produced. Normally, the surrounding muscle and fat provide adequate insulation even when the person may feel very cold. Water carries heat away from the body 100 times faster than air at the same temperature. Therefore, the victim of cold-water immersion should get out of the water and put on some buoyant material as soon as possible even though the water may feel warmer. When body temperature drops from a normal of 37 C (98.2 F) to 34 c (94 F) the victim will be unable to produce enough energy to prevent further loss without active rescue. At 30 C (87 F) coma will ensue as the brain is cooled below its minimum operating temperature. The heart stops beating at a balmy 25 C (78 F) which is above room temperature. The difference between air temperature and water temperature becomes evident since the internal organs filled with fluid would be very cold indeed. Hypothermia in cold water immersion occurs much more quickly, almost sudden when compared to the more gradual onset on land in cold air.

It is unclear how people can break the ice for a swim in winter water near freezing temperature, without harm while others suddenly thrown in cold water and rescued within minutes, can die of hypothermia. The variable in the survivability of immersion injuries is panic and the devastating role it plays. Above all remain calm, stay still in the water unless quick action will enhance self-rescue. The fetal position of the head tucked into chest with legs and arms drawn together will help reduce heat loss as struggling will increase it. The former practice of "drown-proofing" by actively bobbing up and down wastes too much energy, depleting heat stores.

Treatment of Cold Injuries

The victim should be gently removed from the water since a sudden snatching from the water has been linked to death from cardiac arrest. After ensuring the airway, breathing and circulation are intact, wet clothing should be removed, the skin completely dried, and the victim covered in multiple layers of insulating material such as wool. Hot packs, hot water bottles or an electric blanket should be applied to the chest, neck and groin. If these are not available, then a warm naked body should be wrapped around the victim under insulating covers. The presence of shivering is a good indicator that the central nervous system, acting in concert with the heart, blood vessels and skin, warms the body's core. If the person is awake, warm sweet drinks will enhance the treatment (avoid coffee, tea, alcohol). The unresponsive person who continues to appear lifeless must be warmed to 37 C (98.6 F) to be pronounced dead. There are stories of people "waking-up" in the morgue of wintertime northern cities. If one has a choice, it is much better to drown in cold sea water versus a warm public swimming pool filled with bacteria and chemicals.

Frostbite

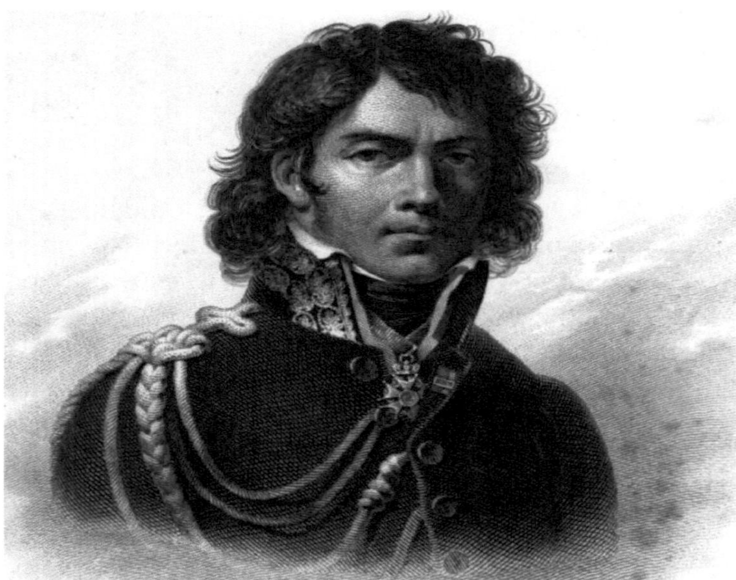

Dominique-Jean Larrey (1766-1842). Napoleon said of Larrey, "He is the most virtuous man I have ever known". He was also one of the greatest military surgeons of the early

19th century and he had plenty of opportunities with the French Imperial armies as they swept back and forth across Europe. He served in 400 engagements and was wounded three times in battle. Larrey developed a system of first aid to the wounded by taking the "hospital" to the wounded in the form of flying ambulances. His treatment of frostbite in the winter retreat from Moscow in 1812 was harmful and unfortunately practiced well until the Korean War. Engraving by Rubirre

Seventy percent of the body is water, and when body parts like fingers, toes and nose are exposed to excessive cold, this water freezes. Ice crystals can form within cells, destroying them, especially if frozen tissue is rubbed vigorously as Dr Larrey recommended. It is unfortunate that for almost 150 years, the advice of Napoleon's chief surgeon was the authority on frostbite. His treatment included rubbing the injured tissue with snow and this treatment was still being administered in the winters of the Korean War. The skin should be warmed by firm, gentle pressure with a hand or other warm body part. Submerging in warm water or blowing warm breath over the frostbite will slowly return circulation to the area and not crush ice-containing cells. This will, however, be very painful! Once the injured part has been re-warmed, treat it as a burn with dry, gentle pressure dressing and antibiotics. Do not thaw if it is refrozen, as refreezing thawed flesh increases damage.

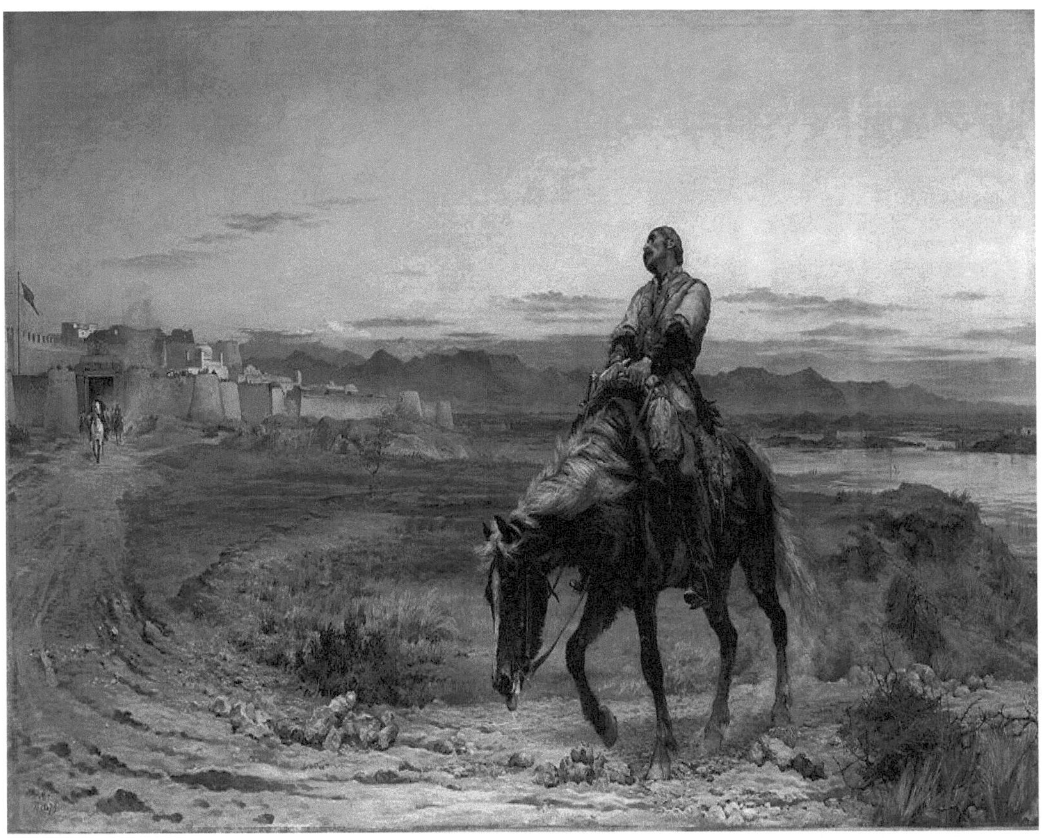

The abandonment of Kabul is considered the worst defeat of British arms until the fall of Singapore a century later. This painting of Assistant Surgeon Dr. William Brydon, one of only a handful European survivor from the winter retreat from Kabul through the Khyber Pass, January 1842. The brutal cold, deadly ambushes and criminally neglectful leadership

doomed an army. Major General Sir Elphinstone along with 16,000 men, women and children's bleached bones littered the road ascending the Khyber Pass for generations. "Remnants of an army" by Elizabeth Butler. A highly enjoyable fictional and largely accurate novel depicting the retreat is found in the novel "Flashman" by George MacDonald Fraser

Field Surgery

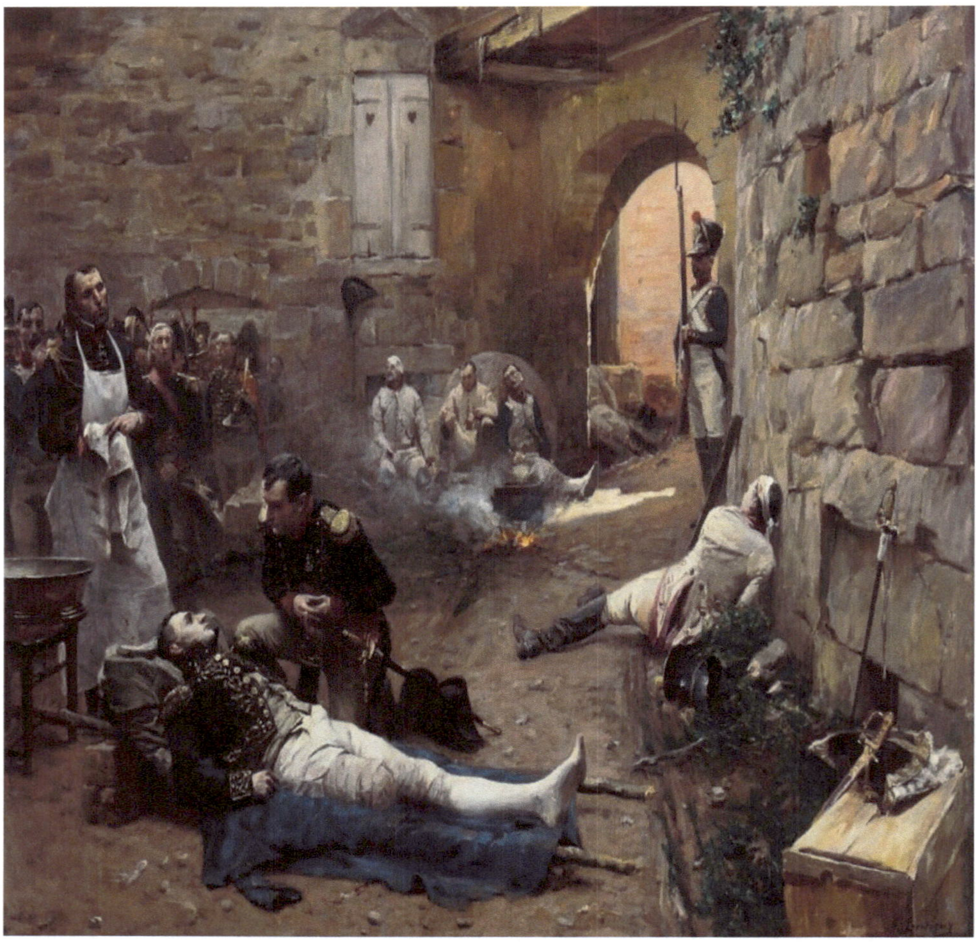

Napoleon at bedside of Marshall Jean Lannes who had both knees mangled by a ricocheted cannon ball. After the first amputation, his 2nd leg was amputated, and Lannes died the painful death of infected wounds over several days. He was one of Napoleon's bravest generals, physically small in stature even in an army of small men. He rose through the ranks from a humble beginning to Field Marshall, fighting as a commander in nine major battles. He was mortally wounded at the Battle of Essling, May 1809. Napoleon: "I found him a pigmy and left him a giant". Standing to the left is Napoleon's Surgeon General Dominique Larrey (one of the author's favorite field surgeons) caring for this special soldier, while in the background are other field commanders looking on anxiously. Napoleon often "led from the front", exposed to cannon and bullets and he expected the same from his generals. Artist Paul Boutigny

Throughout history, almost all wound care and surgery was done in open fields, in barns, under trees and on the decks of ships, often at night after the fighting, with only candles or lantern light. The "cockpit" on war ships was an open surgical theatre, amidships, painted red to reduce the signs of gore. Only recently has surgery moved into the sterile and well-lit operating rooms of modern hospitals. Imagine doing amputations and removing foreign bodies on a heaving operating table in the dark confines of a ship, in an open meadow or poorly illuminated rooms and tents after battles. An important component of a modern field medicine chest are reliable light sources (two to three head lamps).

Surgery as currently practiced, i.e., successful opening and closing body cavities have been a recent advancement. Although there are oblique references to chest and abdominal surgeries going back to ancient Egypt, there are no documented cases of the chest, abdomen or pelvic areas being successfully opened and the person living. In Egypt and later, there are vague terms such as "stonecutters", implying physicians "cut" for kidney stones and the persistent rumor that Cesare was delivered by a cesarean section, surgically removed from his mother's womb. Perhaps in rare cases, an infant cut out of mother abdomen might have survived but the mother's survival would be a miracle. There is documentation that the opacities in eye (cataracts) were surgically excised by Egyptian physicians as well as later Greek, Roman, Hebrew and Islamic surgeons. The movie "The Physician" is a fictional yet excellent story about the juxtaposition of backward European medicine and Hebrew/Islamic medicine in the 11th century. At this time in the West, most surgical procedures were limited to draining abscesses, removing damaged extremities and tooth extractions. Procedures that required limited expertise and simple instruments. Abscess drainage and tooth extraction are discussed elsewhere, while amputations discussed in this text are more of historical interest. Certainly, amputations are still common, especially in diabetics and unfortunately with combat and civilian trauma, but rarely done in the field by non-surgeons, as it was in the past. Wound care has played a huge role in history, often with poor outcomes. Simple procedures have worked for centuries and continue to be important. Cleansing and proper wound dressing are the mainstay of wound care. Following is a review of wound care history, especially in wounds resulting in amputations from lack of knowledge, resources and time.

Wound care requires four basic concepts: examination, cleaning, repair and dressing. Of course, bleeding must be controlled in a wound spilling blood. Direct pressure and careful use of tourniquet are always the first step in wound care when bleeding present. After bleeding has been controlled, examine the wound for its depth, presence of foreign material and damage to deeper structures, such as blood vessels, nerves and tendons. Thorough flushing of the wound with clean water will remove much surface bacteria and debris. Adding an antibiotic soap such as iodine (Betadine) or commercial deodorant soap will also reduce bacteria numbers. A large syringe repeatedly filled with soapy water and flushed into the wound is helpful. After cleaning and removing loose debris, a decision is made to closing the wound. Most wounds heal without sutures and will close over time if not infected. In open and closed wounds, place an antibiotic cream such as silver sulfadiazine, Silvadene (avoid oil-based ointment) lightly over wound. This layer in turn is covered with a non-stick dressing to allow its change with little pain and without further damage. Over these layers are placed cotton sponges (4x4s) to make a soft full covering secured with a lightly firm compressive bandage (ACE). Antibiotics are indicated in most wounds, even for a short time, as infections are more easily prevented than treated.

Wounds such as 3rd degree burns require daily changes while others should be examined and redress at least every 2 days. In the field, antibiotics should be used aggressively since even after thorough cleaning, most burns and deep wounds get infected. Some wounds have healed through the ages without antibiotics, however many perished before the antibiotic era. Third degree burns, deep puncture wounds, animal (especially human) bites and wounds occurring in a dirty environment all require antibiotic treatment.

Burns – cool immediately, give fluids, monitor blood pressure and pulse, place burn dressing in layers as above, elevate extremity, and start broad spectrum antibiotic

Punctures – these wounds often have small entry wound that may have penetrated deeper compartments and require irrigation with syringe and soft catheter (4 inches of IV line) inserted into puncture wound, after thorough lavage place dressing in layers as above, elevate extremity, broad spectrum antibiotic

Animal bites-clean, dress in layers as above, elevate extremity, administer broad spectrum antibiotic

Dressing should be changed when they become soiled or wet. The purpose of the 4x4 cotton gauze sponges over the wound act as a wick, drawing fluid out of wound. Soiled and damp dressings will do the opposite, drawing bacteria from the surrounding skin into wound. The signs of wound infection have been known throughout history, depicted in stone and texts of ancient Egypt. Heat, pain, swelling and redness in and around the wound are still the cardinal signs of wound infection. Until the antibiotic era, wound care was limited, resulting in amputations and deaths. Early use of antibiotics, keeping wound clean, well dressed, and dry will prevent wound infection, saving life and limb.

Amputations have been part of field medicine for thousands of years, especially in time of war which has been much been much of the time; however surviving amputations are a more recent event. There are documentations of successful amputations in Neolithic times, and the earliest written proof in the code of Hammurabi, 1700 BC and later in Greek and Hebrew texts. "The quick death of shock or the slow death of infection" awaited many with shattered limps. Clearly as drastic as amputation was, especially before anesthesia, sometimes it was the only option. Shock and infections were the primary risk with removal of an extremity, and the sooner after injury, the better chance of survival. With the introduction of gunpowder-driven high velocity projectiles, amputations became the primary surgery after sea and land battles. Historically, wounded were likely to die during or after the amputation, however they would surely die without the procedure. Amputations were common because careful cleaning and dressing of wounds require time and materials. On the other hand, amputations are generally quick to perform requiring limited training and tools. The stump is more easily managed when compared to large penetrating wounds contaminated with bone fragments, pieces of shrapnel, clothing and torn muscles. Wounds that are open and dirty or bleeding from deep sources occurred in large numbers of wounded and were best managed by removing the damaged extremity. For centuries medical officers knew that amputated stumps were simple to dress, less likely to bleed and reduced the incidence of infection leading to tetanus and death. Although grisly and usually deadly, on the battlefield or ship, it was the treatment of choice for wounds to extremities.

In the field, the stump was either packed firmly or seared with hot iron to control bleeding. The Greek medical officers of Hippocrates era were the first to record the use of ligatures (sutures), sewing wounds closed. Ligatures reduced discomfort and were efficient in controlling bleeding; however, suturing requires skill and equipment. Most Greek and Roman medical skills and texts were lost to Europe after the fall of Rome. Suturing and other Western Medicine was unknown in the Europe until The Crusades brought Islamic, Hebrew, Armenian and Greek physicians into European courts in the 13th century, yet suturing wounds was not widespread in Europe until 18th century.

With the introduction of gunpowder-propelled projectiles and larger numbers of combatants; battles mass-produced extremity wounds. There have always been fewer surgically trained medical officers than needed in battles, requiring the practice of training field surgeons "in situ" on the battlefield. Napoleon was noted for training his army "on the march", and this was the way most field surgeons were trained in the past. Amputations required simple tools, were quickly taught and on the battlefields until the 20th century, there was unlimited practice. The old medical adage "see one, do one, teach one" certainly applied to battlefield amputations through history. At the beginning of the American Civil War there were less than eighty trained surgeons in the American Army and Navy. With the beginning of war, these men split into two groups, some went north and some south, depending on loyalties. Very soon, a handful of trained military surgeons were overwhelmed in a sea of sick and wounded. Battles involving tens of thousands of men required hundreds of surgeons and surgical assistants, meaning many amputations were being done by men with no formal surgical training. Remember, that until 20th century, most surgeons were trained in the field as apprentices, not in the handful of formal medical schools in the mid-19th century.

During and after the battle of Antietam, September 1862, it is likely that some men who started the day as lightly wounded, who at first carried stretchers into surgery and later restrained men during the surgery. As the wounded mounted in numbers, they first assisted in surgery and by days end, some were skilled enough to become assistant field surgeons in a single day. In the three-day Gettysburg battle, most Union medical services were too far in the rear to serve the front, requiring surgeries to be performed "ad hoc", meaning as necessary with whatever skills and resources available. One of the author's surgeon editors was skeptical that untrained were preforming surgery, however this was common in the British Army during most of the 18th and 19th century. In the journal of Charles Boutflower, a British army surgeon during the Peninsular War describe "Regimental Mates" as soldiers taken out of field duties and given rudimentary training where they were expected to operate on the wounded near the front under fire. Charles Boutflower who graduated from medical school in Edinburgh at the age of 19 was one of the oldest in his class. In the author's class, the average age of medical school graduates was 28, and faced another one to four years of medical training required after successful completion of medical school. Because Boutflowere's family was monied, he bought his commission and joined the British army occupying Malta before moving into the Iberian Peninsula. He reported that on any typical day, 40% of the officers and men were medically unfit for duty. Going into battle without half the force must has strained the generals. Surgeons in the British army and navy were poorly compensated, making about 25% of private practice. Therefore, except for a few like Boutflower and Huxley (*HMS Rattlesnake*), most surgeons in the military were not well trained and not especially competent. Before the advent of general anesthesia and later antibiotics, amputation was an extremely unpleasant experience with a poor prognosis. Without amputation death was almost 100% while amputation was often only slightly better. During the American Civil War (or the War of Northern Aggression depending on one's view) medical officers described gunshot or shrapnel (named for French officer that invented the fragmenting artillery round) wounds to an extremity with this statement "without amputation one would surely die, while with amputation one would probably die".

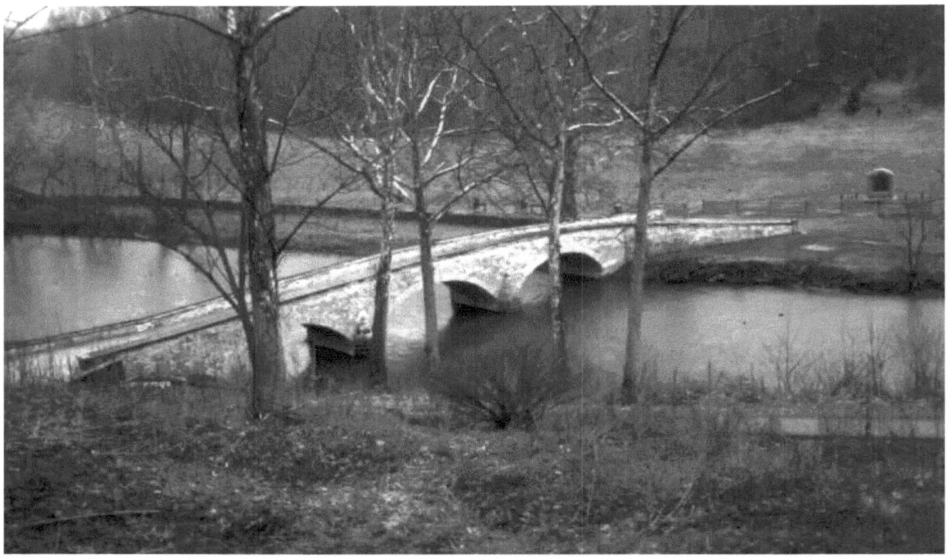

Bridge over Antietam Creek (the single bloodiest day in American history), later labeled "Burnside's Bridge" as his men finally crossed the bridge late in the battle after fighting for hours. After fruitless assaults, Major General Burnside promised extra rum rations when the bridge was taken, and the promise of extra alcohol was enough for Union troops to swarm to the other side. This maneuver flanked Robert E Lee's Army of Northern Virginia and should have led to the confederate Army of Northern Virginia's destruction, but alas the Union general, McClellan proved not up to seizing the moment. He was not known for leading form the front but instead he was drinking cold tea on a shaded porch well behind the fighting. Antietam, September 17, 1862, left 22,730 dead and seriously wounded Americans. Causalities are over four times higher than those on Omaha Beach, D Day June 6, 1944. Medical care at Antietam was more than the military surgeons could handle, requiring help from the local population, regardless of previous medical training. Every home, barn, chicken coop, outbuilding for miles around battle was commandeered for surgery and recovery. These buildings were occupied for over two years after the battle with recovering wounded, many were amputation victims. Photo by author

If the wounded survived both wound and amputation, the great fear of infection was always there. Penetrating wounds with debris such as clothing or foreign bodies increase the risk of deep wound infection. The Minnie' ball (named for the French officer that invented the expanding bullet) of the rifled musket during Civil War attained a velocity of around 600 feet/second, not fast enough to produce sterilization of the bullet (air friction causes heat). This means whatever was on the bullet as it was loaded, i.e., spittle, feces, nasal discharge on the shooter's hands ended up in the wounded. This contamination was added to whatever was on the victim skin as it penetrated, such as clothing, dirt and grime. Standard knowledge at that time was that amputation reduced risk of wound infection and infection is the enemy of the wounded. There are cases where trained medical officers who practiced thorough cleaning, dressing changes and debridement led to saving both patient and extremity. In these rare fortunate victims, the wounded went on to lead normal full life.

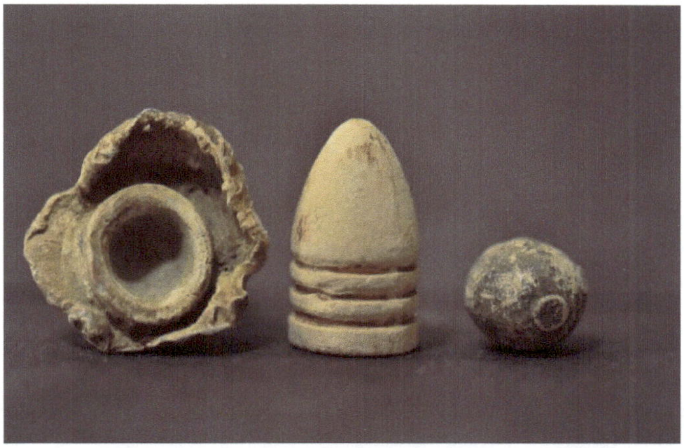

The projectile in middle deforms and expands s it passes down a rifled barrel creating a more damaging wound than the round ball fired from a smooth bore gun. USNPS

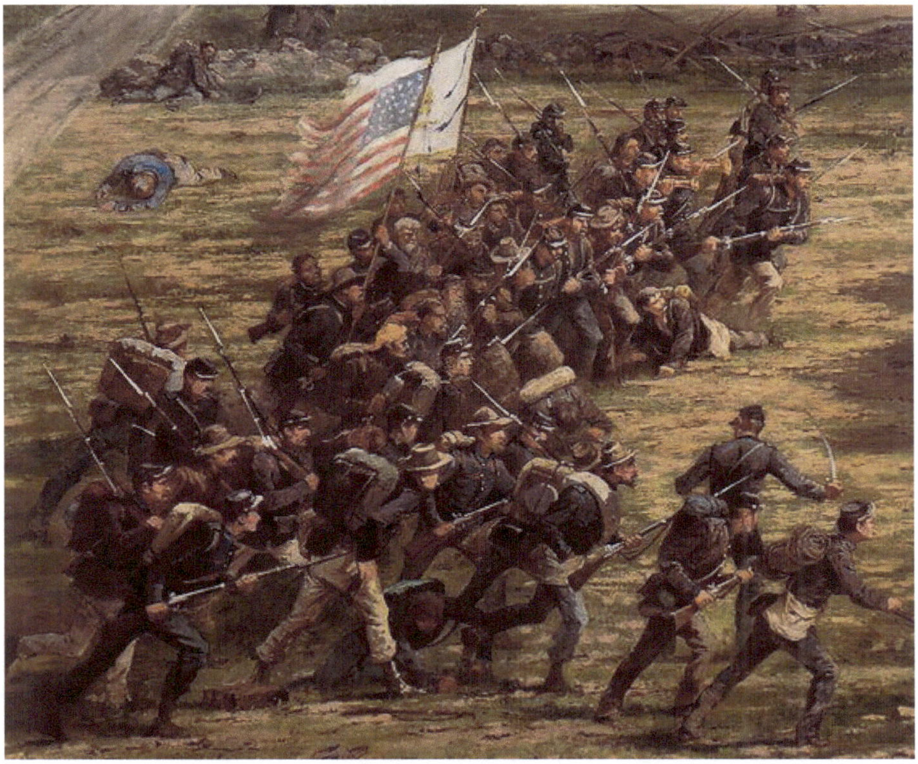

A small segment of painted cyclorama at the Gettysburg Battlefield by Paul Philippoteaux, depicting part of the bloodiest battle in American history. The single most contributions to the Oxford English Dictionary came from an inmate in an English asylum for the

criminally insane. He was an American Union Medical Officer, who became insane after the battle of Gettysburg because of the carnage and amputations. The story is told in Simon Winchester's "The Professor and the Madman". There were 350 Union medical officers present at the battle where 13 were seriously injured and a single assistant surgeon killed in action.

Antibiotics and tetanus vaccine would have saved many more extremities if available, and yet even without these 20th century innovations, there were successful amputations after battles. Success depended on the skill of the medical officer, the overall health of victims and good luck. Horatio Nelson had his arm removed, survived the surgery without anesthesia or antibiotics and went on the win sea battles that changed the course of history at Aboukir Bay (Battle of the Nile), Copenhagen and Trafalgar. He served as the "de facto" dictator of Naples where he had an open affair and child with Lady Hamilton, all with one arm and a single eye. A young Lord Raglan fighting with Wellington at Waterloo lost his right arm to amputation, was alert enough after his severed arm was carried away, to remember a family finger ring and ask for his arm's retrieval. History is filled with individuals who lost extremities to field amputations and went on to full productive lives. However, most field amputations if not leading to death, led to major disabilities and those did not make history.

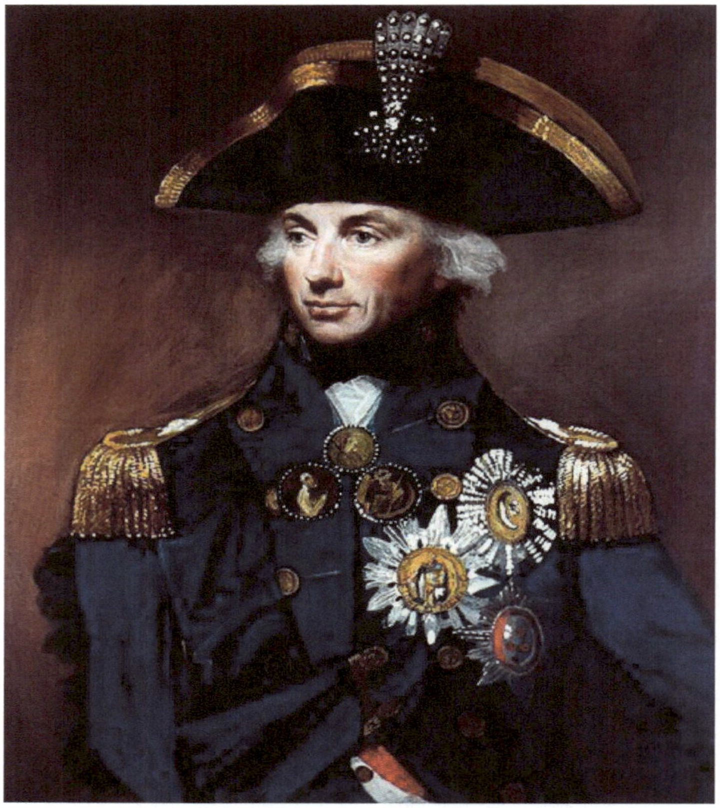

Horatio Nelson, the sixth of eleven children, one of England's most beloved heroes suffered seasickness most of his days at sea. He made captain at only twenty-one but was soon to spend five years ashore on half-pay until the rise of Napoleon. Nelson, like many others adorn the pages in history due to the Corsican and like many heroes, his story ended badly. By time of his death at 42, Nelson had his right arm shattered while leading from the front

in an amphibious landing. The arm was amputated without anesthesia. Earlier, while placing ships cannon on a beach under fire during an invasion of Corsica, he lost his right eye when a shell landed beside him, showering his face with high velocity projectiles of sand. The penetration caused immediate blindness while the injury resulted in a slow progressive loss of vision in his "good" eye. After destroying Napoleon's fleet in Egypt and turning the Mediterranean Sea into an "English Lake", he settled in Naples. Here, he became essentially the Emperor of Southern Italy, making judgmental mistakes not characteristic of his normally astute leadership. Under his watch in Naples, hundreds, perhaps thousands were arrested, tortured and executed by the corrupt King he brought back to the throne. During this period, Nelson entered a long and open affair with Lord Hamilton, England's Ambassador to Naples' wife. Some consider it to be the "scandal of the age". Lady Hamilton and her affair with Nelson has received mixed reviews by historians, strongly holding opposing views. The author believes Lady Hamilton played a larger role in British control of the Mediterranean Sea than any other single person, including Nelson. Her loving respect of the crippled admiral, her massive financial support of his navy, primarily from confiscating wealth from the accused, kept the British navy, fed, paid and equipped. She was one of the most influential people in the Mediterranean Theatre of her time. A truly intelligent, determined, charming, lively, lovely woman. A person the author would have loved to have a dinner conversation. One of many good reads on this story is "The Volcano Lover" by Susan Sontag. After returning to England, Nelson continued to live openly with Emma Hamilton and their infant daughter, much to the chagrin of his wife and King. Leaving his love and their child for the rendezvous with history at Trafalgar must have been difficult for him, knowing knew he would likely never see them again. Nelson was one of those sailors who loved the navy, his King and perhaps even the sea more than the loves of his life. Off the coast of Spain, October 1805 at the Battle of Trafalgar, he sailed into a hollowed place in history. In this battle, he deployed an innovation in naval warfare, where instead of ship's fighting along parallel lines, his ships attacked in two perpendicular lines, piercing the enemy's thin line of ships. Nelson placed his ship, "Victory" in the van and came on deck wearing the full-dress uniform he is wearing in the previous image. Unlike the sea battles in the movies, officers usually dressed "down", appearing as crew to reduce making themselves targets. Officers in a battle are few and valuable targets. His staff pleaded with him to change his attire, but he refused and stood openly in brilliant blue and was struck by a musket ball early in the battle, the bullet piercing his shoulder and breaking his spine. Taken below in his great ship's medical department and gently placed reverently down as the battle raged above. Even though he was in great pain, he refused opium. He had just over an hour to live and learned of the great victory before dying. It was clearly an act of suicide. "Show me a hero and I will write you a Tragedy, F Scott Fitzgerald. Painting by L F Abbot

Burns

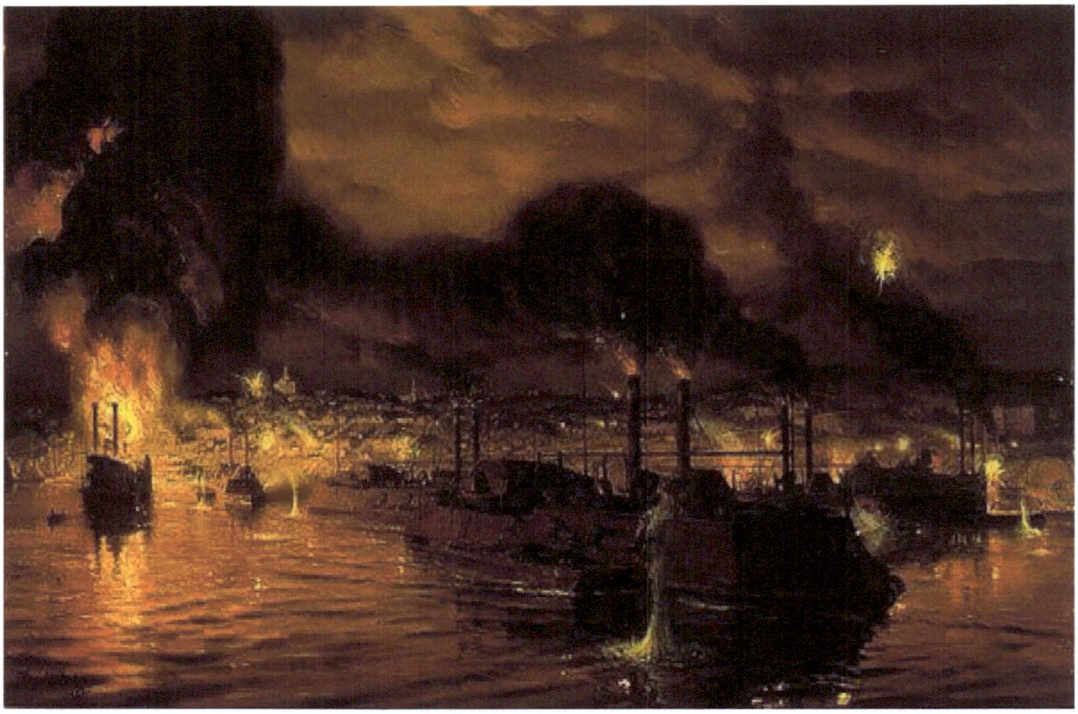

The sea battle for Vicksburg during the Civil War was very much a "fire fight". One sailor remarked "It was as if hell itself were loose". Many a sailor died of burns during the siege of Vicksburg, however for every Civil War death from wounds there were two to three dead from infectious disease. Painting by Tom Lovell

Fatal and disfiguring burns have always been a serious threat to seafarers, especially in wooden ships with open fires for cooking and lamps of wick and oil providing illumination. Naval warfare often employed weapons of fire to burn ship and crew. Greek fire (phosphorus, sulfur and oils of wood pitch or surface bitumen), an early form of napalm had been used in ancient times and continued, until the development of naval gunfire. Medicine chests throughout history carried some type of burn dressing, usually a heavy jell of oil, like modern petrolatum or aloe, poultices of herbs, onions, garlic and animal fat. World War II naval battles saw high numbers of burn victims, injuries that heavily taxed the medical department. Burns are not new to sailors and marines since fire has long been the weapon of choice at sea, but effective treatment is recent.

In early September, a generation before Christ off the coast of Greece, close to where the Persian fleet was defeated by Athens and the Battle of Lepanto would be fought 1500 years later, over 500 ships of war and 80,000 troops of Anthony and Cleopatra slowly closed on the smaller nimbler Imperial Roman fleet. Augustus and his admiral Marcus Agrippa had 250 lighter warships in a light breeze, lured the heavier vessels of the rebel Eastern fleet into the Bay of Actium. Here the larger ships of Anthony and Cleopatra ponderously clumped together with no wind to steer, and many were burned to the waterline by the swifter vessels of Agrippa. Anthony's rebel Romans fought stubbornly since they expected to be executed as traitors if captured. Fire weapons were heavily used in this battle and vessels everywhere were aflame, men roasted alive in armor, many leaping into the cooling water, only to drown or die of shock. Fire swept both navies, killing and maiming, filling the air with the cries of the wounded. Roman ships surgeons left records of the high number of burn casualties in survivors. Cleopatra, fearing that Augusta's forces appeared to be winning the battle, ordered her imperial flagship turnabout and fled the field slowly in the faint wind, remnants of her fleet in tow. Mark Anthony, in one of history's most cowardly acts by a commanding admiral, abandoned his sailors and soldiers to certain massacre and followed her, as would a servant.

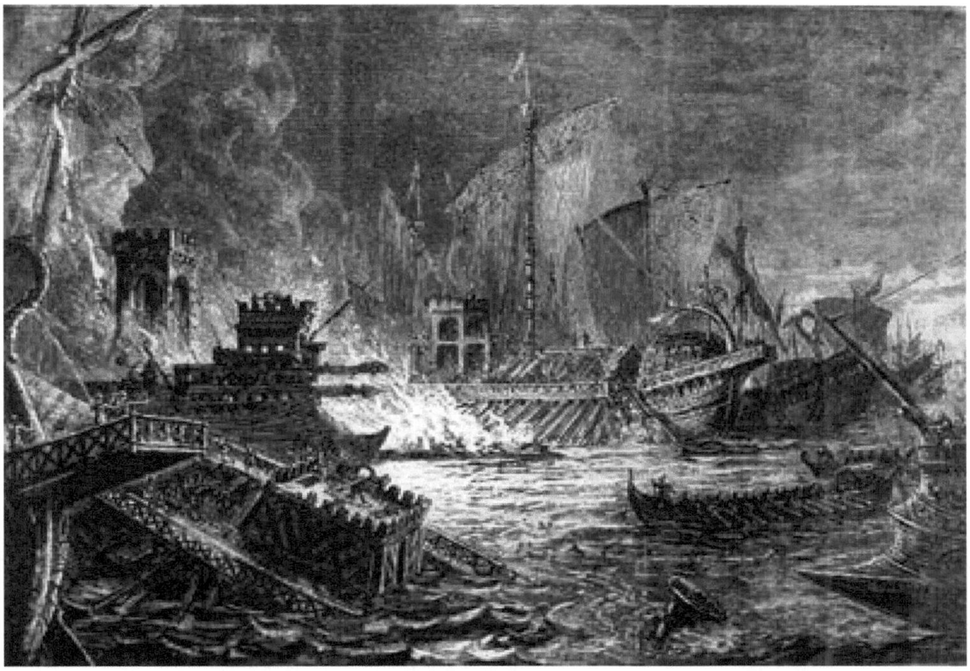

The Adriatic Sea, September 2, 31 BC, off the coast of Actium, was the site of one of history's most important and fiery sea battles. It was here that the young Octavius Caesar, known to history as Augustus, came up against a larger fleet of confederate Roman and Egyptian vessels. Harmsworth

Had Octavius either lost the battle or he been content to leave the eastern part of the Roman Empire to Anthony and Cleopatra, world history could have been much different. Judea might not have experienced Rome's harsh occupation during Christ's lifetime, if Actium had been won by Egypt. Palestine might have revolted against rule from Alexandria and might have gained independence. If so, the oppressive rule of the Rome and the puppet government of King Herrod (who was killing young Jewish male infants in attempt to prevent the prophesized Messiah) would have produced a different history. The novel "Ben Hur" by the former American Civil War general, Lew Wallace was a fictional story of a young militaristic Jewish aristocrat rebel under Roman rule and there were likely young contemporaries of Christ that could have led Judea in a war of independence. The Hebrews were waiting for a King to led them, and reluctant to accept Christ the pacifist, as the promised Messiah. They were expecting a warrior-king, like the fictional Judah Ben Hur created by Lew Wallace, to throw off the shackles of Rome, not one preaching love and peace. Had Christ grew up in a Jewish state ruled from Egypt or an independent nation, as opposed to a state ruled repressively from Rome, his life and history could have been different.

Augustus needed the Roman navy to reach and defeat both Brutus and Mark Anthony ending civil war. When Augustus returned from the frontier of Gaul and came to power in the 1st century B.C., the Roman Empire was rife with civil conflicts following the assassination of Julius Caesar. Farmland and villages lay in ruins, while pirates ruled the sea, disrupting commerce and travel. Trade is dictated by stability and a unified Rome was necessary for trade. The sailors in the port city of Alexandria revered Augustus as a god for driving out the pirates and restoring profitable maritime activity. Augustus, in his final days, traversed the eastern Mediterranean with a young fleet surgeon in attendance, Philippus of Athens. Frequently, they passed ships both merchant and military transports, every vessel saluting the flagship and the emperor. Augustus reflected to the youthful medical officer, that the battles that had truly saved Rome from its enemies were the ones he had fought upon the sea.

As a product of the merchant middle class, Augustus did not have the aristocracy contempt of commerce, instead he embraced it. He established the "Servi Augustales" a knighthood for merchants (mostly maritime) and they controlled every source of salt in the empire. Salt and "garum" a fish sauce made from salted marine products formed a basic pillar of Roman trade. It provided the army and navy with a preserved form of proteins and fats as well as daily salt. He realized that grain from Egypt was more important to the city of Rome than its garrison and the value of Egypt's location and its history of maritime trade from the seaport of Alexandria. Augustus began the construction of the Trajan canal connecting Alexandria's inner harbor to the Red Sea and planned to build a separate Red Sea fleet, from which he could project Roman power into the Arabian Sea and the Indian Ocean. In the British navy, once a man had tasted the salt of the empire he became a servant of the Crown.

For all the good he did for maritime commerce and medicine, it is unfortunate that Augustus was indirectly responsible for one of the great acts of intellectual barbarity in human history. After the battle of Actium, his troops landed at Alexandria and were soon surrounded by a larger Egyptian force. During the battle for the city, fires burned much its great library. It is not known who started the fires and if the great library was burned deliberately on by accident. Some 500,000 scrolls were destroyed, most of this information was never recovered. For over three hundred years the library at the world's busiest seaport had been collecting scrolls as there was a law in the port that any boat landed was required to allow scribes to copy books on board. These hand-copied books were one foot wide and twenty feet long containing about 60 pages of modern texts. These scrolls contained a written record of the western world just prior to Christ, knowledge that could have advanced human culture. In the television series "Cosmos" hosted by Carl Sagan, he stated that of all the losses to human history, Alexandria's library's loss was the most tragic. Three centuries later, the increasingly powerful and narrow-minded Christian population of Alexandria, burned the remaining portion of the great library to destroy pre-Christian literature, completing the loss of one of man's greatest stores of information.

Naval warfare continued to supply serious burn injuries as fire-ships, and explosive oils burned and scalded sailors over the centuries. Burn victims often died immediately from shock, and if they did survive the first day, their wounds became infected, usually fatally. When large areas of flesh have been denuded from their protecting skin, there is no barrier against bacteria invasion and fluid loss. Bums involving the face, hands, feet, and genitalia are major bums, even if small. Burns on other areas of the body larger than a coffee can lid are also major burns. Wounds of these magnitudes deserve aggressive treatment and daily wound care. First and foremost, cool the burn immediately with ice or cold packs if available, give fluids, monitor for shock, administer pain relief and antibiotics, cover with a burn dressing and demonstrate skill in the coming days of burn management. Major burns increase the risk of shock, infection and disability.

First degree burns from over-exposure to sunlight, contact with hot objects and heat sources, cause redness and pain, usually self-limiting, and requiring little care. Repeated first degree from solar injury do accumulate over time and may lead skin cancer. The sun is a giant fusion nuclear reactor and solar radiation, like all nuclear radiation may lead to skin damage and disease. Ice to the area of redness, cool soaks and anti-inflammatory medications are usually employed.

Second degree burns are more damaging to skin, resulting in redness and blister formation. More severe sunburns, hot water, hot metal and steam are common causes of these burns. Ice, cool soaks and pain medications are helpful. Since the blister in second degree burns is the body's own burn dressing, it is recommended to leave intact and not remove. Once the blister has deflated, cover with burn dressing and change as needed. Repeated second degree sunburns are common in malignant melanoma.

Third Degree Burns

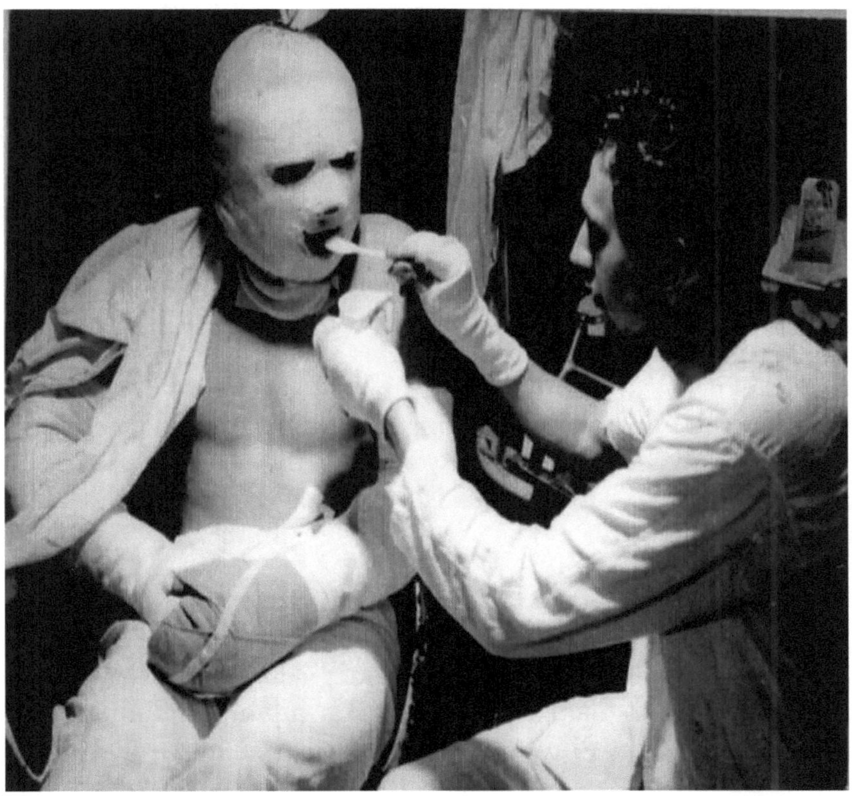

Okinawa, 1945, Kamikaze victim. This type of hard dressing changed infrequently has been replaced by soft, frequently changed burn dressing. National Archives

Third degree burns are the result of heat destroying living tissue, through the full thickness of the skin. The initial damage occurs as heat energy penetrates the skin and later continues when heat is retained under the skin by melted body fat. Underlying the skin of all mammals is a fat layer that provides important insulation, allowing mammals to retain heat in cold environments. This fat layer becomes a major force of destruction when it is converted to hot oil, cooking muscles, vessels and nerves. After removing a steak from a grill or a roast from the oven, the meat continues to cook in its own melted fat found in muscle, bone and surrounding bundles of nerves and vessels. This cooking will last for several minutes. Therefore, all bums should be cooled as quickly as possible by immediate immersion in water followed by ice. Burns should be cooled for at least 15 minutes, during which time airway, breathing, circulation and blood pressures are monitored and maintained.

Major burns are capable of severe damage to the skin and deeper organs by triggering the cascade sequence of shock. Fluid is quickly lost, as formerly protected tissue, wet with precious body water, is exposed. Other body fluids may shift out of circulation, as fluid becomes "hidden" in third spaces for the body's immediate safety. Electrolyte solutions should be given in small continuous sips if the person is alert and able to drink. If possible, start an IV and administer pain medication. Give fluids at the rate of 4-8 ounces per hour until the urine is clear and abundant. Pain relief can be given initially, if available, especially opiates such as morphine, butorphanol (Stadol) or a long-lasting fentanyl skin patch. Relieving pain and anxiety in a burn victim is important in maintaining the person's circulating fluid. Burns are known to deplete circulation, sometimes doing so quietly if the victim's circulating fluid is not supported.

During the period of cooling and pain relief, blood pressure and tilt test are recorded and repeated. Clothes and other debris are removed from the burn, preparing it for cleaning. After 15-20 minutes of cooling and with the victim as stable as possible, the wound is prepared for dressing. First gently bath wound with medicated soap such as iodine or other antibiotic soaps. Any obvious dead tissue should be carefully removed with gloves and forceps. Do not force debris from the wound, only remove what comes off easily. After five minutes of cleaning, dry and cover the entire burn with Silvadene, which is then covered with a non-stick bandage, such as Telfa or even better, Adaptic. Over and around the wound, use fluffed up 4 x 4 sponges held in place by clinging roll cotton gauze. This dressing, when kept dry, functions as a wick, pulling fluid out of the wound. And burns leak fluid. If it becomes soiled or damp with seawater or wound discharge, it reverses the wick action, drawing skin bacteria into the wound. A damp dressing will enhance infection, decreasing the quality of wound care. Wounds are generally better off without dressing if it becomes damp or soiled.

Burn Infections

Antibiotics should be used initially and each day the burn wound is open, since most third-degree burns become infected, even with good wound care. If available, victims of major burns should receive an injection of an antibiotic initially, followed by oral antibiotic (the author prefers an azithromycin). If tetanus shot record is unknown, give .5 cc of Tetanus toxoid. Burn dressings should be changed at least daily, more often if the wound is draining enough to soil the dressing, even if the spot of wetness is small. With each dressing change, remove dead tissue, as it will serve as a food source for bacteria and slow the healing. Scabs keep a wound from healing while they smother living tissue. If not every day, then every other day, dead tissue is gently removed (debridement). Black, green, or yellow material is debrided with clean forceps, scissors and gloves. Some of this tissue may be washed away with soaking and light scrubbing. This is a painful procedure, but one that must be done if the wound is to have the best opportunity to heal. Prior to debridement, a clean 4 x 4 sponge soaked in local anesthesia (lidocaine) can be placed over the open wound and may provide some much-appreciated pain reduction. Oral opiates given thirty minutes before may make the wound care more humane. Soiled dressings can be recycled after washing in soap and air-dried in sunlight. After washing and drying in sunlight, used dressings, even though stained are clean enough to be reused.

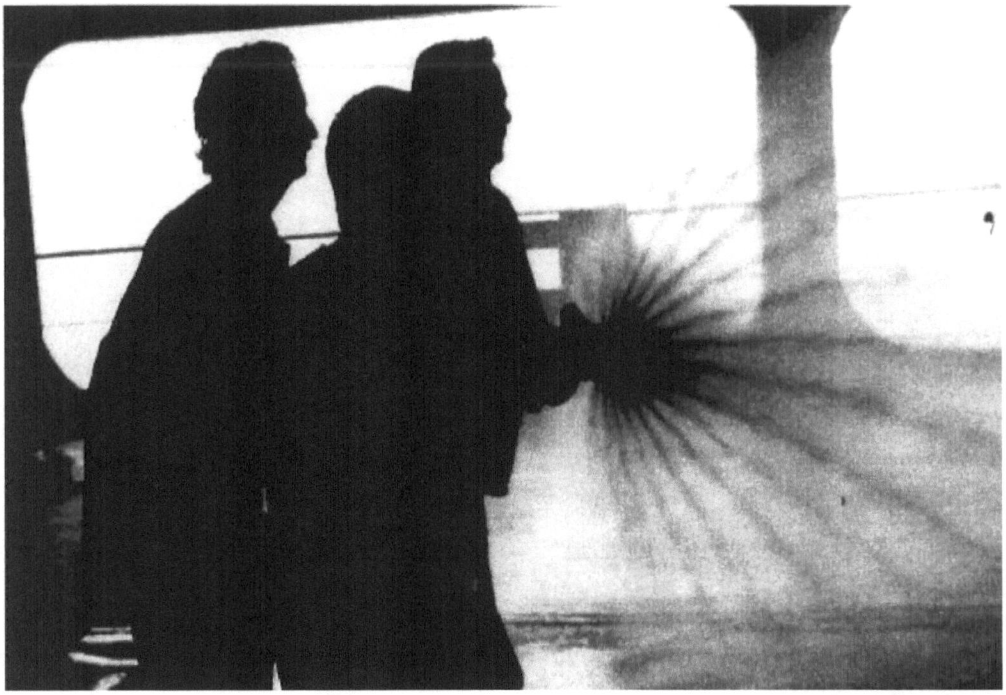

A "fire-drill" the author organized while sailing as supercargo on the SS President Harding. Part of a weekly training exercise on this American President Lines container vessel somewhere in the South China Sea. Every ship spends time practicing and discussing the possibility of fire and other hazards at sea. And every vessel should be prepared to treat burns, as they require a high degree of skill and medical supplies. Cooling, pain relief, shock management and infection control are the mainstays of burn management. A portable medicine chest with a burn kit should be included in fire-fighting exercise and should be available on the scene in case of a real fire. Photo by author

Respiratory Burns

If superheated air enters the respiratory tract, it may convert the high humidity in the lungs and airways into steam, scalding the fragile cells lining these spaces. This can lead to a slow smothering death of respiratory collapse, since the lungs lose the ability to produce a vital substance, surfactant. Lung surfactant is a soap-like liquid that keeps tiny airways and air sacs open (especially in newborns), allowing for the movement of oxygen and carbon dioxide to and from the blood vessels. The presence of singed nasal hair or charred tissue within the throat is evidence of the entry of hot air. There is little treatment for respiratory burns other than supporting the victim with fluids, maintaining adequate circulation and pain relief. Burn centers use steroid injections such as dexamethasone or Solu-Cortef every eight hours for several days after the burn. The same drugs are currently used to reduce respiratory inflammation and death in COVID-19. Oxygen will be helpful in allaying the respiratory distress that signals lung shock.

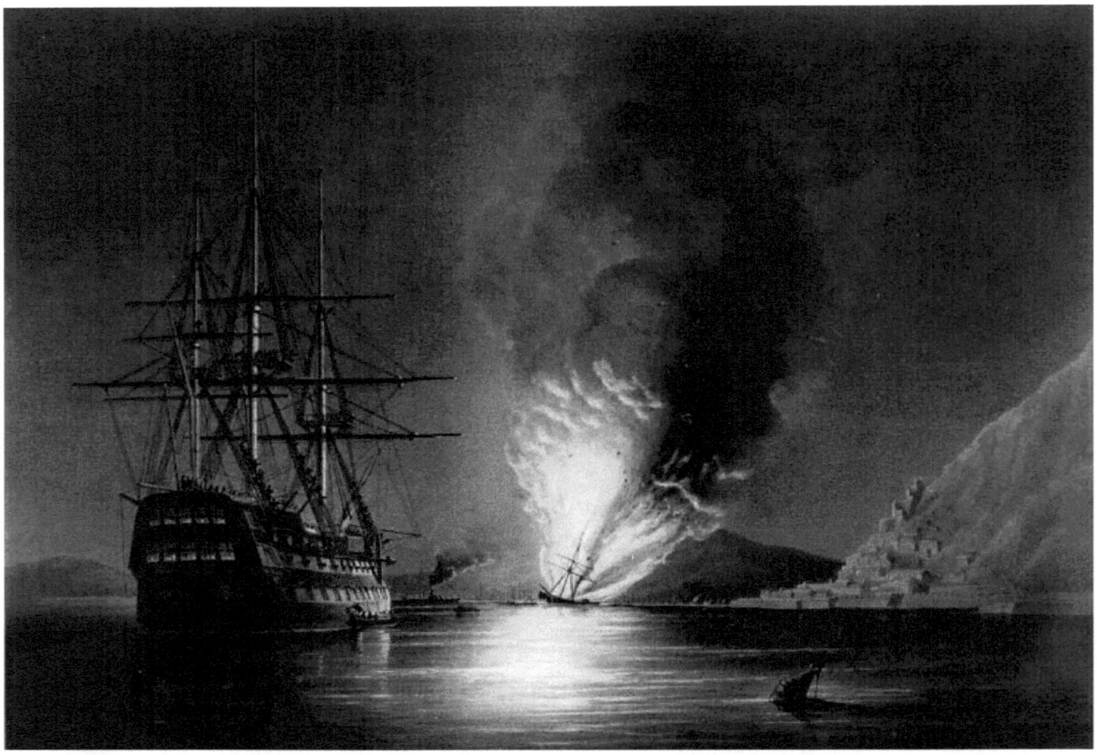

The USS Missouri burning in Gibraltar in 1843, one of the US Navy's first steam powered frigates that accidently caught fire and sank. Sailors fleeing the fire, especially in the engine compartment, certainly inhales superheated air. Although they were injured, no loss of life. The older officers used this as a reason to be skeptical of new coal-fired warships. TG Dutton

Orthopedics

Two words in Greek, "raising children correctly". In Medieval France "to straighten bones"

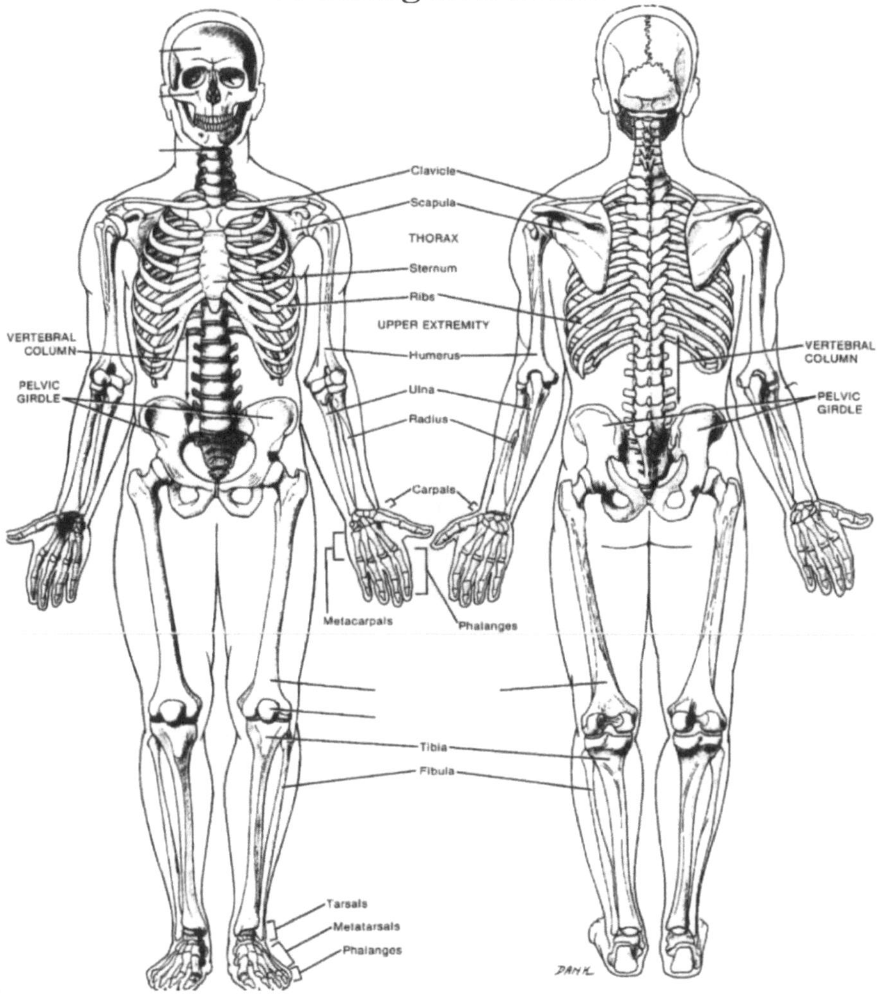

The human skeleton is composed of some 250 bones, the largest is the thigh bone or femur while the smallest are the three bones of the middle ear, the hammer, anvil and stirrup. Vital bone marrow tissue is housed within the large bones of the pelvis, the long bones of the thigh and arm and the flat bones of the chest cage. Bones are held together at the joints by ligaments and bags of connective tissue, the bursas. The exterior of bones is rich in blood vessels and nerves while the interior fossilized and honeycombed to save weight. Most orthopedic injuries are not to the hard bones but the softer muscles, tendons, ligaments and bursa

Sprains, Strains and Trains

Sprains are not a true medical term, nor are "pulled" muscles, however, these terms are in common use. Strain is another term describing soft tissue injuries to flexible components of the musculoskeletal system. Sprains are separated into three grades dependent upon severity of symptoms. Some sprains may appear mild to moderate initially, only to become more serious or chronic over time, especially if the joint is not protected. The following descriptions of injuries and management are for the ankle but can be applied for most joints. The building of the world's railway required the human musculoskeletal system to bend, lift and rotate heavy objects accounting for untold numbers of strains and sprains. Many disabling.

Sprains

In the first-degree sprain, initially there is pain and some swelling while the joint can bear weight with little discomfort. The next day there is typically more discomfort and swelling, especially if ice, elevation and immobilization are ignored. Like first degree burns, the injury resolves over time with minimal treatment. In the first-degree sprain, ligaments are only over-stretched, not damaged. The pain and swelling are completely reversible since tissue is not torn away from its attachments along the bone of the joint border. Although there may be small tears that can be demonstrated microscopically, over time, first-degree recurrent sprains may lead to a weak and easily injured joint.

Initially, place wet thin cloth over the injury with ice, compression and elevation. Later, some type of support-like splint with a conforming bandage (ace wrap) over L-shaped splint that can be made from cardboard. Keep the injury elevated as much as possible and avoid weight bearing for 12-24 hours. Gentle stretching of the joint enhances recovery, by moving the foot in slow circles for 3-5 minutes. Massage and gentle active stretching of the ankle in normal motions by the medical officer will speed recovery of an injured joint.

The second-degree sprain is a more serious injury with increased pain, swelling and bruising (ecchymosis). The injured ankle may not be able to bear weight initially, appearing unstable due to pain. A bruise often develops over 8-24 hours and the affected area becomes stiff. In second degree sprains, ligaments are partially torn from their bone attachments and disrupted blood vessels cause bruising. The overlying supportive muscles respond with spasm, to "splint" the joint, reducing movement and pain (nature's cast). The joint maintains its basic architecture and is stable enough to bear weight, although it does so with pain. Usually the larger the bruise, the more damage.

As with a milder sprain, ice, elevate and immobilize with the addition of a removable splint preventing motion. Analgesic medications reduce suffering, especially anti-inflammatories (ibuprofen, Naprosyn) being the most common used. The author recommends caution in using anti-inflammatory drugs long-term or in presence of hypertension or heart disease. Daily gentle massage to the joint along with passive stretching, will prevent long term stiffness. Ankle sprains should be elevated as much as possible, and some weight bearing is acceptable as tolerated.

Third-degree sprains are severe injuries resulting from sudden opening and over-stretching of the joint. It presents as throbbing pain, swelling, deformity, loss of joint stability and inability to bear weight without moderate to severe pain. A discoloring bruise occurs within minutes to hours, and weight-bearing may take days to recover. Ligaments in these injuries have been completely torn from their bony attachments. These injuries may require months to heal and may be forever an intermittent problem with pain, stiffness and easily re-injured. Treat with ice, immobilization (gently wrapped in splint to allow for increased swelling), no weight bearing for days, gentle massage and more gentle stretching after pain and swelling have been reduced. Keep elevated and splinted until the joint can bear some weight or an X-ray can be done to rule out fracture at the earliest opportunity.

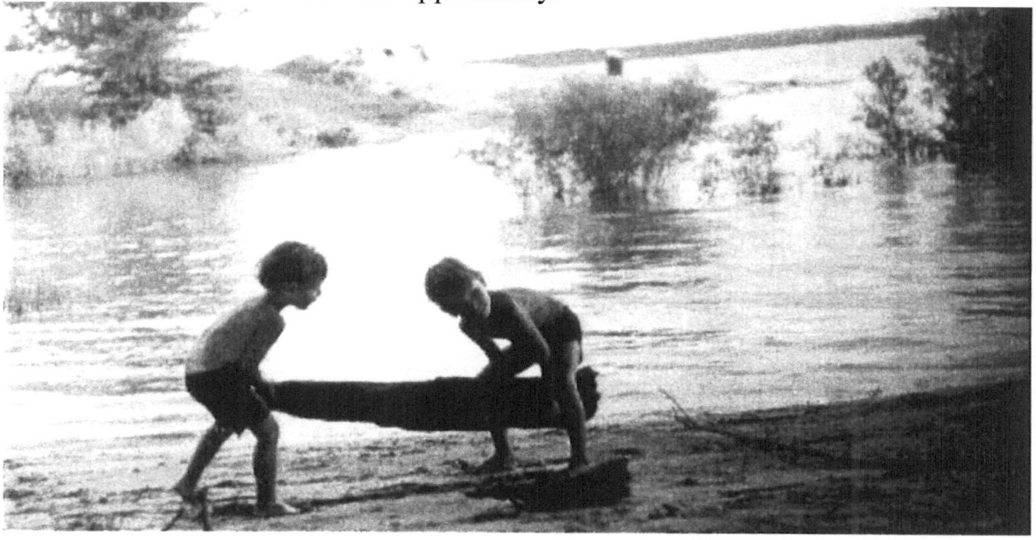

Strains

Back strains are common, accounting for a significant amount of disability in the USA. It usually involves lifting when the back is required to contract under a load. It occurs more often when the back is twisted to one side, the injury on the opposite side when those muscles are trying to contract while the bony spinal column is forcing them to stretch. The pain and stiffness are the result of spasms where muscles or groups of muscles have shortened in response to the injury. Early treatment with ice, gentle stretching and pain relief, if necessary, will reduce disability. The young people above are at little risk of strain, but adults should lift with legs, not backs and begin each day with a few minutes of back stretches. Morning back stretching is proven to reduce the risks of back injuries.

Strains are common injuries, especially in the back, wrist and shoulder. Strains occur when muscles and tendons are over-stretched, responding with spasm. Spasm can be immediate or occur days after the event. Muscle tissue contracts when injured, often recruiting other muscles above and below to participate in the spasm (misery loves company). As the muscle shortens, it closes joints, reducing range of motion causing stiffness. Spasm is generally painful, usually described as sharp and/or cramp-like. In large muscles like those found in the lower back, this natural splinting mechanism can be quite uncomfortable with significant disability. Management of strains includes ice, gentle massage, increasing range of motion and reduced activity usually the time of disability.

The lumbar-sacral strain often prevents the patient from standing straight as most comfortable position is bent forward and sometimes sideways (lumbago). Often, they are "pulled" towards the injured side, creating tilted walk while slightly stooped forward. Pain in the lower back tends to be worse in the morning and improves with motion. Buttocks pain, pain in the back of the leg (sciatica) and a "pins and needles" sensation in the leg (paresthesia) are common complaints. Immediate symptoms of numbness in the foot, especially the little toe side, may be signs of a more serious disc herniation. Back pain alone is usually easier to treat with probable complete resolution, whereas back pain with leg pain is usually more difficult to relieve quickly. Treatments of strains are directed towards increasing the range of motion in the affected area. Stretching is likely to cause some pain at first because the injured muscles are shorter than normal and often stretching will reduce the duration of pain. Stretching is more effective followed by ice for twenty minutes. A good source of therapeutic stretching is found in "Stretching" by Anderson. Gentle massage and stretching the joints through their normal motions is the best therapy for a sprain. Heat may feel good but does little to reduce inflammation and may aggravate swelling. Ice over the painful area will penetrate the skin, reaching injured tissue where the cold helps reduce swelling and inflammation, providing some anesthesia, decreasing the discomfort of stretching. After the ice is removed, the body will flush the injured area with warm blood flow carrying off injured cells and debris while delivering natural healing chemicals (cortisol). Keeping the joint moving after injury by stretching it through its normal range of motion enhances blood supply to the injured joint. A completely immobile joint on the other hand, may promote stagnation and swelling which delays healing.

Trains

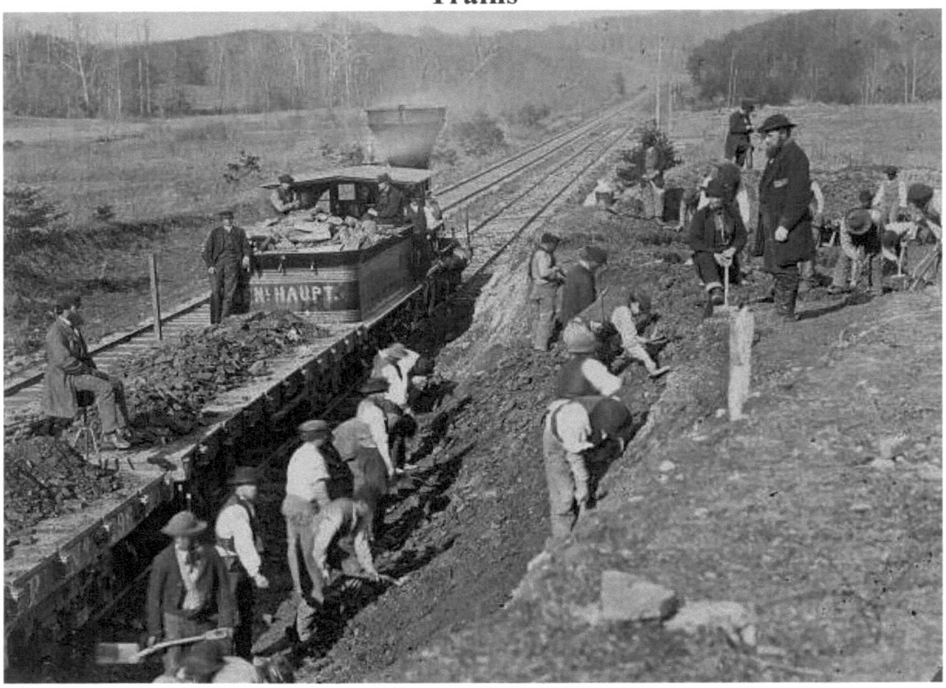

There must have been thousands of back strains, some with permanent disability while building the Transcontinental Railroad. A railroad built largely by recently arrived immigrant males. Imagine the costs of injuries and maiming in the construction of this steel shipping lane. Fractures, dislocations and amputations must have been common and field medicine a necessary ingredient for building the American Transcontinental Railroad, the 19th century's greatest industrial feat along with the Trans-Siberian railroad. National Archives

Anti-inflammatory drugs are commonly used in treating sprains and sprains but can cause side effects, even if used appropriately and be dangerous if used for more than a few days. Aspirin heads a lengthy list of non-steroidal anti-inflammatory drugs, a list that includes over 30 agents. In medicine, when there are more than three or four drugs of one type, it means they are either sporadically effective or have high side effects. For the anti-inflammatory drugs, both are true. These drugs can cause ulcers, gastrointestinal bleeding, kidney damage, high blood pressure, stroke, heart attack and allergic reactions! Despite these shortcomings, they are the most prescribed class of drugs in the world. Probably, because pain is the most common medical complaint in the world. Aspirin is cheap, fast acting and effective. To be effective in musculoskeletal pain however, it often must be taken in high doses and often, which can quickly lead to gut discomfort. Therefore, aspirin is probably best not used for pain. Anti-inflammatory drugs such as Ibuprofen and Naprosyn are longer- acting, more potent and in general, easier on the gastrointestinal tract than high-dose aspirin (which may require doses of 8-12 per day to control the pain). Aspirin can be a life-saving drug in heart attack, and it has been touted as protective of colon cancer, dementia and anti-aging when used chronically in low dose. It may increase bleeding in trauma and surgeons prefer no aspirin use for one week prior to elective surgeries. The author feels that aspirin, 325mg should be part of a field medicine chest for its use in heart disease is based on the anti-platelet effects, as circulating aspirin "poisons" the platelets as they emerge from the bone marrow. Platelets exposed to aspirin are less effective for their entire life. If pain medications are employed, either anti-inflammatory, Tylenol or opiate, use as low a dose as possible for the least amount of time to reduce discomfort. Acetaminophen (Tylenol) has no anti-inflammatory activity.

Dislocations

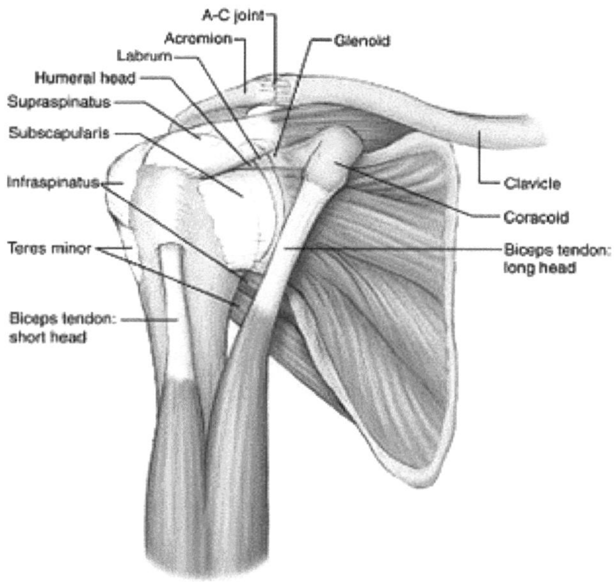

The human shoulder is a complicated composite of bone, sinew, nerve and muscle enabling the throwing motion so necessary for warfare, athletics and survival. NIH

Dislocations, like fractures, cause an interruption of joint structure, producing pain, deformity and loss of function. Small, dislocated joints like fingers and toes can often be reduced with simple grasping traction. Larger joints such as the shoulder require more care. The shoulder is the most dislocated major joint, requiring traction as soon as possible to reduce pain and disability. Controlled traction should be slow and persistent to correct (reduction). Most shoulder dislocations result from a forward fall, driving the ball of the upper arm back and down. The shoulder appears "knocked down" and there is loss of function of the arm usually accompanied by severe discomfort. Although reversible, in some cases the tight bag of connective tissue (bursa) holding the shoulder together may be torn. Once torn, the person may experience future dislocations, each time the bursa (bag of connective tissue that encloses the joint) becomes over-stretched and the shoulder more vulnerable to injury.

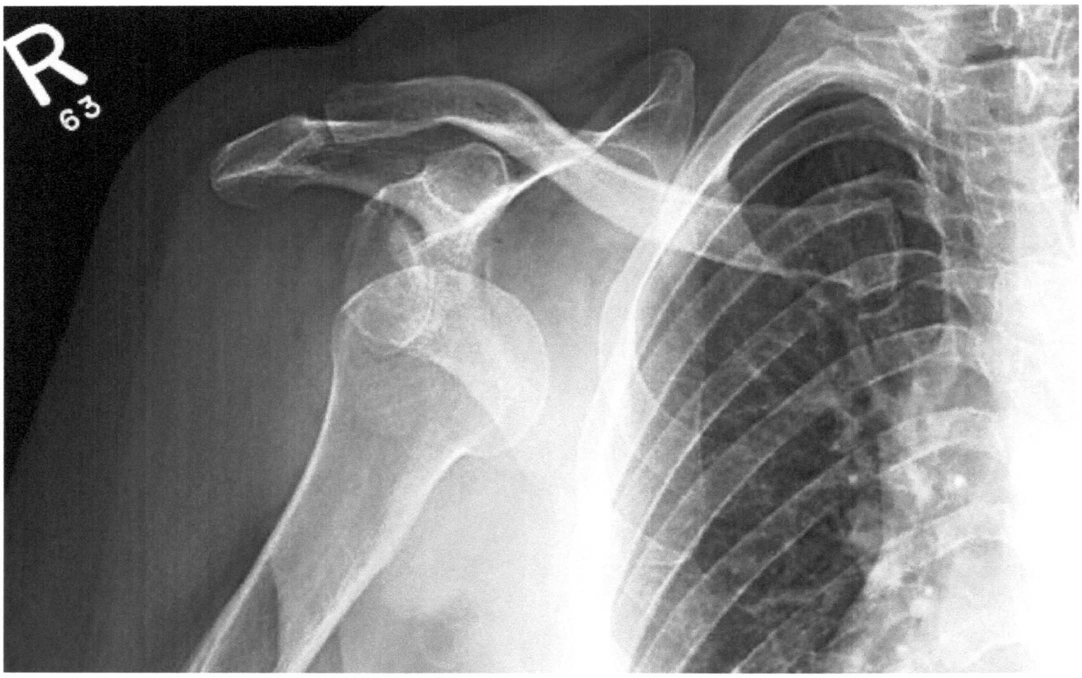

In this x-ray, the ball of the upper arm is clearly not sitting in its socket. Image from files

In reducing the dislocated shoulder or other large joint dislocations, continuous weight is most effective and humane, especially when coupled with pain relief and muscle relaxation. Both may be reduced with an opiate injection. Many separated shoulders have been reduced on battlefields in the past and are still being reduced today on the athletic playing fields by non-physicians using the Kocher Maneuver. With this technique, the medical officer can usually quickly reduce the shoulder manually, and if successful, requires only to secure the injured arm in a sling and immobilize to chest after reduction. With the Kocher maneuver, the arm is grasped firmly just above the elbow, if possible, a sheet of cloth is placed under the armpit with traction applied towards the head. Gentle yet firm continuous downward pressure is applied with this grip as the forearm and wrist are held at 90 degrees. This is done, to pull the ball of the shoulder back under the joint socket. When the downward traction reaches its maximum strength, the arm is brought across the chest, rotating the arm into the chest (internal rotation) while pulling the elbow area to the opposite side from the injury. Reduction is complete when the ball of the upper arm "pops" into its socket. When successful, the arm and shoulder function is returned in a limited fashion and the pain of muscle spasm dissipates. The upper arm will return to its normal position if the medical officer can just get it close to normal position with traction. Muscle spasm and pain are the main hindrance to reducing dislocations and fractures. These forces must be overcome to place a bone or joint back into its normal position (reduction). This is best done with opiates to reduce discomfort, and steady traction to release spasm.

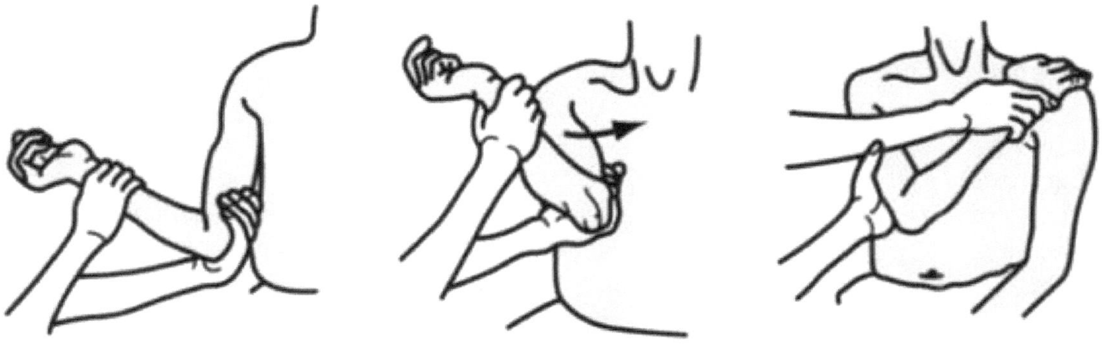

This technique has been in use for centuries, depicting in stone in ancient egypt and later in documents from Greece and Rome. NIH

Another simple, relatively pain-free technique is to place the victim face down on a high table with his hand and wrist taped to a bucket. The suspended bucket is safe and useful not only in shoulder dislocations but also in arm and wrist fractures. This was the preferred technique in Naval Hospital, San Diego during the author's orthopedic training. It is important to make the patient comfortable with pain medications if needed, padding under the injured shoulder with soft pillow and attaching the wrist to the bucket in a non-binding manner. Pain relief, reducing muscle spasm and gentle traction are the keys to successful reduction of dislocations and fractures. The bucket should be wrapped comfortably to the hand with padding. Water or sand is slowly added to the bucket until firm pressure is pulling the arm downward. This can continue for several hours, but generally less time is needed for the shoulder (or wrist fracture) to release and slide into place. The patient, if awake, will often feel the moment the bone or joint is reduced into position. Remember to continue to check for pulse during any traction procedure to prevent the traction from cutting off circulation. There are many forces that can break bones. These include falls, blunt and sharp trauma, projectiles such as bullets, twisting strains, and the concussive force with explosions. Indirect forces such as leverage, traction or torsion can also result in fractures, such as those associated with lifting or moving heavy objects. In any case, the most common complaints of fracture are pain at the site of injury, deformity and loss of function. Physical findings include swelling, tenderness, deformity, bruise (ecchymosis), muscle spasm, loss of motion and possibly a crunching sound (crepitation) with gentle pressure over the fracture site.

The most common human fracture is the clavicle or collar bone, manifested by pain, decreased use of shoulder on the fractured side and usually a tender lump along the clavicle. It can leave alone or treated by placing a figure-of-eight sling that crosses the back under each armpit and crosses the upper chest. This should pull the shoulders back bringing the shoulder blades closer together, allowing the clavicle to heal over a few weeks. Fractures of the shoulder apparatus are possible with more violent dislocation (the shoulder accounts for one-half of all dislocations).

Fractures are more serious than simple dislocation and if patient pain can be controlled, the shoulder should be immobilized and not manipulated. After reduction with traction place the injured shoulder in a sling for 3-4 weeks. The elbow can be fractured/ dislocated with fall onto with outstretched arm. It can be reduced with gentle traction while rotating the forearm away from the body. In hip fractures, the injured leg is usually shortened, and the foot is rotated outward. Fractures of hip and femur are painful, and any leg movement should be limited. These should be carefully immobilized before transport.

Bone is living tissue, rich in blood supply on its external surface, the periosteum is heavily laden with pain nerve fibers. Soon after a fracture, blood gathers at the site (hematoma) which appears as a tender swelling that soon discolors. Fracture pain is a deep pain and sometimes is quite severe, leading to fainting as blood pressure falls. Pain relief by ice, gentle compression, splinting and pain relief are paramount to prevent shock associated with fractures. The author fractured four ribs in a motorcycle accident and experienced the sound of bone fracturing and immediate deep sever pain. In this case, topical ice was augmented with long and short acting opiates, preventing the possibility of shock developing.

Muscle spasm may be the most painful component of a fracture and often hinders the successful reduction of broken bones. Spasm is a defense mechanism to reduce motion and pain in fractures with movement of the injured extremity. In major fractures of leg or arm, the injury should be immobilized before transport to reduce the risk of additional injury and shock. Pain relief early reduces the risk of shock when injured appears in distress. After splint is placed, careful blood pressure readings and tilt test repeatedly to ensure the victim is not slipping into early shock. Cover open wounds with an antibiotic ointment and a clean dry dressing, begin antibiotics if skin broken over fracture site. Give one to two liters of fluid orally or IV along with the pain medication in major fractures.

Local swelling also occurs in sprains, but in fractures it appears quickly and is firmer than the soft swelling of sprains. Fracture swelling discolors early as blood enters the soft tissue. The author has seen deformities of the musculoskeletal system that when viewed, caused swooning of the injured and nausea to the medical officer. It is important therefore, to cover the injury site from the victim's point of view. Crepitation, more common in the small bone fractures of the wrist, ankle and ribs, are felt when the area is gently moved or compressed, producing the sensation of crackles.

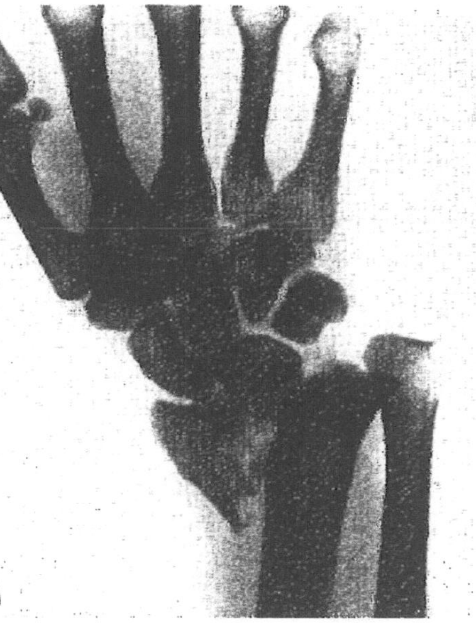

A

This X-ray depicts a moderately severe fracture and dislocation of the wrist. In this case there would be enough deformity that an X-ray would not be needed for diagnosis. If nerve and arterial blood flow are intact, do not try to reduce the fracture. Place ice, immobilize, elevate, give pain relief and continue to monitor nerve and blood flow function. If there is evidence of nerve or blood flow interruption, use gentle continuous traction until restored.

The keys to fracture management include immobilization, elevation, ice, pain relief and antibiotics if the overlying skin is broken. Fortunately, fracture reduction is rarely necessary in the field. When the skin is broken over a possible fracture site, it becomes an open fracture, which is obvious when the bone is sticking out or when a large laceration exposes underlying bone. Less obvious when there is only an abrasion or small cut over an area of swelling, pain and deformity. Any wound with bleeding over possible fracture should be managed as an open fracture. Open fractures should initially be covered with moist clean dressings with layered topical antibiotic agent and later debrided (removal of dead tissue) as dead skin and muscle is "bug" food for infection. Open fractures demand the addition of oral antibiotics with cephalosporins being a good choice. A common undertreated open fracture is from a closed fist strike against hard sharp object, the Boxer's fracture. Too often, this open fracture follows a fight where the fifth metacarpal and the skin over it is broken by bacteria-laden teeth. Because the injury often occurs under the influence of alcohol and goes untreated until the next day. Open hand and finger fractures can lead to a permanent loss of some function if not treated carefully with immobilization, elevation and antibiotics.

The author trained, served and shared "sea stories" with nuclear submarine enlisted medical officers who took every wound seriously, even small ones. Deployed submarine crew are the Navy's healthiest, however problems due arise, usually bumps and scraps. These corpsmen are trained that every wound, even small ones should be examined. In one sea story, a small wound on the little finger of the dominant hand was harboring a fracture later seen on X-ray. The suspected fracture was splinted, examined and dressed every day and given antibiotics. The finger healed and there was no loss of function. The fifth digit, though the smallest, accounts for 20% of grip strength. On submarines, all wounds are examined, cleaned, dressed, re-examined and given antibiotics if warranted.

In large open fractures that do not require reduction, keep the wound covered with clean dressing containing topical antibiotics, irrigate and clean daily while watching for signs of infection, injectable and oral antibiotics are likely needed. In the past, open fractures were common in warfare and treated overwhelmingly with amputation. Historically, amputated limb wounds require less care and less likely infection. Open fractures have been successfully managed in the field with maggots, as the growing larvae only eat dead flesh, thus cleaning the wound. Maggots continue to perform the same maneuver in modern wound care after the larva has been radiated and rendered sterile yet alive.

Fracture Reduction

Fortunately, "setting" or reducing fractures are rarely necessary and can usually be delayed until a qualified medical officer familiar with fracture reduction is available. However, there are times when the fracture is compromising vital nerves and arteries, requiring reduction in the field. Reasons for emergency fracture reductions include loss of blood flow or nerve function to the injured part, especially the hand. The wrist is one of the most fractured sites (the clavicle or collar bone the most common) and the wrist and hand form one of the most complex components of the musculoskeletal system. Normal hand function must be protected, and to ensure that, blood flow and nerve function established beyond the fracture site. Loss of arterial flow or nerve function in the field can cause life-long disability. The author's father-in-law, a retired orthopedic surgeon, believed there is no such thing as a simple wrist fracture. Ice, gently compress and elevate wrist fractures if nerve and arteries are intact. Leave reduction for an expert.

Signs that blood flow is being obstructed by the fracture include pale cool skin past (distal) the fracture site, loss of pulse, and reduced "capillary flush". This is a simple technique to indirectly measure blood flow past a fracture site at the wrist or ankle by using the capillary blood beds under each nail. In a suspected wrist fracture, the victim's fingernail is compressed firmly for several seconds until it is blanched white. After releasing the pressure, the nail bed should quickly return to the same pink color as the examiner's nail beds. A delay or loss in the return of color means the capillaries are not filling, which implies blood brought to the hand by arteries is being compromised by the fracture

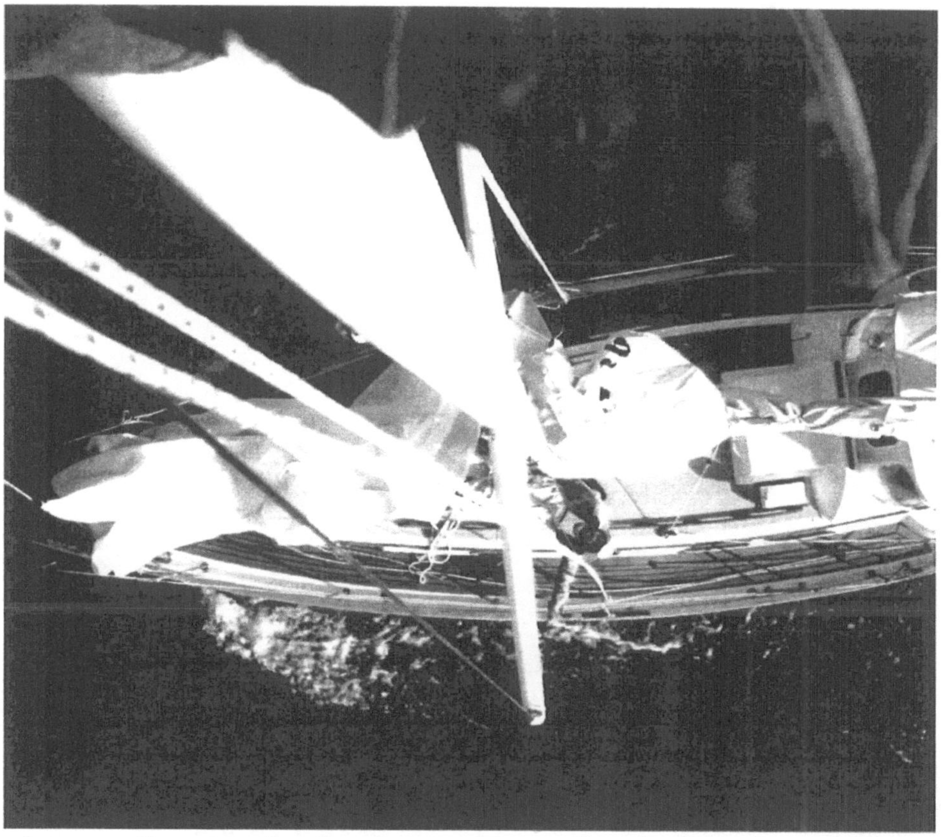

Falls are always a threat on land and sea. At sea, the platform is usually moving and there are stairs, ladders and sometimes a mast negotiated. X-ray capability is not available in the field, so the medical officer must rely on physical exams to suspect a fracture. The author, wearing a canvas helmet is standing directly under wife at the top of the mast with a toolkit of heavy falling objects. Not good engineering by the medical officer.

Once again, pain relief and gentle continuous traction are the mainstays of reducing fractures. An opiate injection is the most effective way to reduce pain, allowing the victim to relax. Fractures are more difficult to manage in an uncooperative pain-filled patient. Other ways to reduce pain at the fracture site are to inject 2-5 cc of local anesthesia (lidocaine) into the swelling around the fracture and the application of ice with elevation. After the victim has been made as comfortable as possible, gentle prolonged traction should be applied. In the wrist, this can be done with the previously discussed suspended bucket or by comfortably anchoring the arm at the elbow while pulling the hand directly away with manual traction (if medical officer strong enough). Ace wraps and padding can be used to strap the elbow and upper arm to the victim's body. In wrist fractures where arteries and nerves are intact, ice splint and elevate, leave reduction for an expert if possible. The function of the wrist and hand are important, so important that injuries to this component of the orthopedic system, they deserve special exam and management.

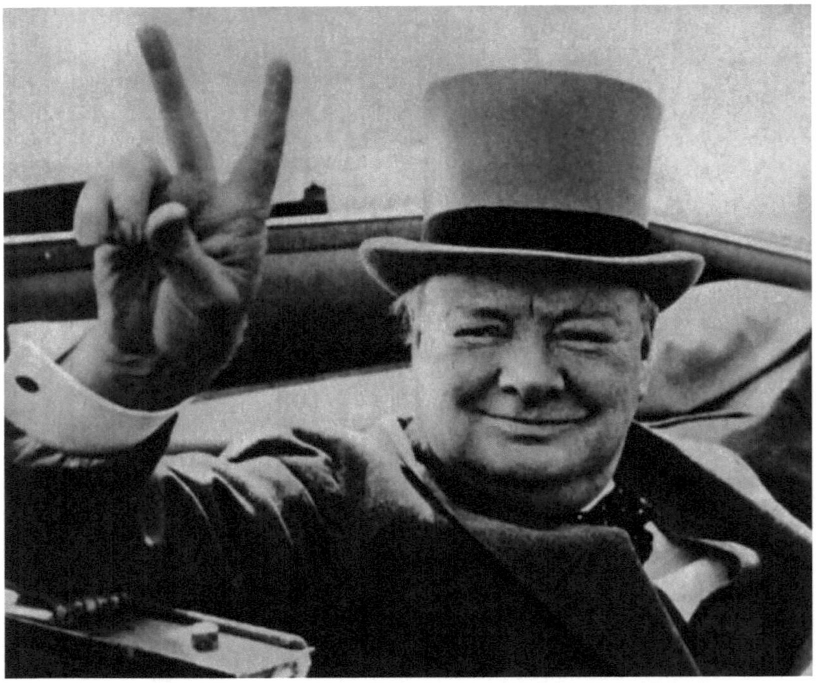

Winston Churchill with his classic "V" for victory sign is possible because all three major motor nerves in his right hand are functional. Churchill overcame a reputation as a poor student, struggling with Greek, Latin and higher mathematics in college. He overcame his early failures to become the First Lord of the British Admiralty at age 36 (youngest by decades) where he was responsible for building the modern Royal Navy, founding the Royal Air Force, designed and pushed for the first produced tanks in the world, survived three major airplane crashes after learning to fly late in life and experienced combat on three continents. An overweight smoker and daily drinker, Churchill was mentally and physically active into his eighties, nullifying the lifestyle medicine recommends. National Archives

The nerve function in the hand can be measured several ways. Pricking the skin gently with a sharp needle and slight brushing with cotton, tests sensory nerves' ability to detect the difference between sharp and soft touch. The most important hand nerves are ones that move muscles (motor nerves). A simple test to confirm motor nerve function in wrist fractures is the ability to form a "V" sign or "peace" sign. If the index and middle finger can be spread while the thumb and little finger are brought together, the three motor nerves, radial, medial and ulnar nerves of the hand are intact.

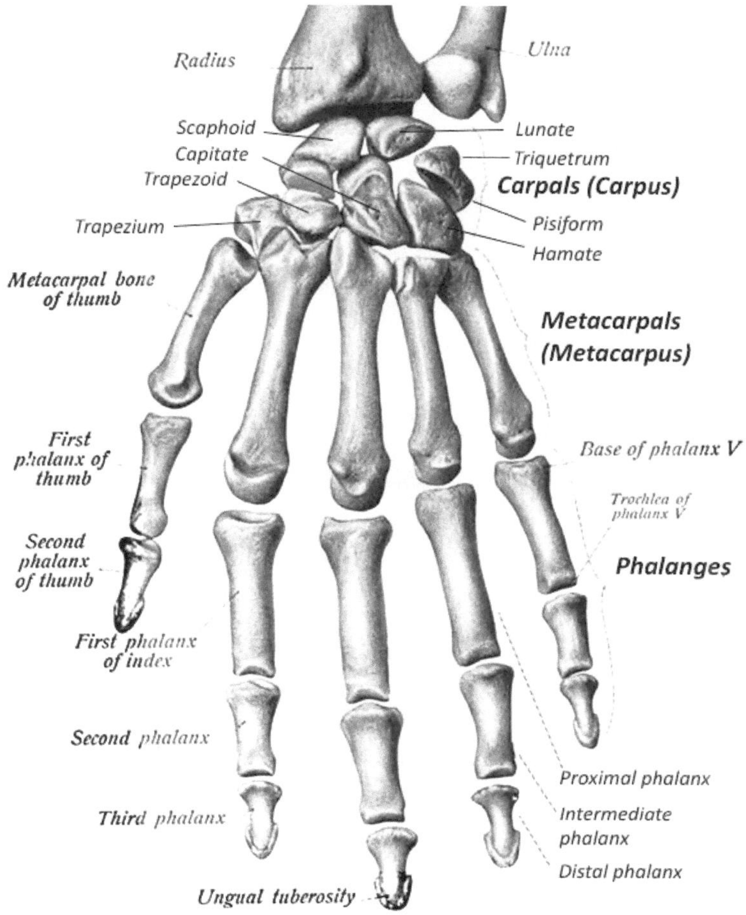

The human hand is so complicated, the author believes it makes the space shuttle look like a stone-age axe. Injuries to the hand demand prompt exam and treatment to prevent long-term disability. Large parts of the brain are dedicated to the hand, and care of hand injuries is an important part of field medicine. NIH

Once again, pain relief and gentle continuous traction are the mainstays of reducing fractures in the wrist, hand, ankle and foot. In the field, ketamine is currently the most common form of pain relief in fracture reduction. If ketamine is not available, narcotic injections have been effective in allowing the victim to relax during fracture management. Opiates such as morphine have been used in fracture management since the American Civil War since just before the war, morphine had been isolated from opium and the hypodermic (below skin) needle was invented. For the first time in field medicine, pain could be treated effectively, however morphine was dangerous if used improperly and habit forming if used too long. “The Soldiers’ Disease”, a new disease emerged following the Civil War, as thousands of wounded veterans came home addicted. Thousands more soldiers became addicted to morphine following France’s war with Prussia, 1870-71

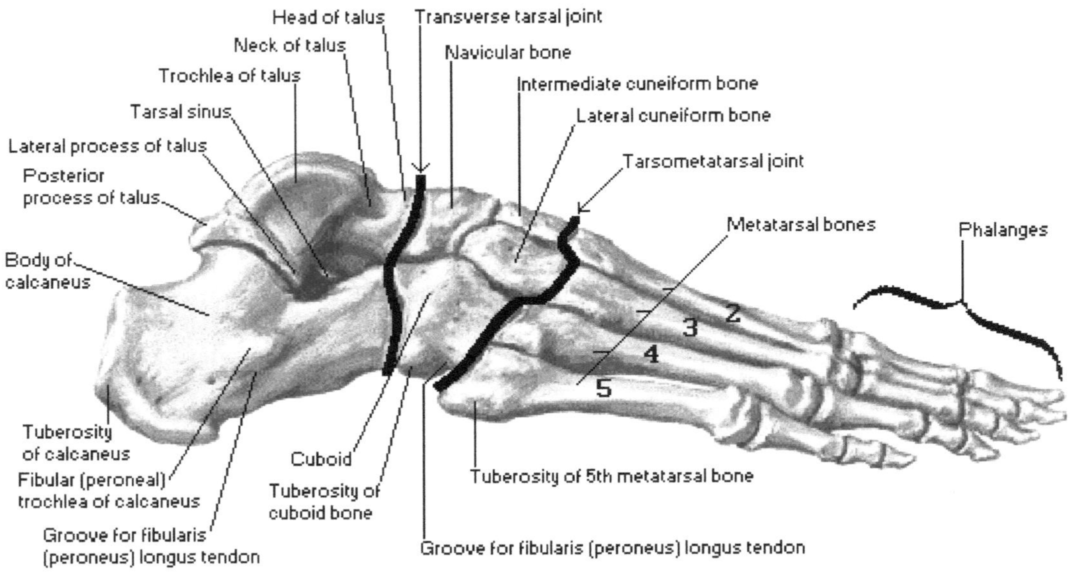

The basic function of the human foot is to bear weight. The structure strongly resembles the hand; however, the function is very different. It is a complicated and durable piece of engineering with injuries and diseases unique enough to demand its own surgical specialty, Podiatry. Proprioceptors within every joint, feeds the brain constantly with information of the joint's position, weight distribution and pressure, allowing humans to walk, climb stairs, dance. Without these receptors, the brain would be walking blind. NIH

Marching has played a huge role in history and marching requires protecting feet. As important as footwear was throughout history, shoes and boots were not manufactured in large amounts nor in multiple sizes until a Union quartermaster developed mass production of boots for the infantry in the American Civil War. General Montgomery Meigs, a graduate of both the University of Pennsylvania and West Point as an engineer, personally assured the Northern armies of Grant and Sherman were well supplied with boots. Meigs' role as quartermaster played a huge role in the success of the Union troops who had food, shelter, ammunition, medical supplies and well-fitting boots. The Confederacy relied on individual footwear suppliers who deliberately manufactured smaller sizes which used less leather and therefore greater profit. Criminal profiteering was common on both sides and was especially painful to the Southern soldiers that marched on bare and bleeding feet to many battles because boots were too small to be worn. One cannot underestimate the value of footwear in infantry. An example was the ill-fitting boots adverse effect on the British infantry early in The Great War (it was not until World War II that The Great War appeared in print renamed as World War I.

When Germany invaded Belgium in August of 1914, Great Britain sent a small Expeditionary Force to the Continent consisting of two under sized Infantry Corps and a Cavalry Division. Most of the men were plucked from civilian life and supplied with new boots among other gear and immediately begin to fight and march. After confronting two German armies of almost one million men, the 110,000 British soldiers begin a hasty retreat down 2,000-year-old Roman stone roads, many barefoot in their new unbroken-in and ill-fitting boots. The lack of proper footwear has cost other armies marching on Roman roads that traversed much of Western Europe. Fighting first at Mons and 200 marching miles later at the river Marne, the sore-footed infantry fought the longest fighting retreat in British history. In just over a week fighting every day, the English infantry with little artillery and almost no automatic weapons, British soldiers armed only with their bolt-action Lee-Enfield rifles fired accurately and rapidly thanks to lessons learned painfully in the Boer Wars. Even though greatly outnumbered in South Africa, the Dutch Boers were successful against the invading English due the accurate fire of the German Mausers carried by farmers and ranchers as 90% of gunshots were headshots. English infantry tactics relied on mass effect of rifles and not accuracy with each shot since before fighting the Boers, they had been fighting small wars against poorly disciplined enemies, some armed with spears and bows. In the early 19th century, the British soldiers trained extensively on accurate firing after the conflict in South Africa. During retreat in 1914, when the British infantry, when the English did turn and fight, many with boots tied to their packs, their fire was so rapid and deadly, the Germans believed it was from machine guns. The British also learned the value of forward medical care in the Boer Wars, where medical officers near the front could triage and return wounded to the fight. Because of this and the bravery of British officers and men, the small British army was able to delay a much larger force playing a large role in saving France.

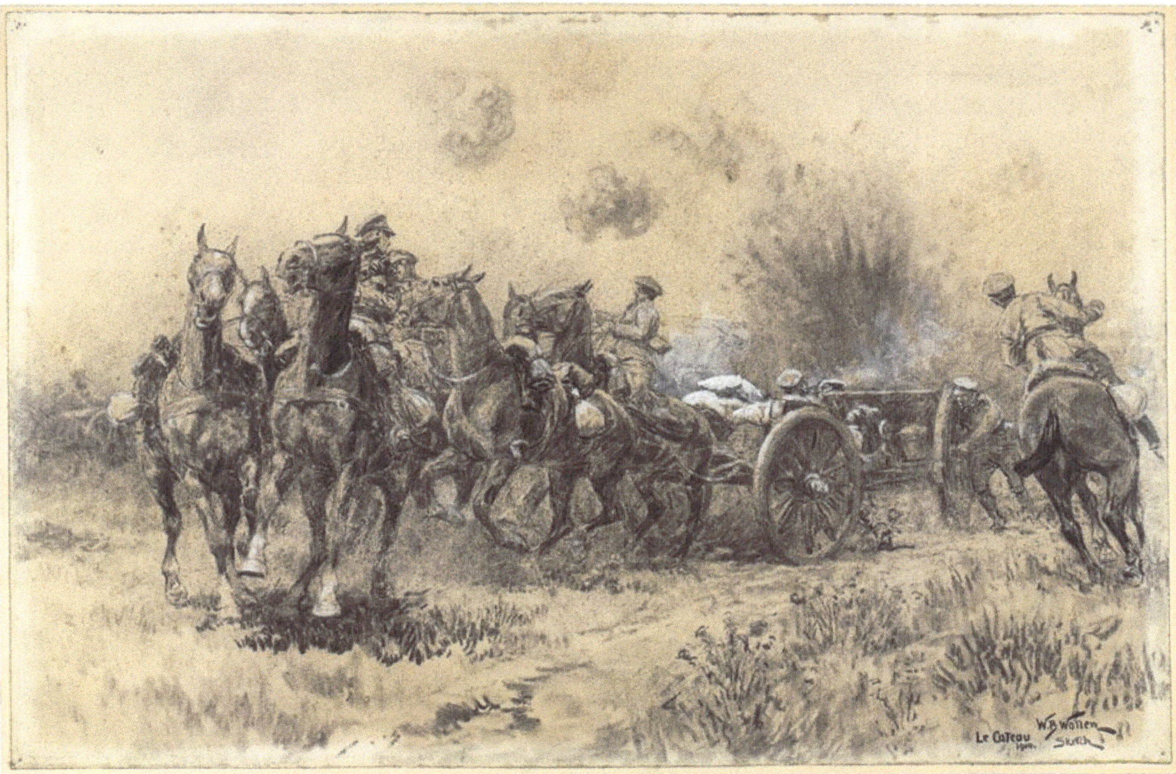

"Saving the guns" charcoal by William B. Wollen at Battle of La Cateau where two Victoria Crosses were awarded for saving some of the artillery although the loss of 36 cannons was the most since the Napoleonic Wars 100 years earlier.

Fractures splinting

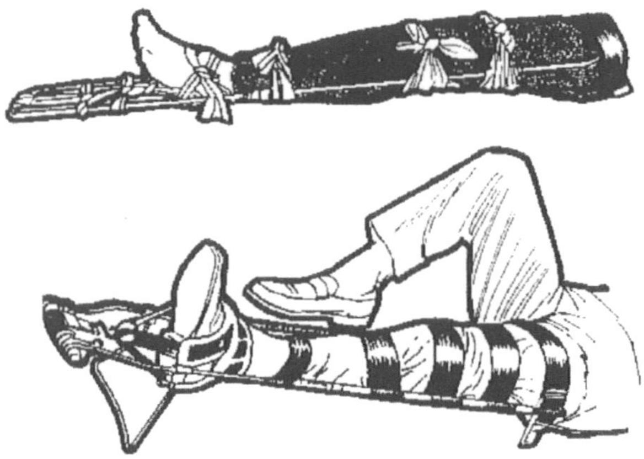

Temporary splints that can be fabricated in the field. USPH

In a suspected fractured femur, it is paramount that the leg be immobilized as soon as possible since motion of a fractured femur could damage nerves and arteries. The above simple yet effective splints should be employed prior to moving the victim. Once the victim has been transported, smaller, better-fitting splints can be placed for long-term care. Immobilization of injuries to the musculoskeletal system is paramount to reducing short and long-term complications and disability. When vascular and nerve function intact, treat conservatively with as little manipulation of the injury as possible. Limiting motion, ice to reduce swelling and pain relief are the mainstays of orthopedic injuries.

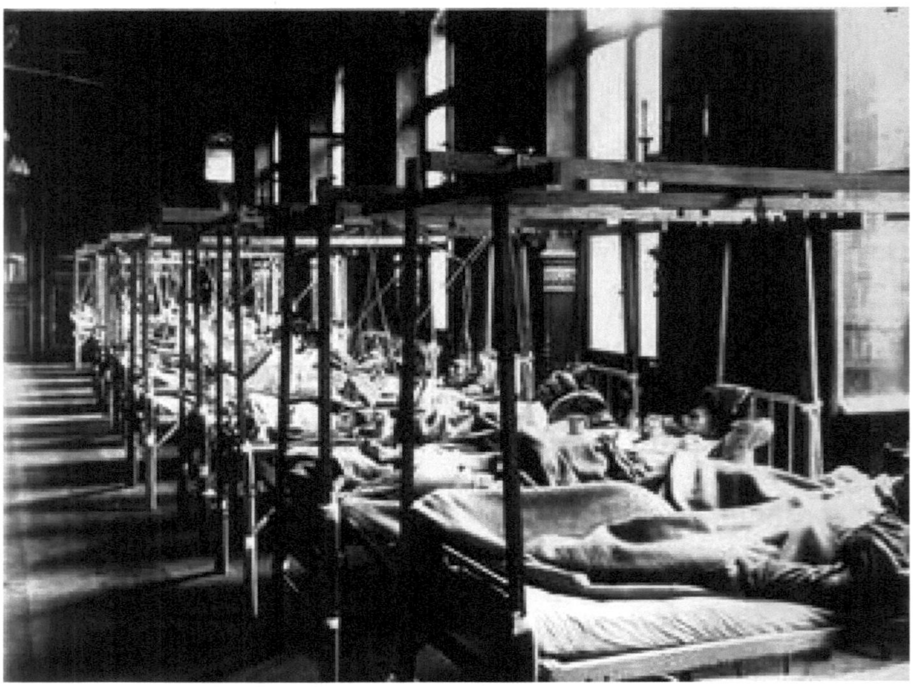

Fractures of the femur (the largest human bone) were so common in World War I entire wards contained rows of men with traction while the musculoskeletal recovered. NWM

Compartment Syndrome

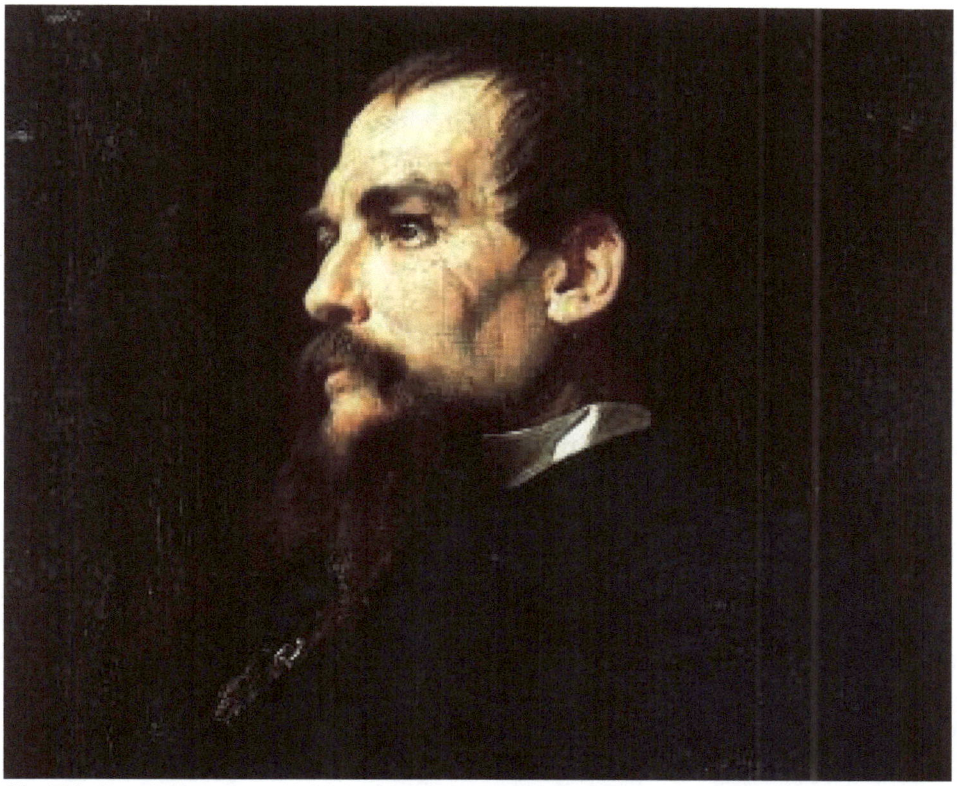

Captain Sir Richard Burton (1821 -1890) was one of the most fascinating figures of the 19th century at least to this author. Soldier, medical officer, spy, scholar, explorer, linguist, a man of incredible courage and endurance. Imagine James Bond with a sword and a story. The scar on his left cheek was the result of an African spear thrust completely through his face in a night ambush. Once, while crossing an equatorial lava field, he developed compartment syndromes in both lower legs, requiring him to take his own hunting knife (every good medical officer always carries a knife) and make multiple vertical lacerations in both lower legs. Without this reduction of compartment pressure, he would have lost both legs and likely his life. At his death, the undertaker found hundreds of healed scars over much of his body, wounds a grim testament to a life fraught with violent dangers. He served Her Majesty's government in India, Egypt, Africa, the Holy Lands and in both South and North America in the tumulus antebellum on the brink of civil war. Burton travelled the United States by train and horse just prior to the American Civil War, likely as a Queen Victoria's personal spy assessing the coming American war. Since textiles were a major part of British industry, textiles solely dependent on Southern cotton. He translated the "Kama Sutra" and "Arabian Nights.", visited Mecca disguised as an Islamic physician, only the second Englishman to do so. He traveled and wrote extensively, was fluent in twenty-six languages, forty if dialects counted. Even though he considered himself a competent physician, he often travelled with a personal medical officer later in life. Burton wrote and published over 50 books, most unpublished work complies in his later life were burned soon after his death by his prudish and vindictive widow, Isabel. Painting by John Cruikshank, National Portrait Gallery

Compartment syndrome is a serious complication of trauma to extremities and has cost many a sailor and soldier an amputated extremity and death. In compartment syndrome, swelling (edema) and or bleeding increases the volume of fluid in the tissue around a fracture, infection or crush injury. Swelling increases hydrostatic pressure within compartments of soft muscle tissue containing nerves and arteries. Do not underestimate the power of water pressure as the hydrostatic pressure within a plant seed can push through asphalt. Layers of tough sheets of connective tissue enclose bundles of muscles into compartments and water pressure can assert enough pressure to destroy tissue. In the arms and legs, these are long capsules with little elasticity. As pressure increases, so does pain. Loss of pulses, cooling and paleness of extremity is highly suggestive of compartment syndrome.

Compartment syndrome is a mechanical injury and medical emergency. It is a hydraulic pressure injury; just as increased intracranial pressure compresses the soft brain and glaucoma compresses the internal eye. As in the life-threatening closed head injury, pressure in the compartment may require mechanical released by opening. The author helped perform a compartment release on a burn victim's chest. The pressure was so great in compressing the muscle compartment of the rib cage, the lungs were unable to expand. Repeated deep slashes over the patient's anterior chest were needed to allow the chest wall to expand again. In the field, this is not to be done without a firm diagnosis and some aggressiveness. Crush injuries to the forearm and lower leg are the most common sites for compression syndrome and these injuries require a more careful examination. In fractures involving compartments, strangulating compression may occur initially or be delayed for several hours. The injured should be instructed to report any sudden increase in pain, pressure, loss of skin color or loss of sensation. The development of pain, numbness, tingling, loss of pink color in nail beds, paleness, cold skin (indicating loss of blood flow), paralysis (poor sign) or any sudden change in the sensations around the injured area should alert the medical officer to the possibility of a compartment syndrome.

Orthopedic injuries are common in the field because the musculoskeletal system is a large target for trauma and fortunately few injuries are serious, even a slight injury can lead to disability. Disabilities, especially on a boat where the need to move about quickly can be required. The author as a submarine medical officer removed crew from the sub if they were unable to climb due to an ankle sprain requiring a restrictive splint. All extremity injuries require an exam after injury to check for function, stability, pain with movement, blood flow past the site and disruption of skin over possible fracture site, immobilization and pain relief are the mainstays of orthopedic injuries.

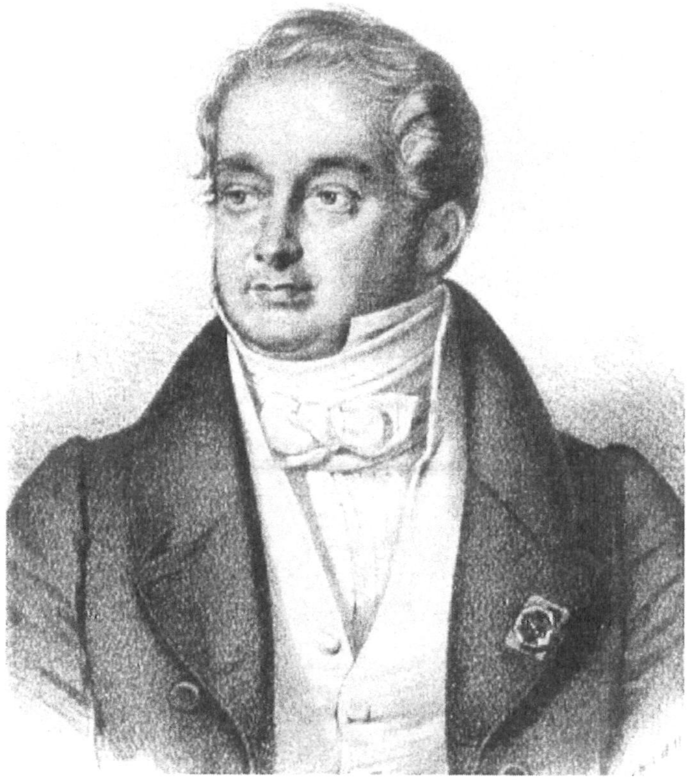

Guillaume Dupuytren (1777-1835) was one of Napoleon's most experienced medical officers and recognized as one of the first European orthopedic surgeons. He was born in poverty unlike most physicians of pre-Revolutionary France and rose to be the most successful surgeon in France, with some 20,000 patients, dying a millionaire and Baron. He developed new orthopedic surgery techniques, and wrote books on war injuries, diseases of the bones and joints. A common contraction ailment of the hands, known today as Dupuytren's Contracture, was treated by surgical release of the contractures by this remarkable surgeon, pathologist and teacher. Unfortunately, he was also cold, unscrupulous and to many, a brigand. He was called "first among surgeons and the least among men" and regarded as nobody's friend. He drew students from all over Europe and was given a prince's welcome when visiting other countries. Illustration from Garrison's Medical History

Arthritis
inflammation of joint

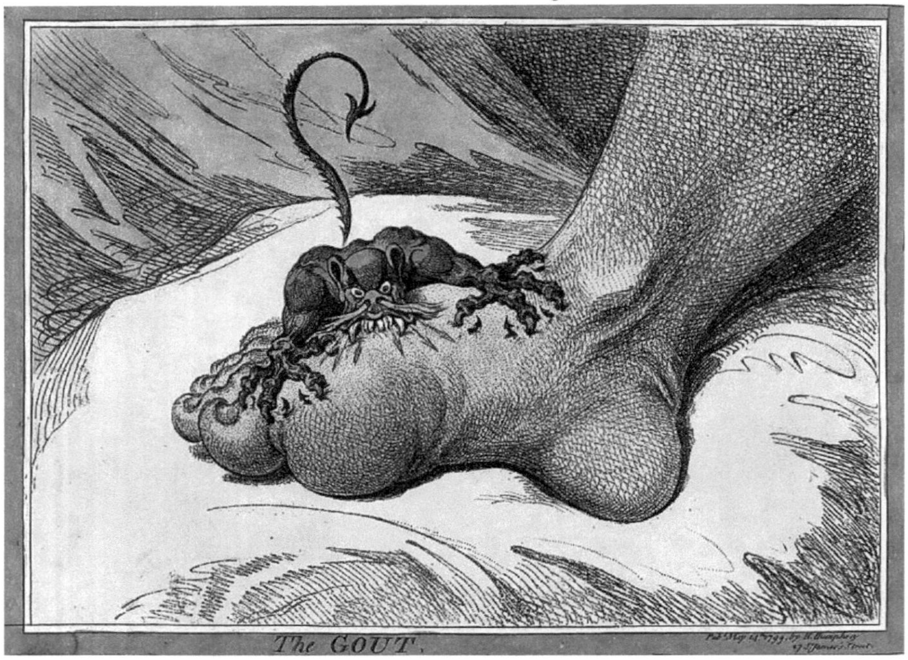

James Gillray (1756-1815) graphic illustration of the painful effects of gout painted in 1799, possibly during an episode of his own gouty arthritis. In the past, only wealthy males suffered gouty arthritis, while now the disease has spread to women and the general population. It often accompanies central body fat, hypertension and type II diabetes. Elevated serum uric acid levels and joint pain are diagnostic for the disease.

There are many causes of joint inflammation, including trauma, osteoarthritis, infection, autoimmune disorders, and gout. Injuries are self-evident and have been discussed earlier. Autoimmune disorders include Rheumatoid arthritis (RA) Systemic Lupus Erythematosus, psoriatic arthritis cause joint pain, swelling and redness and are not discussed in this text. Gout, medieval Latin for *gutta*, meaning "drop", as the disease was believed to be from matter dropping into feet is a common cause of arthritis, primarily involving the great toe, thumb, knees and elbows.

Gouty arthritis has traditionally been more common in males, causing a tender, swollen, red and "hot" joint. It displays the signs of infection, i.e., pain, redness, swelling and heat, however, there is no fever, no red streak, and no wound. Treatment is limited once the joint is inflamed, and consist of fluids, pain meds, elevation of extremity, limited weight bearing, and cherry juice. Colchicine has been used for centuries and is still effective in reducing complaints. "Tincture of time" and restricting purines from diet are the ultimate management. Meats, especially soft body parts such as liver, sweetbreads, animal fats, diary, crustaceans such as shrimp and lobster are high in purines.

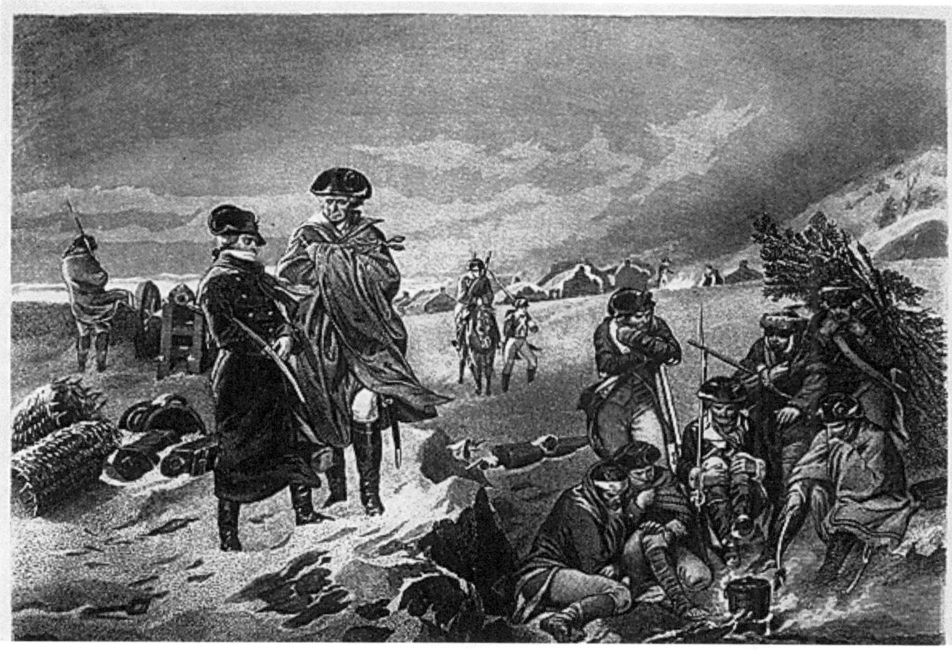

Washington and Lafayette pictured during the bitter winter of Valley Forge, 1777-1778, the nadir of the American Revolution. The twenty-year old Marquis Lafayette was short on military experience but very long on financial assets as he was one of the wealthiest men in France. Thirteen colonies in North America had challenged the greatest military power in the world for their independence even though only one-third of the population supported independence from England. The Americans did have the tenacity of George Washington, the accuracy and range of the rifled musket, French money, the wide and stormy North Atlantic Ocean separating the colonies from Great Britain and unknown to them, an ally in the purine, uric acid. The disease of gout, an abnormal accumulation of uric acid played a larger role in starting and winning or losing the American Revolution depending on one's perspective than any single battle. Engraving by H B Hall

King George III had a malignant form of inherited gout (porphyria), causing uric acid crystals to form, not just in his joints but in his brain, resulting in terrible headaches, some lasting for weeks. During these periods of severe headaches, the pain was so severe to render behavior bordering on insanity. Behind his back, he was nicknamed "crazy" King George by members of his court, the "Mad King" by others. King George's gout was no laughing matter to the British leaders and to the history of the American Revolution. In the years just preceding the outbreak of the War of American Independence, the King's temporary insanity worsened, affecting his ability to make intelligent decisions. Also, during this same time, England's Prime minster, William Pitt the Senior, was suffering severe exacerbations of his chronic gout. Pitt's symptoms became so incapacitating, it prevented him from carrying on duties as Prime Minister, forcing retirement to his country estate and away from decision making in the government. This pleased King George and his secretary for the American colonies, Lord Germain, as they cared little for the Prime Minster, especially his defense of the American colonies and his voice for the common people. Pitt was a staunch supporter of the Americans and strongly believed that it was not in England's interest to saddle them with new taxes, forcing occupying soldiers into their homes for lodging, and the suppression of American trade. Due to Pitt's medical disability, he was replaced by the arrogant and hostile to America, Lord North as Prime Minister. North, the Earl of Guilford convinced the ailing King George to ignore the requests of the American colonies and to suppress them with force.

Lord North had experience in suppressing the rebellious Irish, who had sticks and stones, but the Americans had rifled muskets! The Irish Sea separating England from Ireland is tiny compared to the Atlantic Ocean separating England from North America. North believed England was too powerful after defeating the French, Spanish and Dutch in The Seven Years War for any European power to help the Colonies, leaving them isolated and vulnerable. A mistake by North and his King because England had made powerful enemies eager to help the Americans. King George in his miserable gouty condition did not appreciate the differences between Ireland and America, sided with North and chose force. Pitt had made England the most powerful world power, and King George under North's influence squandered much of that power prosecuting an unwinnable war against the colonies. Many considered the Viet Nam War and the wars in the Middle East also unwinnable for reasons not associated with gout.

The war in America was unpopular in England and others besides William Pitt were opposed to this expensive and far away enterprise. The King had difficulty getting generals and admirals to show enthusiasm, while not enough common men signed on for the overseas venture requiring the Crown to heavily rely on expensive mercenaries, especially Hessians. Voyages to America took weeks and sometimes months of risky sea travel, fraught with storms and diseases. Perhaps a third of the soldiers leaving England landed in the colonies either dead or too ill to take up arms. The final player of this ménage de trois story of the historical significance of uric acid was Admiral George Brydes Rodney. Like King George and Pitt, England's premier fighting admiral was also suffering severe gout in the first years of the war. His gouty arthritis made him too disabled for sea duty and he was enduring self-confined house arrest in France for gambling debts. The American War caught England at her nadir in naval power while France navy without a whiff of gout, was at its zenith.

Cornwallis surrendered the British Army at Yorktown to Washington's small army augmented by French officers and soldiers because the French fleet blocked the Chesapeake Bay denying relief from the smaller British fleet. The British fleet had been reduced in size at this critical time because of Rodney's health and his avarice. It seems the ailing Rodney had finally left France debt-free and in better health, leading warships west from England to bolster the British fleet supporting Cornwallis breaking the French blockade. However, instead of reinforcing the fleet, he sailed to the rich hunting grounds of the Caribbean Sea where he commenced to capture foreign unarmed shipping, seizing these prizes for profit while indulging in rich food and drink, bringing on renewed attacks of gouty arthritis. Feeling too ill to fight, he instead sailed east for home. The missing part of the British fleet gave the victory to France and George Washington's Continental Army. Rodney returned to England richer but with swollen tender joints and blame or credit for the success of the American War of Independence. There was a positive outcome for Great Britain in the loss of America as the incompetence, waste and poor leadership brought about changes in the British Admiralty and Army, making them better prepared to fight France and Napoleon in the late 18th and early 19th centuries. For anyone that has suffered the discomfort and disability of gout can appreciate the effects of this painful condition.

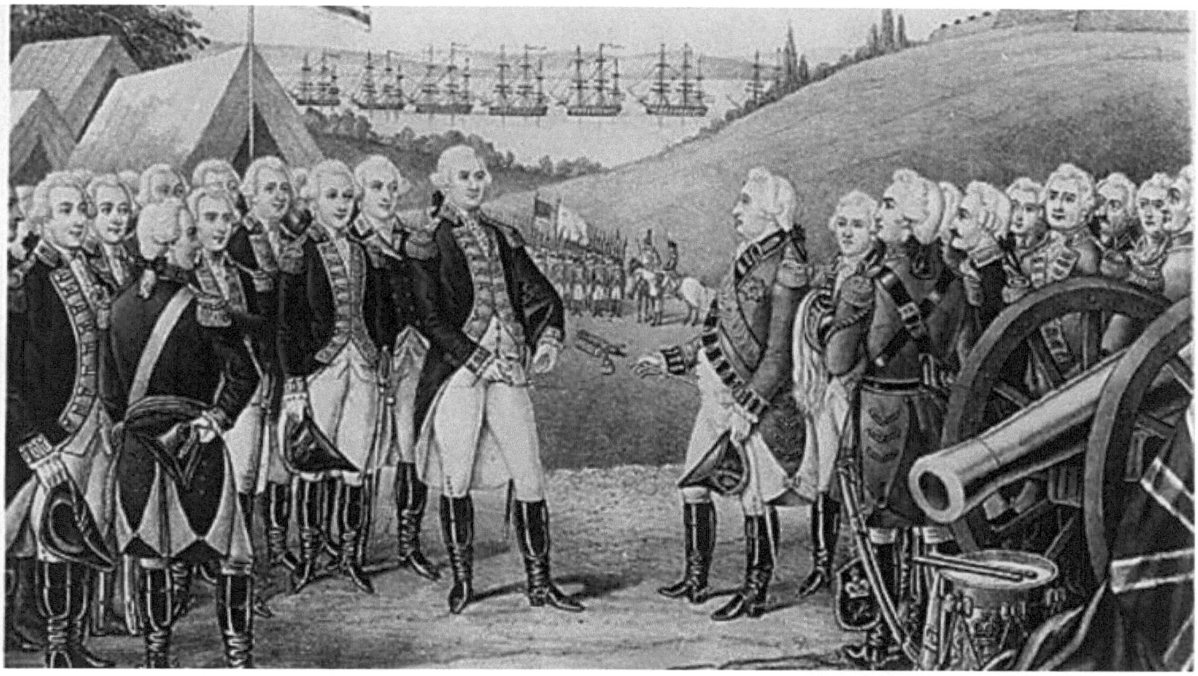

British General Cornwallis surrendering to George Washington surrounded by a large contingent of French army and French fleet in background. So much for Lord North's belief that no major European power would aid the colonies. French assistance to the young United States precipitated the French Revolution and cost the French King his head. Print by J Baillis, National Archives

Joint pain, swelling, redness and heat requires a careful exam to rule out infection versus gouty arthritis. Infections in a major joint is a medical emergency and are usually the result of a puncture wound, however in some cases, i.e., gonococcal infections can occur without direct joint injury. Therefore, any joint with the signs of infection, especially if fever present, should be treated aggressively with antibiotics! If gout suspected, fluids, cherry juice, anti-inflammatory medications such as colchicine and time are the best management.

There is a recent book where the author blames George III's mistakes on severe bipolar disorder of manic depression discounting the metabolic disorder of gout. It is true that he had mood swings but severe headaches and during his "insane" periods with the production of blue urine strongly suggests a form of severe gout. A psychologic disorder could also be present and would add to his metabolic disease. One of the history's greatest medical officers was active during the American Revolution.

John Hunter, Physician, Surgeon, Dentist and Veterinarian

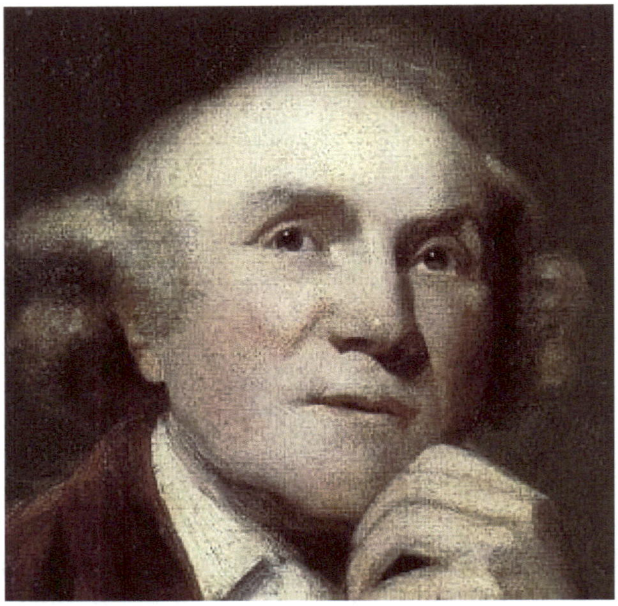

Joshua Reynolds, who painted European and American leaders of the late 18th century captured the thoughtful face of John Hunter, 1728-1793. Hunter performed the autopsy after Reynold's death finding liver cancer metastasized from the eye. Likely melanoma.

John Hunter, the most influential physician of the late 18th century, never attended formal medical training, yet revolutionized surgery and other medical arts into the following 19th century although not officially recognized as a physician during his lifetime. He was the son of a Scottish farmer as was his close friend and world explorer, James Cook. John Hunter learned medicine from a practical perspective, scorning the written word in medicine as in his opinion, the 18th century medical literature was filled with dogma. He followed and taught the scientific method of observation which became the foundation of later medical education. Hunter began his medical training by helping his older Edinburgh-educated physician brother with human anatomy classes in London and soon became an expert in procuring human cadavers. He obtained them from the gallows, fresh graves and sometime from the dark alleys and brothels of the seedier side of 18th century London. His relationships with the underside of the city became a life-long experience and his nocturnal activities may have become the facsimile for Robert Louis Stephenson's "Dr. Jekyll a Mr. Hyde". When the Thames River froze solid one winter, Hunter exclaimed it was "perfect dissection weather". Human dissection forbidden for hundreds of years was a relatively recent addition to medical education and Hunter enthusiastically pursued bodies to dissect, both human and animal. The first known human dissectors were Herophilis and Erasistradatus in 3rd century Alexandria but after them, human dissection appeared to have ceased for almost 1300 years.

Dissecting everything from dead humans to insects, Hunter became the most prolific anatomist in known history. When a dead whale appeared in the Thames River, Hunter climbed aboard the stinking beast, removing tongue, heart and tasted the fluid of the stomach contents, describing it as mildly brackish. Hunter dissected and collected thousands of animals, proclaiming a "regular and continued gradation" of animal to man. His collection of human skulls supported his belief there was no difference in the European and African skull size and shape, that Adam and Eve were negros, the world was much older than the 6200 years claimed by Church experts, there have been several great floods and life changed over time, hinting strongly of the origin of species. Concepts for which Charles Darwin who had access to Hunter's papers and illustrations while spending hours doing research in the library of The Royal Society never recognized in his book "The Origin of Species".

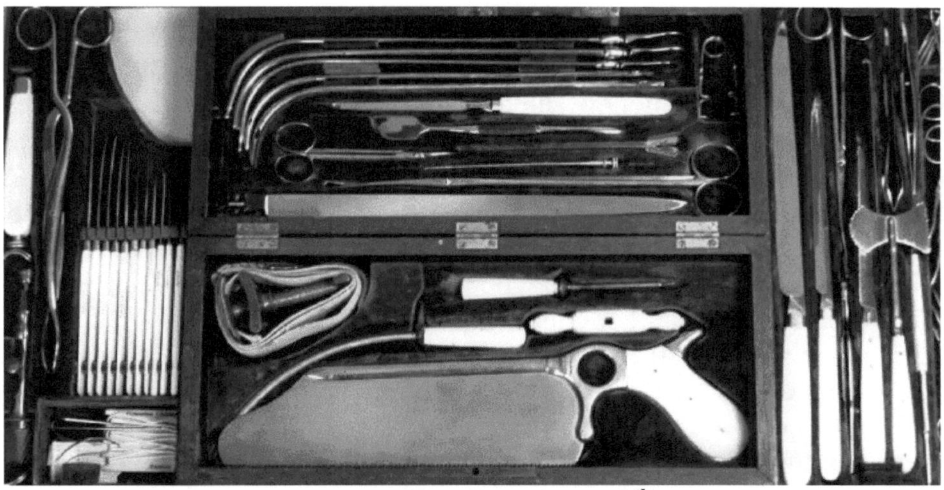

The surgeons' tools of the late 18th century

Heeding Hippocrates, "He who wishes to be a surgeon should go the war", Hunter obeyed the call to arms and joined the British army. Thomas Smollett, an acquaintance and fellow military surgeon described 18th century army camps as places where sewage overflowed from shallow pits, where dysentery, malaria, typhus, smallpox consumed troops and took eight times as many lives as battle. The healthiest troops usually won battles and the reason Islamic armies during the Middle Ages were so successful while Napoleon's victories were in part due to embracement of advanced field medicine. Field sanitation allowed the Ottoman Empire to conquer much of Europe as did the French with significantly less infectious diseases. As an army surgeon, Hunter like Ambrose Pare', recommended restraint with bleeding, amputations, not dilating bullet wounds to extract bullets, cleanliness and the realization that suppuration was evil while encouraging extra food rations for the ill and injured. Hunter's skill in in surgery and his maverick contempt for current military medicine recruited few friends in the army, especially among the army physicians who were paid more than surgeons. Hunter reported the military "physicians" could not use saw or knife were limited to bleeding and administering ineffective drugs were impediments to medical care. However, they could read and write Latin. By the war's end he was appointed to surgeon-general of the regimental hospitals while being paid less than half of army physicians. Hunter entered the army as a staff surgeon in the Seven Years War (The French and Indian War in America) and first saw action in France on Belle-Isle, the island where two of the Musketeers in Dumas's "The Man in the Iron Mask" were marooned. Hunter's competence led to jealously from the medical staff but promotion from combat officers and his competence in field medicine prompted him to be sent to Portugal in the fighting with Spain. England's 16th century treaty with Portugal permitted English troops to be positioned in the country. This treaty allowed Wellington to confront French troops in Spain and in the 20th, century allowed Allied airplanes to be stationed on Portugal's Azores Islands which ended the success of the German submarine warfare in the North Atlantic. A 400-year-old treaty (England's oldest ally) that Churchill dusted off and used to greatly reduce the sinking of Allied shipping. While not treating wounded on the Iberian Peninsula, Hunter continued scientific experiments and proved that fish could hear.

Hunter returned to England after war in 1763 at age 35 and with few prospects living solely on the paltry half pay of an army surgeon took up dentistry for income. In the 18th century, dentistry was in the hands of barbers, blacksmiths, wigmakers and travelling medicine men. Studiously applying the techniques of apprenticeship and observation, he began a new field of medicine. Sugar from the West Indies had greatly increased rates of tooth decay and the need for better dentistry was rampant. Dentistry offered the money Hunter needed and with his battlefield expertise and recommendations from respected associates apprenticed with London's premier dentist, James Spence. Spence and his sons practiced clean, effective oral surgery where Hunter learned not only extractions but filling cavities with gold and in the poor, lead, scaling (cleaning) teeth and making false teeth from ivory. Since ivory from African elephants and hippopotamus was expensive, a popular and abundant source were teeth from poor younger children (especially girls as their teeth were smaller). These children had good teeth because they could not afford sugar. Lady Emma Hamilton (Admiral Nelson's mistress) was a poor young adolescent on her way to sell her front teeth when she was talked out of the procedure. Without her front teeth, it is unlikely she would have entered history as one of the most influential women in the early 19th century. Fresh tooth transplants were common during Hunter's time but were soon abandoned because they were seldom successful in the long term and were a common cause of syphilis transmission. Hunter penned history's first textbook on dentistry, "Treatise on the Disease of Teeth", becoming a best seller enjoying 15 editions. His study of dentation as a comparative anatomist allowed him to declare the skeleton of the kangaroo brought back from Australia represented a new class of mammals.

John Hunter personally trained over 1000 physicians and surgeons, spreading his revolutionary belief that physicians must "think for themselves and only believe what is observed". His students carried his philosophy well into the 19th century around the world. Edward Jenner, the discoverer of smallpox vaccination was one of his most devoted and loved student and John Lister who brought the medical world the concept of handwashing and modern wound care considered John Hunter as his model physician. Fortunately, few of his students copied his blunt manners and contempt for those in unearned positions.

17th century Europe was rife with sexually transmitted diseases and Hunter was all over it. He needed money for the animals, both living and dead, he collected. His museum and zoo at his residence included 14,000 specimens, becoming the most complete in the world near the end of his life. His patients, both the rich and poor, came to him for his skill in treating syphilis and gonorrhea (he mistakenly believed both were the same disease). His patients included James Boswell, Giacomo Casanova, dukes, counts, ambassadors, masters and their servants, vicars and other men of the cloth. He believed syphilis crossed both placenta and breast milk, a discovery at a time when men believed sex with virgins cured the disease. In the 17th and 18th centuries, 75% of the income of physicians came from treating venereal diseases. Hunter's "A Treatise on Venereal Disease" became another best seller, recommending treatment with mercury, penis stricture dilation, abstinence and the use of Dr. Condom's invention of a sheath made of pig or goat bowel tissue secured with silk thread. The same Dr. Condom was the personal physician of George III, the "mad king". Inspection of the lady in question for signs of disease was highly recommended in his text. Sir Richard Burton, a medical officer and explorer in the mid-19th century likely owned Hunter's treatise and used candlelight to inspect his consorts before indulgence.

Hunter formed an informal lecture group that became the premier science gathering in London, at least as impressive as the "the Royal Society" ruled over by Sir Isaac Newton. Newton would not have fit with this group as it required humility and sustained abuse in the form of pranks on the members. Hunter's group included Sir Joseph Banks (botanist, British Lord, passenger on the HMS *Endeavor* and premier botanist of his day), James Cook (perhaps the greatest British explorer), James Watt (steam engine), Edward Jenner, Frederich Herschel, the royal astronomer who discovered Uranus and other luminaries. Fifteen years after beginning his practice of surgery he was finally formally accepted into the Academy of Surgeons and, like Ambrose Pare was not allowed into the realm of physicians as he could not read nor write Latin.

Hunter provided medical care for his own large animal population and often his patient's pets, prompting him to establish the first school of veterinary medicine in England. Not only did Hunter become the premier surgeon of the late 18th century, but a competent dentist and possibly the England's best veterinarian. He wanted to "sweep away all past unproven doctrines and taught his students medicine grounded in life sciences, further alienating the learned trapped in moribund Latin. In 1790 he was made Surgeon-General of the British Army although still not recognized as a physician. When war broke out with Revolutionary France, he attempted to modernize military medicine but the old guard and the Church he had antagonized blocked him. When the same people attempted to destroy his teaching method in the hospitals, he finally lost his temper and in an outburst of anger against the dogma he battled his entire professional life, dropped dead from a heart attack. He had suffered anginal attacks for years for which he took daily doses of opium and likely became addicted to the drug in his last years as was Benjamin Franklin and the great American surgeon, William Stewart Halsted. With his four hours of sleep at night, marginal eating habits, workaholic lifestyle, his heart, not Hunter, gave up the fight. Few medical officers have played a larger role in medicine.

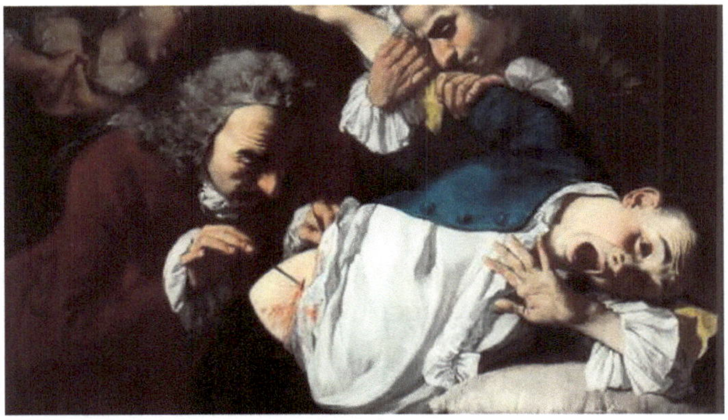

"The Operation" by Gaspare Traversi depicts John Hunter in action before general anesthesia. Opiates were often employed to dull the pain and render the patient less difficult to restrain. "The Knife Man" by Wendy Moore is an excellent study of a remarkable medical officer.

Abdominal Pain

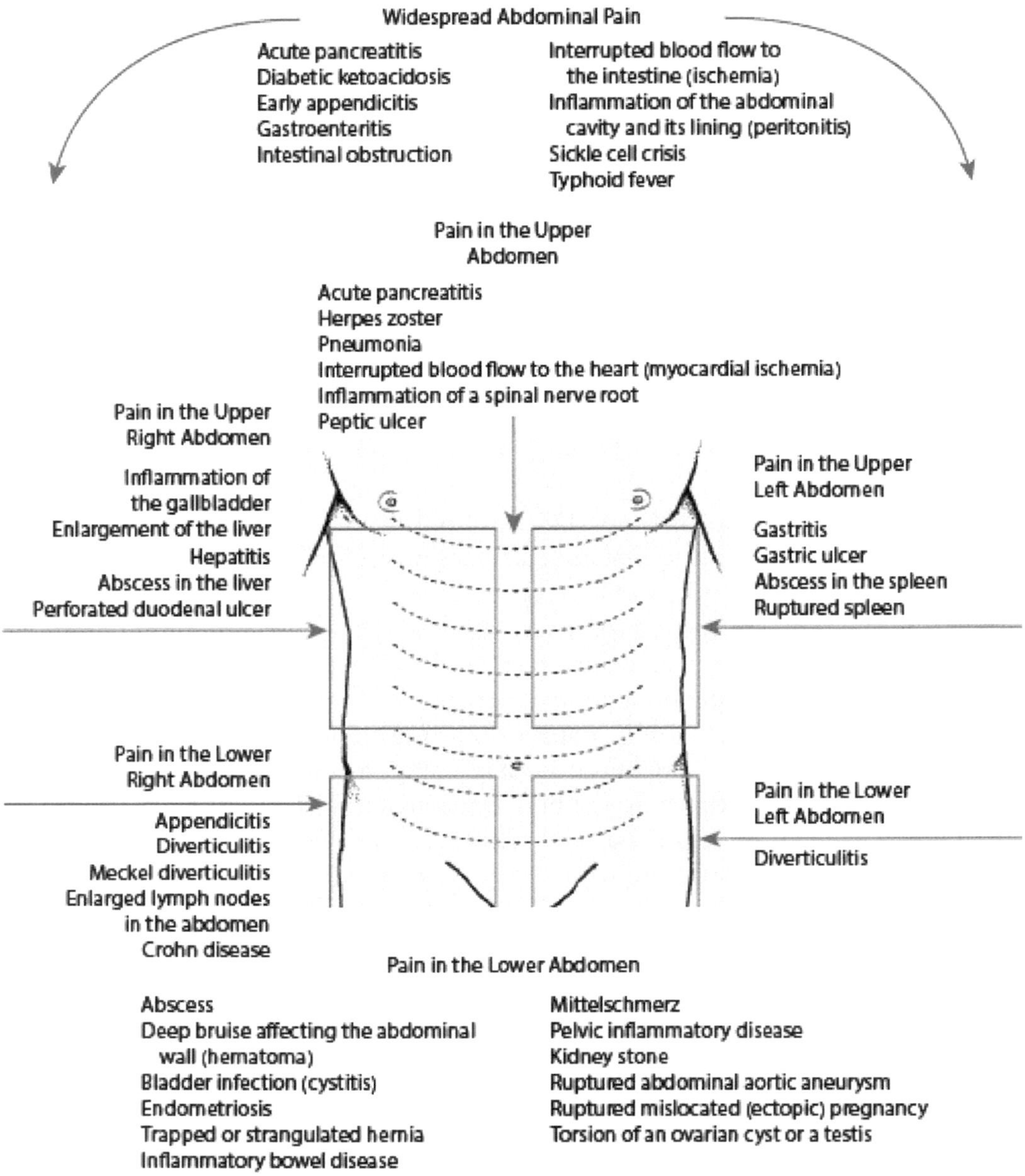

Although there are many causes of abdominal pain, most resolve with minimal treatment. Taking a good history, performing a careful physical exam, understanding anatomy of abdomen and deploying field lab tests help identify if any of the above are the problem. NLM Note: the above term of Mettelschmerz is pain with ovulation when a small amount of blood is deposited in the lower abdomen.

Among the causes of abdominal pain, fortunately only a handful are life-threatening, and in many cases, even serious causes can be effectively managed in the field. This was not true in the past, as intractable abdominal pain was managed by little more than hope and perhaps prayer that the pain would pass. The fear of abdominal pain at sea is a common concern of those who leave the safety of shore and over the years of lecturing, the author believes being able to manage abdominal pain in the field makes students more apprehensive than any other problem. To allay their anxiety, the author stresses that today a lay medical officer has access to effective drugs and diagnostic tools in the management of abdominal pain not available until recently. A proper medicine chest and an officer comfortable in using it, enhances the safety and pleasure of travel, especially in the cases of abdominal pain. Diagnosis is based on the history of pain, physical exam and lab tests. Treatment is directed by an assessment based on history and thorough exam. When abdominal pain steadily increases without relief, it is likely serious and requires vigilance.

Causes of Abdominal Pain

Sudden onset-deadly-(instantaneous)-Treat like shock

- **Perforated Ulcer-pain lower mid chest**
- **Ruptured ectopic pregnancy-lower abdominal pain**
- **Ruptured major artery (aneurysm)-crushing, no response with opiates**

Rapid onset (minutes to hours)

- **Perforated bowel**
- **Strangulated bowel**
- **Pancreatitis**
- **Ectopic pregnancy**
- **Obstructed gall bladder**
- **Appendicitis**
- **Diverticulitis**
- **Reflux/Heartburn**
- **Angina**

Gradual Onset- (hours to days)

- **Constipation-number one cause of abdominal pain**
- **Appendicitis**
- **Ulcer**
- **Inflamed gall bladder**
- **Pelvic inflammatory disease**
- **Bladder infection**

Diverticulitis

Bowel obstruction

Kidney stone

Ectopic pregnancy

The Patient's History in Abdominal Pain

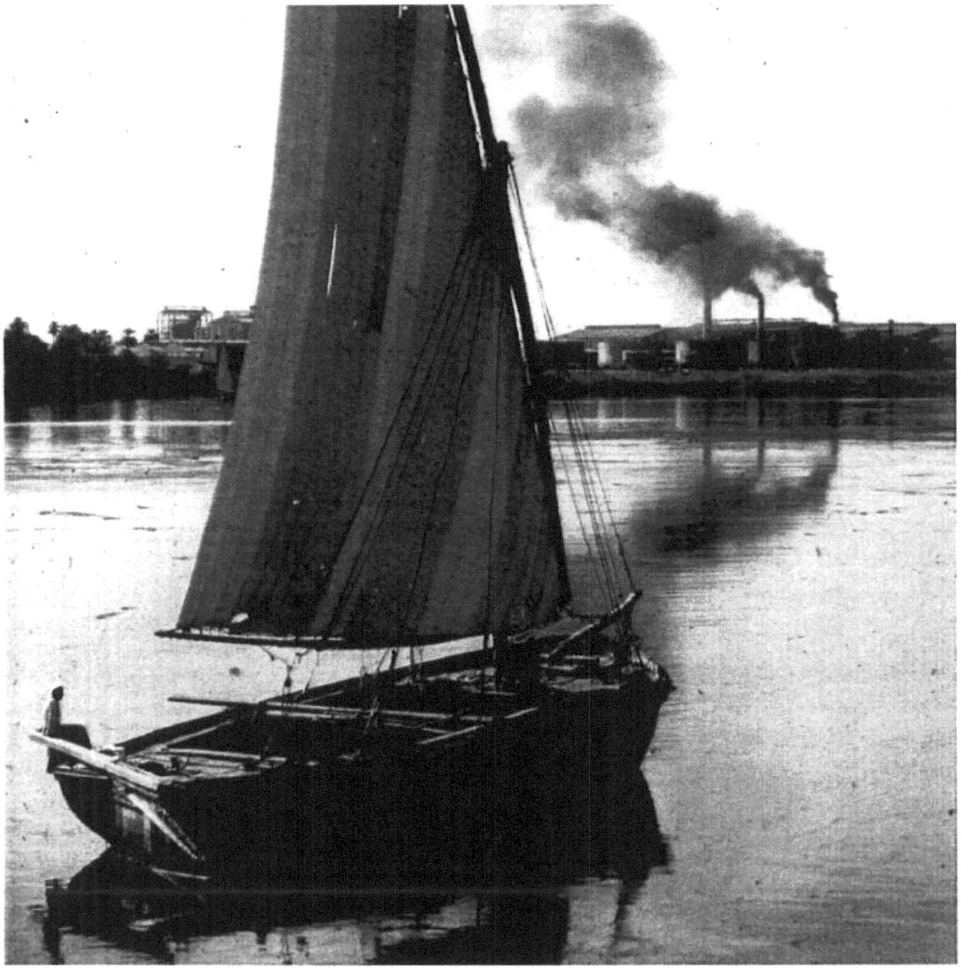

Dhows are sailing vessels with a pointed bow, deep hold and lateen sail, allowing them to sail down-wind and to weather on the Nile, Mediterranean, Red Sea and Indian Ocean while carrying large loads. Vessels like the one above have changed little over twenty-five hundred years of continuous use, just as the written descriptions of abdominal pain in the acute abdomen have changed little over the centuries. Photo by author

The medical history or the story is important when evaluating abdominal pain. A good history serves as a navigational aid just as a compass and accurate charts are helpful in plotting a course and the history is likely the most important part in deciding on action in abdominal pain. History of previous similar abdominal pain and past treatment, the pattern of the pain's onset and what aggravates or relieves the abdominal pain are very helpful. The presence of vomiting, diarrhea and fever are critical to manage while deciding on management. The history combined with exam and simple laboratory tests are major components in arriving at a plan.

Most causes of abdominal pain will resolve with simple treatment, requiring little more than resting the gut by giving clear liquids until the discomfort has passed. Viral infections, increased bowel gas, cramping, constipation, parasites, ulcers, kidney stones, bladder infections, pelvic inflammation, menstruation and a host of others can cause abdominal pain, and all are manageable in the field. The more serious causes represent a tiny fraction of abdominal pain, even though the list in this chapter is lengthy. Pain that comes on rapidly and increases in severity over a short period of time is always a concern. Fortunately, it is extremely rare. Pain that begins and steadily increases requires careful exam, thoughtful consideration of causes and early management. Even in cases of serious abdominal pain, there is usually enough time to formulate a plan that will help the patient's own body deal with the problem.

The term "**acute abdomen**" is medical slang for an abdomen harboring a serious problem. A problem, that without medical intervention may result in death. Historically in the acute abdomen, the pain continues to increase, the bowel sounds normally heard in the abdomen become quiet, the patient's condition deteriorates as fever, vomiting, delirium and finally death occurs without intervention. Stagnation is the enemy of the gut and a common cause of acute abdomen. Healthy digestive function requires constant motion towards its exit and bowel sounds are generally always present, even though faint. Medical officers are trained to listen for 30 seconds in four areas of the abdomen (quadrants) before declaring the abdomen quiet and their absence is a poor sign. To determine the presence of bowel sounds, gently place the stethoscope over a suspect abdomen as firm pressure may artificially induce gas movements creating bowel sounds as will pressing into the abdomen with hands. Therefore, listen before palpation.

There is often a history of previous similar attacks in ulcers, gallstones, diverticulitis and appendicitis, especially with chronic constipation. Ulcer-caused abdominal pain is often relieved by food, whereas gallbladder pain aggravated by eating (especially fatty foods). People with a history of abdominal surgery have an increased risk of abdominal pain caused by bowel obstruction from scar tissue resulting in strictures which can strangle the softer bowels. Normal ovulation can result in abdominal pain (Mettelschmerz). Women with an ectopic pregnancy, the "Deadly Pregnancy", generally have missed a period, experienced a small amount of vaginal bleeding (spotting), complain of painful intercourse and may have other signs of pregnancy, including morning nausea, breast tenderness and enlargement. Gallstone attacks (cholecystitis) and pancreatitis have a history of intermittent (colicky) pain associated with fatty food intake. Colicky abdominal pain is pain that slowly increases and then resolves for a brief period before returning.

Abdominal pain can at times be sudden, as in a rupture of some hollow organ or cyst. However, abdominal pain usually follows a slow, more deliberate course of several hours, as is the case in appendicitis, cholecystitis, peritonitis, intestinal obstruction, diverticulitis and acute pelvic inflammatory disease. With pancreatitis and the ectopic pregnancy, there can be sudden flushes of irritating fluids leaking into the nerve-rich peritoneal cavity (peritonitis) resulting is sudden severe pain. Peritonitis usually develops steadily over hours, relentlessly becoming more painful without the intermittent easing of pain associated with the other causes of abdominal pain.

Abdominal pain that follows a course of steadily increasing without abating is always serious and should be managed with all available resources!

Appendicitis

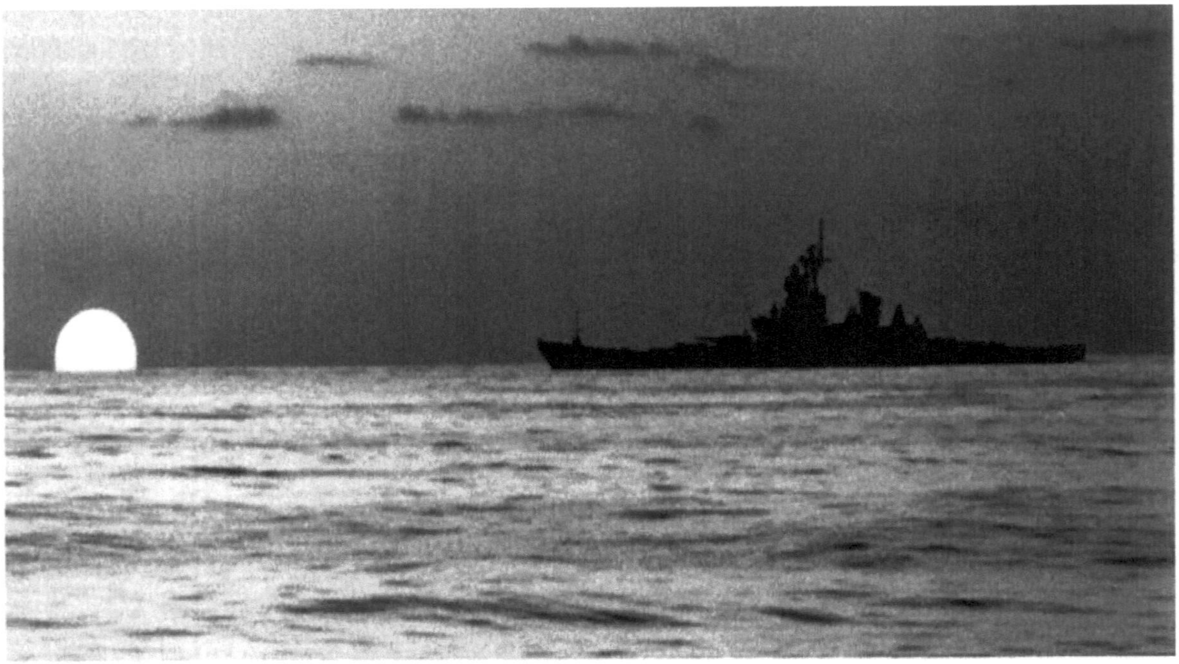

The USS Missouri on station in the Indian Ocean during Operation Desert Storm, 1992. Her decks witnessed, Kamikaze attacks at Okinawa, the Japanese surrender in 1945 and with upgrades, has served intermittently from the Second World War into the 1990s. Her sixteen-inch guns fired accurately for twenty miles, and she is home for thousands. Battleships carry a full complement of medical staff with medical officers trained in chest, abdominal and trauma surgery, an anesthesia department, nurses, the works. Resources are seldom available in the field. A battleship carries the staff and equipment to diagnosis and treat abdominal pain at sea. Fortunately, even a small vessel can do some of what the larger battleship can, short of surgery. By knowing the structures underlying the pain, obtaining a history of the pain and doing some simple shipboard lab test, a field medical officer can diagnosis and successfully treat almost all causes of abdominal pain at sea. Photo by Lt. Joe Cobb

All medical officers will see appendicitis, since it is not rare. The incidence of appendicitis is higher at sea, especially for neophytes. In the Soviet Submarine Corps, the incidence is as high as one in ten as new sailors are taken from land to sea for the first time without acclimation, exposed to new diet and wave motion experience increase risk of stagnation within the gut. Vomiting, lethargy, and reduced fluid intake can lead to constipation and reduced hydration. Appendicitis is often preceded by constipation, as over-firm stool blocks the normally free-flowing appendix. Most cases of appendicitis in the United States are managed with surgical removal. However, in many countries and in the field, it is managed with early antibiotics, fluids and resting the gut. Since any abdominal pain with a fever could be appendicitis, the author recommends giving antibiotics early in abdominal pain when accompanied by fever. Robin Graham, the skipper of the vessel *Dove* was the youngest person to sail solo around the world at age 16, nearly died of appendicitis while sailing in the South Pacific with his parents prior to his solo circumnavigation. His appendix ruptured just before getting to a hospital in Tahiti, and even though he received surgical treatment, it was nearly fatal. A simple course of oral antibiotics early in his disease probably would not have placed him so close to death.

Among the causes of life-threatening abdominal pain, appendicitis is common and therefore, knowledge of how appendicitis reveals its possible deadly course is an important part of this text. The pattern of pain can be unpredictable, especially in young children or the elderly. Fortunately, in most cases, it follows a charted course, a story that begins like a fairy tale; "In the beginning" the pain is mild and centered around the umbilicus. Nausea, mild fever, diarrhea or constipation and loss of appetite are also classic early symptoms. The first stage of symptoms could mimic many other problems, such as the common stomach flu. However, if the vessel has been to sea for several weeks, flu is unlikely since its spread requires contact with new people.

In the second stage of appendicitis, the pain shifts to the right lower abdominal quadrant, an area known historically as McBurney's spot, halfway between the umbilicus and the upper right groin. The site likely overlying the appendix. Abdominal pain that follows this pattern over several hours is all but diagnostic for appendicitis, since imitation of this course of symptoms by other conditions is rare. The finding of rebound pain confirms the diagnosis, as rebound is associated with an acute abdomen. Rebound is an historical physical finding revealed by the sudden release of hand pressure, after slowly pressing into area of pain. Increased pain when pressure withdrawn is caused by the abdominal wall "rebounding" and sending waves of motion through the inflamed peritoneum. At first the pain is cramp-like and intermittent, later in the third stage becoming constant, steadily and cruelly increasing until the sudden or prolonged emergence of even more severe abdominal pain, heralding rupture of the hollow swollen appendix.

At the time of surgery, infected appendixes appear an angry, red, foul-smelling clump of tissue, swarming with bacteria. As the walls of the appendix begin to breakdown, bacteria and inflammatory fluids leak from the stricken stagnant organ causing peritonitis, the fourth stage. The subsequent flooding of the sterile peritoneal cavity with colon bacteria from a leaking appendix (ruptured) was universally fatal until the development of anesthesia, modern surgery and finally antibiotics.

Antibiotics, fluids and bowel rest are the foundations for management of abdominal pain and fever in the field. In the early stages of appendicitis almost any antibiotic should be effective, but the emergence of rebound should increase apprehension and prompt the use of stronger antibiotics including an injection. Few should perish from appendicitis in the field, as treatment is simple when deployed early. Even though the urine test will not diagnosis appendicitis, it is a good plan to monitor urine every few hours to ensure the person is receiving adequate hydration. A comment by a mature Naval surgeon the author remembers from surgical rounds was "in my experience, patients with appendicitis always lose two things, their appetite and their sense of humor".

Stages of Appendicitis

Stage I
abdominal discomfort around umbilicus
fever, usually low-grade around 100 degrees F (38 C)
diarrhea or constipation loss of appetite, vomiting

Stage II
abdominal pain, centering in right lower abdomen continued fever, slowly increasing, decreased bowel sounds, slight rebound

Stage III
Increasing abdominal discomfort, increased rebound, increasing fever, few if any bowel sounds

Stage IV
signs of shock, falling blood pressure, decreased alertness, perhaps delirium, elevating fever, raising to 104 degrees, rigid abdomen and extreme abdominal pain

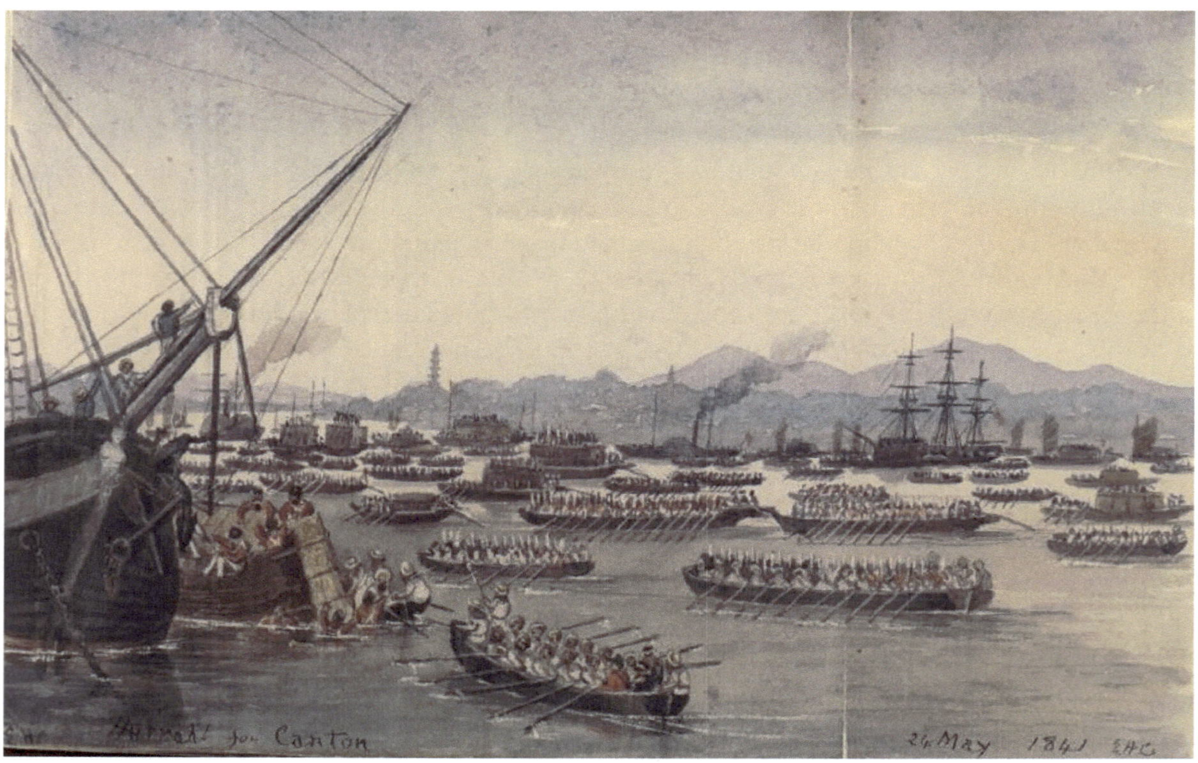

Another Dr. Cree image illustrating an amphibious assault on the Chinese during the Opium Wars. The British Navy with long range military transport could bring the Royal Army halfway around the world and attack military and commercial centers on the

Chinese coast at will. Rome built roads to move its army to project power distantly, the British used ships. In the Far East, many sailors, marines and soldiers in this theatre died of abdominal pain.

Ulcer Pain

In stomach ulcer or more commonly gastritis (inflamed stomach lining), the abdominal pain is perceived in the upper middle abdomen or low chest (above umbilicus), just under the sternum. It tends to be constant in nature, somewhat relieved by eating or antacids. The pain is often described as "boring" or "gnawing" through the chest to the back. Gastritis causes some bleeding, although the blood is so slight may be only detected by a field lab test. Even small amounts of bleeding will be detected by the stool guaiac test for occult (hidden) blood. Ulcer or inflammation pain is relieved in the short turn by opiates and in the long run by acid blockers. Nicotine significantly increases stomach acid production, while inhibiting the action of acid blockers.

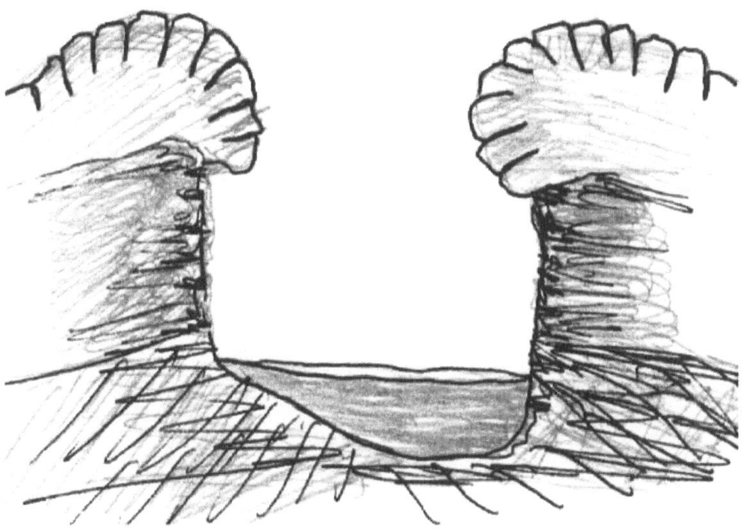

In this author's illustration showing a pool of stomach acid that has broken through the protective mucus layer, pooling in a crater. Here it has "eaten" its way down to blood vessels causing bleeding which in the beginning will be tiny amounts. If it goes undetected and untreated, it may cause significant bleeding, resulting in black stools or coffee-grounds vomit. The ulcer sometimes avoids contact with pain fibers in its corrosive trenching and bleeding can occur without much discomfort. In severe cases, an ulcer can perforate the stomach or small bowel and enter the peritoneum resulting in life-threatening peritonitis.

Ulcers are more common in the first part of the small bowel (duodenum) than in the stomach, because while the stomach's lining is suited for an acid environment, the small bowel is not. Excess acid reaching the duodenum will injure its fragile lining causing pain and bleeding. Black stools, vomiting "coffee grounds", paleness and severe bleeding, low blood pressure are signs of bleeding ulcers. Acid blockers such as Tagamet, Axid, Zantac, and in the smoker, Carafate have been replaced with the newer proton pump inhibitors (omeprazole) drugs with scientific names ending in "azole" are the mainstays in the treatment and prevention of ulcers. In the presence of black stools (melena), give vitamins with iron to replace lost blood for several weeks, restrict nicotine and alcohol while monitoring the stools for continued blood loss.

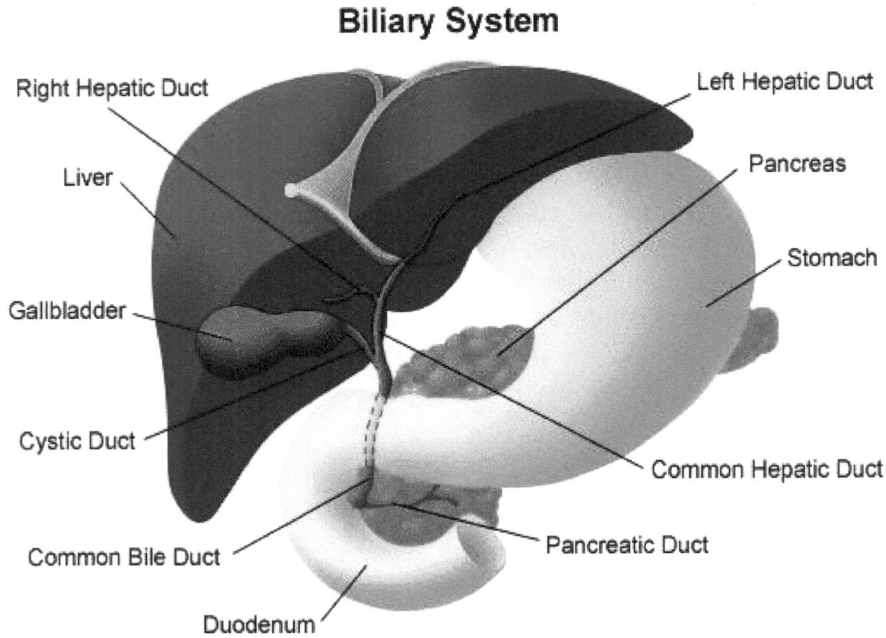

Lots of things happen when the gall bladder, pancreas and small bowel get together. NLM

Gallstone pain

When a gallstone becomes obstructed in the long slender neck of the gall bladder, the pain is intermittent (colicky) and located in the right upper quadrant of the abdomen or the lower right chest, often radiating through the deep chest to the right shoulder blade. Belching and rectal gas are common, with nausea and vomiting. It typically occurs after meals high in fat content, such as pizza, cheeseburgers, gravy, fried dishes and the like. The attack can last one to six hours, is relieved by bowel rest, fluids, anti-spasmotics and future avoidance of fatty meals. Alcohol and dehydration increase the risk of a gallbladder attack. Gallstones can cause milder symptoms such as intermittent nausea and mild abdominal discomfort after meals. Persistent nausea after meals could be caused by gallbladder disease or pancreatic disorders. Gallstones can be diagnosed with abdominal ultrasound and suspected gall bladder, or pancreatic complaints should be investigated. Gallstones can be removed by surgery or by a gallstone-dissolving drug (Actigall). Although painful, the attacks usually resolve with fluids and bowel rest. However, when fever accompanies gallstone-like pain, start antibiotics.

Most gallbladders lie silently on the underside of the liver only becoming vocal with gallstone obstruction. Large stones are of little concern as they cannot gain access to the narrow neck of the cystic duct. It is the small multiple stones that aggravate the gallbladder or worse, the pancreas. Nausea after meals is the first sign of gallbladder or pancreas disease and should be evaluated by an abdominal ultrasound if it persists. Current therapy for gallstones includes a low fat diet, possibly surgery and an ancient drug to dissolve the stones. Ox gall was found in Egyptian medicine chest 4500 years ago used for abdominal pain and Actigall, like its ancient predecessor, is made from gallbladder contents of cattle.

Pancreatitis Pain

Pancreatitis is one of the more severe causes of abdominal pain, especially when appearing suddenly and continuing with constant severe discomfort. Nausea, vomiting and pain in the left upper quadrant with radiation across to the right and through the back to the left shoulder blade are highly suggestive of pancreatitis. The severe pain is due to swelling of the obstructed pancreas and the leaking of its destructive enzymes. This is a serious condition that is sometimes fatal even with the best medical care. It is managed with bowel rest, antibiotics, fluids and narcotics for severe pain. It is commonly preceded by a period of low hydration when a large fatty meal is consumed with alcohol. Many have died over the centuries after a celebration feast. "Survive the fight, to succumb to the party". Nausea and left upper abdominal pain after meals could be due to chronic mild pancreatitis or pancreatic cancer, which can be diagnosed with an abdominal ultrasound. An orthopedic surgeon, the author worked with experienced an attack of pancreatitis when yard work on hot summer day interrupted by a cheeseburger, fries and two beers. A few hours later abdominal pain began and worsened resulting in hospitalization. He never completely recovered, had difficulty keeping on weight, chronic diarrhea and was forced to work part-time. Pancreatitis can be avoided by avoiding fatty meals, alcohol and dehydration.

Pancreatitis is almost always due to obstruction caused by stagnation, although it can be the result of abdominal trauma. It is serious and not well treated even in a modern hospital. Pancreatic juices are the body's most destructive chemicals if they escape the gut and enter other parts of the body. Modified versions of these digestive enzymes are the chemicals found in viper venom.

Peritonitis

Peritonitis the most serious causes of abdominal pain. Inflammation and infection of the peritoneal lining of the abdomen was often the cause of death in abdominal pain before antibiotics. The pain of early peritonitis, regardless of its cause, is described as constant, moderately severe and with hand pressure or with body movement, the pain is felt over a large area of the abdomen. Bowel obstruction causes a rapid increase in pain with cramp-like "griping" waves and may subside completely until the next spasm. A tubal or ectopic pregnancy was known as the deadly pregnancy since its rupture and subsequent peritonitis was fatal before modern surgery. As the growing fetus stretches the hollow Fallopian tube, the pain becomes steadily severe, originating in one of the lower abdominal quadrants, increases with movement and is only slightly relieved with opiates. Large ovarian cysts can rupture and present with peritonitis.

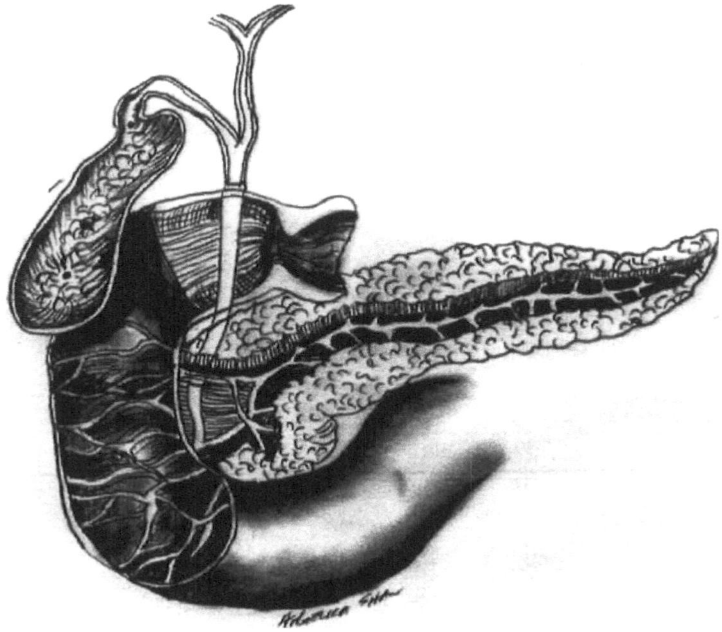

The above illustrates the merging of the stomach, small bowel, gallbladder and pancreas. Much happens here, including problems. Stomach acid, food, pancreatic juices and gall bladder emissions converge on the first part of the small bowel. Pain from this area is perceived in the upper abdomen. Ulcers, gall stone attacks and pancreatitis are possible causes of pain from this cluster of hollow organs. AM.

Urinary tract pain

The urinary system may produce abdominal pain and, in most causes produce a positive urine test for infection (white blood cells) or stone (blood). Pain radiating from the back through the abdomen into the groin, strongly suggests the urinary system. Abdominal pain associated with painful or frequent urination, the presence of blood and/or leukocytes (pus) in the urine should be treated as an infection. Another urinary cause of abdominal pain is the kidney stone (renal calculus), where pain is intermittent (colicky) in nature and the urine contains blood. An infection or stone in the urinary tract usually causes more back pain than abdominal pain. Urinary infections cause fever, nausea and vomiting. In all cases of abdominal pain or back pain, collect urine for a dipstick test, since in almost all cases of problems within kidneys and other components of the urinary tract, the urine test is helpful. The author recommends prophylactic antibiotic use in kidney stone.

Vomiting (emesis)

Emesis may emerge during most conditions discussed previously; however, it can be absent. In appendicitis, diverticulitis and ectopic pregnancy, it usually occurs early and then may cease. With continued emesis, fluid will turn from yellow to green as bile replaces stomach contents, indicating that small bowel material is now being forced backwards into the mouth. In bowel obstructions the vomitus turns fecal, foul smelling and stool-brown color. Sudden unremitting emesis with few if any other abdominal complaints, think increased intracranial pressure. This is especially true if vomiting gives no relief of nausea, and a headache is present. Increased intracranial pressure could follow a head injury or be associated with brain tumors.

Bowel Movements

Constipation is the rule in the acute abdomen, although small amounts of loose stools is often seen early, escaping around firmer stool. In serious cases, as abdominal pain becomes more severe, bowel sounds become quiet, indicating the cessation of movement of fluid and even gas through the bowel. The presence of gas passing through the rectum (flatus) means the bowel is still open and is always a hopeful sign. The reappearance of the lowly fart after a bout of abdominal pain or surgery is the indicator that the bowel is recovering, alive and moving! Constipation is the most common cause of abdominal pain.

Examination of the Abdomen

The normal abdomen is soft on exams, filled with sounds and contains no firm masses. Abdominal infection results in the abdominal wall becoming tender and usually firmer, as muscles tighten, in an effort, to reduce irritating movement in the underlying tissues. Bowel sounds, noises created by gas and fluids passing through the hollow gut, in some conditions become more prominent (gastroenteritis) but in the more serious cases, become silent. On examination, the abdomen is divided into four quadrants, the umbilicus being the center point. The lower chest and pelvic area are included within the confines of these quadrants. Their underlying organs are listed by quadrant in the preceding pages and include components of the gastrointestinal tract, urinary tract and lungs.

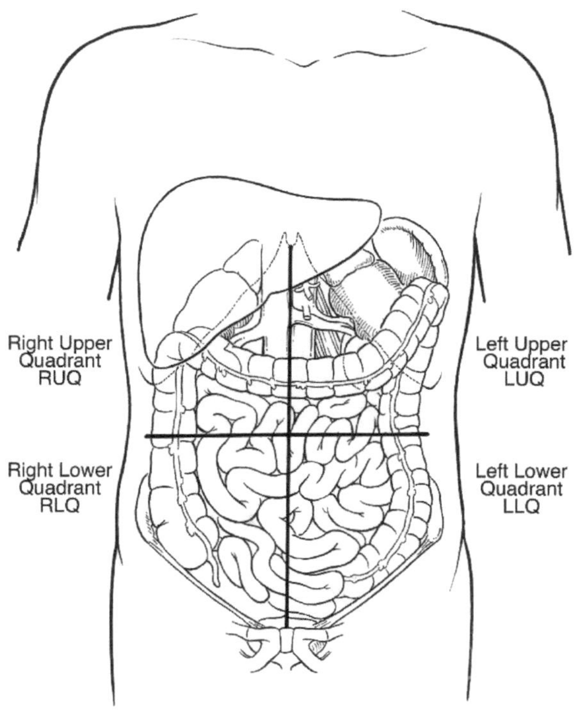

When describing abdominal pain, these four quadrants are navigational aids. NLM

Listening (Auscultation)

The abdominal exam begins by listening to the bowel sounds with a stethoscope in all four quadrants. The presence of bowel sounds in even just one quadrant assures some flow. Hyperactive bowel sounds (loud and frequent) often represent bowel irritability, evidenced by diarrhea or excessive gas production. The loss of bowel sounds is due to bowel paralysis, and is a poor sign, especially when associated with fever. Some infections within the bowel cause irritation, increasing bowel sounds, sometimes explosive and painful. If the infection escapes the hollow gut's interior and enters the sterile cavity that surrounds the gut (peritoneum), it will cause the bowel sounds to diminish, and if untreated, bowel sounds may cease all together. Peritonitis without antibiotic treatment is fatal.

Palpation (Latin for touch)

The normal abdomen is only tender with deep pressure. Any other tenderness indicates some type of problem, usually one that will be resolved. If tenderness increases, especially in one site, it increases the likelihood of something more serious. The finding of **rebound** tenderness is always significant, prompting aggressive therapy. Rebound is a term for the sensation of pain when the peritoneum is inflamed or infected. If there is more pain upon taking the hand away quickly after pushing deep into the abdomen, it is rebound pain. The pain is created as the inflamed tissue "rebounds" away from the sudden release. It represents a problem that prior to modern surgery and the development of antibiotics, was common cause of death after battles, where swords, arrows, bullets, shrapnel, wood splinters and spikes penetrated the soft thinly muscle-covered abdomen. Penetrating abdominal wounds could be unusually cruel, killing slowly over days, sometimes weeks, with peritonitis. President Garfield died the slow agonizing death of peritonitis after being "gut shot".

To detect rebound, one can apply deep steady pressure to the site of abdominal pain and then suddenly release the pressure. If the patient has fever and reports that the pain on release is greater than the pain on downward pressure, rebound and peritonitis are presumed. Another test for rebound is striking the heel firmly, producing jolting waves into the abdomen. If peritonitis is present, the patient will feel pain at the site of peritoneal inflammation with "heel strike". The finding of rebound should initiate aggressive therapy consisting of two antibiotics, an injectable and oral medication from a different class of antibiotics and bowel rest.

Field Lab Test used in the Assessment of Abdominal Pain

Urinalysis, examination of stool for blood and in the fertile female, a urine pregnancy test should be done in evaluating abdominal pain. When these lab tests are combined with the history and physical examination, the medical officer can assess and manage conditions physicians were unable to diagnose and treat a few decades ago. All cases of abdominal pain, back pain and fever should warrant urine tests. The urinalysis may aid diagnosis while reflecting hydration status (specific gravity) and monitor the effects of treatment. As the urinary tract infection clears, so should the urine clear of leukocytes and blood. The successful passage of a stone from the urinary tract should be followed by the urine becoming negative for blood. Pregnancy testing is not only useful in abdominal pain but also useful before dispensing drugs that may be harmful to a developing fetus.

Pregnancy test-+ within weeks of pregnancy
+blood-infection, kidney stone, trauma, if no other symptoms, suspect cancer
+WBC (white blood cells)-infection
+nitrate-infection
+bilirubin-hepatitis
+protein-infection, kidney disease
+glucose-diabetes
+ketones-fasting
pH-measure urine acidity, often increases with infection
specific gravity-compares urine to fresh water, higher the #, more concentrated is urine

Dangerous Animals

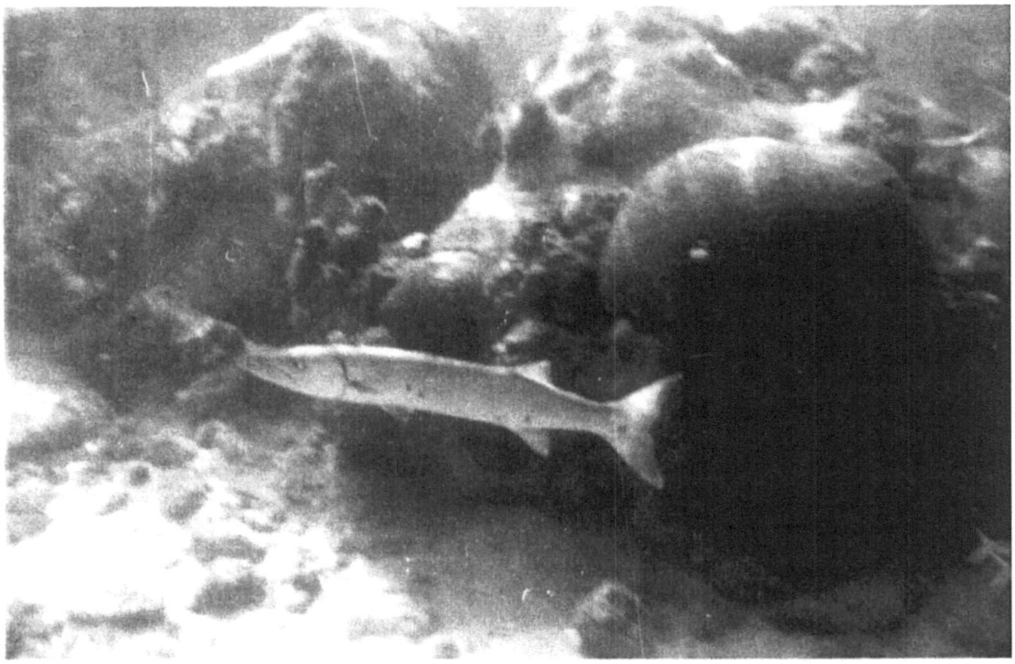

Barracudas are common in much of the Caribbean where they sedately swim among divers posing for pictures. They seldom attack without deliberate provocation. Photo by author

There are many ways animals can harm human beings. Some can inflict mechanical injury by tearing or crushing tissue, others are venomous, capable of injecting a poisonous substance. A few animals possess a toxic chemical when ingested, which can cause disease. Some animals are capable of injury through more than one of the above mechanisms, like the stingray containing venom, electric shock and a formidable spear. There are over one thousand marine animals and scores of others living in closely related ocean environments that are known to be harmful to man. Few, if any deliberately stalk mankind, but inflict injuries in self-defense when disturbed. They range in size from the tiny, but deadly, cone shells to the great white shark.

One of the earliest records of the possible toxic effects of marine animals comes from the Old Testament. Exodus 7: 20-21"and all of the fish that were in the river died and the river stank, and the Egyptians could not drink the water of the river and there was blood through-out all of the land of Egypt". This may refer to a "bloom" of toxic dinoflagellates, known today as a red tide. Huge gatherings of a microscopic organism so concentrated they create mass mortality of fishes and other marine animals. Another ancient report of hazardous animals comes from the Greek scientist Pliny in "Historia Naturalis" on the topic of stingrays... "So venomous is it, that if it be stuchen into the root of a tree, it killeth it, it is able to pierce a good cuirae (protective chest plate) or jacket or buffe or suit-able as if it were an arrow or a dart launched..." Although rays can inflict serious wounds, Pliny is certainly guilty of at least overstatement, if not exaggeration.

Venomous Animals

The venom of the animals varies widely among different species. However, several generalities can be made. Venom is a complex solution of proteins, enzymes and amino acids. It commonly contains serotonin which in man is a potent pain stimulator and promotes histamine release. Marine venom is chemically fragile, denatured by heating (heat labile). This is fortunate for the victim, since it can be partially destroyed by applying moist heat to the wound, reducing the injury from marine venom. In small animals it is paralytic while in man usually results in pain, swelling and redness at the wound site. In rare cases, it can be fatal, since any foreign substance injected into our circulation may precipitate anaphylactic shock. In general, suspected envenomation is treated with hot soaks, antihistamines (diphenhydramine) and pain relief.

Coelenterates

Greek koilos - hollow, enteron - intestine

Coelenterates are hollow body animals that may possess poisonous tentacles or spines that can penetrate intact skin. Very few of these animals are harmful to man and then only through accidental contact. Jellyfish inflict injury using the same mechanism by which they capture prey. Attached to their long flowing tentacles are nematocysts, saclike structures containing chemicals that penetrate and paralyze small marine animals. In man, this results in painful, red, raised welts. Larger jellyfish such as deadly sea wasps and Portuguese-Man-of-War can inflict more serious injury because they carry greater numbers and more potent nematocysts. It is not uncommon for swimmers to drown after contact with these jellyfish as large muscles become paralyzed. Increased sweating, salivation, mental confusion and possibly anaphylactic shock indicate a severe reaction to the animal's toxin.

Initial care consists of mechanical removal of any intact nematocysts. This is best accomplished by gentle scraping with a knife edge or by carefully rubbing the skin with sand. Some authors, especially fiction writers have romanticized the use of fresh urine for pain relief. However, more traditional analgesics such as opiates/NSAIDs may be more appropriate for pain relief. Meat tenderizers have been effective in relieving pain when sprinkled over the wound. Diphenhydramine (Benadryl) may reduce symptoms of nausea, anxiety and welting. It may also help prevent the development of shock by blocking the adverse effects of massive histamine release.

Due to the risk of anaphylaxis, the victim's vital signs should be monitored every five to ten minutes along with tilt testing if the person appears in any distress. Airway management may become necessary due to vomiting, increased salivation or coma. Keep the victim dry and warm to reduce shivering. Opiate injection may be necessary for severe pain using a shallow injection since intramuscular injection could cause deep bleeding due to anti-clotting chemicals in some marine venom. If possible, an IV should be placed if the victim appears in respiratory distress. Remember, an IV is much more likely to be successful in a person with good blood pressure and veins filled with blood than later when the victim develops shock. Considering whether to start an IV is like considering shortening sail as wind increases. It is better to do it now than later when conditions have worsened.

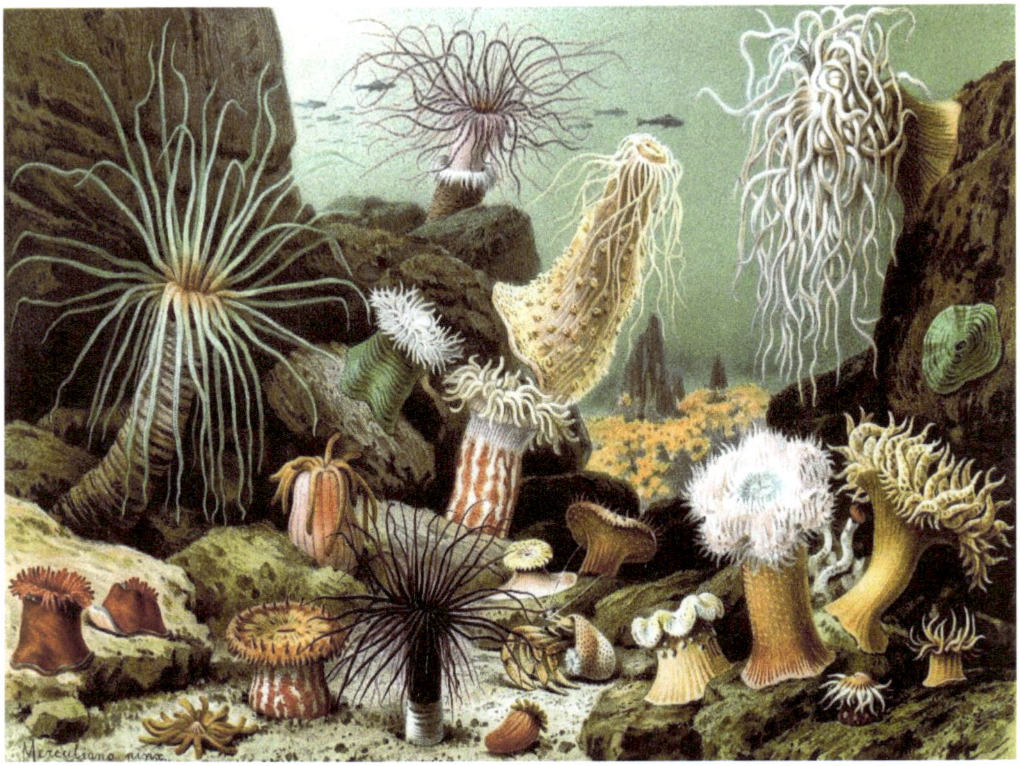

An 1893 print by Giacomo Merculiano representative of the beauty and variety of anemones representing an animal constructed by an alliance of many-celled animals.

Sea anemones injuries (sponge divers' disease) are not uncommon wounds in curious swimmers if they inadvertently handle poisonous sponges resulting in pain, redness and ulcerations where tentacles have touched the skin. Wounds may become infected, especially if the water is contaminated with human waste. Treatment consists of warm compresses for twenty minutes followed by cleaning the wounds with antibiotic soap. Antibiotics may be indicated if the wound shows signs of infection, i.e., redness, swelling, heat and pain.

Mollusks

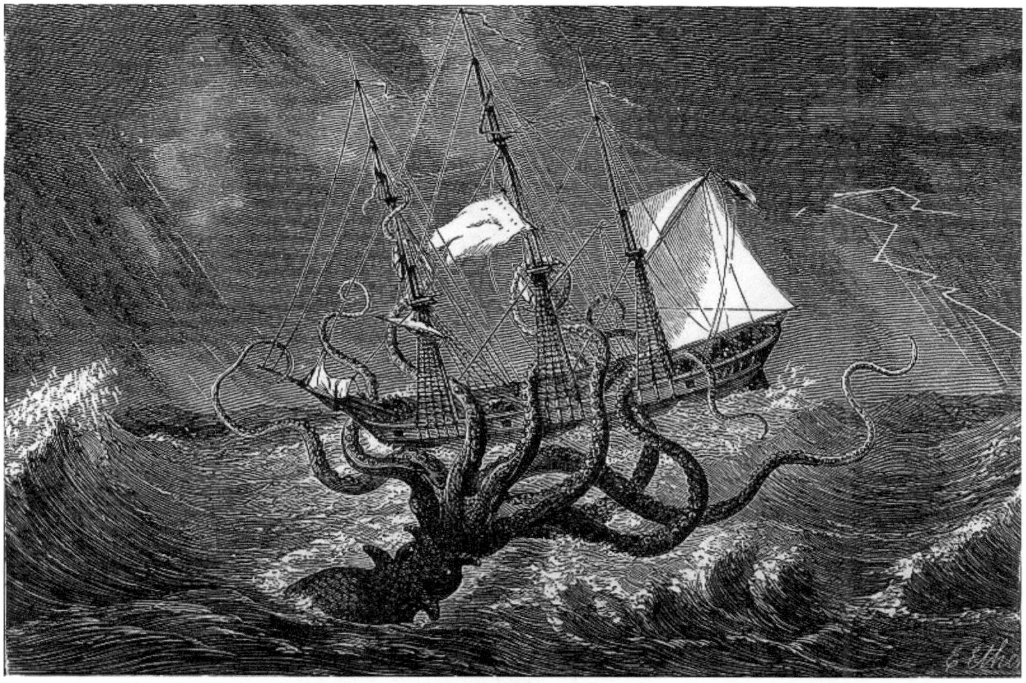

Sailors for centuries believed that huge mollusks (Krakens) were awaiting them in the deep dark oceans. Fear of Krakens kept many sailors from leaving the Mediterranean and venturing into the Atlantic. Woodcut by Edward Etherington

The world contains over 80,000 species of mollusks, with only 85 known to be toxic to man, either by bite, injection or more commonly when a toxin ingested. The most dangerous mollusks are the cone shells, carnivorous snails possessing hollow darts. Their venom apparatus is attached to poison sacs that rupture on contact, injecting both dart and venom as a hypodermic needle. They use their darts to hunt and kill other snails, thankfully only rarely inflicting humans as some species mortality is reported at 15-20%. Symptoms include pain and redness at the injection site initially, followed by muscle weakness, convulsions, paralysis, and perhaps shock in severe cases. Treatment consists of incision, lavage and suction of wound, using clean technique such as suction from a syringe, not one's mouth. This is followed by soaking of site for thirty minutes in hot water or hot compresses. To reduce the risk of an allergic reaction, give an oral antihistamine like Benadryl. Antibiotics can be used to prevent bacterial infection at the wound site, especially if an incision is made. The pain is so severe, victims report little relief with injected morphine.

Octopi as a group are shy and retreating animals. However, they are equipped with a powerful beak, which in rare instances can inflict painful bites if accidentally or deliberately provoked. The bite, like other animal wounds can become infected. The blue-ringed octopus of Australian coastal waters is unique among its species in that it is deadly poison. Mortality rates of 25% are reported. One of these creatures was pulled from Australian coastal waters in a Brisbane marina where the author's former students were staying. As with other wounds, treatment consists of clean excision and lavage of wound site with hot clean water followed by hot compresses or emersion. Consider giving Benadryl in anaphylaxis suspected.

Echinoderms

Word derives from the Latinized Greek word for porcupine, sea urchin

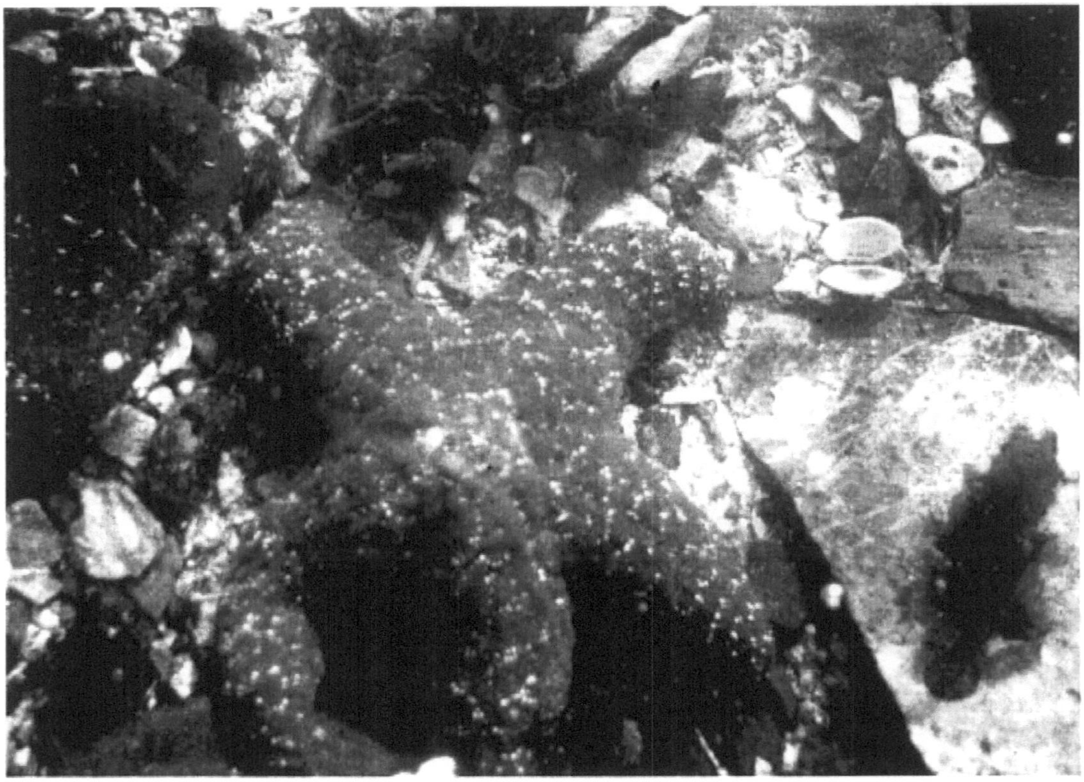

This cold-water starfish of Alaskan waters enjoys the many clams found in the Pacific coastal waters. These creatures may end up taking a fishing hook where they can inflict mild wounds as the hook is removed from their mouth on the underside. Urchins are much more likely to cause injury than starfish as the author experienced. Photo by author

Sea urchins, starfish and sea cucumbers are included in this group. Sea urchins are covered with projecting spines that can penetrate unprotected skin and discharge venom. Once in the Caribbean, the author was pushed into a bed of sea urchins by an unexpected large wave. After the encounter, over thirty spines were imbedded completely through both feet, primarily through toes and distal feet. Although extremely painful for several hours, the wounds healed without sequalae. Since open seawater is considered sterile and the projectiles were imbedded, little wound care was required. The puncture wounds tattooed skin with purple discoloration of the spines slowly faded. If signs of infection appear after any puncture wound, use hot soaks, elevate area to promote drainage and give oral antibiotics for one to two days after infection appears resolved.

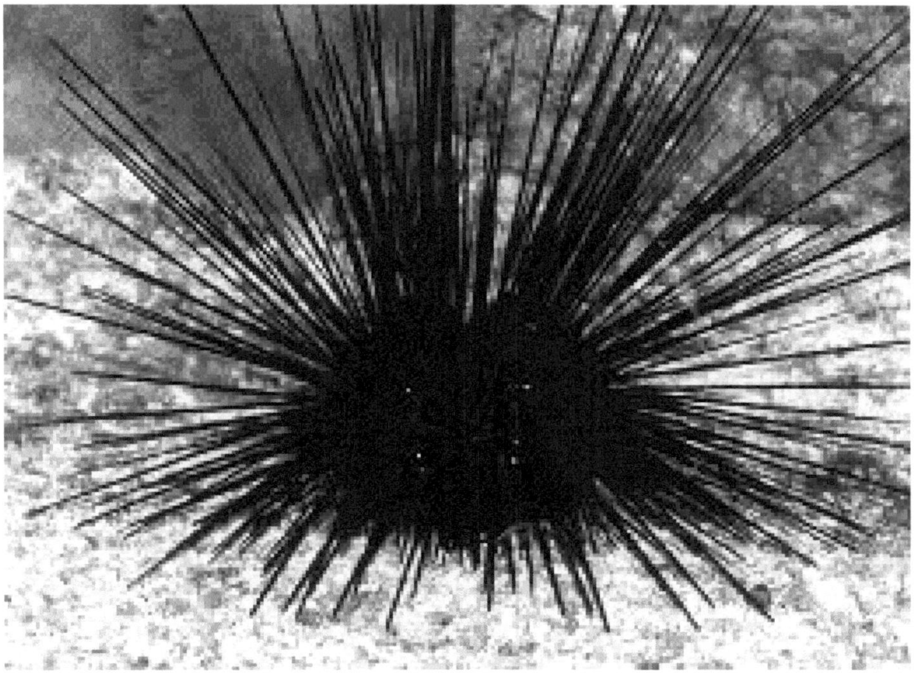

A well-protected creature with spines that easily penetrate soft flesh. Photo by author

Signs of echinoderm injury include pain or intense burning and redness at site. Treatment consists of pain relief, soaking in hot water and removal of spines with forceps if they can be grasped. Excision is not recommended as it increases the risk of infections, and spines will dissolve over time. Give antibiotics at the time of the wound if occurring where boats discharge human waste. Punctures occurring over a joint or in people with a history of skin infections and diabetics deserve more aggressive care. By giving one to three days of an oral antibiotic, wound infections may be avoided.

Venomous Fishes

Over 200 species are known to be dangerous to man, many found in the coastal waters of California, Florida, Gulf of Mexico and the Caribbean. These fish contain apparatus can penetrate deeply into skin and underlying blood vessels, causing mechanical injury while capable of injecting venom. As previously mentioned, marine venom is a complex solution of proteins, enzymes and amino acids easily dismantled by moist heat to the injury site. Antihistamines such as diphenhydramine (Benadryl) reduce the risk of allergic reaction. Envenomation varies from simple pain, swelling and redness at the wound site, to the extreme of possible death from venom-induced shock. The primary players in the venomous fish are stingrays, scorpion fish, fire fish zebra fish, stone fishes, weavers, toadfish, stargazers, certain sharks, ratfishes, catfishes and sturgeon fishes. Wound by these animals should be treated with moist heat for thirty minutes and antihistamine by mouth. If sudden signs of anaphylactic shock appear such as shortness of breath, hives or falling blood pressure, give 0.3 cc of adrenalin (epinephrine) by injection every 15 minutes until the risk of shock has passed. Pain relief is important in preventing pain-induced fainting or falling blood pressure. An infection is possible in any wound, prompting thorough wound cleaning and possibly antibiotics.

Spine fish contain some of the nature's most lethal venom. This group includes turkey fish, lionfish and the deadly stone fish (found in reefs of Indian and Pacific oceans). Stone fish resemble rocks while lying motionless, hidden among rocks and kelp forests, as well as buried in the sand. Along the back of spine fish are long slender hollow spines, natural hypodermic needles. The primary symptom of envenomation is intense pain at the wound site, lasting twelve to twenty-four hours. The venom is so potent, the skin and underlying tissue at wound site rapidly becomes swollen and discolored. In addition to severe pain, symptoms include nausea, vomiting, diarrhea, breathing difficulties, possible convulsions and falling blood pressure. Shock is not uncommon, and death is certainly not rare in stone fish encounters. Treatment is aimed primarily at pain relief and prevention of shock, which is paramount to reducing mortality. The wound site frequently develops a large ulcer of dead flesh, increasing risks of later infection, prompting early use of antibiotics and good wound care for several days.

Stingrays

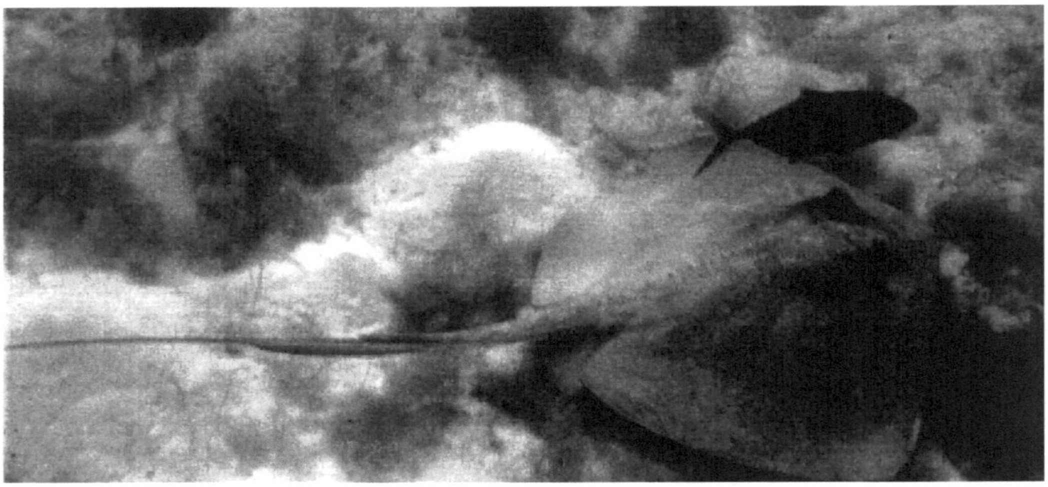

The small Caribbean ray above was disturbed by snorkeling just above its sandy retreat. Even a ray this small could cause injury to an ill-placed unprotected hand or foot. Diving gloves offer significant protection but are not often worn in warm tropical waters. Photo by author

These bottom-feeding fish do not attack man or any other animals, its venom apparatus is purely defensive. Injury almost always occurs in shallow water when waders unknowingly step on a resting animal, causing the ray to suddenly "whip" its defensive tail into unsuspecting flesh. Two of the author's former students were simultaneously injured by different rays while stepping out opposite sides of the same dingy. The term "stingray" does not come from the animal's tail, but the ability of some rays to suddenly release an electrical charge. This bioelectric system is used at lower voltage to detect prey. Stingrays, especially large ones, can inflict significant wounds. These wounds are not only mechanical injuries but also may deposit venom.

The ray's venom apparatus is encased in a fearsome piece of engineering. The long whip-like tail terminates into a bony spine, which in an average animal is 5" long 1/ 2" wide, and 1/ 4" thick, rock hard and possesses back-slanting barbs on two sides. This defensive weapon was fatal for the "crocodile hunter", Steve Irwin, when the ray he was handling, suddenly thrust this spine into his chest cavity. As the spine is lashed across skin it lacerates and punctures flesh, creating wounds sometimes deep enough to severe vessels and nerves. Stingray spines were utilized by American Indians and in the Pacific islands as points on fish spears.

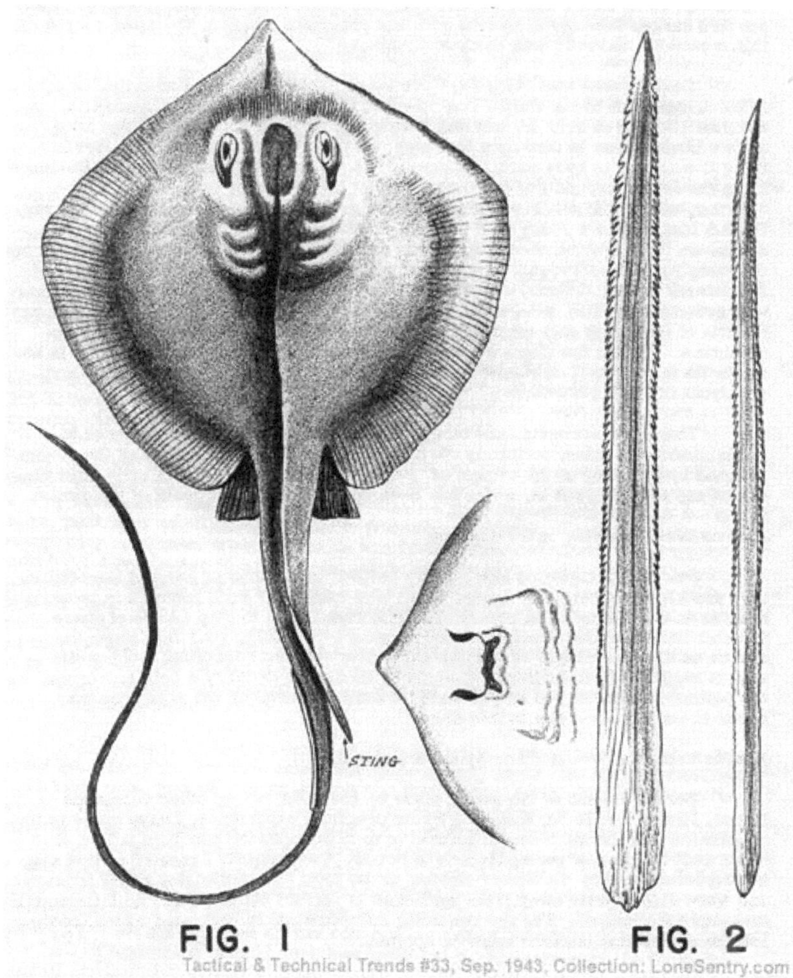

Image from a US Army publications about hazards troops may encounter when fighting in the South Pacific, 1943. Figure 2 depicts the ray's sword-like bone

In the living ray, the spine is surrounded by thousands of small poison glands that rupture on impact. Bleeding will be followed in a few minutes by intense pain within four to ten minutes. Pain will spread from the wound site, along with expanding swelling. This will normally peak in one to three hours and be gone in six to forty-eight hours. In larger more poisonous wounds, muscle weakness, shaking chills, nausea and vomiting, sweating, paralysis and shock can occur. Death is rare and limited to cases where the spine has entered a body cavity or when anaphylactic shock develops unchecked. Treatment consists of pain relief, wound lavage, hot compresses to denature toxin and removal of the spine if impacted. Place a pressure dressing of Silvadene, cotton sponges and roll gauze. Large lacerations should be closed with sutures and antibiotics used early if wound shows signs of infection. Give Benadryl 25-50 mgs to reduce allergic reactions.

Snakes

"Upon thy belly shalt thou go and dust shalt thou eat all the days of thy life."

Genesis 3:14

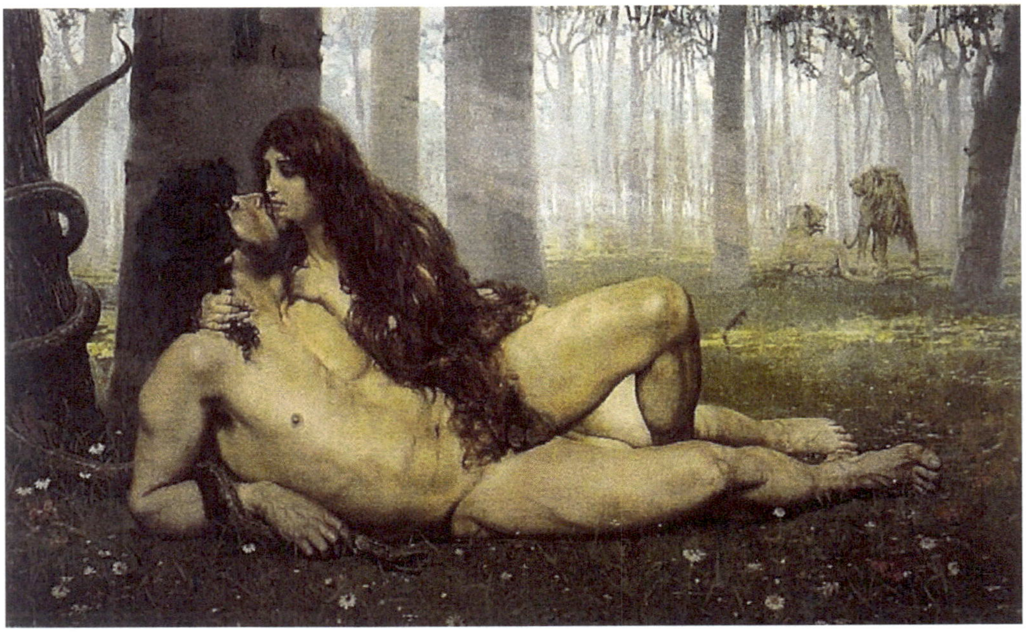

"The First Kiss" Salvador Viniegra's painting as he imagined the Adam, Eve and snake story.

The serpent has long been depicted in the Judea-Christian texts as a bearer of evil and the seducer of Eve, causing them to be driven out of the Garden of Eden. Because of this, snakes have been feared and scorned by most western cultures and some animals. Carl Sagan says that young primates have only two fears, those of falling and snakes. In many cultures the serpent is revered, even though deadly. Among ancient ruins on the Indian subcontinent and throughout the huge ruins of western Cambodia's Angkor Wat, venomous snake images are found on many structures. In ancient Egypt, a giant serpent is depicted as swallowing the sun at night, giving birth to it again with the new day. The Greeks made the image of a snake the emblem for medicine, an image still in use in military field medicine.

To early Greeks, the snake represented the spirit of healing and other positive attributes. The Greeks named the healing serpent Asklepios (the Romans Latinized it to the modern name of Aesculapius) and by the 8th century BC had erected over 300 temples to the sacred mystic snake god. Temple sites were usually built on high ground away from the insect-infested swamps, founded around ancient medicinal springs. From these waters, priests and priestesses made mixtures of minerals, animal parts and herbs that were given to the ill and injured.

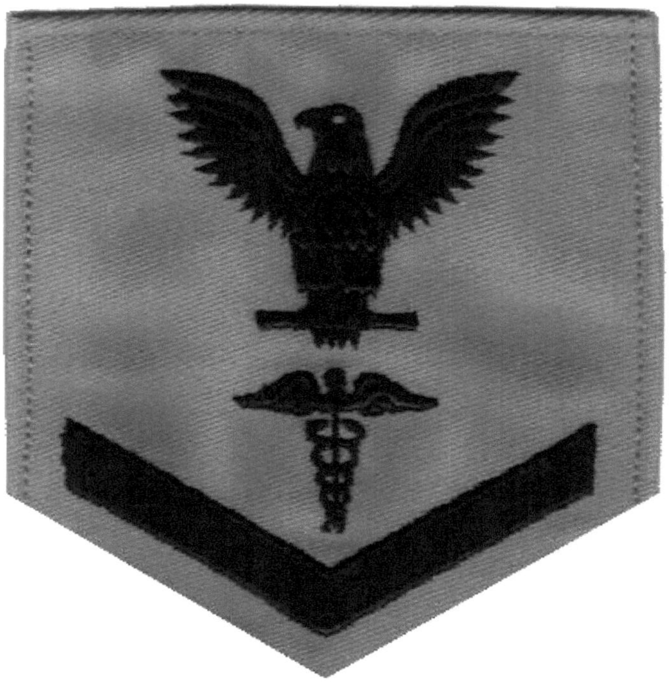

This is patch worn by navy corpsman, Aesculapius emblem signifies United States Navy medical department, and the chevron under snake indicates the rank of 3rd class petty officer. This person would have hundreds of hours of class and supervised experience, passed examinations both written and oral, to wear this patch. Navy corpsmen serving with the marines and sailors are addressed respectfully as "Doc".

Greek temples contained not only statues of snakes but real live snakes. The temple snakes most sought after by the Asklepieia were the large yellow reptiles of the Hieron Valley. Temple snakes were well cared for, long-lived and encouraged to lick the wounds and areas of pain of the patients. The early Greeks referred to the Asklepieia as the Giver of Children, Restorer of Health and the All Wise. Another myth concerning the snake was the mythical Theriac, an elixir that supposedly cured many maladies while imparting long life. It contained a long list of secret ingredients including the flesh of poisonous vipers (thus the name theriakos, Greek for reptile). According to Pliny the Elder, the formula for the true theriac was inscribed in poetic verse on the wall of a cave under temple of Aesculpius on the island of Cos (the birthplace of Hippocrates). During the Middle Ages, generations of European physicians and alchemists reported their rediscovery of the secret formula for theriac. Apothecaries (early pharmacist) and the traveling medicine men of the American west, claimed to have formulated this ancient theriac. Thus, the term, "snake oil salesman" used to describe the trade.

Snakebites

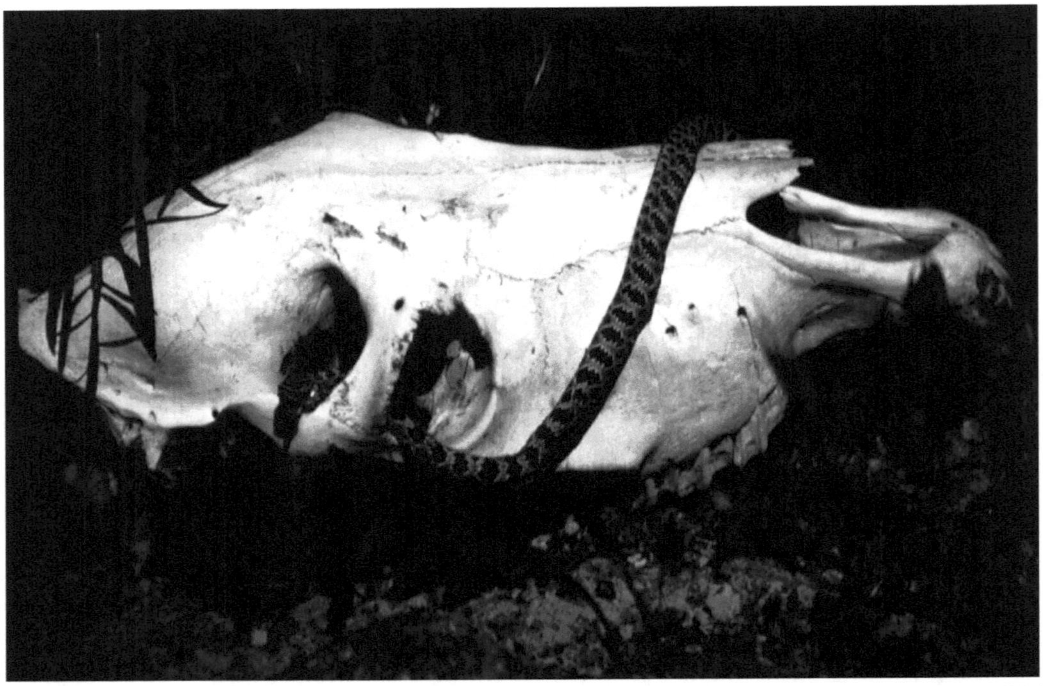

The snake coiled around a wooden staff has long been the emblem of medicine. This is the desert version of Aesculapius, a Western Diamondback rattler curved around a wild horse skull. This is the most dangerous snake in North America. It is aggressive, especially the smaller, less mature rattlers like the one above. It is unlikely to be encountered in the marine environment but is not uncommon in California and other western states in coastal countries. Photo by author

The author has an interest in snakes from a distance. Growing up in Oklahoma, there were many snakes, most were harmless, only with a rare encounter with rattlesnake, water moccasin or copperhead. Snakes play important roles around the author's farm and if possible, left alone. While backpacking in the desert and summer mountains of the west, one will encounter rattlesnakes, and given time and space, a respectful distance is achieved. Making plenty of noise while walking by kicking rocks gives rattlesnakes time to retreat or to make that characteristic sound warning. Watch where feet and hands are placed and make lots of noise.

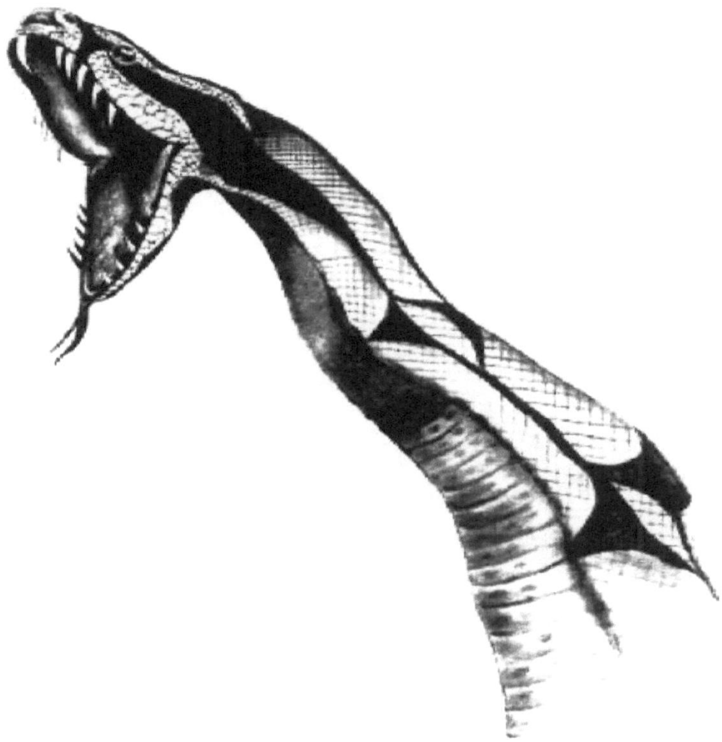

This is an artistic image of a venomous snake with an attitude. Snakes are some of nature's most successful predators, eating only other animals and are the only non-microscopic creatures capable of eating animals as large as themselves. Large meals allow some snakes to consume only four meals in twelve months. Digestive juices found in snakes are nature's most powerful and snake venom is a modification of these digestive enzymes. Snakes, pound for pound are the strongest animals in nature and some venoms remain poisonous for decades. Snakes have lost external ears, replaced by as many as 300 boney vertebrae (tuning forks) connected to the ribs resting on the ground. Snakes hear with vibrations transmitted from the ground, through their ribs and onto their internal ear. These hundreds of ribs give snakes their unique, near silent and frightening locomotion.
Angelica Mager

Only a minority of snakes are harmful to man, however, it is often difficult to differentiate poisonous from harmless snakes. Therefore, all snakes and snake bites should be handled as venomous. Poisonous snakes are found worldwide except at high altitudes, Antarctica and on islands of New Zealand, Iceland, Ireland, Crete, Madagascar, New Caledonia and most of the Caribbean islands. One venomous species even resides within the arctic circle, while almost all snakes in Australia are poisonous.

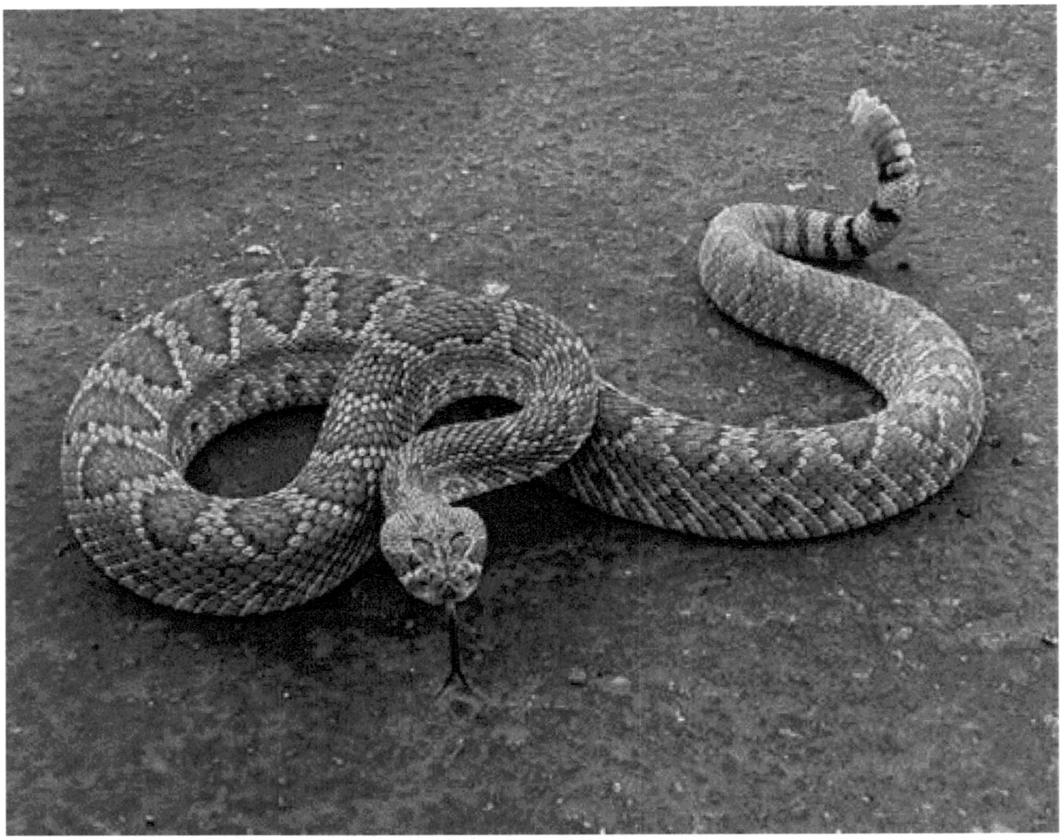

CDC photo of rattlesnake, the triangle-shape head usually denotes venomous snake. The Western Diamondback rattlesnake above could be carrying enough venom to kill forty-seven adult humans.

Snakebites primarily occur in rural areas of the tropics, especially in the jungles of Third World countries. India has reported annual mortality of 20,000 for the past century. Periodic hurricanes causing flooding greatly increases the numbers of snakebites as humans and snakes are compressed into small islands above the rising floodwaters. In west central Africa, Burma, Central and South America snakebites cause a significant number of deaths. Whereas, in the USA only a handful of deaths are reported, and these almost always occur while handling the snake. Death is not always the result of envenomation, but shock brought about by terror.

World Distribution of Poisonous Snakes

Listed below is a partial list of harmful snakes, by location, common name and scientific Latin name, important because these are the Latin names used internationally in medicine and treatment, especially when using anti-venom.

Area/Scientific (Latin) name	Common name
North America	
Crotalus atrox	Western diamond back rattlesnake
Cr. adamrnteus	Eastern diamond back rattlesnake
Agkistrodon piscivorus	Cotton-mouth moccasin
Agkistrodon contortrix	Copperhead
Micrurus tener	Coral snake
Central America	
Cr. Durissus	Rattlesnake
Bothrops asper	Terciopelo
South America	
B. atrox	Fer-de-lance
B. jararaca	Jararaca
Cr. Durissus terrificus	Rattlesnake
Europe	
Viper atrox	Viper, adler

V ammodytes	**Long-nose viper**

Africa

Echis carinatus	**Carpet viper**
Bitis arietans	**Puff adler (Cleopatra suicide)**
Naja nigricollis	**Black cobra**
N. Haje	**Egyptian cobra**
Dendroaspis	**Mambas (most aggressive viper)**

Asia/Middle East

E. carinatus	**Carpet viper**
Viper lebetina	**Levantine viper**
V. palistinae	**Palestine viper**

Southeast Asia

E carinatus	**Carpet viper**
Naja naja	**Asian cobra**
V. Russeli	**Russel's viper**
Callosasma	**Pit viper**
E. schistose	**Sea snake**

Far East

N. naja	**Asian cobra**
Trimersurus flavoviridis	**Habu (ten step viper)**
T. mucrosquqmqtus	**Chinese habu**

Australia and related Islands

Acanthophis antarcticus	**Death adler**
Notechis scutatus	**Tiger snake**
Pseudonaja textilis	**Easter brown snake**

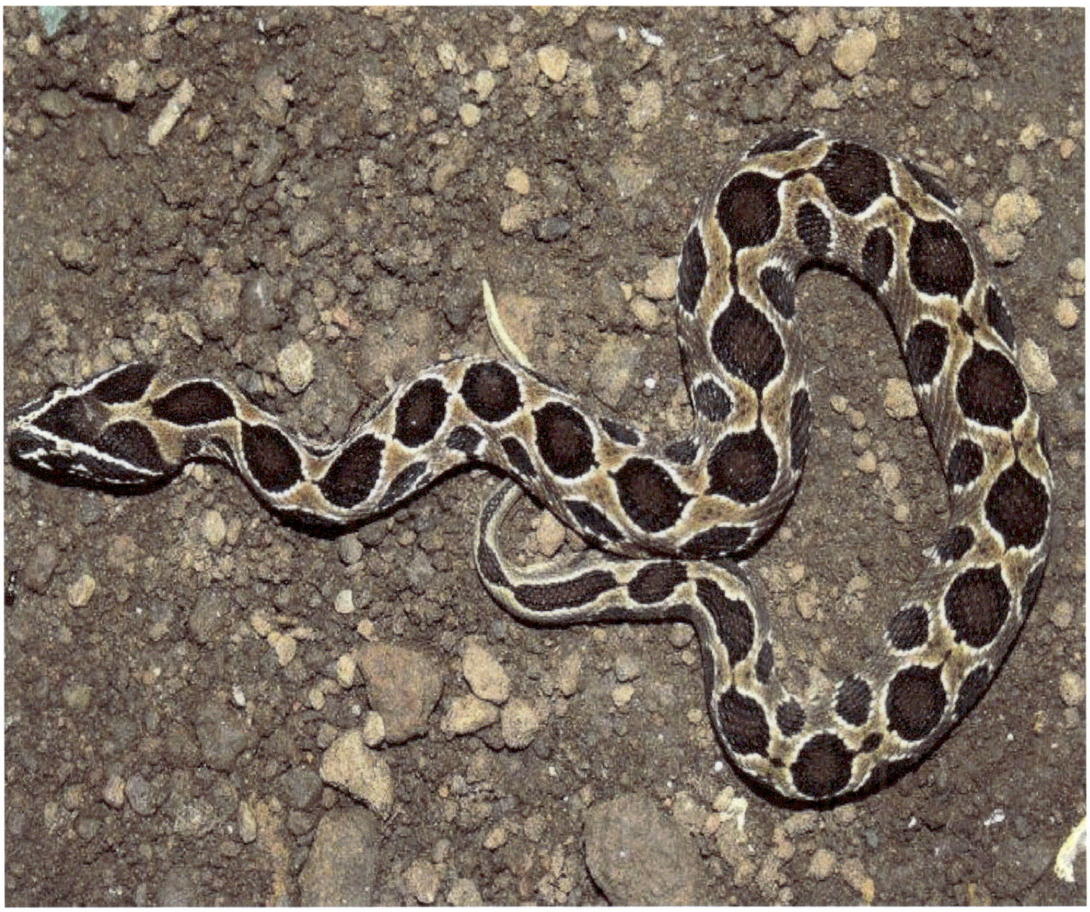

Russel's viper, one of the most deadly and beautiful serpents. CDC

The treatment of snakebites should always begin with maintaining airway, breathing and circulation, especially since anaphylactic shock is possible when foreign protein is injected directly into circulation. Initially, immobilize the area with splint or sling and apply moist heat to denature the protein and increase blood to the area to dilute any venom. Tight tourniquets are of questionable value. They are effective in reducing blood flow to the wound site which may decrease the amount and concentration of venom reaching internal organs. However, by decreasing blood flow to the wound site, the injected poison remains localized, increasing tissue damage at the site of injection. Remember, snake venom is modified digestive juices, designed to break down tissue and tissue destruction enhances the risk of infection. If a tourniquet is used, it should be released every one-half hour for five minutes and should not be used for more than two hours. This author discourages the use of tight tourniquets, although other text may continue to recommend its use. Current research also discourages ice, since it too will reduce blood flow to the wound, increasing tissue destruction.

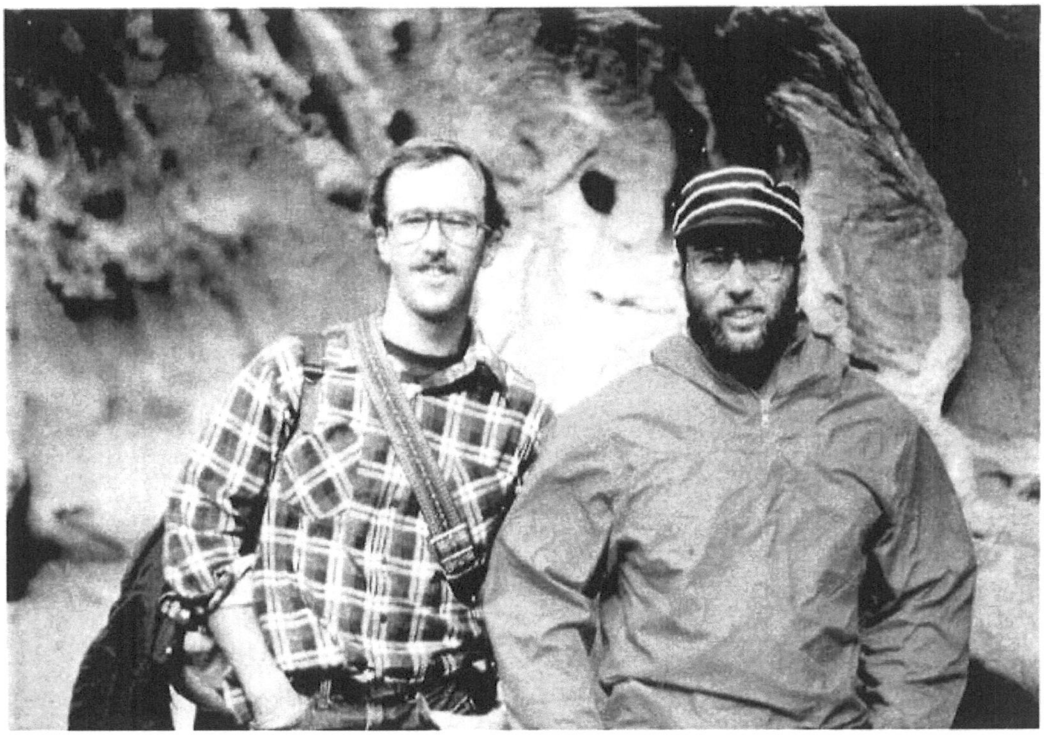

Michael Stolpe to the left of the author in Utah's east desert, became the Army expert on pit viper envenomation while stationed in El Paso. His recommendation is to remove as much venom as possible from the injection site. Clean suction or extraction using a rubber suction cup or syringe-like extractor along with a loose tourniquet to impede lymphatic flow and the avoidance of ice is helpful in reducing tissue damage at the wound site. Moist heat is less useful in desert dwelling snakes, as their venom is less likely to be inactivated by heat. Dr. Stolpe has seen hundreds of snake bites and in almost every case, the victim was handling the snake.

It is currently recommended to remove venom with clean suction at the wound sites. This is best accomplished with a syringe or the old fashion Boy Scout red rubber suction device. The mouth, although more dramatic, is too dirty to apply to wound, and increases the risk of getting venom into circulation of the rescuer. Pain and anxiety relief are important in preventing shock which can develop from excessive nervous system discharge with panic and fear. Snake venom contains blood-thinning chemicals, ensuring that the venom will not be walled off at the wound site but enter circulation and be widely dispersed. Aspirin could further thin blood and should not be given. For the same reason, no deep intramuscular injections are used since the needle could puncture vessels and cause internal bleeding. Opiate and/or diphenhydramine (Benadryl) injections, if necessary, should be administered with a short needle just under the skin. Benadryl is a useful drug for many reasons in snake and other venomous bites as it may prevent anaphylactic shock, which can cause sudden death in some victims. It may be helpful with nausea and vomiting commonly associated with snakebites (because of the high risk of vomiting and aspiration, the victim should be placed on their side). Benadryl will impart a slight tranquilizing effect as well as enhancing any opiates that is used.

Marine Food Poisoning

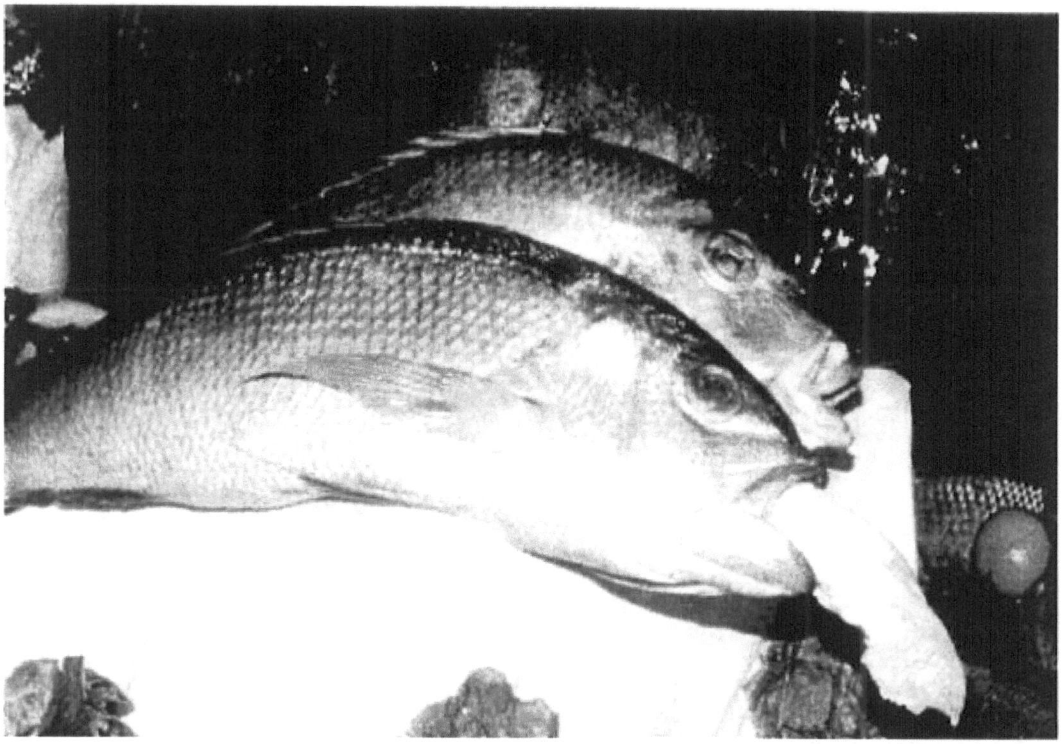

These fish are fresh from the Red Sea and are safe to eat. In much of the world, one must rely on the expertise of the locals in consuming fish, as tainted fish often look the same as those that are free from human and natural toxins. Photo by author

Ciguatera is one of the most studied but least understood seafood poisonings even though fifty thousand poisonings are reported each year. It may be encountered in reef fish in the Pacific and West Indies when large fish either eat the reef or feed upon other reef fish. The onset of symptoms is from four to thirty hours, depending on the amount of toxin absorbed. Nausea, vomiting, diarrhea, abdominal pain, increased salivation, dilated pupils and restlessness have all been reported in victims. Mortality is usually rare but has been as high as one in ten. Some residual problems may last for six months. Treatment in suspected cases, is to induce vomiting, administer a laxative to enhance the gut in clearing the toxin and if the victim becomes agitated, sedation such as Valium (diazepam) may be helpful. Local knowledge is consistent with when to consume reef fish. A test of fish flesh for Ciguatera has been promised but the author is unaware if commercially available to be used in the field.

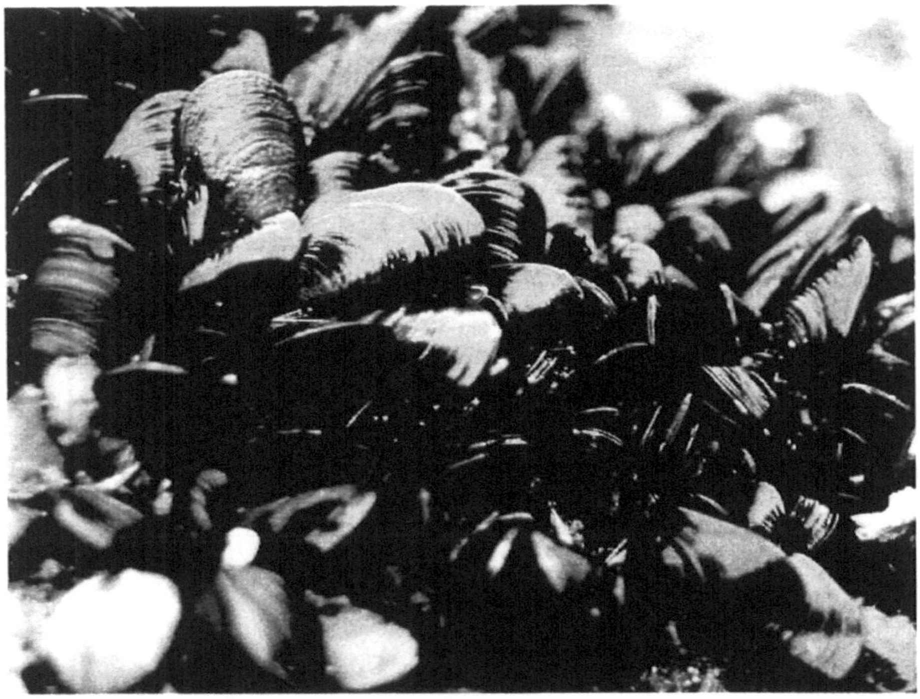

These Alaskan mollusks are easy to pick up by the hundreds when the tide drops and are safe to eat if there is no human activity around to pollute the water. Mollusks feed by filtering passing water and will concentrate on some human pathogens such as hepatitis and cholera. Along California and other coasts, mollusks are not always safe to eat as they concentrate toxic organisms (red tide) during certain times of the year. Local knowledge is important when gathering this food source. Photo by author

Shellfish poisoning is common and usually self-limiting, causing nausea and vomiting, abdominal pain, passing in eight to twelve hours. In some people, it causes a more severe allergic reaction, beginning with itching and hives within minutes to hours after ingestion. This allergic reaction can be severe, requiring a bee sting kit to be carried by the vulnerable in the accidental ingestion of even small amounts of shellfish. Another form of shellfish poison is paralytic, a toxin resembling the curare neurotoxin of South America poison darts. Paralytic shellfish toxin causes paralysis beginning with numbness around the mouth, spreading to face, trunk and extremities. Weakness and instability with walking preceded the more serious paralysis. Mortality is low, ranging from one to seven percent and full recovery is the norm.

Tetrodotoxin is one of the most potent and interesting poisons in nature, being fifty times more potent than strychnine or curare. It has been written about for centuries, being mentioned by ancient Egyptians and in the Old Testament. "These ye shall eat all that are in the waters; all that have fins and scales shall ye eat; and whatsoever hath no fins and scales ye may not eat; it is unclean unto you" Deuteronomy 14:9-10. Tetrodotoxin-containing fish have scales, although they are quite small. Captain Cook and crew experienced this type of food poisoning on the islands of the Coral Sea. The Japanese have long used potions made from the organs of this fish for poison in suicide and political murders. James Bond was nearly "neutralized" by this toxin. Tetrodotoxin has been found in voodoo potions used to induce the "living dead", a zombie-like state in Haitian folklore. Fish that contain Tetrodotoxin include the common puffers, blowfish and globefish.

These fish can be safely eaten if extreme care is observed in preparation. Japan consumes large amounts of pufferfish, prepared by specially trained chefs who know which species of fish are safe, depending on the season of its capture and sex. They are further skilled in cleaning the fish, not allowing the safely eaten flesh to be contaminated with toxin found in eggs, ovaries and livers. Victims of puffer fish poisoning do not have long to wait, with symptoms beginning within thirty minutes. These include headache, sweating, numbness around the mouth, increased salivation, followed by nausea, vomiting, abdominal pain, weakness, difficulty in walking. Death results from paralysis of respiratory muscles, occurring in sixty percent of cases, although in some cases poisoning results in lifelong mental deficits. Treatment is limited to inducing vomiting along with giving sodium bicarbonate or antacids (since these will reduce body acid, inactivating some of the toxin) given by mouth and sedation if needed. Recovery can be expected in survivors within twenty-four hours.

Scombroid poisoning is caused by eating spoiled tuna or mackerel-like fish. Incomplete freezing or improper canning causes bacterial contamination, giving the afflicted fish a "peppery" taste when eaten, followed by headache, hives and generalized swelling beginning in three hours. It is treated with an antihistamine like Benadryl, with recovery in a few hours.

Leeches

These blood-sucking creatures are usually confined to fresh water or brackish swamps. They contain suckers forward and aft by which they attach themselves securely to a warm source of blood. In the process of feeding, they regularly inject their own body fluids into the host, which prevents the blood from clotting and terminating the meal. These injected fluids may contain bacteria and parasites infecting wounds created at the sucker attachments, as well as cause body-wide infection or infestation after entering the blood stream. Treatment consists of removal of the leech quickly with either a hot object or table salt. All leech sites should be thoroughly cleaned, and antibiotics used if sites develop signs of infection or fever.

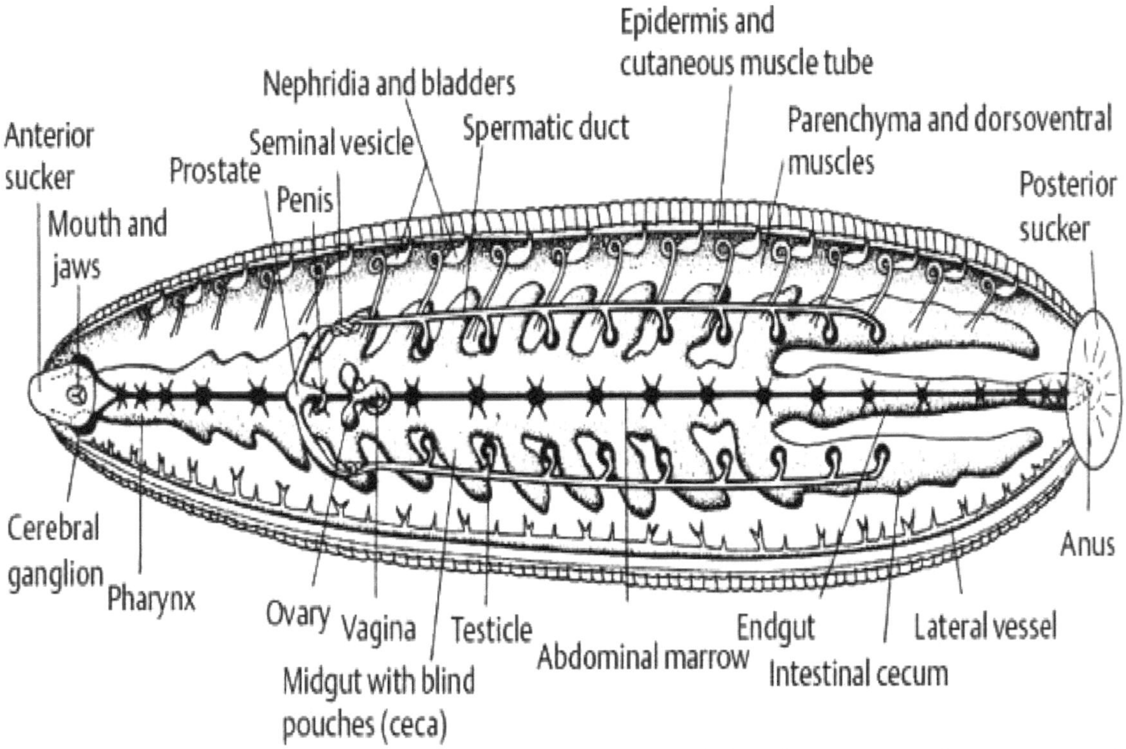

A complicated creature that has been used in field medicine for thousands of years. Leech saliva contains some one hundred pharmacologically active substances like hirudin, hyaluronidase, vasodilators, anesthetics, antibacterials and collagenase, and agents injected into the human body while sucking blood. The proteins in leech salvia helps numb pain and reduces swelling and was a form of wound care extensively during the American Civil War. Currently, thousands of leeches are dispensed every day for post-operative surgery where fingers and toes are reattached and in some plastic surgeries the leeches remove blood at surgical site and reduce hydraulic pressure. Before placement, they are radiated to sterilize and prevent reproduction. Another creature from past medical history used today are fly larvae, maggots. These are also irradiated and placed into wounds where they eat dead flesh, essentially debriding or debulking wounds. CDC

The Systems

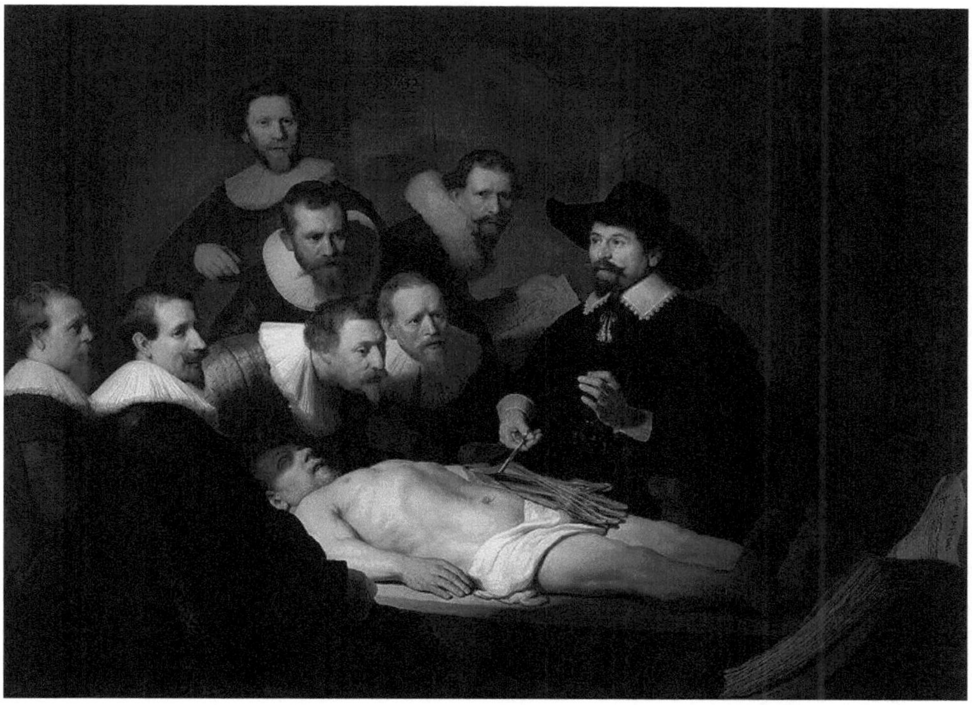

"The Anatomy Lesson of Dr. Nicolaes Tulp," Rembrandt 1632. Protestant Netherlands had finally fought off Catholic Spain, releasing the repressive educational system from the Church, especially dissections.

Human dissection is a foundation of modern medical education; however, since ancient times, dissection was banned through Western Civilization until the last four hundred years. Galan, the best-known medical officer of the Roman Empire, illustrated his human medical anatomy texts with dissections of North African apes. Galan's care of injured gladiators and soldiers with opened body cavities, exposed him to the interior of human bodies, however he was not allowed to dissect human cadavers. Hebrew, Greek, Roman, Moslem and Christian cultures all displayed an unexplained aversion for human dissection since earliest recorded medicine. Early human anatomists took risks, endured persecution and were sometimes executed for the practice of human dissection. Michelangelo and De Vinci along with other artists, used illegally obtained bodies for dissection in creating their life-like sculptures and paintings. Human dissection reveals the body in illness and health and its prohibition damaged medical education for two thousand years.

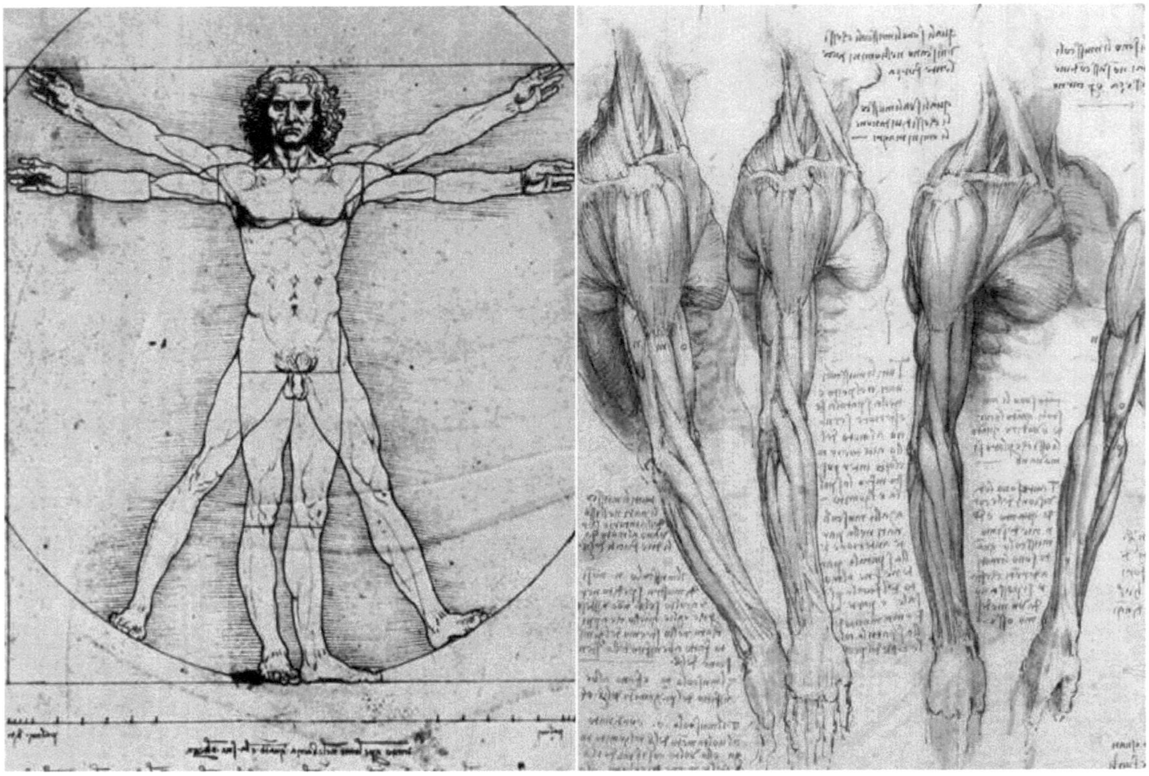

The detail of Leonardo de Vinci's anatomy drawings required cadavers and hours of dissection and study. Had he been inclined; he would have made a good surgeon.

The medical school the author attended used a novel method of teaching medicine at that time where basic sciences and clinical medicine were woven with the body's systems from the first day. Traditional training taught basic sciences first, followed by clinical medicine. This System approach combined medical sciences with clinical medicine and has been used by the author in lectures and this text, whereby the anatomy, physiology, pathology and pharmacology are discussed within each system. This blending was useful to the author during the long hours of lectures and was useful in training those at sea. The Orthopedic system is included in trauma and not discussed here. Once again, the author has combined and simplified concepts in the interests of the reader.

The Ear

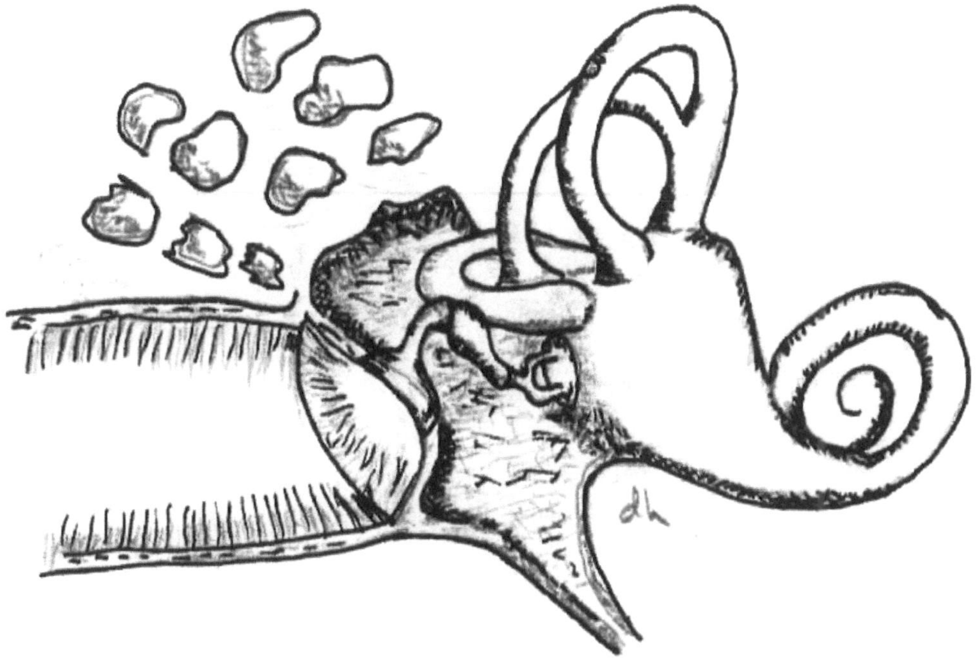

The author's drawing used during lectures to expose the internal ear

The ear serves several masters connecting the outside world to the central nervous system while tying the upper respiratory tract together. For the central nervous system, the inner ear serves as a listening post to the sounds around the body and provides the mechanism whereby the body maintains equilibrium. The external ear is part of the skin's blood and lymph circulation and in some animals, elephants and humans, it is important in heat radiation.

All vertebrae (segmented bony spine) animals share some characteristics of a middle and inner ear, especially the three semilunar (semi-circular) canals. Only mammals have a "coiled" cochlea. The most primitive mammal, platypus has only a .25-inch turn, while a whale has 1.75 inches of coil, man 2.75 inches, a cat 3 inches and the pig, a full 4 inches. Reptiles have a middle ear except for snakes, which instead of hearing sounds through an external ear detect vibrations with a segmented column of bone connecting the ear to the first vertebrae and thus to the long chain of hundreds of vertebrae. This links hundreds of "tuning forks" to the snake's nervous system, each vertebrae a listening post resulting in a sensitive replacement for sound-wave hearing, instead based solely on vibrations transmitted through the ground into the skeletal system and perceived by the snake nervous system. This allows the snake to identify the size, distance and direction of prey. The vibrations of a large animal not appropriate for food allows the snake to evade or in the rattlesnake, issue a warning of its presence.

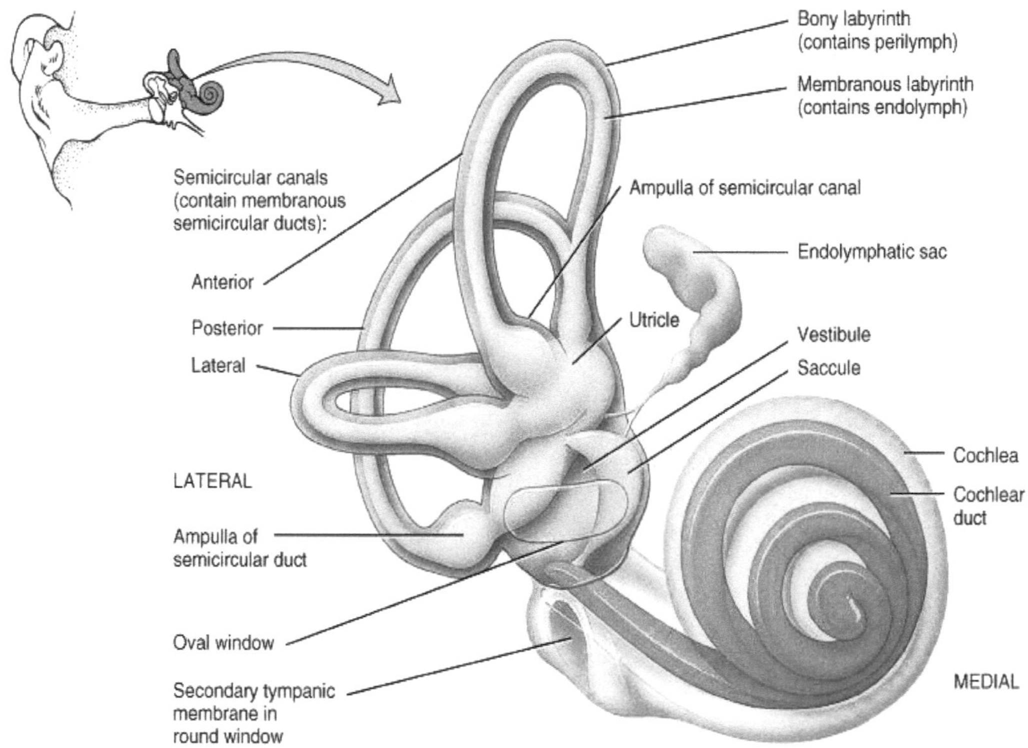

Image from NLM shows the relationship of the plumbing of hollow bones

Three interconnected hollow tubes form the labyrinth or vestibular system found in all animals with a segmented spinal cord (vertebrae). Sharks, rays and sturgeons have a cartilaginous notochord instead of segmented boney spinal cord have a vestibular middle ear and use iron to carry oxygen. Mollusca, especially the horseshoe crab and arthropods use copper to carry oxygen in blood and when exposed to oxygen turn blue instead of the red of humans. Mollusks are the true "blue bloods" of animals. The labyrinth is an elaborate plumbing system connected to a central reservoir of fluid, the ampulla. Within this swelling, created by an enlargement of the canal, resides the cupula. A complicated piece of plumbing that senses the orientation of the animal to the earth's center and is paramount to maintaining balance. Dizziness with spinning, which rapidly moves fluid through the cupula results in loss of balance. Alcohol intoxication also confuses the system, frequently leading to loss of balance. In migratory animals, it must be a major component of their navigational system. Head movements cause lymphatic fluid in the tubes to move, the motion bending tiny hair-like cilia which sends that information to the brain. Because the cilia are evenly matched on each side of the skull, like the stereo vision of two eyes.

Vertigo

A story from the author's medical training explains the difficulty in understanding and treating the complaint of "dizziness". Dizziness has many causes, but true vertigo has only a few. Many people confuse "lightheadedness" with dizziness, and both are vague complaints whereas vertigo is defined as a sense of rotation when no rotation is present. While doing ophthalmology training during internship, the author had the option of spending one day with the US Naval Hospital, San

Diego's expert in vertigo. Arriving promptly at 0800 at the medical officer's clinic and given a brief thirty-minute discussion on using a finger to diagnosis the presence of **nystagmus** (pupil bouncing after prompting a lateral gaze). This simple test is performed by having the patient look straight forward and follow the medical officer's finger with the eyes only as it quickly moves towards each ear. Normally when moving outside of eye orbit, the pupil may bounce back and forth once or twice. If the pupil enthusiastically bounces back and forth more than three "beats" of motion or the patient complains their symptoms worsen with this maneuver, this is diagnostic for true vertigo. The Navy's expert on vertigo then recommended a brief course of doxycycline for vertigo and upon removing his hat from the door, told me I knew enough about vertigo to see the patients coming to his clinic today and walking out. The author was only three months out of medical school and yet for a day was the expert on vertigo in the US Navy's largest and busiest medical center! Surprisingly, the two dozen vertigo patients seen accepted the author as an expert. Vertigo is a common complaint and yet is difficult to diagnosis and treat. Medications that may reduce the complaint include antihistamines such as diphenhydramine, scopolamine patches and perhaps doxycycline if an inner ear infection is suspected. However, it is a difficult and common complaint to manage in many cases.

Equilibrium

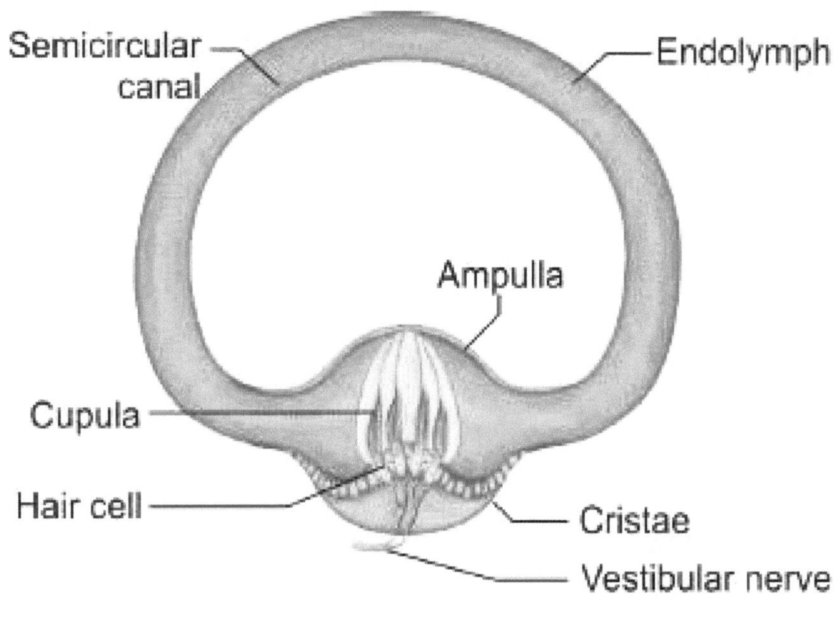

This drawing depicts only a single tube. NLM

Pitch, roll and yawl are motions monitored by labyrinth system, movements often encountered by pilots and seafarers. The system can be stimulated by running in circles, stunt flying, irregular motion, i.e., ship at sea, spinning on ice and the dance floor. Many nausea and seasick medications are designed to affect the vestibular system as it is likely responsible for the nausea of sea sickness. The vomiting control system in the brain is located near to inner ear. Pilots and astronauts go through extensive evaluations of their sensitivity of the labyrinth apparatus.

The Outer Ear

The outer ear is the visible part and composed of flexible cartilage covered with a thin gland-punctured skin. It is exquisitely sensitive to pain, effective in radiating heat and if injured, bleeds easily under the skin. Bleeding in the outer ear usually requires draining, otherwise a deformity known as a cauliflower ear may develop. If a discolored lump (hematoma) appears after ear trauma, it is best drained with a large bore needle, 16-20-gauge needle. Often 2-3 holes must be placed into hematoma to drain, and moist heat placed several times each day until fully drained. After incision and draining, continue warm soaks to encourage wounds to weep fluid and start antibiotics.

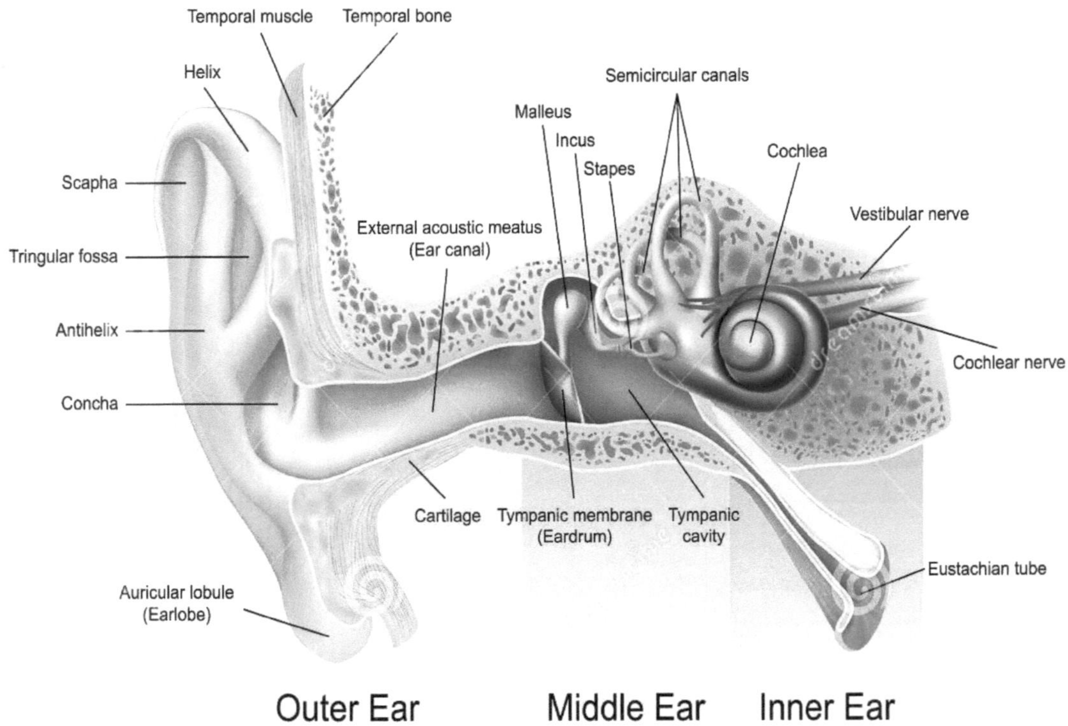

The outer ear is divided from middle ear by tympanic membrane and the middle ear separated from the inner ear by the tiny round window (pictured but not labelled) from the inner ear. NLM

Otitis externa, often called "swimmers' ear", causes pain, discomfort and sometimes discharge from ear. The ear canal contains glands that secrete the thickest oil of the body, cerumen. This heavy oil protects the easily injured external canal from trauma. Otitis externa is treated with antibiotic ear drops or a solution of vinegar and rubbing alcohol, applied 2-3 times daily. This common malady is seldom caused by swimming, but by invasion of the ear canal with an instrument. It is not a good idea to place anything smaller than the elbow into an external ear canal. In the case of African explorer Lieutenant John Speke, it was nearly fatal. In the 19th century, the search for the source of the Nile River had captivated Queen Victoria's explorers, the most famous were Speke and Sir Richard Charles Burton. Spending months in the East African bush was dangerous and Burton's training as a medical officer saved both their lives several times.

One night, an insect crawled into Speaks' ear and began to bite the exquisitely tender tissue. Burton was going to pour hot wax into the ear, but Speke panicked, grabbed a sharp object, and plunged it into his ear. This act resulted in traumatic perforation of his ear drum and a subsequent deep infection. In the age before antibiotics, this nearly killed him. Over the next weeks, Speke was so ill with fever, he had to be carried.

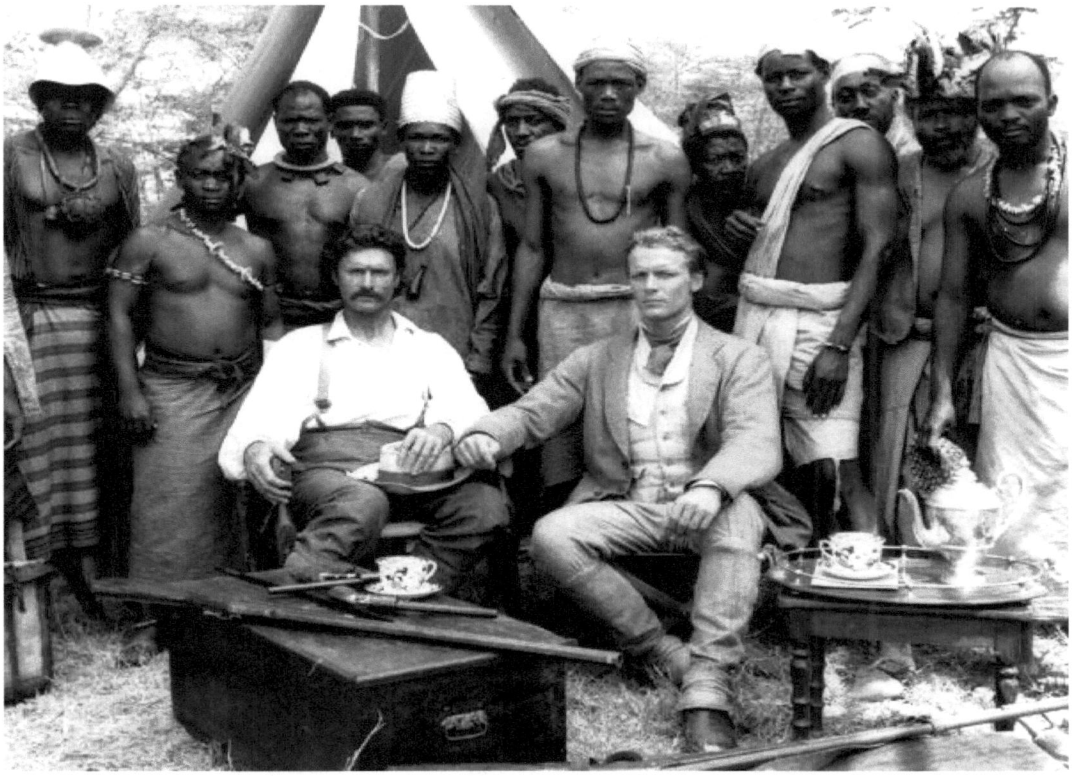

A still from the movie "Mountains of the Moon". Seated are the actors portraying Richard Burton and John Speke. An excellent movie and generally respects history except for a fictional meeting between Burton and Dr Livingstone.

The Middle Ear

On each side of the bones of the skull, connected by air passages, are a pair of air-filled cavities, the middle ears. These two cavities are embedded in bone, surrounded by hundreds of smaller cavities (mastoid air cells), enhancing the ear's acoustics. This honey-comb system is duplicated in many recording studios and similar structures are found in large stone cathedrals, designed under a dome with multiple floors opening into adjoining rooms. The Middle Age stone builders designed these structures for their acoustic properties, unknowingly imitating the human ear. Mastoid air cells not only improve reception of sounds, but they also aid in producing clear sounds. Hollow spaces within skull enhance and magnify the quality and resonance of the voice in singing and speaking, allowing amplification without distortion as well as making the skull lighter. The middle ear and its surrounding air cells are connected by a collapsible ventilation shaft, the eustachian tube, to the posterior mouth. This tube opens and closes throughout the day unnoticed, its periodic opening is important for a healthy middle ear and normal hearing. Unfortunately, this tiny canal surrounded by bone is readily blocked, leading to middle ear disturbances. It is the

Eustachian tube opening that causes the "pops" with pressure changes and sometimes achieved by clearing when diving or flying as pressure changes. Infections of the middle ear begin with blockage of the Eustachian tube, allowing collection and stagnation of mucus, which is quickly colonized by bacteria.

Blowing gently into the nose with its openings pinched closed (Valsalva maneuver), yawning widely, and gum chewing are methods to encourage a plugged Eustachian tube to open. Nasal spray containing decongestants or steroids are useful in treating and preventing Eustachian tube dysfunction. Prophylactic nasal sprays should be employed when pressure changes (diving, flying) are expected and the person with a previous history of ear discomfort.

Hearing

Suspended in the middle ears are the ossicles (bones) of hearing, the three smallest bones in the human skeleton. The malleolus (hammer), incus (anvil) and stapes (stirrup) form a lever-like bridge of three bones connecting the tympanic membrane (ear drum) to a much smaller window-like membrane on the other side of the middle ear. As sound waves strike the ear drum it oscillates back and forth moving first the malleolus which then strikes the incus (hammer on anvil). This motion produces oscillation of the stapes, which is connected to a footplate, the round window, which is located on the far side of the middle ear.

On the other side of the thin flexible round window is a wafer-thin, (snail-like) tube of bone, the cochlea (Latin for spiral), filled with a special type of lymph fluid. As the round window moves inward and outward with the plunger action of the stapes, fluid waves radiate into and through the cochlea, like ripples in a pool. The cochlea contains an extension of the central nervous system, the Organs of Corti, which contain the auditory receptor cells. To the author, the cochlea appears as a vast microscopic underwater kelp forest, some 55,000 separate nerve fibers swaying back and forth in the currents of a tiny sea. Movement of the fibers stimulates the nerve endings at the base of each hair embedded in the cochlear wall, converting fluid wave energy into electrical energy. These waves of generated electrical current are carried by the acoustic nerve to the brain where it is processed into music, birdsong, spoken words, thunder, waterfall, pin dropping, amazing! What a piece of engineering.

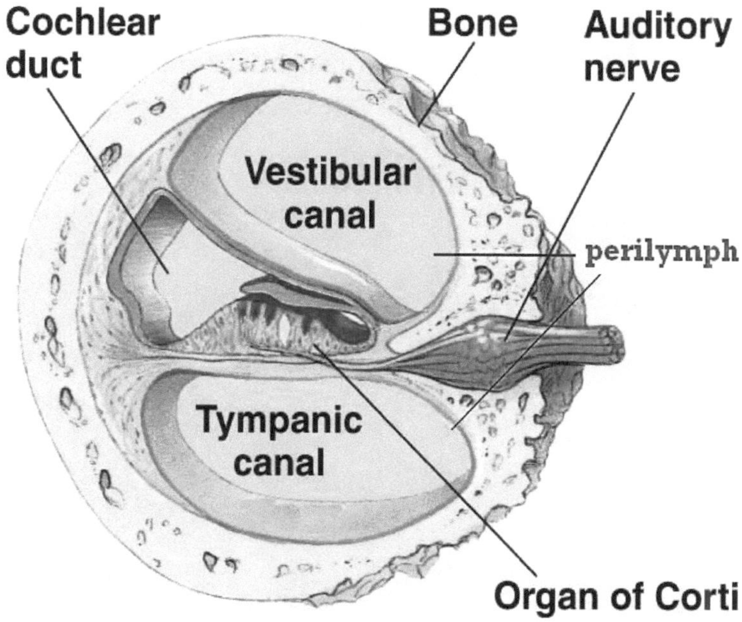

An artist's rendition of the site where mechanical energy converted to electrical. NIH

This microscopic energy transfer system, whether the result of evolution or a single act of creation, is capable of amplifying sound waves some thirty-three-fold, providing the ear is healthy. This amplification is almost distortion free because of the apparatus' suspension within the walls of the tiny air-filled acoustic cathedral of the middle ear. The acoustic chamber itself is surrounded and connected to the echo chambers of sinuses and thousands of mastoid air cells. Hard to believe this system was not designed.

The inner ear, with its network of canals, is responsible for balance as well as hearing. The system is formed of three hollow half circles of bone, the semilunar canals, oriented in 90-degree angles to each other. Through a series of nerves, both centers are in direct communication with their twin system on the other side of the skull. These hollow tubes, like the cochlea, contain a form of lymph fluid, which moves back and forth in the canals with head motion. Fluid movement is detected by fine hair-like nerves whose tops are embedded in a gelatinous membrane (which decreases sensitivity) and atop this layer sat microscopic rocks of calcium (otoliths-Latin for ear rocks). The author believes that people with larger otoliths probably experience less seasickness as the heavier rocks suppress motion of the hairs with semilunar canals. The size and number of these hairs bent by the current, communicate to the brain the direction and velocity of movement, orienting the brain to the direction of the Earth's center, allowing the body to remain in balance.

The most common complaint of inner ear dysfunction is a loss of balance or dizziness. Dizziness is the sensation of rotational movement when there is no movement. To a medical officer, this symptom is vertigo. Many people confuse dizziness with lightheadedness which has many causes. Vertigo usually has only one cause, inner ear dysfunction. True dizziness can be brought on by sea motion, excessive body spinning, infection, circulation problems, fear of heights, multiple sclerosis, and drugs such as alcohol. If it comes on suddenly, it is probably an infection. On the other hand, if the complaint is intermittent, it may be due to poor circulation or other equally vague causes (Meniere's disease). Vertigo is a common complaint, especially with aging with a poor chance of relieving it with current therapy. Antihistamines such as Benadryl or scopolamine patches can be employed if there is a fear of falling

The Nose

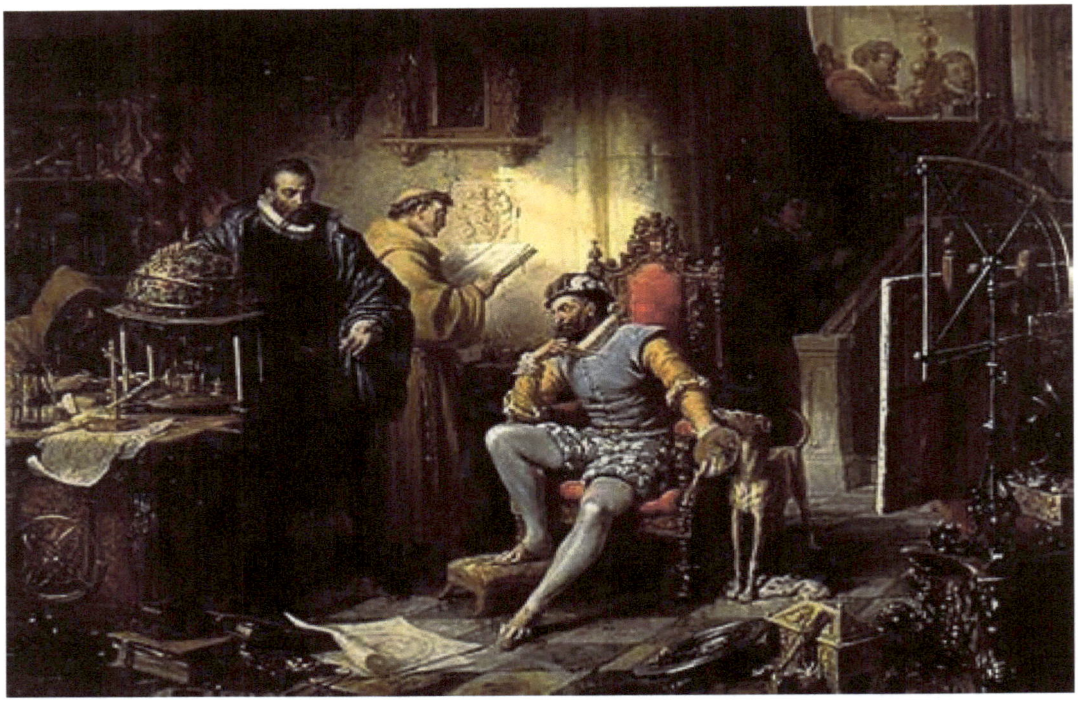

Eduard Ender (1822-1883) painting of Brahe Tyco (seated) delivering his handmade the globe to Emperor Rudolf II of Austria in the late 16th century. In this painting, Tycho still has a nose. Later he wore a silver nose piece to cover his lost nose, claimed to be the result of a duel where it was "bitten" off, however, many noses were lost in the 16th century due to syphilis. Tyco designed some of Northern Europe's most impressive forts of his day, some withstood 20th century assaults. The almost blind mathematician, Johannes Kepler, Tyco's assistant spent years trying to obtain the planetary observations Tyco had accumulated. Kepler needed the dates of planetary positions over several centuries to prove his math equations for the planetary motions. Kepler near blindness led him discover that light passes through the lens creating vision and invented corrective lens.

Noses have several functions in man and other animals, especially in those depending on odors for hunting or defense (especially sensitive to smoke). The nose is best known for its sense of smell provided by an elaborate olfactory system whose primary function is detection and identification. Some snakes evolved an olfactory system, the Organ of Jacobson that can smell airborne chemicals delivered on the tongue. In humans, smell is less important for survival and the nose serves its primary function as guardian of the respiratory tract. It is important in humans for food taste, sexual arousal and the identification of possible harmful odors. Mechanically, the olfactory system and the surrounding nose is connected to the skull by a complex system of suspended ligaments and highly mobile facial muscles.

Under normal conditions, most air enters the airways through the nose, allowing it to filter, warm, humidify and condition air brought to the lungs in nature's perfect sauna. In the roof of the nasal cavern at the back of the nose, odors are brought to the brain via tiny sensory nerves penetrating the thin cribriform plate at the base of the skull. The cribriform bone is the thinnest and most fragile skull bone. Inside the nose there are spiraling thin plates of bone, the turbinates, covered with moist mucus-secreting glands. This convoluted corrugated surface of the internal nose provides a large surface area where debris can be trapped, preventing many particles from reaching the lungs. This large surface allows drugs such as nasal sprays to be absorbed. The interior nose surface area when added to the capacity of the sinuses, provides ample space for mischief such as allergies or infections. Lining the sinuses are moist walls, thick with glands, draining outward to the back of the nose. Imagine a network of thousands of microscopic springs in hundreds of dark damp warm caverns well-ventilated and with running streams. These caves and passageways lined with a soft living carpet-like moist tissue, tall columns of cells of the respiratory tract and is like the lining of the vagina.

Where the respiratory tract meets exterior skin along the nose's entrances, lie areas prone to infections. Borderlands in human history were sites of friction (especially between England and Scotland) where conflict and injury were common as is the borders of the nose, where respiratory moist mucosa meets normal dry skin bacteria serves as sites for infection. Most infections caused by opportunistic infections (normal flora). Skin infections in and around the nose are minor wounds usually caused by unwashed fingers brought into the nose. Frequent nose-wiping with the runny nose of a cold can injure skin and lead to infection by normal bacteria. The most common cause of nasal lining injury is nose picking, where skin bacteria are traumatically introduced to the delicate mucosa via the evacuation by fingernail. Infections around the nasal openings such as impetigo will cause a red raised tender sores covered with yellow scales. The presence of a green discharge, foul odor and fever should alert to a deeper nose or sinus infection. Skin infections around the nose are treated with gentle bathing with medicated soap and topical antibiotics (Silvadene) along with oral antibiotics such as erythromycin if not responding to topical therapy.

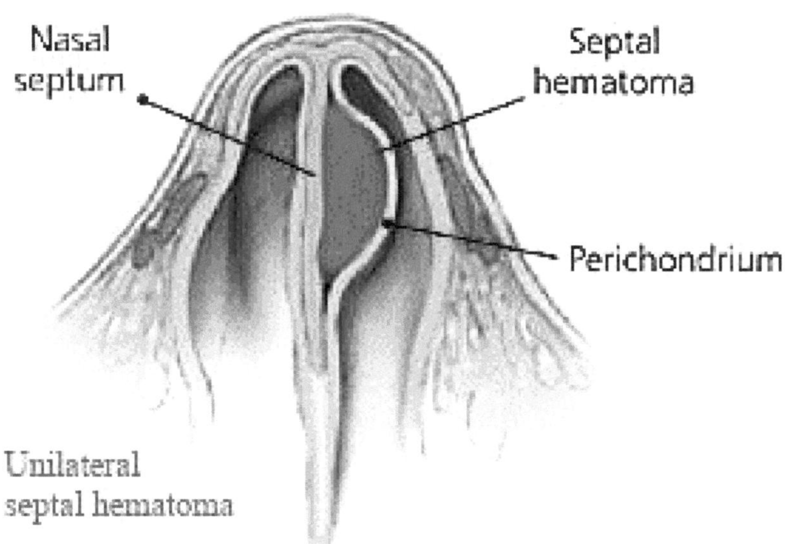

Like the hematoma of the outer ear, septal hematomas must be drained, and infection prevented, or deformity of nose will be permanent. NIH

Blunt trauma to the nose can fracture the nasal bone, a short thin shelf of bone in the upper nose between the eyes. In addition to swelling and bleeding, trauma can deform the cartilage that forms most of the nose. If nasal fracture is suspected, treat with ice and fix later. A septal hematoma, where blood forms around the central pillar of cartilage that separates the nose into two compartments, must be treated surgically and soon after injury. In examination of the nasal openings with a bright light, a septal hematoma appears like a bright "cherry-red" bulge in one side of the medial nose. This should be opened with a large needle or small knife and the blood removed as soon as possible, as failure to do so within a few days of the injury can lead to permanent deformity. Use antibiotics if a hematoma is drained or if there are visible wounds along with hot soaks.

Nosebleeds

This is a common event that normally is more of a nuisance than a serious medical problem. However, recurrent nosebleeds may indicate a more severe underlying problem, i.e., cancer, bleeding disorder, infection and in rare cases, life-threatening blood loss. One of the more famous deaths attributed to a nosebleed (epitasis) was that of Atilla the Hun, a nosebleed of significance in the history of Western Europe. Over generations, the Huns had violently migrated from plains of central Asia, raiding and displacing people in their path as they moved west. Atilla which translated as "little father" had spent time as a young man with a Roman aristocratic youth hopefully to reduce Hun aggressiveness. As an adult and senior chief of the Hun tribes he appeared in the year 451 with a huge, mounted army on the bulwarks of the Roman Empire. The rulers of Rome and its clinging Empire had been paying annually in gold to prevent Huns from attacking the militarily impotent empire. Atilla was no uneducated barbarian, he spoke several languages and was literate in Latin. The Roman youth he grew up with became general Aetius who confronted him in Gaul and though Aetius knew Atilla and Hun military tactics, Atilla was confident his army was larger and more mobile. The Hun was surprised when the Roman army he faced included Rome's arch enemy, the Visigoths under Theodoric I. Somehow Aetius had formed a temporary truce with an enemy increasing both the size and mobility of the allied forces. Atilla reluctantly engaged the larger than expected Roman forces in a battle on the bloody Catalaunian Plains near the city of Chalons in present day France, leaving 162,000 men dead and unburied. Both armies were so mutilated, there was no further enthusiasm for conflict. Medical records are scant from this battle, the scantiness mutes a great deal of suffering of the wounded. After the battle, Atilla returned to his chieftains affirming his leadership among the Hun clans after his first defeat. He begins recruiting an army estimated at one-half million and plans to invade Italy following the winter. Considering the weakness and dissention within the remnants of Rome and knowing he would not face the Visigoths again, he could have likely taken both the city and empire, sweeping away much of the vestiges of Roman Europe. Except for a timely posterior nosebleed, the history of the western world could have been much different.

Atilla, facing the lonely winter months and eager to appear manly and warrior-like among the tribes feeding his army, married a young nubile maiden, Ildico, the daughter of a local chief. To celebrate the union and to entertain his captains, he presided over a large feast complete with heavy wine consumption (unusual for the normally sober Atilla). After the party, sometime during the nuptial rites, a blood vessel burst in Atilla's posterior nose and owing to a combination of excitement, sexual bravado and intoxication, the mighty "little father" bled to death. The morning after the wedding, found his young widow crying over a cold stiff body. Deprived of leadership, the army scattered, leaving an important enclave of western civilization intact for a few more decades.

Anterior Nosebleeds

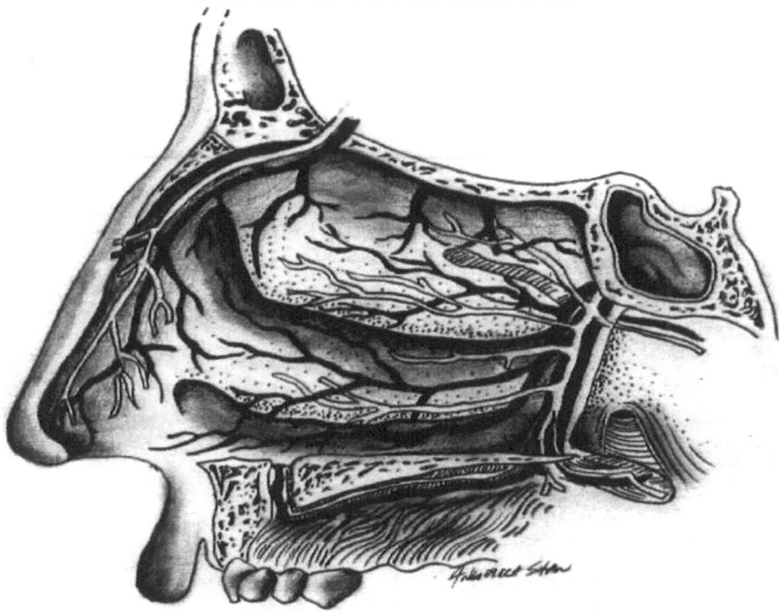

The nose is well supplied with blood by large numbers of veins and arteries flowing along the damp nasal passages. The moist surface of the internal nose can bleed profusely if injured or if blood vessel ruptures. Bleeding in the back of nose can be difficult to manage. Nasal mucosa contains erectile tissue over the turbinates that swell as capillaries fill with extra blood. A common side effect of erection-inducing agents (Viagra) is nasal congestion. The internal nose is an excellent place to absorb medicines and drugs such as decongestants, pain medications and hormones as nasal sprays. Angelica Magar

There is a site in the anterior nose on each inboard side of the middle pillar (septum) that divides the nose into two openings (nares), where many small blood vessels lie close to the surface. The mucosa here is thin and easily injured when dry. Dry heat, excessive nose blowing or more commonly, nose picking, are the most common causes of nosebleeds of this area known as Kesselbach's Triangle.

In the anterior nosebleed, bleeding is bright red, limited to one side and usually appears worse than it is (especially if a white shirt or towel is used to staunch bleeding). Bleeding is best controlled by pressure, ice and gravity. This is accomplished by pinching the nose, tilting the head back, and applying ice to reduce bleeding and swelling. Drugs such as aspirin should be avoided since it increases risk of bleeding. The appearance of recurring nosebleeds should alert to other more subtle underlying causes such as infection, hypertension, blood clotting abnormality, cancer, and in children, a foreign body. Bleeding that persists should be evaluated at the earliest convenience by a physician.

After bleeding has subsided, the nose should be checked to identify the bleeding site so that a small amount of nosebleed ointment can be applied. The recipe for this poultice in equal parts; Silvadene cream, petrolatum (Vaseline), steroid cream (hydrocortisone 2 ½ %) and estrogen cream (Premarin). The authored prepared and dispensed this nose-bleed salve hundreds of times in practice. Silvadene acts to reduce bacteria, controlling infection. Petrolatum forms an air barrier reducing drying. Anti-inflammatory steroid lowers the amount of inflammation, while estrogen thickens the skin overlying the vessels in the Triangle of Kesselbach (as it moistens and thickens vaginal mucosa in menopause). This preparation should be applied 3-4 times each day for at least seven days following the nosebleed. It is effective if used occasionally to prevent bleeding, especially if the area feels dry or inflamed.

Posterior Nosebleeds

Unlike anterior bleeds, these are rare events, occurring when a large vessel in the back of the nose suddenly ruptures or when a series of smaller ones begin to spontaneously leak. Possible causes include facial trauma, concussion, injuries from explosions, penetration of nose with a sharp object or in many cases, occurring with no warning or obvious cause. The blood is bright red, flowing freely from the nose, often on both sides and sometimes through the mouth. With head tilt and pressure, the blood is forced into the throat causing choking. Within minutes enough blood can be lost to initiate the cascade of shock.

If a posterior nosebleed is suspected, treatment must be rapid and effective. Historically, bleeds emanating from the posterior nose were difficult to manage even by trained medical personnel. Ear, nose, and throat surgeons were often called to the emergency room to place cumbersome packs of sponges through the mouth and pulled into the posterior nose. This takes time and expertise, things not readily available in the field. Fortunately, there is an effective and relatively easy procedure for packing the posterior nose with pressure dressing, accomplished with a modern balloon urinary catheter. Use of urinary catheters were developed and successfully deployed by innovative corpsmen during the Viet Nam War. These enlisted medics (field medical officers) developed life-saving techniques in field surgery with no anesthesia. Working far from surgical support, with simple drugs and little equipment, they saved lives and limbs. One of these techniques is placing a pressure pack in the posterior nose to staunch bleeding.

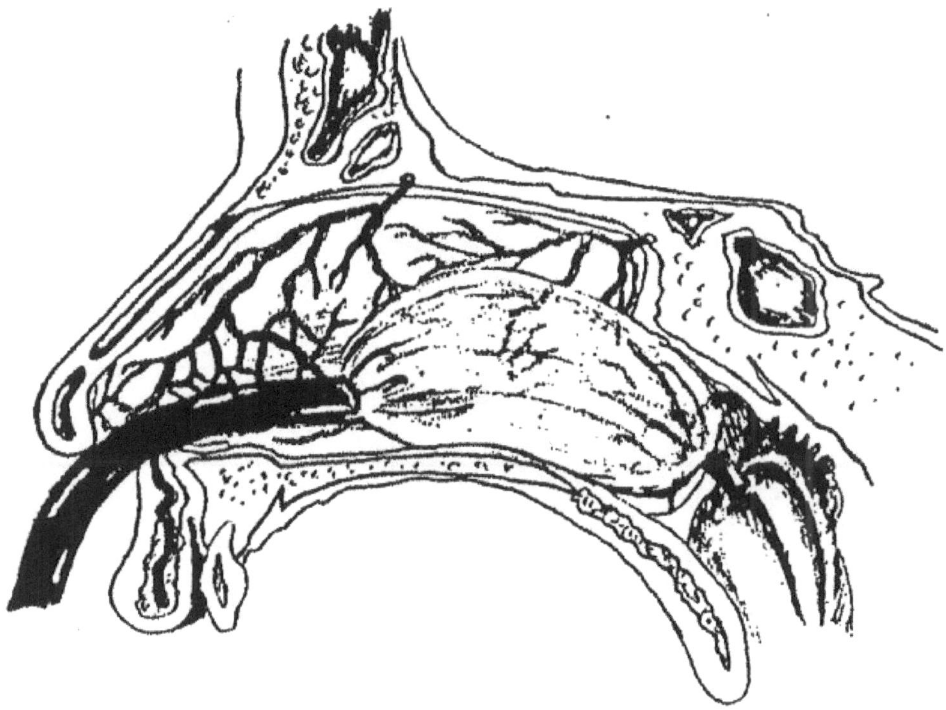

The competent placement of a urinary catheter in the internal nose should quickly reduce bleeding in a posterior nosebleed. There is some concern with filling the balloon with water as there is a small risk of the balloon rupturing and causing a near drowning. For this reason, some believe air might be a better choice to fill the balloon, however in the field, the author would use heavier water to fill.

The patient should be made comfortable, while briefly describing what is to be done and why. Two urinary catheters should be accessible in the medicine chest. These should be pre-lubricated with a water-soluble lubricant such as K-Y jelly, do not use petroleum base lubricates (Vaseline) as they can get into the lungs causing severe lipid pneumonia. Check the balloons quickly for leaks by filling fully with water and deflating them. The amount of water needed to fill the balloon is printed on the catheter, usually 30-50 cc. Since blood may be visible from both sides of the nose, choose the most likely side first. Insert the catheter gently through the nose until the tip is visible at the back of the throat. The balloon is then inflated to the cuff volume that is stamped on the side of the catheter. At least 30 cc of volume is needed to firmly fit the irregular walls of the posterior nose. Apply traction on the catheter pulling the filled balloon from the posterior throat firmly into the back of nose. If bleeding continues, secure this first catheter, and catheterize the remaining side. These catheters should be left in place for three days to prevent re-bleeds. The patient is placed on antibiotics to reduce the large numbers of bacteria that stagnant blood and pooled mucus will attract. At the end of three days, the catheters should be deflated and gently worked back and forth to dislodge a catheter anchored with dried blood and mucus. Nosebleed ointment should then be applied gently to the chafed, inflamed areas around the nasal entrances that the catheter will leave behind.

The Sinuses

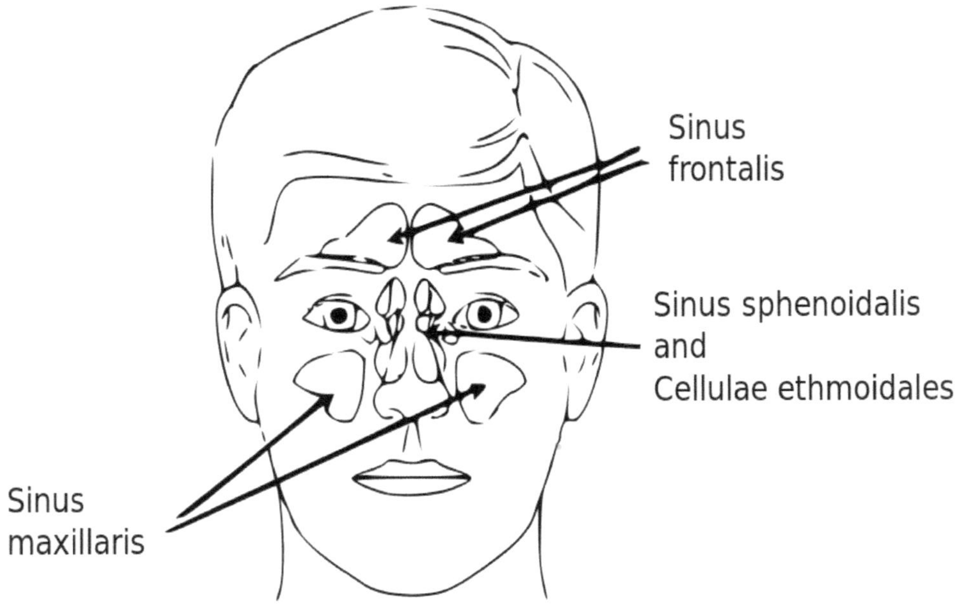

The human skull, especially the area behind the face, is honeycombed with air-filled cavities. Cavities that seem to have little use except to torment them with congestion, discharge and pain. However, they are important for humans to maintain health and for human history. The sinus system has played a major role in human development, for without the sinuses, civilization might not have happened. Sinuses are barely present at birth, growing larger and more complex as the head increases in size. The largest sinuses are found behind the face and via the Eustachian tube are connected to the air-filled middle ear. The middle ear in turn communicates to hundreds of tiny sinuses in the bone surrounding the ear (acting as acoustic chambers enhancing the quality of hearing). The sinuses are covered with tall column-shaped cells that secrete a thin film of mucus that is gently "whipped" in the direction of the sinus's exit by microscopic hair-like cilia. If this flow is blocked, it becomes an ideal site for bacterial infection. Sinus infections can be triggered by allergies, a cold, smoke, air pollution and dental problems. The infection is manifested by headache, face pain, green cloudy mucus, a bad taste in the mouth (especially in the morning) fever and foul breath. Sinus infection can trigger wheezing in people with asthma.

Examination in suspected sinusitis may reveal tenderness or pain relief with firm finger pressure over the sinuses. The voice may sound nasal, changing the quality of speech and often accompanied by “muffled” hearing. When X-ray is not available, the sinus can sometimes be visualized through the thin facial bone with a bright light in a dark room. Place a bright penlight firmly against the skin at the base of one eye directing the light downward. With the mouth open, compare the amount of light penetrating the roof of the mouth under each eye. Decreased light on one side may indicate the maxillary sinus is fluid-filled. Another method is to press the light up from the roof of the mouth with the eyes closed and ask if the sensation of light is greater or diminished on one side. These techniques may help determine which of the sinuses is filled with fluid and can be used to monitor the progress of treatment.

Steamy showers or mist machines are helpful in thinning sinus fluid, allowing for normal flow of mucus secretions to their exits. The use of antihistamines and decongestants, especially nasal steroid spray, may also be helpful in clearing the obstruction. Antibiotics are needed to treat or reduce the risk of infection, which because of its proximity to the brain, could lead to a life-threatening infection. Useful antibiotics are amoxicillin, erythromycin, cephalosporins, Sulfa and doxycycline. Due to its single dose for three days, the best choice is azithromycin (Zithromax).

The largest of the facial cavities are the maxillary sinuses lie on each side of the nose below the eyes. There is a smaller, but important cluster between and above the eyes. When combined with the complex system of air sacs around the middle ear space, these echo chambers and humidifiers provide a large surface area allowing the human voice to be greatly amplified. All these cavities are interconnected to each other, the throat and the nose, providing a significant air-filled volume for projection of the voice in public speaking, singing, and in times of anger or assault, for yelling. An example of the survival effects of the sinuses can be found in another mammal that, like mankind, has a significant sinus system. This animal is the small rat-like rodent found in the rock islands of the Serengeti plains of east central Africa. The hyrax lives in deep burrows among these rocky mounds in a world of darkness. It has many enemies with few tools to protect itself. Its most important protection is its loud growl for its diminutive size which is due to a skull filled with echo chambers, producing a snarl that sounds like it belongs to a much larger animal. The ability to produce a loud noise in a dark tunnel is effective in discouraging would be hyrax-eaters. Enhanced vocalization was surely helpful when humans were hunted at night in the treetops or in caves and the production of a loud voice likely saved predation.

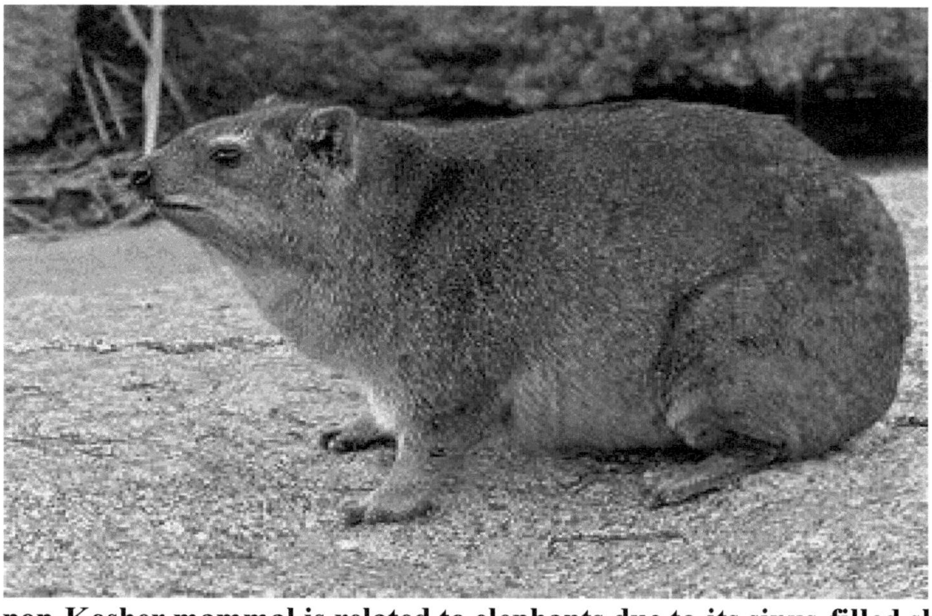

This tiny non-Kosher mammal is related to elephants due to its sinus-filled skull. Like elephants, its skull design enables loud, long-carrying vocalizations. Elephant trumpeting can be heard for miles and is the loudest vocalization of any mammal. Animals Library

The ability to vocalize to hundreds or perhaps thousands of people was important in inspiring armies, directing warfare, building complex structures such as the Pyramids and the Greek Parthenon, giving orders on a large sailing vessel and the rise of religions. The bone chilling "rebel call" that echoed from the throats of Robert E. Lee's 12,000 troops at Gettysburg on the 3rd day of battle was possible because thousands of sinuses resonating with similar pitched screams. Some Union soldiers claimed the sound was worse than the bullets. The Sermon on the Mount would have been less effective without the sinus system, otherwise Christ's voice would have only been heard by those standing close to him and the range of sounds available would have been quite small. Diminished sinus capacity (as in upper respiratory infections) reduces both the quality and volume of voice used in speech and song. In addition to amplifying voice, sinuses serve the respiratory tract by warming, humidifying and filtering the incoming air to the lungs.

Located in the front of the face, above between and below the eyes, these air-filled spaces make for the lighter, larger skull that is supported by a comparatively small human frame. The sinuses are lined with respiratory mucosa that produces some 500 cc (16 oz) of mucus each day. This mucus drains into the upper rear part of the throat, an area that becomes irritated when mucus membrane becomes inflamed. Sinuses can become congested causing pain and pressure, sore throat and headache. Sinus mucus, if allowed to pool and be stagnant, will breed bacteria within a closed space, sometimes causing intense pain and pressure behind the face. Although antibiotics are helpful in sinus infections, the problem will not be clear until the sinus is once again open and draining. In the pre-antibiotic era, sinus infections were more than a nuisance, they were chronic, foul smelling, disfiguring and sometimes fatal as bacteria penetrated the protective bone and entered the sterile brain. Even if non-fatal, it could become a life-long infection, destroying the tiny bones of hearing, producing a constant foul breath, and distorting the underlying structure of the face. Chronic sinus infection along with syphilis, smallpox and leprosy were common causes of facial deformities.

Headaches

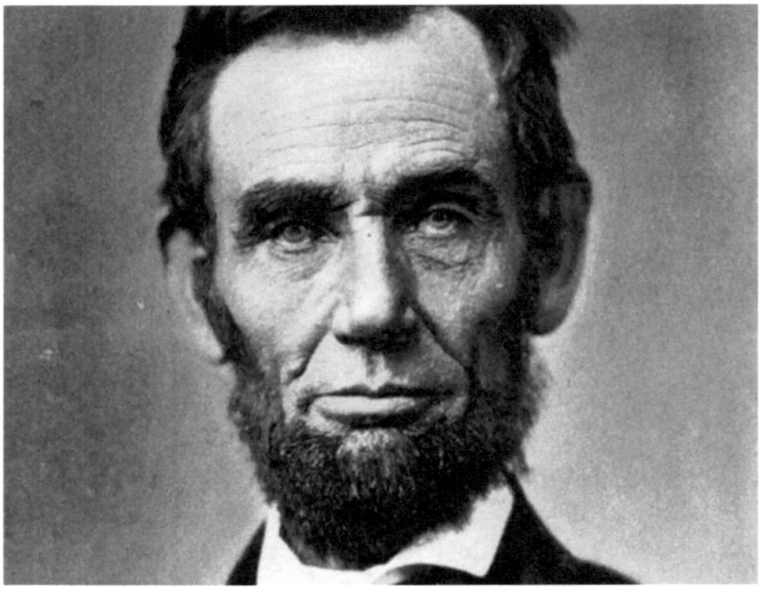

One of American history's most famous chronic headache victims. Pain and the stress of four long bloody years of war show in his face. Prior to his election as president, Lincoln was retired after only a single term in Congress since he was one of the very few

Congressmen to oppose the American Mexican War, believing the war was immoral. Ironic that he opposed a very popular war and later directed an immensely unpopular and bloody conflict between the States. National Archives

This common malady has long plagued humans, continuing today as a major cause of pain and the most common reason of referrals to neurologists. Headaches have many causes, including infection, allergies, muscle spasm, dilating blood vessels in the brain that increase intracranial pressure (classic migraine or vascular), stress and eye strain. Other, rarer causes are increased blood pressure, cardiovascular accident (stroke) and tumor. Although nausea and vomiting are common with severe headaches, if vomiting becomes unrelenting, look for the danger signs of increased intracranial pressure; a dilating pupil and decreasing alertness. Many headaches can be treated with success if the proper diagnosis is made. History of previous headaches and treatment are helpful in determining the probable cause and selecting the proper treatment. Headache therapy usually involves some mechanical components such as ice, heat or massage combined with medications. Headaches often have more than one mechanism causing pain; therefore, many headaches have mixed causes and therefore do not perfectly fit the following descriptions. Do not be surprised if the history, symptoms and physical findings of headaches overlap two or more of the headaches types.

Muscle Tension Headaches

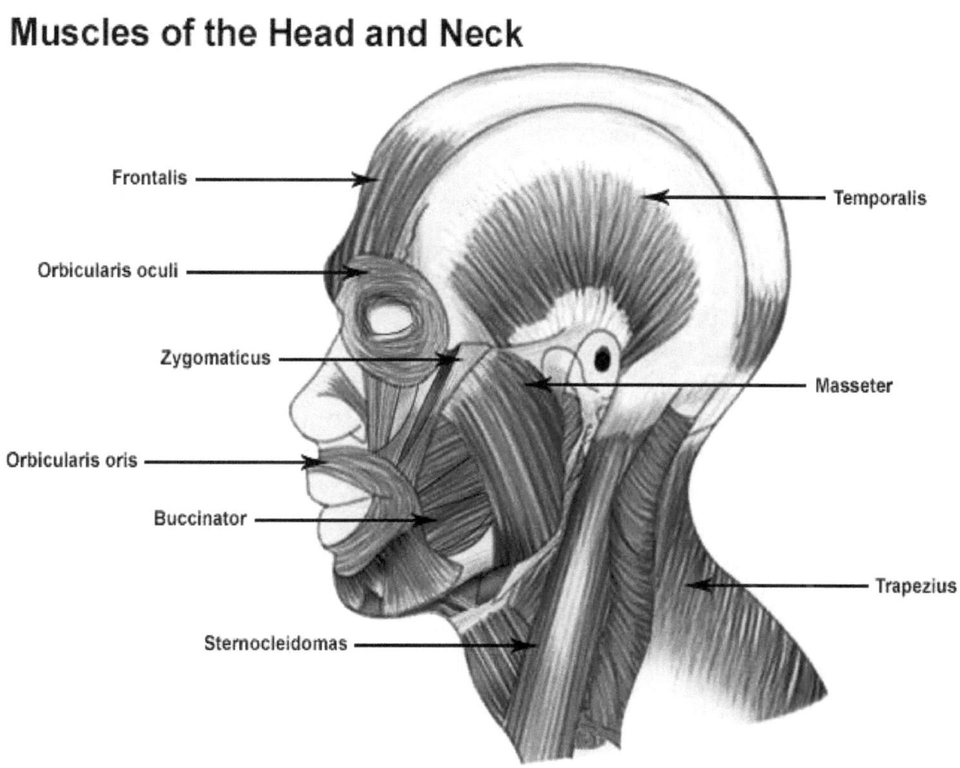

Head muscles tend to be long and thin, capable of sustained contractions, leading to pain. NIH

The head and neck are completely sheathed in muscle fibers, tendons, and sheets of thin strong connective tissue. These are arrayed in groups, allowing for head and neck movement as muscles contract and relax. Pain results in when muscles, normally soft and relaxed, become firm, shortened and tender. If muscles contract in a sustained spasm, they reduce motion in joints and begin to put tension on the scalp, causing a headache that may begin in the upper neck, spread over the top of the head, and settle behind the eyes. The pain is aggravated by head movement, especially when neck muscles are stretched. Often there will be small tender firm "bumps" or swellings along the back of the neck and tender areas at the skull's base. Gentle pressure over these tender sites followed by equally gentle stretching of these areas often results in decreased pain. Ice placed over the back of the neck and at the base of the skull will also decrease pain. Aspirin, Tylenol, anti-inflammatory drugs and opiates may reduce the discomfort. Mechanical treatment includes ice for 20 minutes, followed by gentle traction to the base of the skull and gentle stretching of the head forward on the chest with side-to-side motion until the patient reports reduction of pain.

Migraine Headache

It is believed that in a migraine headache, arteries within the brain dilate, increasing blood flow which translates as increased pressure to the brain tissue. The reason for this vascular dilation is not understood, but in the classic migraine it produces an "aura" or visual hallucination, such as streaks or flashes of lights before the pain begins. This is the most effective time for treatment before the actual headache begins. Blood vessel constrictors such as ergotamine and caffeine are useful, but only in the early aura stage, not after the headache begins. The pain is normally one-sided and is associated with light sensitivity, nausea, vomiting, scalp tenderness and perhaps some temporary loss of vision on the side of headache. Chocolate, alcohol, ice cream, nicotine, exhaustion, anxiety and emotional distress are known to trigger migraine. Commonly used drugs in the management of migraines are the ergot alkaloids, drugs derived from lowly fungus and the newer 5-hydrotryptophan blockers as well as beta blockers, anti-inflammatory drugs, opiates and seizure medications.

Ergotamine was a mainstay in migraine headaches during much of the author's practice while having an interesting medical history. Ergot is produced by fungi (*Claviceps purpurea*) invading the ovary of a grain, especially if poorly dried and damp. Contamination of grain, especially rye, produces a hard-purple ball (purpurea). When humans began cultivating grains, ergot became part of the human story. Consumption of spoiled grain was known to have an adverse effect on humans for thousands of years, especially in pregnancy, as it caused constriction of the uterus, killing the developing fetus. One of the sacred books of the Parsee (Zoroaster-worshippers Persians) from 400 BC: "among the evil things are noxious gasses that cause pregnant women to drop the womb and die in childbed". Skilled physicians and midwives had used ergotamine compounds for centuries for abortions and to staunch bleeding after birth. Its most notorious stories come from the dark Middle Ages when entire villages were stricken after eating moldy grain. It was known as St. Anthony's Fire as severe blood vessel constriction turned limbs black as charcoal, along with agonizing burning pain. Limbs would fall off like dead tree branches. In 15th century Europe, authors report some villages where hundreds were seemed to be dancing in pain, "Saint Anthony's

Dance", a few losing both arms and legs, producing a helpless living trunk, to be cared for by family or church.

Lysergic acid (LSD) is a water-soluble chemical produced with this plant-fungal ergot combination and has historical implications. Eating grains contaminated by fungi may contain enough psychoactive products to induce hallucinations (dreams while awake). Some believe the Salem Witch Hunts were driven by mass hallucinations of imagined witches because the village consumed lysergic acid in bread made from spoiled grain. Joan of Arc and her army experienced mass communal dreams the nights before overcoming larger English forces as she did at breaking the siege of Orleans. Some have attributed her vision and her army's success to eating bread tainted with LSD. Joan's success help end the English-dominated One Hundred Years War and like many heroes, her life ended in tragedy. Armies need food and often were reduced to eating moldy bread, possibly contaminated with psychoactive chemicals. Another story of shared dreams may have played a role in battles found in the Bible. Two examples were the dreams of Prophet Elisha and the Army of Angels in the Book of Kings and again in Gideon's 300 men against the Midianites in the Book of Judges. God told Gideon to reduce his army from 32,000 to only 300 men who consumed "barely bread and shared common dreams before the battle where the tiny Hebrew army routed an army of thousands. Perhaps there was only enough LSD for 300? LSD in low doses is now successfully used for PTSD by the Veterans Administration. "Foods of the Gods" by Terrence and Dennis McKenna is a fascinating and informative story of the biodynamics of plant-fungi interactions with humans. Most of the anti-depressants from fluoxetine (Prozac) to its many selective serotonin reuptake inhibitors (SSRIs) derivatives have been described as "detuned" LSD.

It is common practice in migraine headaches to give the patient an injection of opiate with promethazine (to reduce pain and nausea) hopefully to promote sleep. Most migraine sufferers will be awake without the headache if a restful sleep can be induced. Ergotamine drugs should be avoided in patients with possible heart disease, as they could precipitate a heart attack. Several new nasal sprays (butorphanol) are available for migraine and the most useful medications now include drugs containing the base chemicals called "sumatriptans".

Sinus Headaches

Pressure within the sinuses or middle ears can produce constant or intermittent headache. The pain is around the face and ears, usually associated with congestion or productive cough and perhaps low-grade fever. Placing thumbs over the sinuses and applying pressure will often cause pain if the sinus is infected. Hot showers or steam offer some temporary relief, as well as decongestants and antihistamines. Difficulty in clearing the Eustachian tubes (plugged ear), a foul taste or odor in the mouth (especially in the morning), and green mucus from the throat or nose are other signs of a sinus infection. In addition to steam, decongestants nasal sprays, antibiotics should be employed if this type of headache is suspected. Azithromycin 500 mg each day for three days is the author's favorite treatment.

Bell's Palsy

Pain on one side of face and head, followed by paralysis and dropping of facial muscles on the painful side is diagnostic of Bell's Palsy. This is not a rare condition as the author has seen dozens of cases. A condition of unknown cause that almost always resolves slowly without treatment over several weeks. Bell's Palsy can be temporarily painful and disfiguring, more frightening than dangerous. Reduced hearing and dizziness can be associated with this condition, some recommend short use of 60mg prednisone each day for three days and pain relief is helpful with anti-inflammatory meds of opiates. Although frightening for the patient, it usually resolves without sequelae, and in the author's experience, the first complaint is a dry eye in the mornings since the eye lid is not completely occluding the eye on affected side during sleep. Later, in may appear as a stroke (cardiovascular accident) due to flaccid appearance of the affected side of face. The major difference is the acuteness of a stroke verse the slower development of Bell's Palsy. The man who labelled this condition is another sea story.

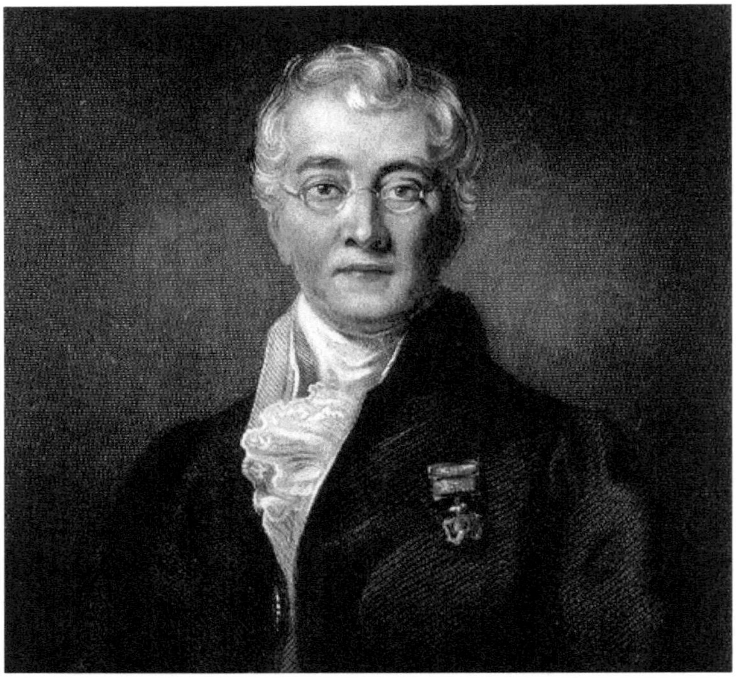

Sir Charles Bell, 1774-1842, born, raised and educated in Edinburgh, Scotland came from a privileged and well-educated family. His three older brothers served as professors in medicine, literature and law. Bell was a rare combination of surgeon, physiologist, artist, premier anatomist, philosopher, and was keenly interested in neurology. He helped establish the medical school in Kings College but soon resigned as his concepts of medicine clashed with older dogma. England's wars with Napoleon brought Bell into the army as a military field surgeon in 1809 and he served until Waterloo near the front under fire. Even though brave, he faced harsh criticism from other British medical officers for poor surgical skills. After the battle of Waterloo, Bell operated continuously for three days and nights on wounded French soldiers, primarily doing amputations. His 90% death rate in amputations was probably why he was not treating British wounded. Clearly, he was a better teacher, artist and anatomist than a field medical officer. Painting by Granger

Lymphangitis

A tender, soft lump in the soft neck tissue often accompanies infections in the head and neck, i.e., facial pimples, ingrown hairs, upper respiratory tract infections and in rare cases, cancer of the lymph nodes. Persistent lumps in the neck should be evaluated by a physician as should any chronic discomfort in the neck and throat. The larynx is a box-like structure containing vocal cords and can be an access port in an upper airway obstruction. In the field, tender, enlarged lymph nodes are treated with antibiotics. The author recommends azithromax as the drug of choice.

Head and Neck

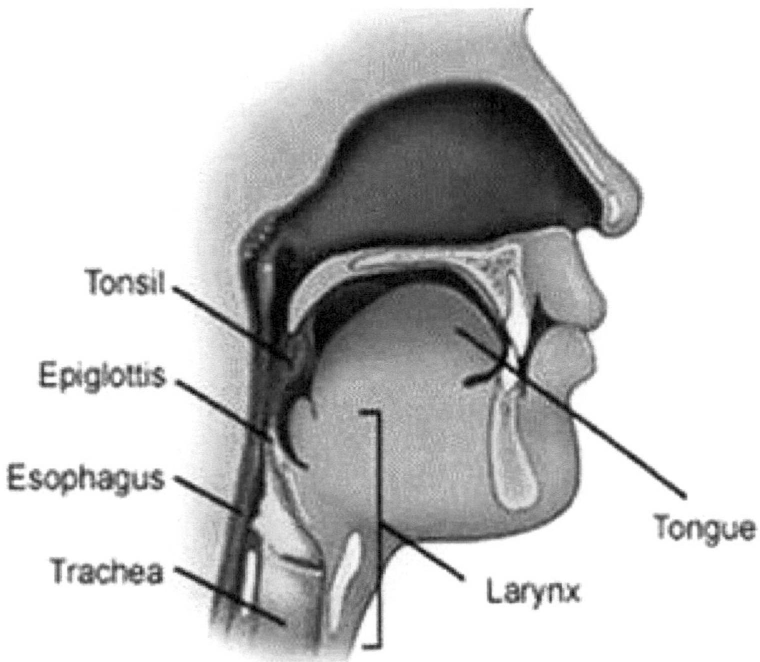

Major structures of the neck and throat. NLM

The neck is primarily composed of soft tissue surrounding the cervical spine bones. Outside the bony spine, the tiny bones and cartilage of the larynx are the only firm objects palpated in the soft neck. The upper respiratory and gastrointestinal tract share a common opening, however, are quickly divided by epiglottis. Hoarseness, cough, pain and bleeding may have their cause in the neck and throat. Sore throat with fever and illness is usually caused by viral agents which are self-limiting. Strep throat, caused by a streptococcus bacteria can cause throat pain with fever, rash and generalized illness. Throat cancer is usually presents with coughing, sometimes with coughing up blood (hemoptysis), hoarseness and ear pain as ear canal and larynx shared common pain fibers. Weight loss, chronic sore throat and voice changes are common. Finding tender and non-tender lymph nodes in the neck indicate infection and too often cancer.

Epiglottis is a rare condition, primarily in children, that can be lethal if not treated with antibiotics. The symptoms occur quickly with high fever, difficulty in breathing, drooling and painful swallowing. For centuries, diphtheria was a deadly etiology of sore throat and primarily a killer of children. In diphtheria, the throat develops a thick white membrane caused by a toxin the diphtheria bacteria discharges. The membrane spreads and thickens, slowing choking the victim to death. A long and painful death, agonizing for patient and parent. Diphtheria is rare now because of immunizations; however, it is still around and an immunization for diphtheria should be given with tetanus every 10 years (dT).

The Cricothyrotomy

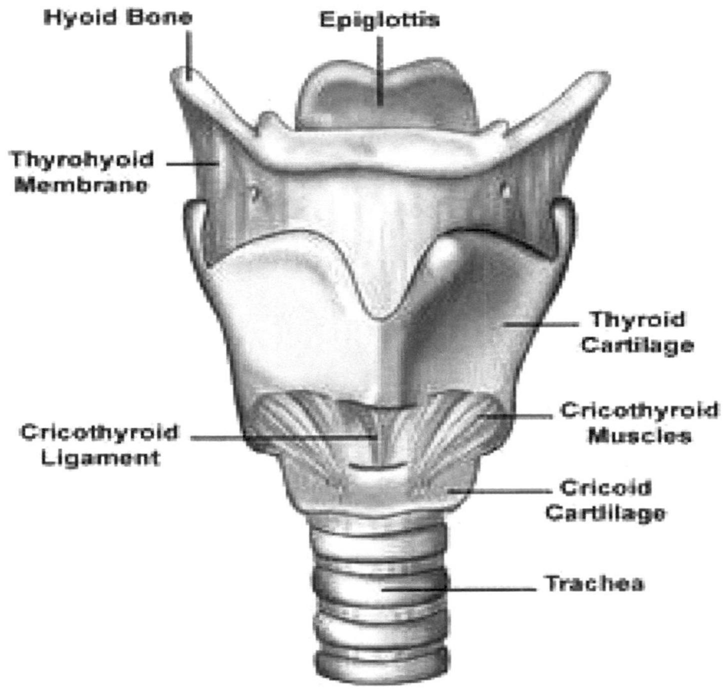

The cricothyroid membrane gives access to the upper airway in field surgery. NLM

Corpsmen in Viet Nam encountered upper airway obstruction in firefights that could not be cleared without field surgery. Tracheostomy is complicated, requires some type of anesthesia and is too difficult to do quickly in the field, especially under fire. A quick entry into the obstructed airway entry was needed to open the trachea in the field. Corpsmen innovated the concept of inserting a large hollow needle through the cricothyroid membrane, avoiding blood vessels and requires only a basic knowledge of anatomy and accomplished with a single surgical tool. In another type of cricothyrotomy, a vertical incision in made in the cricothyroid membrane and then the surgical blade is rotated sideways (horizontal) and the blade left in place while a hollow tube, i.e. straw or ink pen barrel inserted along knife blade. The blade is removed and hopefully an airway is established. A quicker, one-step procedure is the placement of a large bore, 14-gauge needle through the cricothyroid membrane. Following this procedure, antibiotics are administered.

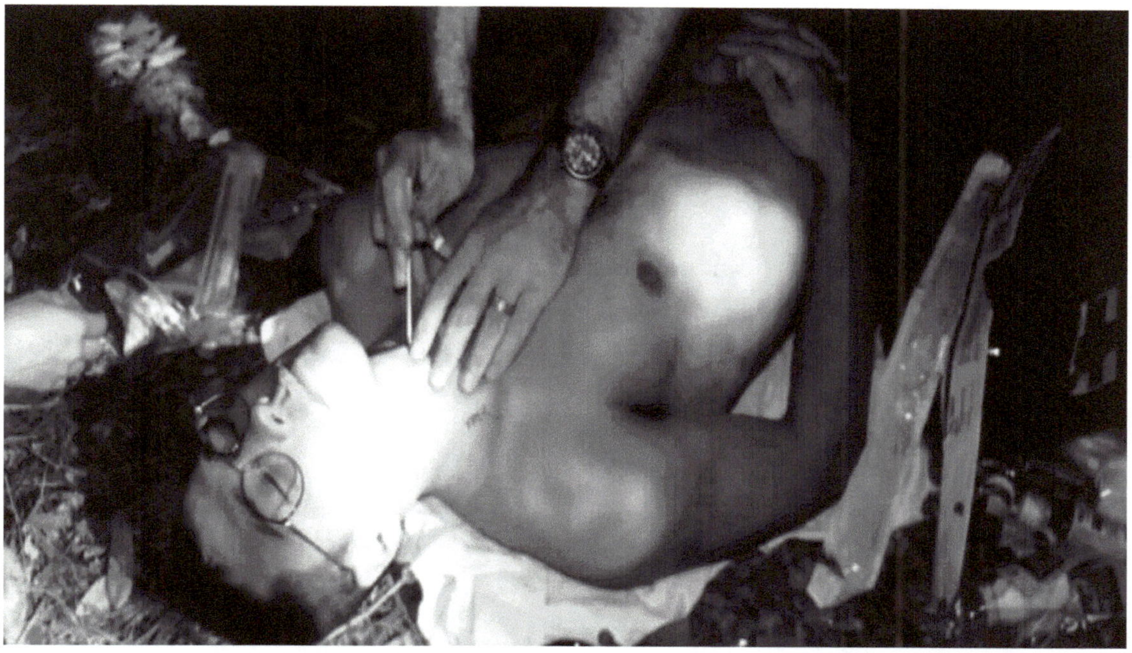

In an emergency, the cricothyroid membrane located in the mid lower larynx and a large bore needle (14 gauge), straw, barrel of ink pen or any hollow tube is pushed through the membrane and into trachea. When performed properly, this surgical procedure is bloodless and quick. Photo by author

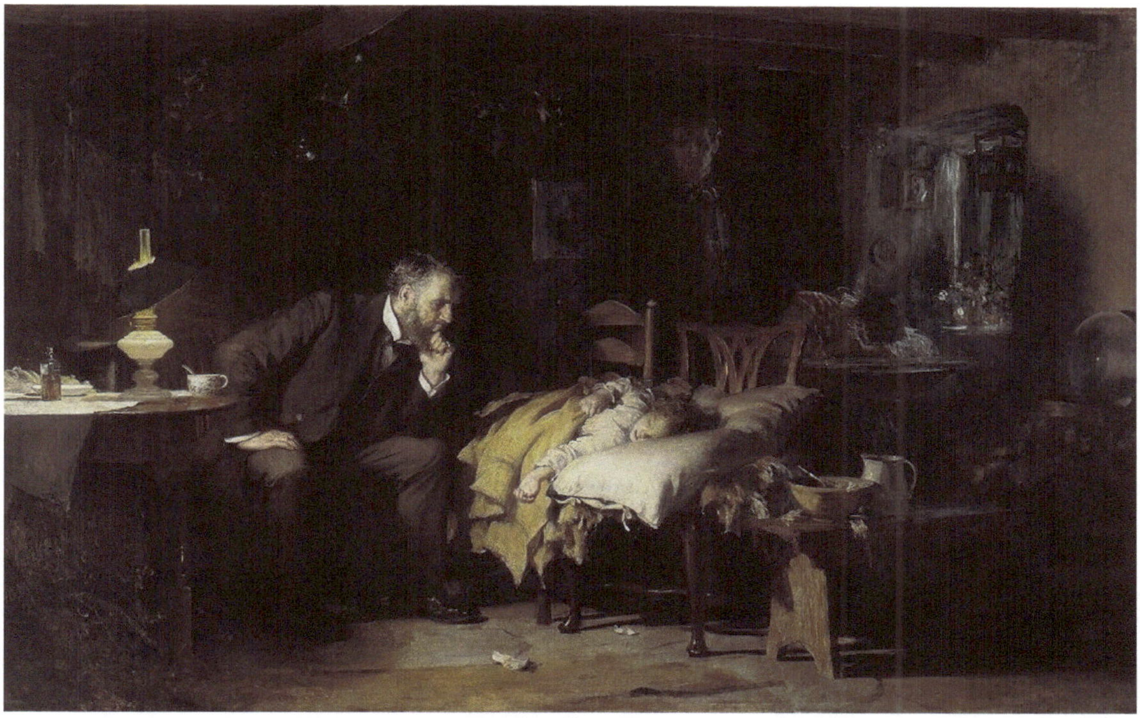

"The Doctor" by Luke Fildes illustrating an ill child, grieving parents and the doctor with little to offer besides his presence. Many a medical officer watched a patient die slowly of the upper airway obstruction with the swelling and "bull neck" of diphtheria, with nothing to offer but caring observation.

The Eyes

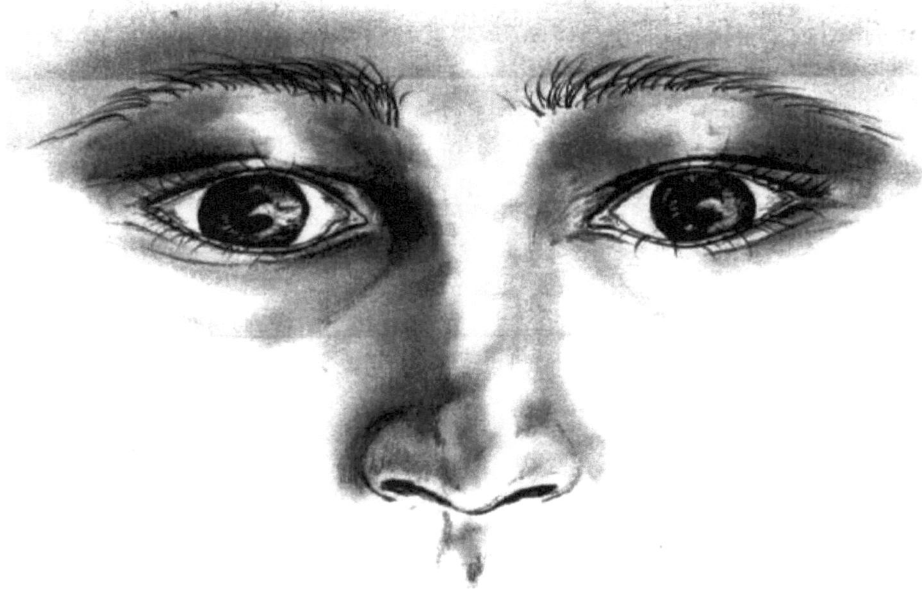

The eyes may reflect what is going on inside the body and have much to tell a medical officer. An example was late in the nine-hundred-day German siege of Leningrad (St. Petersburg), where hunger stalked the population, and thousands died of starvation. In weight loss, the eyes appear larger and farther apart while in weight gain, eyes will appear smaller and closer together. During the siege, those with small eyes closer together and ruddy complexion marked them as cannibals, since these few had access to meat. Art by Angelica Mager

The eye, like other human organs, is a composite of several systems requiring perfect harmony to produce vision. The eyeball is sturdy and well protected, covered with a tough fibrous bulb of connective tissue set deep into a bony socket formed by seven different bones. The lens divides the eye interior into two main chambers. The posterior half is lined with blood-rich tissue, the retina, while the front of the eye is transparent, allowing light to reach the retina unimpeded. The iris (colored part) surrounds the lens and is made of two sets of pigmented muscles, one dilates while the other constricts the pupils, functioning like the erectile tissue found in penis and breast. Suspended in a central defect of the iris is the lens, the purist pristine collection of proteins found in the body, composed of six-sided crystals, laminated layer upon layer with a glue as clear as the finest optical glass. These crystals are encased in a transparent capsule, its shape changed by contractions of the muscles encircling the iris, focusing the lens.

Human eyes have been described as living gems, containing protein crystals in the lens and multicolored muscle fibers in the iris. Looking into the multilayered pigment muscles of the iris with a microscope, it is not difficult to imagine a tropical reef with its crevices of bright colors and flowering shapes. Regardless of the dominant eye color, the ring of the iris contains a rainbow of other bright and pastel colors scattered with flecks of pigment. So important is vision, perhaps one-third of tissue in the cerebral cortex is dedicated to vision with two million separate fibers in each optic nerve carrying light-stimulated nerve impulses to the posterior brain. The eye is durable and designed to last a long lifetime if protected from injury, infection and sunlight. Visible light is the energy source that triggers vision when it strikes a kinked wire-like chemical derivative of ingested vitamin A. The collision of light and certain chemicals causes the structure to suddenly straighten starting a series of chemical reactions that result in stimulation of the vision center at the posterior of the brain. Seeing "stars" is much more common when the blow is to the back of the head, directly stimulating the visual center.

Vision is so important to human life; blinding was a common form of punishment in the past. One of the most profound episodes occurred during the reign of Basil II, the longest ruler of Byzantine in the late 10th and early 11th centuries. Known as the "Bulgar-Slayer" for his successful wars in the Balkans and the deliberate blinding of 15,000 Bulgar prisoners. Groups of one hundred prisoners of war were blinded in both eyes and a single prisoner only blinded in one eye led the other 99 back to their king who upon return of his defeated and blinded army died of a heart attack.

Vitamin A-the vitamin of vision

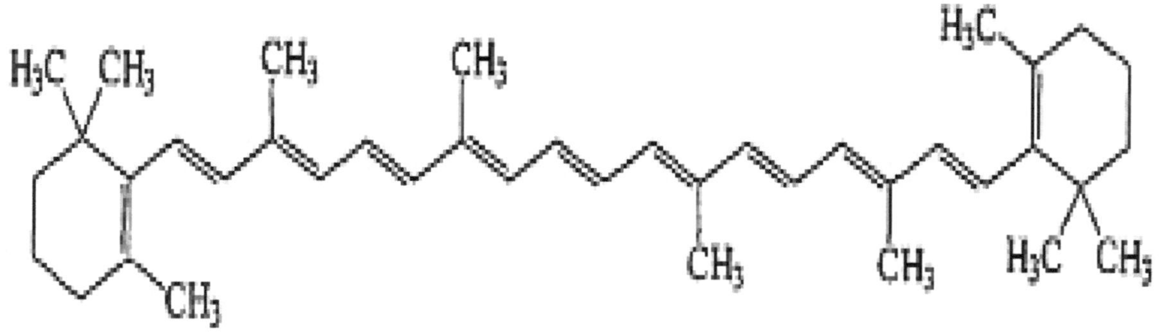

Beta carotene, one of the light-changeable molecules responsible for vision. NIH

Beta carotenes responsible for vision are chemical cousins of hallucinogens found in the spices nutmeg, mace, cloves as well as the alkaloid purines DMT and MMDA (ecstasy). These structures are the reason all hallucinogens produce visual effects. Carotenes are molecules with carbon chains bookended by ring structures, structures repeated throughout nature in certain plants and animals. A tiny sliver of wavelengths released by solar radiation, 400-700nm strikes the ground unimpeded by the earth's atmosphere, triggering the reactions in the eye to produce vision and photosynthesis in plants. The same wavelengths convert vitamin D to its active role in bone formation as the light passes through transparent skin and strikes circulating vitamin D.

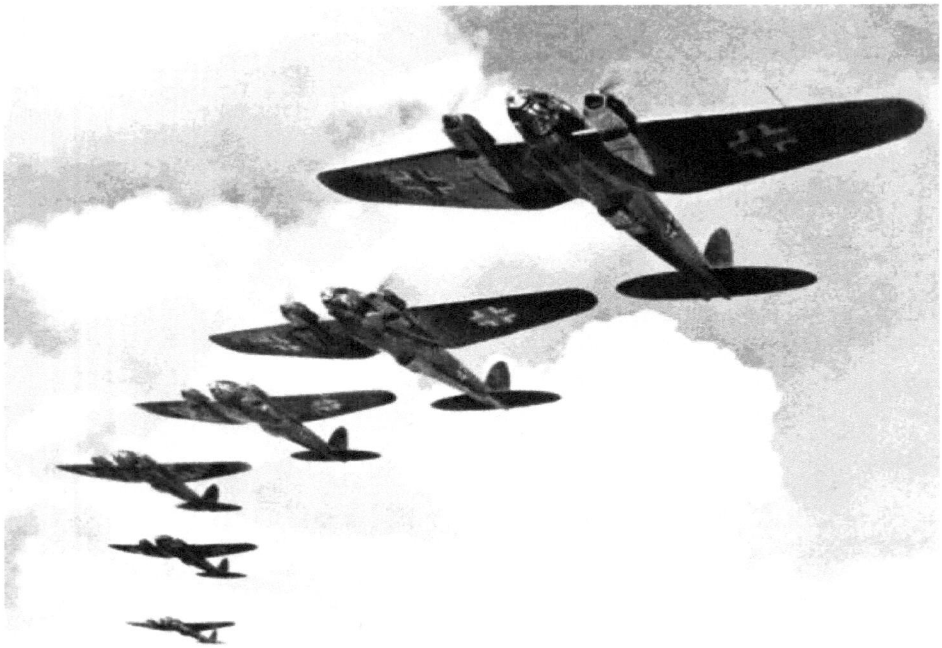

The Battle of Britain was fought in late summer 1940 with most of Europe under Hitler's control. Only Great Britain held out and the Germans believed they could force England's surrender by bombing from the air. Unfortunately for Hitler, the British had a secret weapon, enhanced vision. National Archives

Pigmented vegetables, especially carrots and yellow squash, are high in beta carotenes (type of vitamin A). Eating large amounts of yellow carotene-containing vegetables can turn skin yellow but not the whites of eyes (as it does in hepatitis). Since carotenes were discovered and touted to enhance vision early in the 20th century, the British government used this widespread knowledge to confuse the attacking Germans. To hide the ability to see incoming aircraft by newly discovered and secret radar, the British Government broadcast propaganda that they were feeding the English people and soldiers' high amounts of carrots to enhance their vision, especially at night. The author's good friend Reginald was born in London in 1933 and lived through the terror of German bombing as a child remembered the carrot story in the late summer of 1940. He does not recall getting any carrots but remembered hunger during this period as food was strictly rationed due German submarine warfare. Germany had also experimented with radar but instead pursued using radio beams from the French and Dutch coasts to bisect over targets in England shrouded by clouds or darkness. While British radar allowed interception and destruction primarily of daylight bombers. The English scientists attempt to "jam" these German radio signals led to a navigational error that changed the war when this jamming resulted in German bombers accidently striking a purely civilian target. Churchill responded by deliberately bombing civilian targets (against the laws of war) and all sides continued bombing civilian targets throughout the war in Europe. Ultimately leading to the atomic bombs dropped on Hiroshima and Nagasaki.

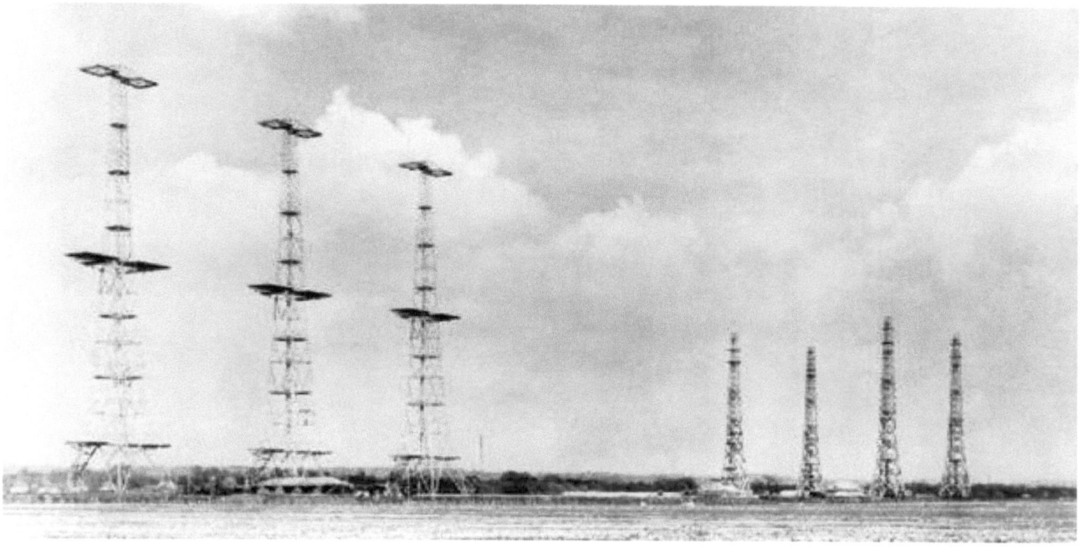

Thousands of German planes flew over these radar towers not aware of their significance. National Archives

This misinformation was done to hide the effects of radar which was still a closely guarded secret during the "Battle of Britain". Perhaps because of this "lie", the Germans were late in discovering the purpose of the new towers along the coast that were really "seeing" the approaching aircraft. By the time Germany targeted these radar transmitters it was too late, and the air battle was won by Great Britain. An example of how effective fake news can be.

Vitamin A, fat-soluble chemicals, are not a single entity, but a group of light sensitive compounds that animal cells have harnessed for their ability to change their shape and function when exposed to light. The adaptation of these chemicals by animal cells gave rise to vision. How the central nervous system perceives images, colors, shapes, motion is not completely understood and what is known of vision is beyond the scope of this text. Whatever the mechanism, vision begins when light penetrates the eye and results in a series of chemical reactions dependent on carotenes. Because vitamin A is concentrated in certain animal tissues, strict vegetarians sometimes suffer from reduced night vision because there is less light and less vitamin A available to trigger visual reactions. Carotene vitamins usually contain yellow, or orange pigment found in plant and animal oils (highest safe concentration in cod liver) and contain rings of carbons connected by chains of carbohydrates. Fat soluble vitamin A is the only known toxic vitamin, even fatal in high doses. Polar bear liver is the highest concentration in nature and consumption of even a small portion can be fatal, as early artic explores discovered and the natives knew better.

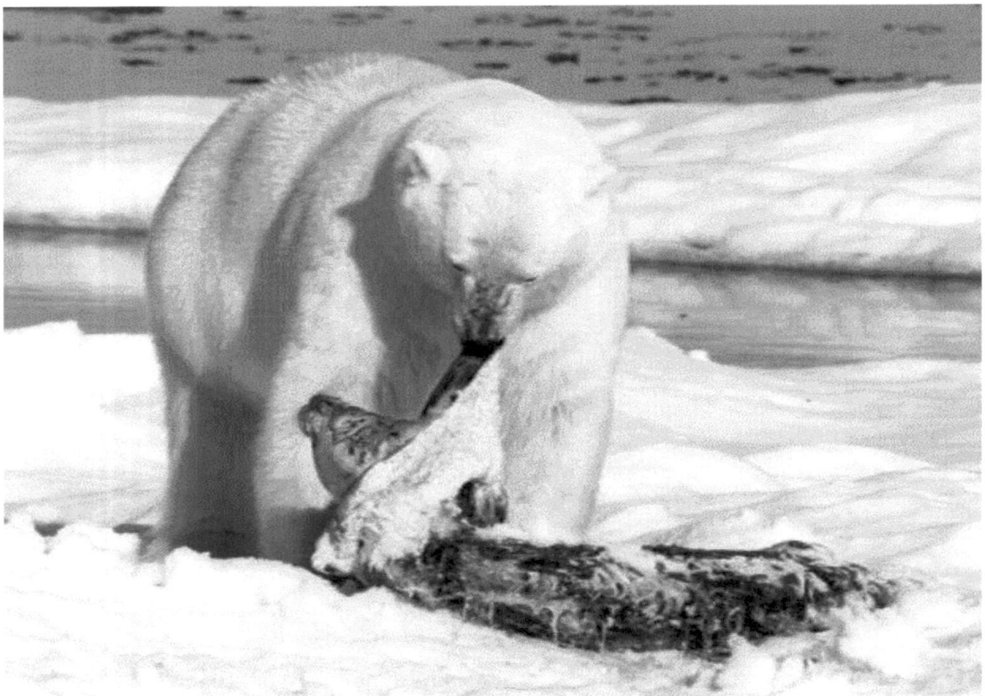

Polar bears eat nothing but fat and protein, since there is no vegetation on the arctic ice. They concentrate vitamin A in their liver to remarkably high levels, likely for enhanced night vision in long Artic night. National Archives

In the retina, a chain of chemical reactions begins when light strikes a carotene molecule coupled with opsin (visual protein), reconfiguring its structure to rhodopsin. Vitamin A has other uses in growth and repair of cells and is used to treat skin disorders as it is important in repair of DNA molecules. This repair of DNA is responsible for the "rejuvenation" of skin with topical Retin A.

In the pupil, a "defect" in the central eyeball functions like the lens of a 35 mm camera. For close focus, requiring a narrow, sharp field of focus, the pupil dilates, increasing the amount of light entering the eye through the lens. In bright light and far focus the pupil relaxes to a small, constricted state (becoming pinpoint). Eye strain develops more readily when reading, watching television or peering into a radar screen, since the eye must maintain constant near focus with dilated pupils. With distant vision, daydreaming and under the influence of the central nervous system depressants such as opiates, pupils are small, pen point in a resting state. Dilated pupils can occur in low light, with stimulating drugs such as cocaine and amphetamines and when the body's "fight or flight" system has been activated, releasing its natural catecholamines.

Age and sunlight combine to make the eyeball stiffer (presbyopia) and the lens less transparent, becoming opaque (cataracts). In the marine environment, sunlight is more intense, both direct and reflected off water. Years of bright sunlight will denature and break down proteins in the lens creating areas of cloudiness, cataracts. Just as a clear egg white, turns opaque when cooked. Cataract formation is related to the amount of sunlight passing through the eye, and on the water, sunlight reaches the eyes even in the shade. The slow loss of night vision is a sign of less light passing through lens, a common complaint with cataract formations. Wearing sunglasses significantly reduces the risk of cataracts and should become a life-long habit, beginning in childhood. As applying sunscreen gives the skin a longer healthy life just as dark glasses give the eye longer life.

The External Eye

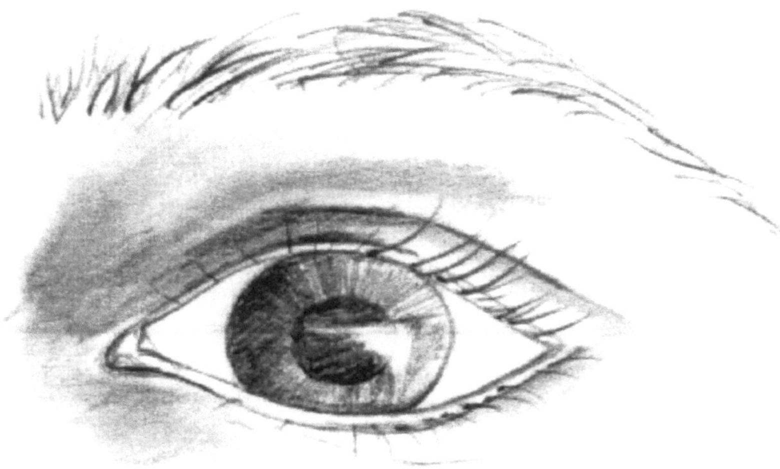

Note the reflected light on the outside of the pupil. The position of this reflection should be the same in both eyes. After facial trauma, an asymmetrical light reflection is a sign of disruption of the bony eye socket. Angelica Mager

The external eye is the target of many agents. The eyebrows, eye lashes and lids offer protection by trapping debris and preventing many insects and foreign bodies from reaching the eyeball. If this fails, the tear duct can pour rinsing fluid over the eye at a moment's notice. Sunlight passing through the external eye can not only cloud the clear lens but cause melanoma of the retina. Sunglasses are effective even in the shade.

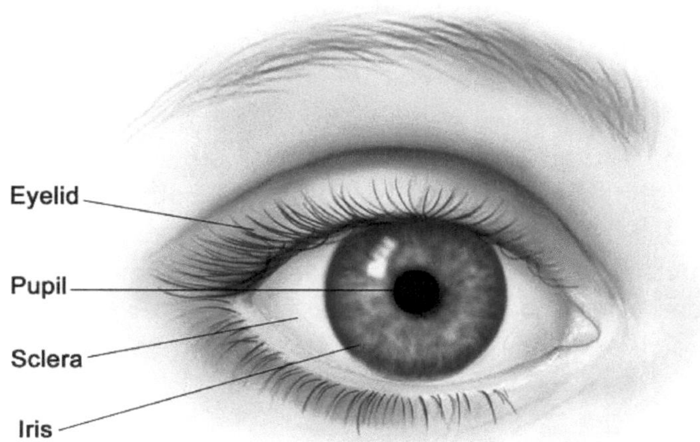

The main parts of external eye, the normally white sclera turns red with injury, allergy, and infection. The border where sclera meets iris is the limbus. The iris is composed of bands of pigmented muscle fibers that function as erectile tissue that by swelling change the shape of the lens giving the eyes the ability to see up close and at long range. NLM

The visible part of the eyeball is composed of the white conjunctiva, and more sensitive cornea (the nerve rich skin covering the colored part of the eye). Within the cornea resides numerous and highly sensitive pain fibers, making injuries by burns or abrasions especially painful. The external eyeball is serviced by several different glands located in the eyelids and within the skull, producing oils, lubricants and tears. Tears are a complex fluid rendered in separate glands, that when mixed on the eye's surface, provide lubrication, moisture, protection and elaborate emotional experiences. The fluid stored in a shallow bay at the nasal side of each eye, the lacrimal lake, and drain through to the back of the nose. Most of the liquid forming tears comes from the large lacrimal gland, located in the skull above the inside of each eye. The gland is a sac-like structure connected to the eye by a long slender neck. The secretion produced here is a form of lymphatic fluid, a diluted version of blood serum, high in immune cells such as leukocytes. With conjunctivitis, tear fluid becomes thick with white blood cells, dead bacteria and debris, producing pus in the eye. Conjunctivitis is common and highly infectious, prompting frequent handwashing.

Human eyelids are retractable shutters composed of a lamination of five layers. Most animals have lids, one exception is the snake, which protects eyes with a clear external lens, goggles. This is a much better system for an animal that survives by hunting low to the ground, driving its body through bush and bramble. Without the need to blink for protection, the snake can keep its prey in sight. Over time, scratches cover the snake's lens decreasing vision, requiring the lens to be shed periodically with the rest of the skin. With each skin shedding, the snake obtains a new set of goggles. In humans, the lid is highly specialized skin coated in layers over a shield of flexible tarsal bone in the form of a plate, unconnected to the rest of the skeletal bones. Embedded within the lid are glands producing the oily secretions found in tears and coating the eyelashes.

The retina is a matrix of ten layers formed in the shape of an amphitheater in the back of the eyeball. Within these layers reside the rods and cones, specialized nerve endings containing a protein derivation of vitamin A, retinol. When exposed to light, retinol undergoes a chemical reaction releasing minute quantities of electrical energy. The amount of area stimulated, the type and magnitude of the light, and the parts of the retina where the light is focused determine the response in the brain's visual center. In a poorly understood process, the eyeball converts light energy to electrical energy, which when passed onto the central nervous system is converted to colors, shapes and motion. The blood-rich retina is responsible for red eyes that often appear in flash photography and in the "flash" of wildlife eyes in headlights. After injury, this reaction should be present, unless the internal eye has been damaged. The presence of the "red reflex" on eye exam assures the internal eye is free from bleeding. This requires a special instrument, the ophthalmoscope, and a dark room. If a flash of redness is seen, the anterior chamber, the lens and the vitreous chamber are clear. The loss of the red reflex after injury could be from bleeding within the eye, a hyphemia.

The Internal Eye

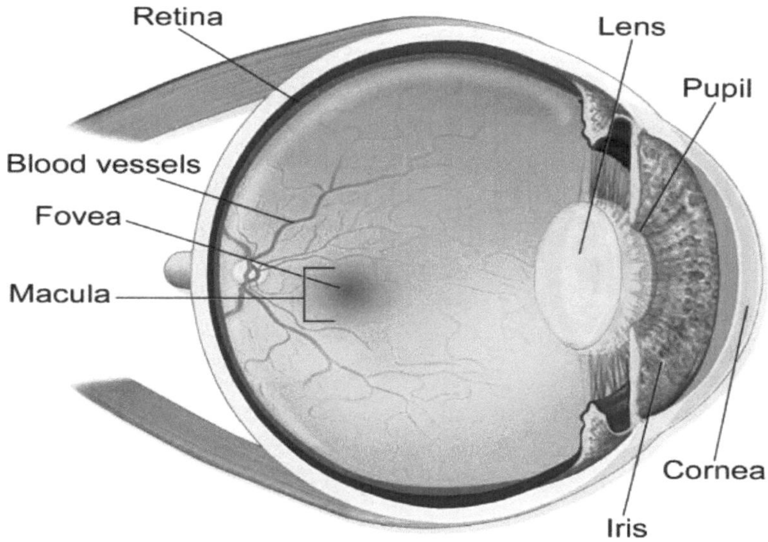

The central nervous system's window to the visual world while at the same time, the eye allows a medical officer to see what is going on inside the body. Conjunctiva turns yellow in liver disease, pales in anemia, signs of diabetes and heart disease are seen in the retina. The eye in the physical exam can reflect much about the body in health and disease. Beautiful in function and design. NLM

Eye strain and aging lead to abnormal eye shape and stiffness. In nearsightedness (myopia), the front part of the eye becomes egg-shaped, longer and thinner, instead of the normal round ball-like shape. Myopia reduces the eye's ability to focus objects clearly onto the retina, requiring corrective external lenses. The surgery (radial keratotomy) for myopia involves cutting slits completely through the outer eye allowing the eyeball to return to its normal spherical shape. This invasive surgery has been replaced by resurfacing the eye with laser, Lasik. However, very few ophthalmologists have the surgery themselves.

The inside of the healthy eye is a crystal-clear fluid-filled ball with the lens separating the smaller anterior chamber from the amphitheater of the retina. The anterior chamber and the lens are designed to focus images onto the retina, if the anterior part of the eye is egg-shaped, the image falls short of the retina as a blurred object. Glasses and contact lens in a near-sighted person are designed to move the focus of the image backward, where it becomes crisp. Watching TV or radar screens for long hours and reading in low light seem to increase the severity of near-sightedness (myopia).

The Red Eye

The red eye has many causes, most self-limiting requiring little or no care. However, some causes of red eye must be diagnosed and treated appropriately to preserve vision. Redness in the conjunctiva indicates increased blood flow seen in injury, infections, allergic reactions and in rare cases indicates increased intraocular pressure.

Eye Injury

The eyes represent only 0.27% of the body's total surface area but account for 10% of all injuries requiring medical attention in emergency rooms and urgent care. In the field, on the water and in warfare, the incidence of eye injuries is higher. Protected by a powerful blink reflex and a surrounding ring of bone, the eye is generally not easily injured and can withstand some trauma without ill effect. It is the medical officer's responsibility to examine every eye carefully after injury. Trauma to the eye, either by sharp or blunt injury will cause redness and pain. The colored part of the eye, the cornea, contains many pain nerve fibers while the conjunctiva is less sensitive. Therefore, corneal injury is much more painful.

The conjunctiva is largest part of the external eye and will bleed if vessels rupture, creating a red-purple discoloration under the clear covering of the eye, the sub-conjunctivae hemorrhage (it looks worse than it is). Conjunctival injury usually does not affect vision but does result in pain with eye movement, i.e., side to side and up and down. This same hemorrhage can occur with retching, hard coughing spasms, bleeding disorders (thin blood) and often, for no apparent reason. The patient should be examined by a physician at the earliest opportunity to rule out a more serious problem. Aspirin intake increases the risk of these bleeds.

Foreign Bodies and Corneal Abrasions

Injury to the cornea is much more painful than injury to the conjunctiva and requires treatment. Corneal injuries occur with foreign bodies such as metal filings, wood splinters, excessive eye rubbing, contact lens lacerations, sand and tree limbs are all capable of "scratching" the colored part of the eye. When the cornea is damaged, there is the persistent sensation of "something in the eye" even after the offensive object has been removed. Scratches or abrasions over the cornea are best seen with fluorescent stain under a black light where defects fill with stain revealing a crater or scrape on the cornea. Large abrasions may be seen using only plain light and magnifying glass.

The first step in eye injuries when a foreign body is suspected is lavage of the eye with large amounts of clean water. A gentle stream flowing over the entire surface of the eye rather than application directly on the cornea will be better tolerated. It is important that the eye be open and using an eye cup will provide a greater chance for washing off the foreign body. If this fails to dislodge the object and medical help is far away, the eye should be rendered "asleep" with eye anesthesia drops. After eye anesthesia, the object may be removed gently with a wet Q-tip or if metal, with a small powerful magnet. An eye loop of monofilament fishing line or flexible plastic can be used to safely sweep off an embedded object. If these measures fail and sea conditions are calm, the object is best removed with an eye spud. The medical officer should have some skill in the technique of lifting an embedded object off the cornea with a tiny needle. This should only be attempted when the other medical care is far away and the medical officer has a firm, steady platform to work on. If the foreign body is not dislodged, it can discolor the eye with a rust ring if metal, and wood, especially treated lumber splinters can cause infection. The hand holding the spud is braced against the patient's face with the needle held bevel up along a low angle to the cornea. Using short gentle strokes, the needle is used to scrape and lift the imbedded foreign body out of its hole where it can be washed off with lavage. After removal of the foreign body or any time the eye is anesthetized, it is best to place topical ophthalmic antibiotic and cover eye with a patch to protect it, as the blink reflex is lost. This patch should be placed for 12-24 hours. If on removal, the next day the eye still has the sensation of a foreign body, the process is repeated. Lavage and patch if abrasion is seen, rechecking the next day. In class, students practiced with a hard-boiled egg as it has the same constancy as the external eye.

Chemical Burns

The external eye is tough, covered with a protective membrane that resists injuries from most chemicals. A common chemical irritating in the eye is battery acid and, in most cases, causes little damage after prompt lavage. However, some chemicals can "porcelainize" the eye, rendering the soft transparent covering stiff and opaque. This is especially true of alkaline agents such as lye, a chemical found in some cleaning products, like drain cleaners. If these agents should be replaced by non-lye containing cleaners.

In chemical injuries, irrigation should be done immediately with whatever clean water is available, even seawater. Irrigation should be continued with at least 500 ml (1/2 quart) of a clean solution such as intravenous fluid if available. Irrigation fluid should be gently directed onto the white of the eye with the lid held open. A small eye cup allows an individual to rinse by opening the eye looking into the fluid filled eye cup. After lavage, antibiotics should be placed in the eye and covered with a patch to reduce blinking. Recently, Vitamin A dressings have been used on chemical burns with encouraging results. In the unfortunate case of scarring, corneal transplant is required to restore vision.

Thermal Burns

Fortunately, in fires, the suddenness of the blink reflex prevents most injuries. The more common eye burns include welding lights, sun and snow blindness, burning the uppermost layers of the eye's skin (oculokeratits). Treatment of eye burns like corneal abrasions include application of topical anesthesia, antibiotics and gentle pressure dressing, upon closing eye lid. Artificial tears may be helpful if mild irritation persists after the dressing is removed. In more severe burns there is the risk of scarring, and these should be seen by a physician, preferably an ophthalmologist, as soon as possible. Until aid is reached, keep the eye moist with frequent drops of artificial tears or other lubricating solution and instill antibiotic eye drops every 4-6 hours. Keep eyes patched between treatments. If the skin around the eye is burned with the use of oral antibiotics with appropriate burn dressings.

Hyphemia

As with other blood-rich tissue, the eye may bleed internally when injured. Bleeding into the eye following trauma creates a "veil-like" effect to vision and producing a decreased or absent red reflex in the injured eye. The hyphemia differs from bleeding into the conjunctiva (subconjunctival hemorrhage), in that it obscures vision and reduces the red reflex. After the examination, keep the victim at rest with the eye protected by a shield or patch and the head elevated. This will allow gravity to help the eye remove the blood. Avoid aspirin and physical activity kept at a minimum.

Glaucoma

Glaucoma is caused by increased pressure within the eye which commonly develops slowly over years and is diagnosed by measuring the pressure. Increased pressure in a closed space of the eye as in other spaces within the body, compresses tissue and if untreated, pressure destroys tissue. Increased pressure over time will permanently damage vision and glaucoma, like hypertension requires treatment. Beta blockers lower blood pressure and when applied to the eyes as drops, lower pressure within the eye. Acute glaucoma, a sudden increase in intraocular pressure is an ophthalmological emergency! In the field, pilocarpine eye drops may keep pressure low, until an eye surgeon evaluates. Pilocarpine is the only treatment for acute glaucoma in the field and the author placed in every offshore medicine chest.

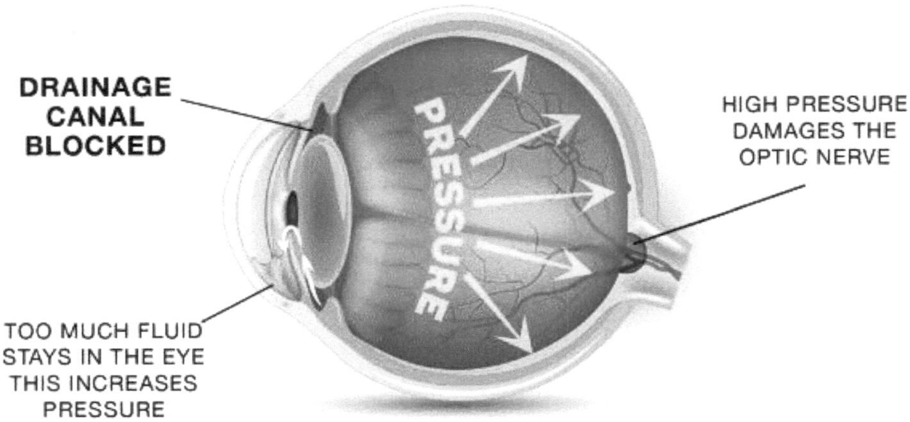

This eye condition is a serious eye emergency and fortunately rare. The author has seen only one case of acute glaucoma over 40 years. Another example of stagnation leading to increased pressure within a closed compartment. NIH

Retinal detachment is a common disorder (the author has experienced bilateral detachments) manifested by a sudden "veil" in vision in one eye, "a curtain over part or all of the visual field". There is really no treatment in the field, and it should be evaluated and treated as soon as possible to prevent vision loss. The retinal has been described as a wet piece of tissue paper and therefore naturally fragile. Retinal detachment can occur with trauma but in many cases occurs spontaneously.

Eye infections

After trauma, the most common causes of red eyes are allergies and infections. Both can present similar complaints in the beginning of redness, irritation, discharge and discomfort. Allergic reactions in the eyes are often associated with sneezing and itching with clear discharge. Infection causes more pain, discolored discharge and more swelling. Even though many eye infections are viral, the author was trained to place antibiotics and warm soaks. Eye infections like conjunctivitis are highly infectious to others. Antihistamines will reduce allergic complaints while antibiotics for infection are placed in both eyes three times a day for two days after eyes clear of symptoms. The author prefers erythromycin as ointment in eye infections as it is less irritating than sulpha drops. Ointment remains in contact with eye tissue longer, although solutions are easier to administer. Topical antibiotics should be applied three to four times daily for one to two days after clearing of eyes.

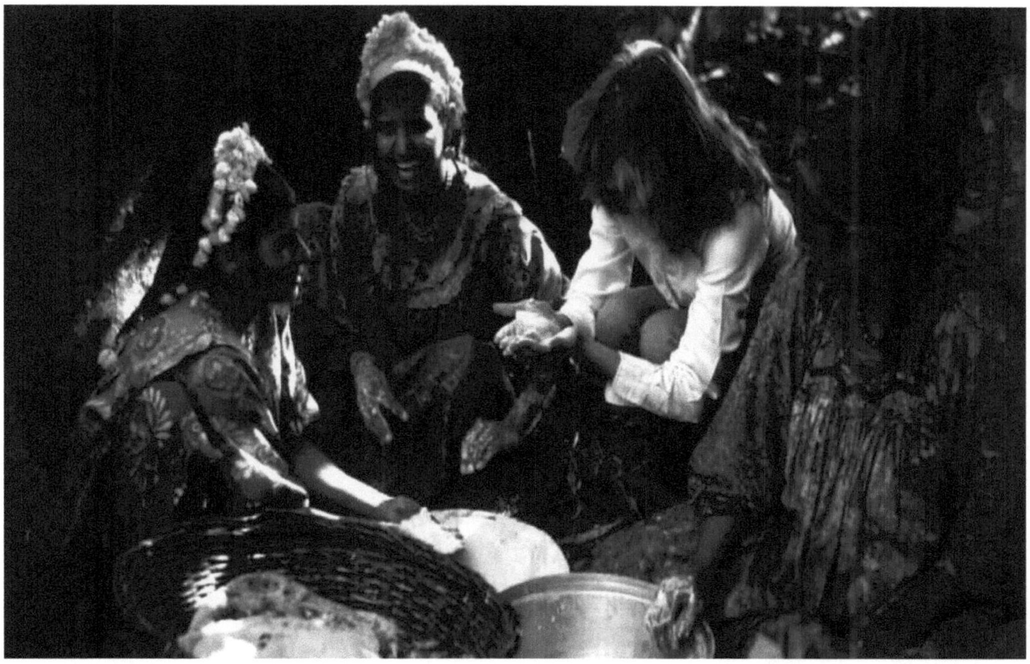

The author's wife making bread in the rural Egyptian delta. Although the oldest female in image at 25, Gail is the only woman with sight in both eyes. The other ladies have trachoma, the leading cause of blindness in the world (in the USA, it is diabetes). Blindness in trachoma is caused by mechanical abrasions "scratched" into the clear cornea by the hard, tiny razor-sharp eggs laid by flies among the eyelashes. As the lid rises and lowers, the cornea is repeatedly scraped, rendering it opaque after years. Trachoma is an extreme example of corneal abrasions, abrasions prevented with screened windows and antibiotic ointment. Screens, unknown in Egypt prevents flies from entering bedrooms, classrooms, churches, mosques and businesses, greatly reduce incidence of trachoma, however in the time the author spent in Egypt, even the hospitals lacked screens and flies were part of every procedure, particularly spinal taps.

Dental

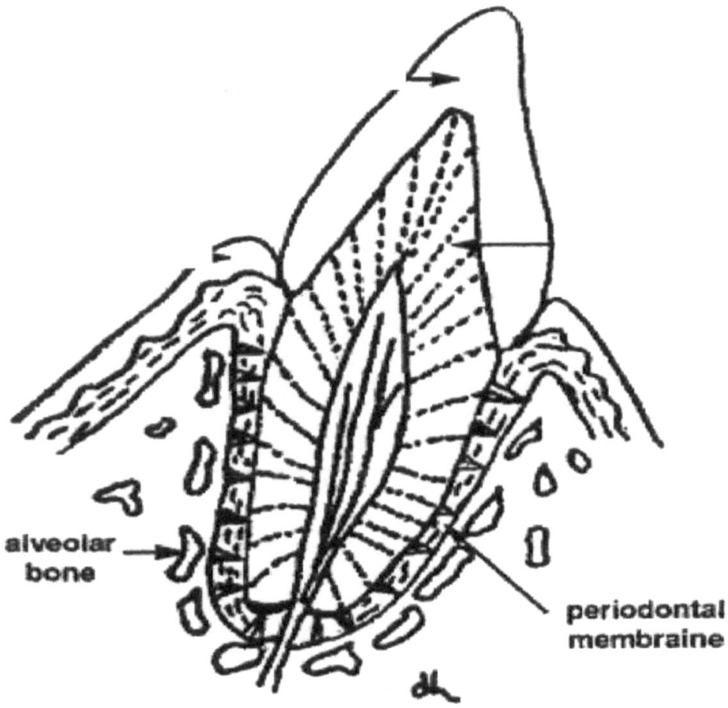

Each tooth is set into a bony cavity lined with a living membrane, separating the teeth from the bones of the jaw. Tooth enamel is the densest, hardest substance in the body and can last for centuries, with ivory from mammal tusks being thousands of years old.

Toothache is one of mankind's oldest and most common medical complaints. Modern dentistry has reduced human suffering much and is one of the primary reasons for longer life. Only recently has the pain and suffering of tooth disease been brought under control with antibiotics and dental surgery. In the past, dental pain and infections were primarily treated with tooth extraction, performed in Europe by barber-surgeons for a thousand years. It was not until late in the 18th century that in both England and France, the barbers and surgeons were separated into separate guilds, with surgeons agreeing not to cut hair while the barbers agreed to limit surgery to dentistry. Dental problems have always and continue to be common aboard ships and in other isolated environments.

The US submarine force during World War II experienced a high rate of dental casualties and when the author served in the submarine community, a tender for a submarine group will carry one physician and three to four dentists. During the 1939 Byrd Expedition to Antarctica, Dr. Russell Frazier; the expedition physician, reported "the most common and most painful malady encountered was toothache". In the past, the non-surgical field management of tooth ache was clove oil dipped in gauze and held against the painful tooth. If this failed, it was followed by extraction in most cases. Certainly, removing the painful infected tooth was often effective, but thankfully this invasive treatment is seldom necessary. Dental problems in the field may be common and likely preventable by good oral hygiene, brushing and flossing with cleaning (scaling) at least every six-twelve months. In the author's experience, most dental pain is reduced with oral antibiotics until dental care is rendered.

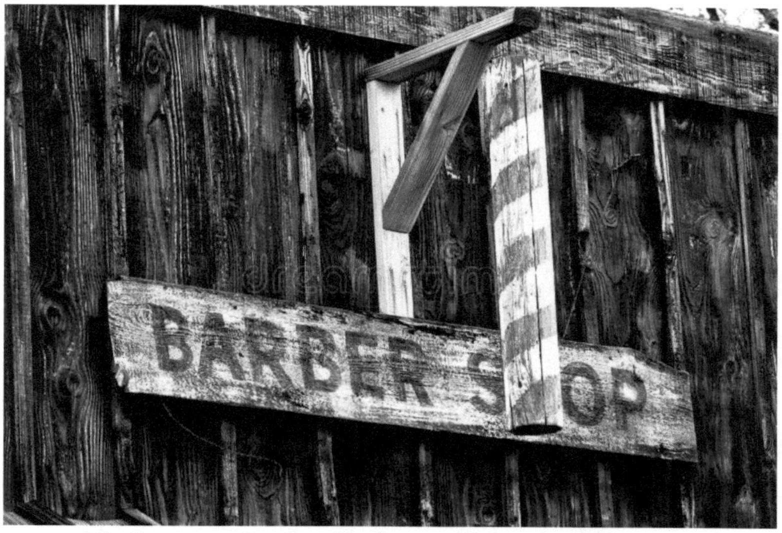

Barber-surgeons provided most of what little medical care was available in the early and late Middle Ages of Europe. A recent remnant of the barber-surgeons is the red and white-striped pole used in America for a barber shop. Throughout the 19th century in the American West, a pole with white bloody rags indicated this barber could remove teeth.

Under normal conditions, the mouth is teaming with many types of bacteria, that during chewing, are injected into circulating blood. This increases with dental procedures, requiring those with artificial heart valves to take preventive antibiotics. Fortunately, even though they gain brief access to the internal body, they seldom cause infections. A mouth cursed with bad teeth and inflamed gums allow larger numbers of bacteria to be "seeded" into the blood stream with each meal. Sterile blood that flows through the mouth can become heavily laden with bacteria if the barrier of tooth enamel is breached by cavities (caries) or the gums become loose and inflamed (gingivitis). Saliva, in addition to rinsing teeth of bacteria, does carry infectious components of the blood such as hepatitis, prompting the use of gloves in examining or treating the mouth. Wounds created by the human mouth are potentially the dirtiest wounds encountered, and quickly become infected. Human bites, especially to the hand (a closed fist to the mouth) require aggressive care, including irrigation, antibiotics and warm soaks.

Continuously flowing saliva keeps the numbers of bacteria low, as saliva laden with bacteria is swallowed or spit away. If pockets develop in the mouth, bacteria will gather in the stagnant fluid, causing local infections. A chronic infection in the mouth can lead to a more serious internal infection if bacteria are chronically spilled into passing blood. Sites for such infections include the potential space between the gums and teeth, the root of the tooth and the interior of the tooth itself. Under normal conditions teeth are covered with bacteria, but seldom cause infections because enamel provides an almost impregnable slick barrier to bacteria. The gums are normally adhered firmly to the teeth, but with poor cleaning and plaque build-up, they loosen and breach by foreign bodies such as small chunks of food. Gum inflammation leads to bleeding, discoloration at the foot of the teeth and are painful. Both caries and gingivitis can lead to deeper tooth abscess in the root of the teeth. Normal teeth can fall from the mouth if gingivitis is not controlled.

There are four major types of human teeth: incisors (knife-like), canines (dog), premolars and molars. The sharp frontal teeth are for tearing while the flat thick back teeth are for grinding. Teeth are not held rigidly in place but set in a socket of flexible bone filled with tiny air cells (alveolar bone). Teeth are not anchored to this bone, but instead are suspended in the alveolar bone by a network of fibers forming a continuous ligament, the periodontal membrane. This piece of bioengineering allows teeth to move ever so slightly in their sockets during chewing which enhances the grinding action of mastication. Damage by trauma, poor care or infection, leads to permanent teeth being lost. The gingiva (gum tissue) covers both bone and periodontal membrane while enveloping the base of the teeth, forming a tight protective cuff. The periodontal membrane is so important, dentist specializes in its treatment as periodontist.

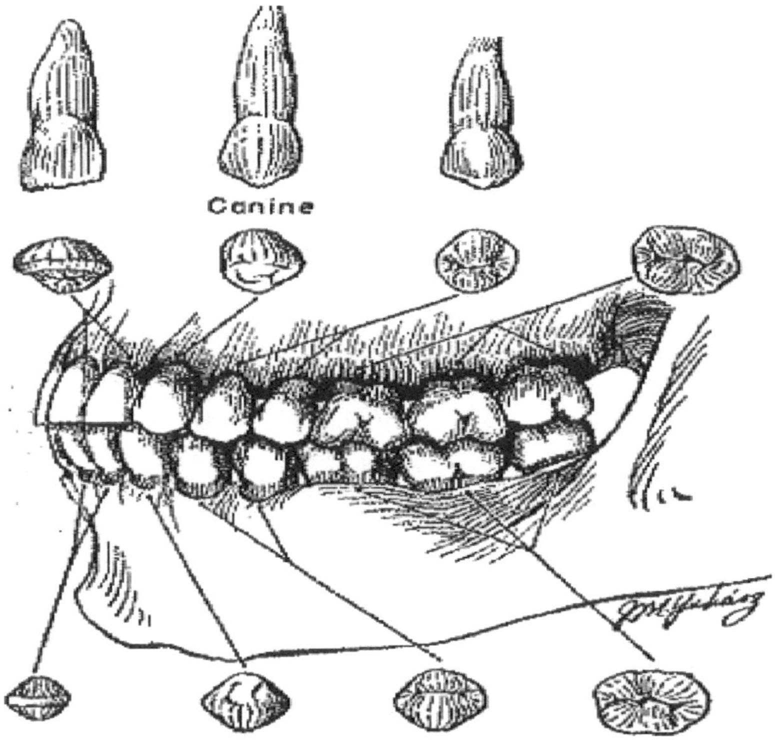

The human mouth contains a variety of teeth, the most found in nature, allowing humans the extensive possible variety of food.

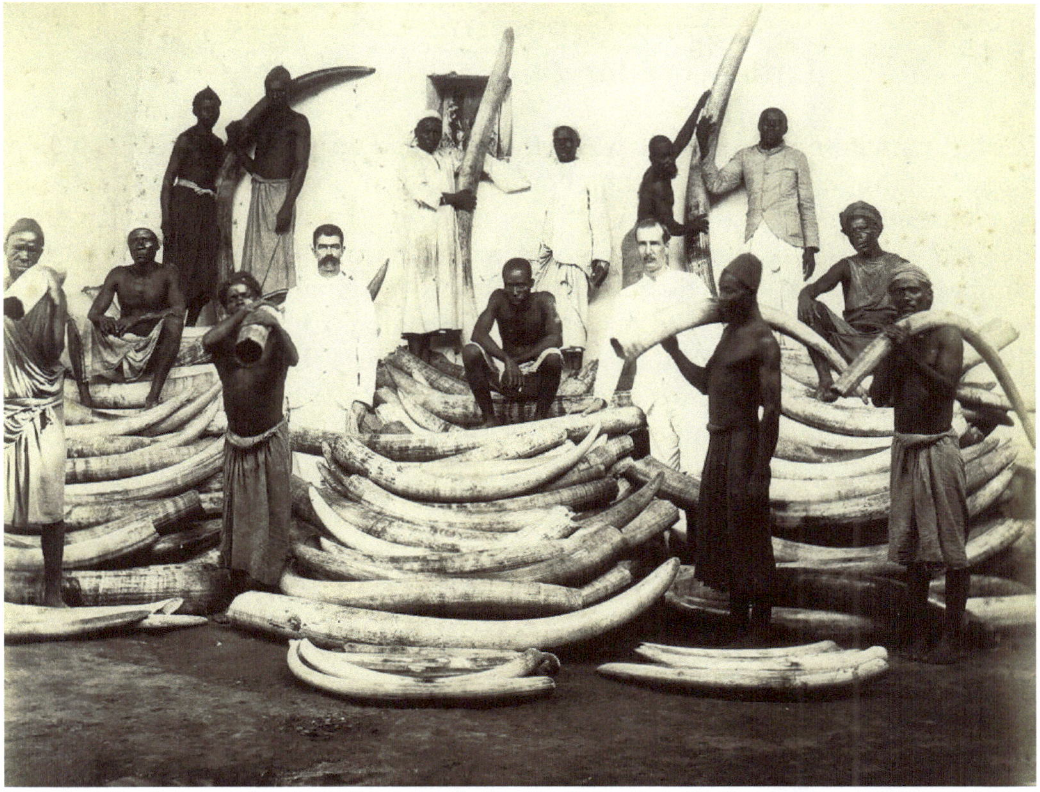

Enamel, in the form of sub-Saharan elephant ivory tusks has connected Africa to the Western world as a major trade item for thousands of years. The durability and beauty of enamel has made it a lasting form of artwork and its harvest has wrought much cruelty and heartbreak to both the animals and humans. Tons of African ivory, rubber and gold was coming out of the Belgian Congo when this picture was taken, while only guns, bullets and axes going in. Belgian King Leopold II, 1835-1909 personally owned the Congo, it was the King's private property, subject to no oversight. Leopold used the press, who accepted his generous donations to their publications, to print stories lauding many fake awards Leopold was garnishing for his humanitarian accomplishments in the Congo. The King's primary agent on the ground in the Congo was a newspaper correspondent and African explorer, Henry Stanley. Stanley as a respected member of the press was an important part of the scheme telling the wonderful things being done in the Congo, touting enlightenment, medical care and education to natives of the Congo. This entire time, the natives were being enslaved, raped, murdered and maimed, their resources plundered for no return. Still today, the Congo is one the richest places on earth containing almost every valuable natural resource, abundant water, precious metals, diamonds, timber, oil, jungles containing medicines undiscovered and the source for the radioactive uranium used in the first atomic bombs. And yet continues to be one the most violent and impoverished nations on earth. Image from 1880

Gingivitis
Latin word for gums + inflammation

Gingivitis is inflammation at the borders where the gums and teeth meet. Bleeding after brushing, gum pain and swelling are common symptoms. Treatment includes cleaning (scaling), more thorough use of toothbrush, flossing or even a toothpick and oral antibiotics to help prevent more serious infection. Gingivitis can produce chronic symptoms of fatigue, fever, and a general sense of not feeling well (malaise). It is difficult to feel healthy if gingivitis and dental caries present. Symptoms will resolve with the resolution of the inflammation. Chronic gingivitis can lead to loss of normal teeth. In scurvy, gingivitis is an early symptom, followed by teeth dropping from inflamed gums. Long-term inflammation of gum borders creates deep fissures, offering sites for stagnation and bacteria overgrowth. Periodontal (around the tooth) abscesses form in these pockets, causing pain and swelling at the abscess site. Treatment is simple incision and drainage of the tender swelling. Often just releasing the gum edge at the tooth with a toothpick or dental exploring probe will allow the pocket of pus to drain.

Cavities (caries)

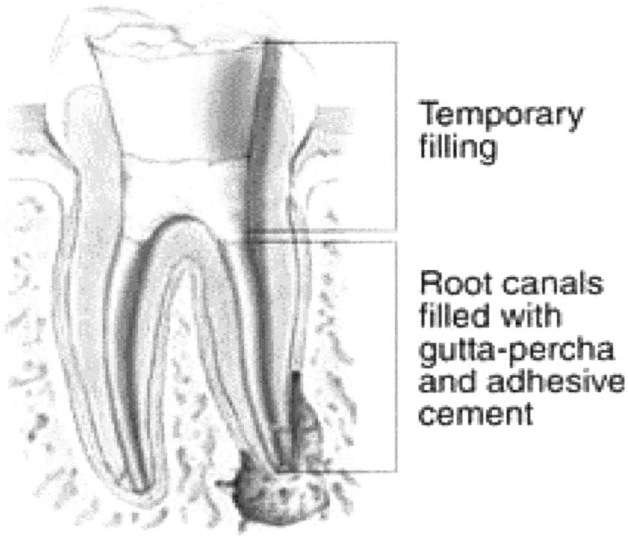

A temporary filling seals off the living tooth from a mouth filled with bacteria. Early golf balls were made from gutta-percha. NLM

The most common dental disease, the cavity, has long plagued humans and a great debt is owed to modern dentistry which has greatly reduced this affliction. Cavities occur when the protective covering enamel of the tooth is broken down and bacteria invade the soft interior. One mechanism of this injury is the deposition of a waste product of bacteria, plaque, which allows bacteria to adhere to the normally slick surface of a tooth more easily. Plaque can be prevented with good oral hygiene. It is composed of acids and other waste substances that each generation of bacteria deposit on the tooth's surface, slowly eating away the barrier. Not unlike generations of sea birds depositing guano on rocks. Once the enamel is dissolved, bacteria will invade the soft tooth pulp, produce decay and eventually cause pain.

The treatment of cavities in the field requires the use of temporary tooth filling. The most effective is ready-mixed tubes of soft, clay-like material (Cavit) or can be crafted from mixing clove oil and powdered zinc oxide. A dentist at a "Safety at Sea" conference recommended sugarless gum. In any case, the cavity must be gently cleaned with lavage from syringe to remove the softer infected debris bone and then dried. The filling must adhere to air-tight bonding to prevent further decay. Failure to completely dry the cavity will lead to poor adherence of the filling. Drying can be accomplished with paper/gauze sponges to absorb saliva or with dry air from scuba tank regulator blown directly into the cavity. After drying, the filling material is packed firmly into the cleaned defect repeatedly, and then smoothed to the tooth's contour with a finger or burnishing tool. When using zinc oxide and clove oil, mix the filling to the consistency of soft chewing gum. By compressing the teeth together while the filling is still soft, excess filling can be removed, reducing the chance of a rough area catching on other teeth. These rough areas will also serve as sites of new bacteria colonies. The new filling should be as smooth as the surrounding enamel.

Tooth Abscesses

This is a deep infection, which, if left untreated can spread to bone, sinus and blood, causing more than dental problems. The infection occurs in the tooth's pulp or roots, causing symptoms of a closed space infection, localized pain and fever. The pain can radiate behind the face or trigger headache as a sinus infection might. Often a tender firm mass (lymph node) arises in the neck on the side of tooth abscess. Treatment is oral antibiotics (amoxicillin a good choice) until a dentist can diagnose the cause with X-ray. Rarely does the infected tooth need to be extracted in the field, since antibiotic use will control infection and reduce the symptoms. Antibiotics may not clear the infection, only subdue it until professional dental care is available.

The Chest

The Chest Pain of Heartburn

Esophageal reflux or heartburn is probably the most common cause of chest pain and can so closely mimic angina or heart attack to be indistinguishable from life-threatening heart disease, especially in the field. Heartburn, like angina, can be associated with sweating, shortness of breath, paleness, nausea, it can radiate to the left arm and for all practical purposes appear very like the pain of angina or even a heart attack. Unlike angina, it is not associated with irregular pulse or low blood pressure but instead elevates heart rate and blood pressure. Heartburn is the result of normal stomach acid that has "leaked" through the protective mucus layer onto the sensitive lining of the esophagus. The pain commonly occurs after eating and lying down, allowing gravity to help in dispersing acid from the stomach into the lower esophagus. The pain is usually an hour in coming, described as intense burning, lasting longer than 15 minutes, even hours. Spicy foods, caffeine, tobacco and alcohol all increase the incidence of reflux of stomach acid.

In the field, it may be possible to separate heartburn from angina with the use of a "heartburn cocktail". By combining an antacid like Maalox with a liquid local anesthetic such as Viscous Xylocaine (lidocaine), the esophagus is rendered almost pain free in several minutes. If effective, the long-term treatment of reflux (heartburn) is aimed at reducing acid production with acid blockers, removing chemicals that increase acid such as caffeine and tobacco and having the person stay upright for at least 2 hours after eating. Remember that aspirin-like drugs (ibuprofen, Advil, Motrin, etc.) will all increase the risk of heartburn, especially in the person with a history of attacks. Chronic heartburn can lead to esophageal cancer and should not be tolerated.

Chest Wall Pain

Underlying the external chest are the ribs, muscles and connective tissue of the rib cage, the lungs, heart and several digestive organs including the stomach, pancreas, liver, gall bladder and some of the bowels. The softer organs of the chest cavity are well protected by the sturdy chest wall, especially in the back. Thick posterior ribs, stack of thoracic vertebrae, large back muscles and the plate-like shoulder blades make the back the strongest shield of a body cavity. Examination of the chest is best done in a systematic method of observing the manner the chest moves with breathing, feeling for areas of tenderness, lymph nodes in the armpit and lower neck and listening to the breath sounds and heart sounds. A medical officer should be able to perform a simple chest exam and determine if there are abnormal findings that could explain a patient's complaints. Remember that the chest contains organs of digestion, not just the heart and lungs.

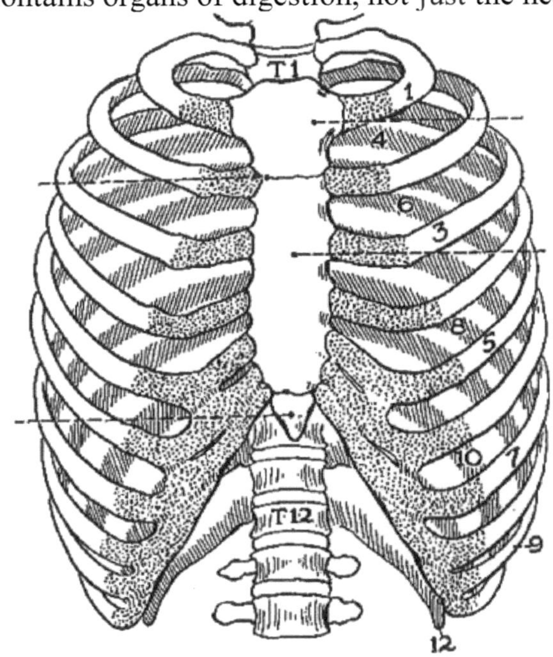

The bony chest is strong, flexible, protective and lovely. Seven thoracic ribs connect the spinal column to the sternum with cartilage-lined joints.

Chest wall pain is common and an attempt to separate the more dangerous angina from other causes should be attempted. **Pleurisy** (Latin for painful breathing) is chest discomfort from inflammation of the lining of the chest wall, aggravated by deep breathing and coughing. Musculoskeletal strains are common in the chest wall and more painful than serious. Chest wall pain usually increases with deep breathing or coughing, with the body in certain positions and associated with a tender spot is found somewhere on the chest wall. Tenderness around the sternum is common since this is the site where multiple ribs and muscles attach to the breastbone. Pain that increases with the finger pressure over the sides of the sternum is not coming from the heart, but the bones and sinew of the chest wall. Pleurisy, chest wall pain and muscle strains are treated with anti-inflammatory medications such as aspirin or ibuprofen and time.

Using both hands to gently compress the chest wall causing tenderness indicates injury to muscle, joint or rib. Compression of the sides of the chest will often illicit pain at the sternum when inflammation develops in the joints where the ribs and sternum meet. Rib bruising or fracture causes tenderness over the injury site with both direct pressure and side compression of ribs. These injuries should not be managed with tape or rib belts, even though by decreasing chest wall movement they will reduce discomfort. During the author's training, any sailor coming into the ER with chest bound after a rib fracture caused the emergency room supervising physician to "flip-out" and if possible, would contact the medical officer that placed the binding for a "chewing-out" (providing he outranked the offending officer). Although pain reduction is achieved by splinting the ribs with a belt, it increases the risk of pneumonia as fluid and airflow becomes stagnant. Even though painful, the person must deep breath and cough and therefore pain relief with opiates, acetaminophen and anti-inflammatory medications is important.

Chest Exam

The chest exam begins with noting any respiratory distress in the patient. Signs of respiratory distress are rapid or labored breathing, the use of neck muscles contracting in breathing and in severe cases, a bluish tint to the skin (cyanosis). If fluid is present in the chest, it may be felt by placing the hands over the chest and feeling for vibrations or rattles with breathing, noted as **fremitus** and sometimes called the "death rattles". The modern stethoscope allows the examiner to detect abnormal sounds that do not transmit through chest wall.

Listening to the Chest

Physicians have been listening to and tapping on the chest for centuries. What is known about the Greek medical school on the island of Cos founded by followers of Hippocrates is limited but chest examination was documented 2500 years ago. Students were taught to feel the chest, to listen or auscultate the chest for abnormal breath sounds, with ear to chest wall and tap the hollow lung as one would test a hollow container for fluid levels. Two millennia later, a French physician working at a Spanish Naval hospital, developed the modern technique of tapping the chest to diagnose fluid levels. Leopold Auenbrugger published a textbook on his techniques in 1761 based on his experience. His method of percussion was learned from his father, an innkeeper who tapped on the sides of wine barrels to detect their level of contents. Percussion was used extensively at sea to measure the level of drinking water and fluid in other casks kept in ships' holds. Keeping careful records of a long-range sailing vessel's water supply was an especially important task of the vessels' chief Bosun in the British Royal Navy. Another French physician, Jean Corvisart, who later became one of Napoleon's personal physicians wrote an even larger book (over 500 pages) about the art of percussing the chest to diagnose and follow the progression of chest diseases. Without stethoscopes, the hands were major diagnostic tools in the past.

The sounds of air moving in and out of the lungs (breath sounds), should always be heard with a stethoscope, if not with the ear pressed onto the chest. As air is brought into the chest by active contraction of the muscles of respiration, making more noise than the more passive exhalation, as the muscles of respiration relax. Normal breath sounds are soft and clear, the stethoscope hearing only dry, unimpeded airflow. The author describes normal breath sounds to students as sounding like "a slight breeze through dry leaves". Inspiration is normally louder than exhalation in the healthy lung but in bronchitis and asthma exhalation become nosiest. Healthy flow and sounds change when fluid collects in the lung's air sacks and airways, distorting breath sounds from soft dry noises to ones that sound wet, almost musical. These sounds include crackles, honks and whistles.

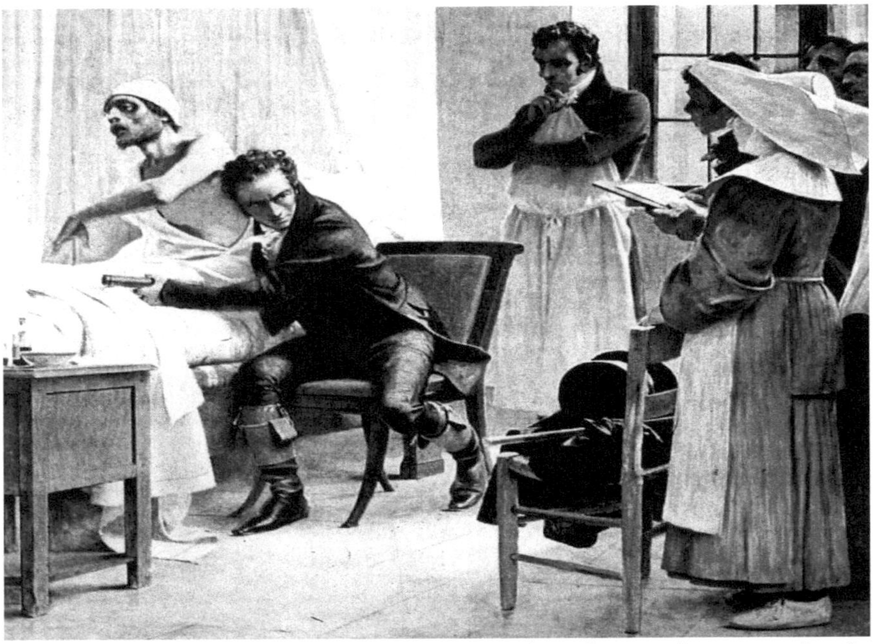

Renne Laennec (1781-1826) is credited with inventing the stethoscope, in the beginning a simple hollow wooden tube. It was no accident that the inventor of the stethoscope was an accomplished flutist as the instrument requires perfect hearing to play. He carved his own wooden flutes, invented the words, rales, rhonchi, fremitus. Painting by Theobold Chartran

Air flow meeting fluid within the air sacs creates crackling sounds, rales, described like crumpling cellophane close to the ear. Rales are multiple, intermittent "popping" sounds heard in one area of the lung or lungs. They are heard on inspiration, as incoming air "pops" open tiny fluid-filled airways and clusters of air sacs. Rales may be the result of several causes, depending on the circumstances and where they are heard in the lungs. If associated with chest pain, fever and cough, rales confirm the diagnosis of pneumonia. Since pneumonia is a potentially life-threatening disease, treat with antibiotics, both injectable and oral. When rales are found in heart diseases, with swelling in the ankles, the fluid is likely caused by heart failure (pulmonary edema). Heart failure is treated with salt restriction and diuretics to remove fluid from overloaded circulation by increasing urination. If rales develop quickly in a suspected heart attack, treat them with injected furosemide (Lasix) into a vein.

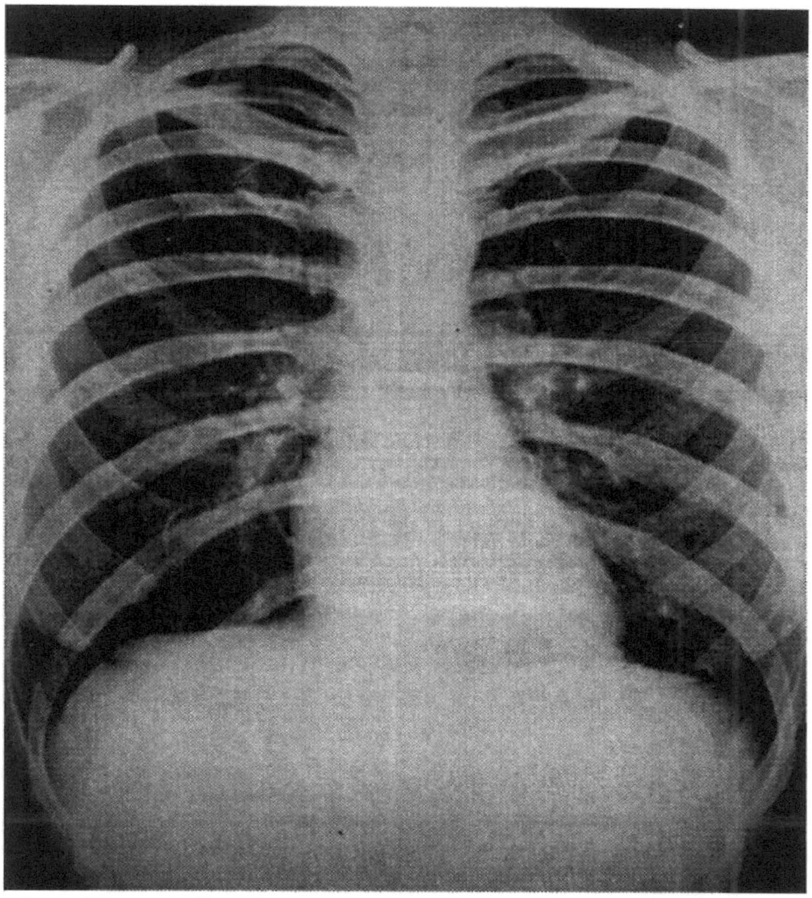

This is a normal chest X-ray. The dark areas within the chest are air filled lung spaces with the solid white heart in the mid chest, lying slightly on the left side. The oval white areas at the bottom are the domes of diaphragm lying atop the liver. The right lung is shorter because of the underlying liver. In pneumonia the dark areas become fluid filled and will appear white. In asthma and emphysema, the lungs overfill with air and the diaphragm pushed lower and flatter. The diaphragm acts like a pair of pistons dropping during inspirations and raising during expirations. A chest X-ray is done at maximal inspiration to reveal more of the lung tissue. Photo from file

Another abnormal sound often heard within the chest is rhonchi, sounds created as expired air passes through a partially obstructed airway. Unlike rales that are heard on inspiration and usually in one area, rhonchi appear during exhalation and occur over the entire lung or lungs, front and back. Rhonchi are generated as air "whistles" within an airway constricted by the spasm of asthma, or in the case of bronchitis, a collection of infected thick mucus. Both conditions, along with emphysema, create airway obstruction. Obstruction occurs primarily during exhalation since airways are held more widely open during the more active inhalation. Asthmatic and bronchitis chests sound similar, with asthmatic rhonchi usually more high-pitched whistles, while bronchitis is lower, more rumbling. Bronchitis causes chest pain and fever, asthma does not. Asthma tends to cause more shortness of breath than bronchitis. Bronchitis and asthma are both treated with bronchodilators and antihistamines, along with increasing clear liquids to reduce the thick respiratory mucus associated with it. If fever is present, antibiotics are indicated, such as an erythromycin, doxycycline, amoxicillin, sulfa.

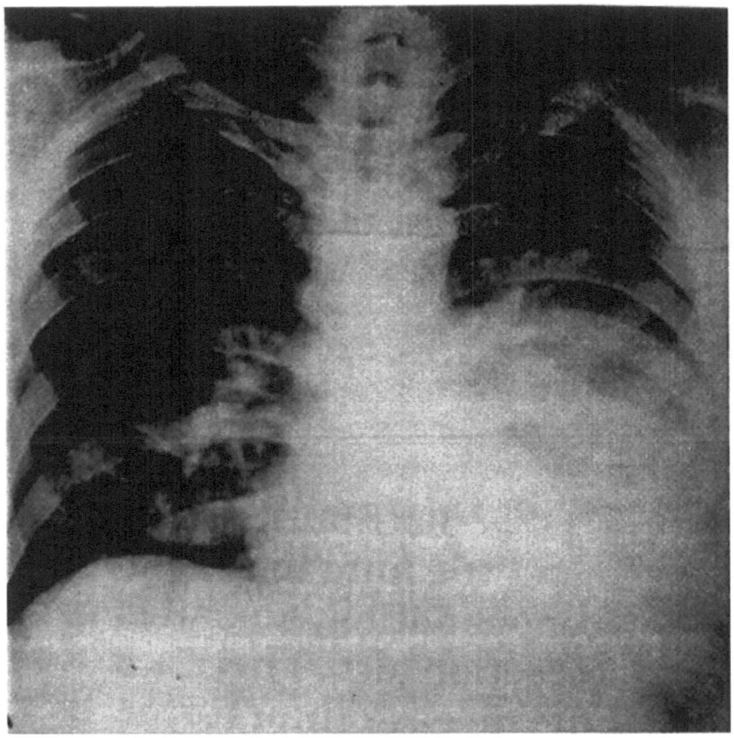

This X-ray depicts a left lower pneumonia. The white area in the left lung has obscured the heart shadow as fluid has replaced air in the lung. This person would have a fever, shortness of breath and rales along with decreased breath sounds over the left chest. With proper care including multiple antibiotics, fluids, rest and probably oxygen, the pneumonia should clear. Remember that pneumonia even in a young, previously healthy person can be fatal with-out proper care. Photo from files

Chest tightness and dry cough are more subtle signs of asthma, and rhonchi (wheezing) may not be heard under normal conditions, requiring exercise or a forced, hard exhalation to induce wheezing. Chronic smokers usually develop emphysema, caused by lung tissue destruction. Destruction results in soft, distant breath sounds hard to hear under normal conditions without a stethoscope. Emphysema usually produces rhonchi all the time, worse when the disease intermittently flares. It is treated like asthma with bronchodilators and fluids. When asthma or emphysema are accompanied by fever and/or green mucus, antibiotics should be used. Inhaled steroids are useful in treating lung diseases of asthma, emphysema and bronchitis since they enhance the lung's ability to clear mucus. These include inhaled steroids, Azmacort, Aerobid, Beconase and others. Inhaled bronchodilators are useful for the short term and will improving breathing and force of cough.

The loss of breath sounds is a poor sign. In severe pneumonia, no air moves through that section of lung. In pneumothorax (collapsed lung) airflow diminishes in the affected lung, and in the life-threatening tension pneumothorax, breath sounds disappear altogether. The most severe sign of respiratory distress is cyanosis, a blue tint to the skin. Cyanosis always indicates that inadequate oxygen is being delivered to the blood passing through the lungs. Give oxygen, completely examine the chest, and call for help if cyanosis appears. It can be seen in cold exposure and has little to do with lung function.

Chest wall injuries can lead to lung damage and pneumonia. When the flexible rib cage is forcefully misshapen in a fall or blow, the lung is bruised (contusion). Fluid collects at the injury site and because it is too painful to cough, the fluid becomes stagnant and then infected. Pneumonia was often fatal before antibiotics and continues to kill young healthy people today. Pneumovax immunization reduces the risk of pneumonia and wound infections. Stonewall Jackson died of pneumonia complicated by arm amputation. He might have lived had the stretcher bearers carrying the wounded Jackson to medical care had not dropped him on a tree root contusing (bruising) his lung.

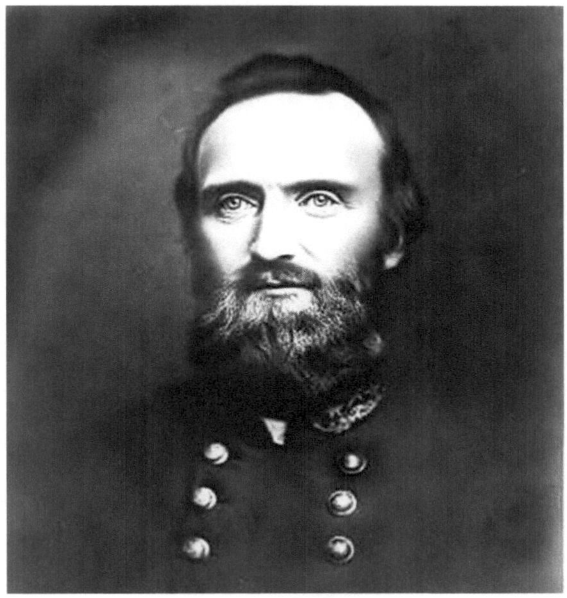

Thomas J. Jackson, better known as Stonewall Jackson for the way his brigade fought at the Battle of First Manassas (Bull Run) or for how slow he was at the Battle of White Oak Swamp. Jackson died of pneumonia days after his left arm amputation. Pneumonia likely the result of the stretcher barriers dropping him after he was accidently shot by his own troops. After turning the Union flank at Chancellorsville, Jackson was leading from the front in the gathering darkness, when troops from North Carolina fired on him. Days after the wounding, as he was dying of pneumonia and being a devout Christian (some would say, a religious fanatic), was pleased to pass on the Lord's Day, Sunday, May 10. Jackson's death prevented him from being present for the Battle of Gettysburg, where many historians believe Jackson would either have taken the high ground the first day of battle or agreed with Longstreet that it was a bad choice to attack the Union forces on the high ground. Loss of Jackson and the author's belief that Lee suffered a heart attack during the battle of Chancellorsville were major reasons for the Confederate defeat at Gettysburg. Stonewall Jackson is almost revered like a god to the South; however, he was a heartless killer to the enemy and his own men. Jackson executed more soldiers in the two years of his command than the German Army executed in four years of the Great War and drove his men ruthlessly before and during combat. Jackson's infantry was called "foot cavalry" for their ability to cover more distance in marching than any other troops. This was due in part to their dearth of medical care Jackson provided for his men. Although he travelled with a personal medical staff, he allowed only a single wagon of medical supplies for an entire division (3-5,000 men). He sacrificed logistics for speed. National Archives

The Cold
viral upper respiratory tract infection

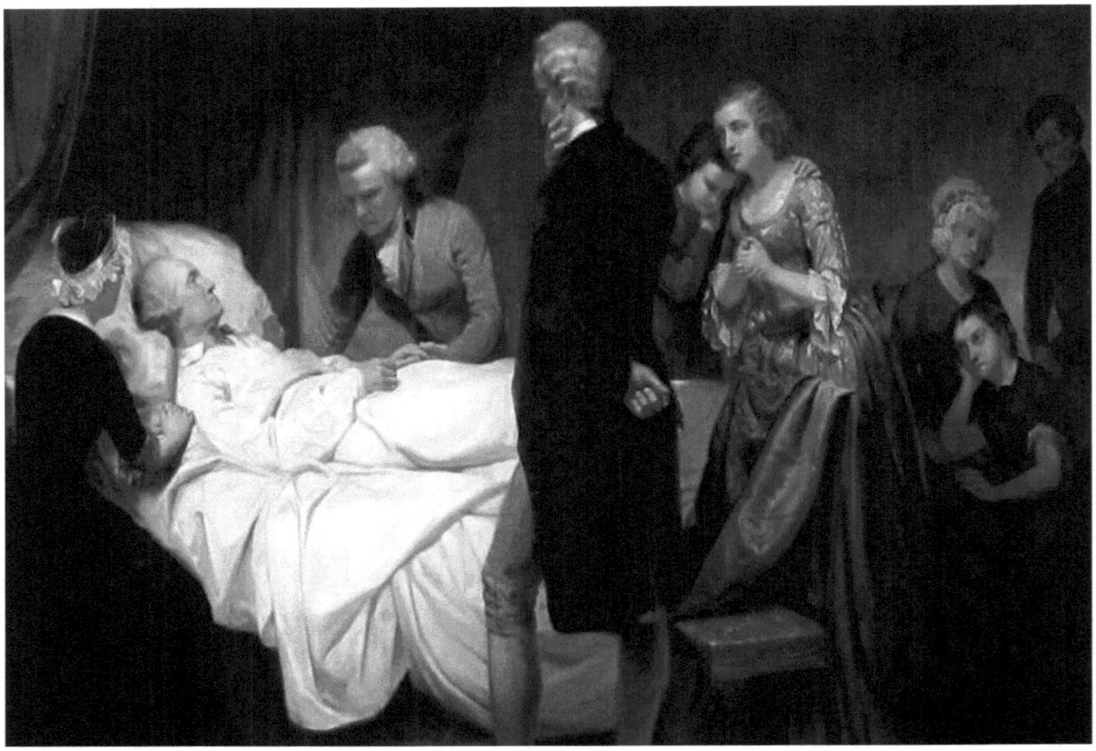

George Washington on death bed dying of pneumonia, painting by Junius Brutus Stearns. At least eighty ounces of blood was removed by his physician and likely contributed to his death.

Becoming chilled and "catching" a cold has long been associated with serious consequences. This fear certainly discouraged most of western civilization from bathing until recently. Viral respiratory infection is more common in the very young, the elderly, the already sick and the foolish. A sudden and sustained cooling of the body may inhibit the immune system, allowing viruses to reproduce, triggering congestion, which can lead to the collection and stagnation of fluids. Sinuses, middle ears and lungs then become more vulnerable to bacteria, leading to deeper more serious infections like pneumonia. During a winter coach ride in the 17th Century, Sir Thomas Bacon (1620-1697) became fascinated with the concept that ice could preserve flesh. Being a scientist, he had the coach stop at a farmyard, where he commissioned a hen to be killed and cleaned, while he stood outside on a cold, wet, windy evening stuffing the fowl with ice. He later caught a chill and shortly joined the ice-preserved chicken in death. George Washington, insisting on his daily horse ride, even in winter, was caught in a sudden wet snowstorm. On his return, wet and shivering, he took to his bed with a chill, was bled repeatedly in the medical tradition of the day, and died, having never left his bed following his last ride.

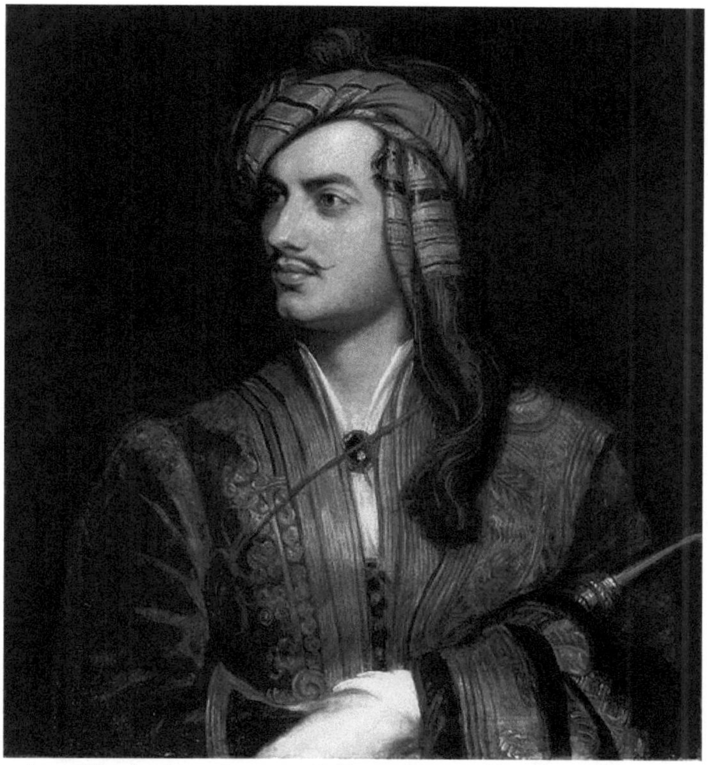

Lord Byron in Albanian Christian dress while a Crusader by Thomas Phillips (1770-1824) born with a club foot he developed a shuffling gait to disguise his disability

Lord Byron who in 1823, with his own money outfitted a warship, stocked it with seasoned marines and sailors, and sailed to the Ionian Sea to aid the Christian Greeks in their war of independence against the Ottoman Turks. The Greeks spent more time fighting each other while Lord Byron sat helplessly not knowing which faction to support. Against his physician's advice, he went for a horse ride in a heavy downpour, caught a chill and died of pneumonia, just as countless other would-be crusaders had done before him.

Colds are best managed by warming the person with heat, insulating clothing and hot drinks. A good hot drink is raw apple cider vinegar since all vinegars contain acetic acid, antibiotic, which kills viruses and bacteria. Increasing fluids will keep secretions watery and therefore less likely to plug the airways. Aspirin or Tylenol will reduce the aches and fever of colds, but a low-grade fever is perhaps helpful in containing the viral infection. Since bacterial infections can follow close on the heels of a cold, antibiotics should be considered if the person is at risk of respiratory infections. People with diabetes, emphysema, chronic diseases, the elderly, infants and heavy smokers are likely candidates for early antibiotic use. Symptoms of bacterial infection include productive cough (especially if green or bloody sputum is produced), fever, fluid sounds (rales) within the chest, decreasing alertness, loss of appetite or normal color, shortness of breath. The consequences of these signs warrant aggressive use of antibiotics. The best antibiotic management of suspected pneumonia is erythromycin-like antibiotic, azithromycin and cephalosporin injections.

Antihistamines, decongestants, and cough suppressants are sometimes helpful in making the patient more comfortable, but in no way replace the use of antibiotics in preventing and treating pneumonia. Good warm nutritious food such as chicken soup, vinegar on fresh vegetables and extra vitamins all enhance the immune system's ability in protecting and ridding the body of infection. Pneumonia continues to kill today, even striking healthy people. Fever and chest pain accompanied by shortness of breath should encourage early use of antibiotics and the pneumonia vaccine administered every five years reduces risks of death or disability.

Examination of the Heart

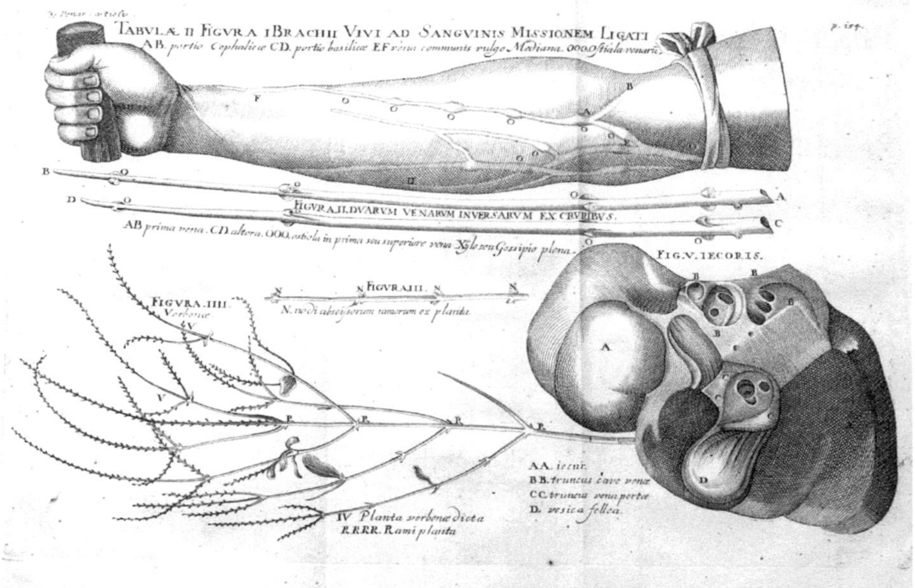

Illustration of William Harvey's lovely work, proving the heart pumps blood to the arteries and blood returned via the veins.

The heart is a fist-sized muscular pump found deep in the chest, surrounded by bone, fat and a tough connecting tissue (pericardium) giving it excellent protection, while making it difficult to examine directly. It can be indirectly examined by measuring the strength and regularity of the pulses, listening to the heart sounds and recording blood pressures. Pulse is normally regular and strong. Weak "thready" pulses may indicate reduced heart pumping volume which occurs in shock or heart failure. Irregular pulse is normal in some people, but its development during and after chest pain may indicate problems with the heart's electrical system. A slow steady strong pulse usually indicates good physical conditioning, since an athletic heart pumps strong and slower. On the other hand, a fast (greater than 90 pulse) at rest often indicates poor conditioning. Pulses less than 50 can be dangerous unless the person is a world-class long-distance runner. Low pulses are particularly worrisome after a possible heart attack, indicating damage to electrical behavior. Beta-blockers drugs often used around suspected heart attack can lower pulse, but usually not below 50.

In the days of Hippocrates, exam of the heart was done by feeling the pulse, laying hands upon the chest and watching for pulsations in the large neck veins (jugular). These are still useful in the field, combined with stethoscope and blood pressure device. The pulse can be monitored at several sites, the most common are radial pulse on the thumb side of wrist, the mid arm in the crease of the elbow (brachial artery), the neck (carotid), groin (femoral), behind knee (popliteal) and just behind the lateral ankle bone (posterior tibialis). Normally, the heart rate is measured by locating the pulse and with light pressure of the index and middle fingertip pads, gently press down. Count the pulse for one minute and that equates the heart beats per minute. Most medical officers count for thirty seconds and multiply by two or for fifteen seconds and multiply by four. Normal heart rates vary widely depending on health, age and sex of patient. Certain medical problems may be reflected in the heart rate. Normal heart rate is somewhere around 72 beats per minute; however, this number can range from 50 to 90 and is considered normal for that person.

Normal heart rate is regular, beating at exact intervals. Irregular heartbeats can be regularly irregular or irregularly irregular. An example is when every 3rd or 4th heartbeat is missing and often followed by a stronger pulse, this is common and caused by an electrical heart block. For some, this is a normal heartbeat and causes no symptoms. However, an irregular heartbeat emerging after an episode of chest pain is significant and is a physical finding of a heart attack. The most common irregularly irregular heart rate is atrial fibrillation, a common condition in millions of people who walk around without treatment. However, atrial fibrillation increases risk of strokes (cardiovascular accidents, CVAs) and some patients are placed on blood thinners to reduce stroke risk. Blood thinners increase the risk of bleeding in trauma.

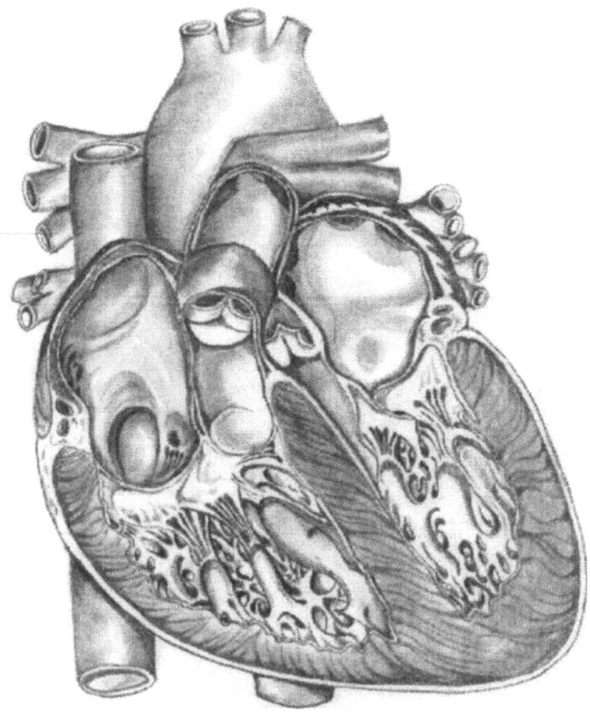

The human heart is a complex mixture of muscle, connective tissue and specialized nerves. Under normal conditions it should last for 100 years beating some 100,000 times each day of a life. The right side of the heart receives blood from the body and pumps it through the lungs where it exchanges carbon dioxide for oxygen. After it returns to the left side of the heart, it is pumped throughout the body. In the adult, 5 liters of blood passes through both sides of the heart each minute at rest. This amount greatly increases with exercise or when

the heart is exposed to adrenalin in the "fight or flight" reflex which increases not only the heart rate but also the force of contraction. If the heart is required to pump against higher pressures for long periods of time, the left side of the heart overstretches and becomes less effective as a pump, leading to congestive heart failure and shortened life. Angelica Mager

Blood pressure readings reflect the strength of heart contraction and pressure within the arterial system. High blood pressure is expected in pain and anxiety since, the body releases adrenalin, elevating blood pressure by stimulating the heart while at the same time contracting blood vessels. Low blood pressure is seen in shock as there is reduced blood volume to fill the interior of the arteries. A single blood pressure reading is not adequate to evaluate heart function. Repeated blood pressures are part of a thorough exam, taken lying and sitting. Low blood pressure in a suspected heart attack is a poor sign since an elevated pressure would be expected if the heart undamaged.

Listening to the heart sounds requires some experience and a quiet setting. These sounds have been heard over thousands of years, first with the ear pressed against the bare chest and recently with the stethoscope. Although we know much about heart sounds, the actual cause of the heart sounds remains a mystery. They may be the sounds of the heart valves opening, closing or simply the blood being pushed quickly through the constricted spaces of the heart. Under normal conditions, heart sounds consist of a first, S 1 and a second S2 sound. The first sound occurs when the large ventricles of the heart contract (systole) and is usually the louder of the two sounds. The second heart sound heard during diastole follows quickly after S1 and the two together have been described as "lub-dub", "lub-dub", "lub-dub". A heart murmur is a variation of heart sounds. Instead of a crisp "lub-dub" one hears a slurred sound or a low-pitched rumble. Many people have an innocent systolic murmur, heard during the first heart sound during the ejection phase of the heart's contraction. More worrisome murmur is one during diastole, and all diastolic murmurs are considered pathological and not innocent. The development of a murmur during and after chest pain in a person with no previous history of a murmur likely indicates a heart attack with now dead heart muscle. This dead tissue is now causing new turbulence within the heart. A murmur strong enough to be felt through the chest wall is a **thrill**, a term from an old English word, *pyrlian* meaning to perforate or pierce, in medicine comes from word for shivering.

The Thrill

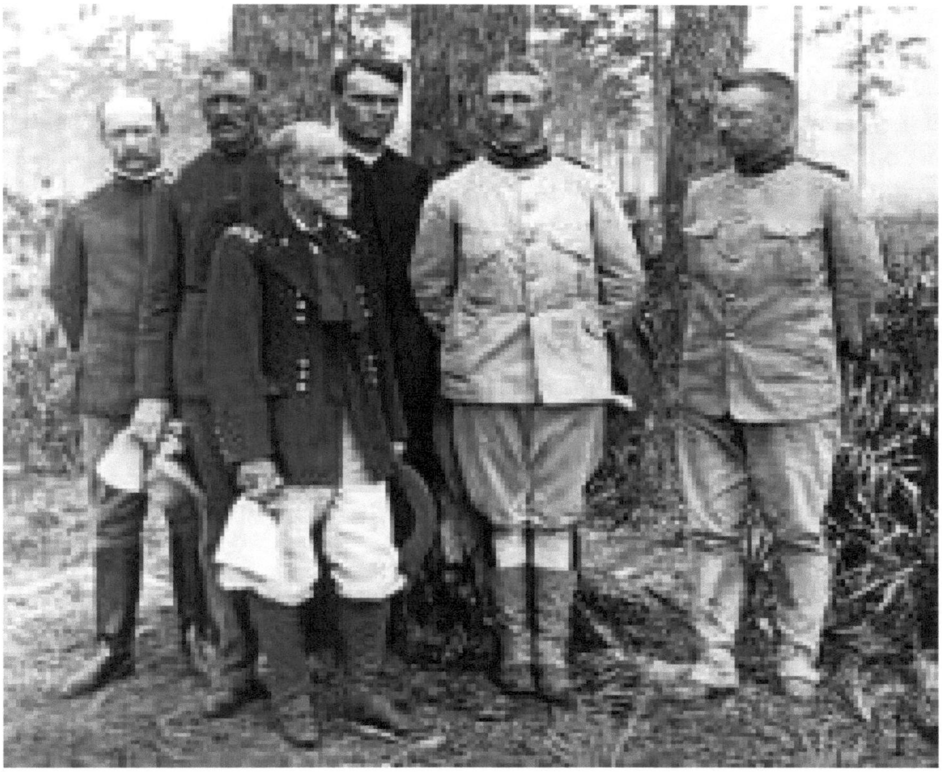

Brodie, 2nd from left, the significantly shorter Wheeler in front with Wood and Roosevelt on the right. Four major players in American history in the late 19th and early 20th centuries. National Archives

Alexander Oswald Brodie, Army officer and engineer (like Robert E Lee), 1870 grad of West Point, served with 1st Cavalry in the West (the unit commanded by Lee before the Civil War), direct descendant of Robert III King of Scotland (descendant of Robert the Bruce made famous by the movie "Braveheart" and "The Outlaw King"), fought in the Apache wars (where Leonard Wood, MD won the Medal of Honor) and Chief Joseph's War in the Pacific Northwest, served in Benicia California Arsenal, home of the author. Brodie is credited with saving the lives in combat of both Theodore Roosevelt and Leonard Wood, acts which changed history.

Joseph Wheeler is fascinating piece of history, and the author uses his story to explain the medical term, a thrill. Born in Georgia, raised in Connecticut and graduated at the bottom of West Point class 1859, where he was just tall enough to be accepted. Wheeler fought in most major Civil War battles in West, including Shiloh, Perryville, Stones River, Chattanooga and Atlanta. He was captured by the Union's Maj Gen George Stoneman, becoming the highest-ranking Confederate officer prisoner of war. During the war he was wounded three times, had thirty-six staff officers killed beside him and sixteen horses shot out from under him. After the Civil War he was elected to the House of Representatives 9 times by Alabama and served as chairman of Ways and Means Committee when Spanish American War was declared. In the late 19th century, Joseph Wheeler was the most powerful man in Congress and second to the President, the most powerful man in Washington.

At the peak of Wheeler's political power, war with Spain was nearing. The press led by William Randolph Hearst was screaming for war and continuously encouraging hostilities. Exactly the behavior of British and French press igniting the Crimean War. Along with Hearst, Teddy Roosevelt, the Undersecretary of the Navy pushed the United States into war. President McKinley was reluctant to declare war between the United States and Spain for several reason. The President was himself a combat Civil War veteran and knew the human costs of war. The war was unpopular requiring moving thousands of federal troops, many of them black soldiers, through the South, still unsettled after decades of occupation by federal troops and there was concern the South would feel they were being invaded again. Most importantly, McKinley needed Wheeler and other Southern democrats to fund the war.

To secure Wheeler's support for the Spanish American War, McKinley gave him a commission as a Major General and a combat command at the age when most officers were retired. Joseph Wheeler is the only former Confederate General to be later made a United States General. During fighting in Cuba, while leading from the front, another his horse was shot dead under him. When slowly getting back on his feet, he was reported to say, "It's been over 30 years since I had a horse shot out from under me, it's still a thrill". At one point when the Spanish troops broke before an American charge, Wheeler yelled, "we have the Yankees on the run", forgetting he was now a Yankee. He later fought in the Philippines under Douglas MacArthur's father, served with Leonard Wood MD who now commanded all American forces in the Philippines and his daughter Anne Early Wheeler served in WWI as a Red Cross nurse. He had a role in one of the first motion pictures, "Surrender of General Torel" in 1898 and is one of a few confederates buried in Arlington National Cemetery.

Discovery of a thrill after an episode of chest pain, like Wheeler's last horse, is a "thrill" of a physical finding. The appearance of a thrill or murmur during an episode of chest pain is diagnostic of a heart attack in the field. Normally, when the hand is held lightly (palpation) over the heart with flat palm or back of hand, contraction is felt through the chest wall. The strength of contraction can be roughly measured with palpation, along with beats per minute and regularity. An irregular heartbeat is more concerning if it appeared after episode of chest pain. Murmurs created by high flow aberrations in heart structure can be turbulent enough to be felt. If there is enough turbulence, it can be felt through the chest wall as an intermittent "rattle" transmitted to the medical officer's hand. Thrills are significant and usually associated with leaky or stiff valves or by dead cardiac muscle "banging" back and forth in a ventricle. Whatever the cause, a thrill emerging after an episode of chest pain is significant.

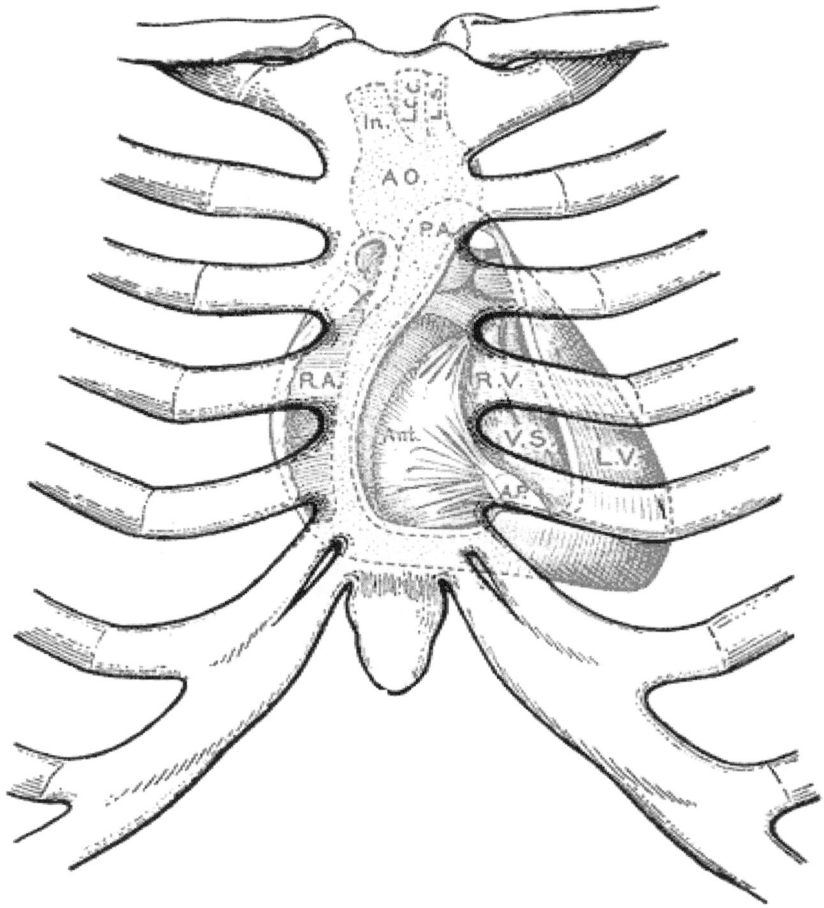

The heart in most people is just offset to the left mid chest. Placing the hand over the heart area should give the medical officer a "feel" for the heart function. Contraction of the heart should be felt except in conditions such as shock or in very thick people. In heart disease, especially heart valve disease, turbulence with the heart and major blood vessels can be felt. These vibrations are transmitted through the chest wall, producing a thrill of shivering felt in the well-placed hand. NLM

The Skin

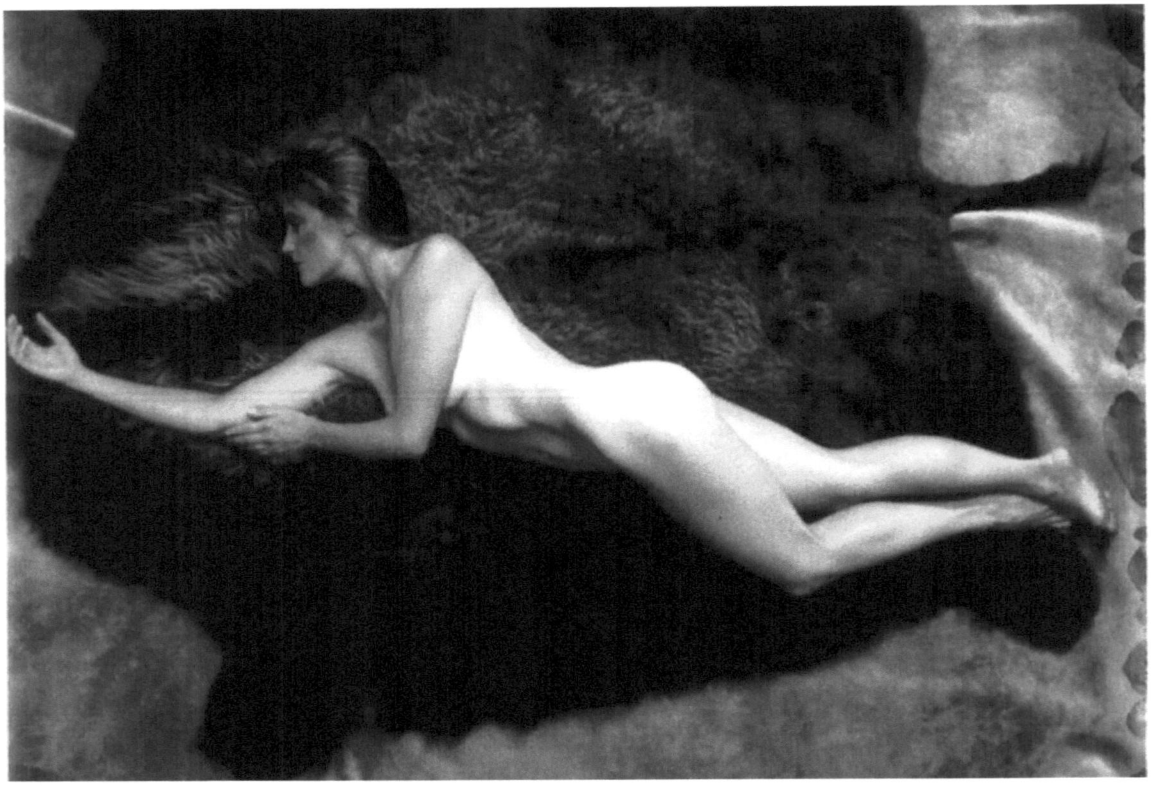

Stretched over the bones and soft organs of mammals, fish, fowl and reptiles, is a tough yet pliable membrane, known simply as skin. In humans it varies from a microscopic thinness 0.5 mm over the eardrum to a ten-fold increase in thickness of 5 mm (1/8 inch) over the palms of hands and soles of feet. Thin special modifications of skin form the lips, eyes, genitalia, rectum, and line the mouth, upper respiratory tract and vagina. Averaging a surface area of six by three feet, the human skin is considerable protection from a surrounding environment hostile to the body's fragile interior. The buffalo skin and that of the young woman above, biological engineering producing both beauty and durability. Photo by Dave Bush

The surface of the skin (epidermis) is composed of layers of dead cells connected to the deeper living tissue (dermis) by thin interlocking projections. The dermis is home to nerve endings, tiny complex organs for sweat and oil production, blood vessels, lymph channels and hair roots, all protected under an outer shield of tightly packed skeletons of former living cells. Opposite of a reef composed living animals atop layers of dead ancestors.

The primary function of the skin is protection, blocking the entrance of toxic agents and microorganisms, while reducing the amount of penetrating ultraviolet radiation generated by the sun. Skin insulates the body's interior from temperature extremes, mechanical forces and the loss of body fluids. But the skin is much more than a simple protective envelope. It is an elaborate communication system connecting the internal organs with constant information from the skin. Nerves within the skin measure temperature, detect tactile (touch) sensations, hear sounds and classify mechanical forces as painful or pleasant. Much of the stimulation of the sexual centers comes from the skin. Skin is filled with tiny lymph channels and blood vessels imbedded and coursing through its layers, constantly patrolled by specialized white blood cells (leukocytes) that detect injury or invasion. At the site of the skin's breach, circulating "scouts" or sentinels of the immune system release chemical markers into the lymph system, bringing immune cells to the battle site of breached walls. These chemical messengers communicate to the body's entire immune system the details of the type and severity of injury. Cytokines are chemicals released that "control" behavior of other immune cells, chemokines are chemicals that attract immune cells to site of battle and CDs (cluster of differentiational) are chemicals imbedded in wall of white blood cells that dictate their response to injury. CD4 helps stimulate B cells, while CD8 acts like a "bangalore" explosive tube knocking holes in walls of invaders. Healthy skin has a remarkable ability to repair itself, many times with little or no scarring. It secretes its own natural antibiotics and provides protective oily secretions to cover hair, coat feathers and lubricates eyes. As a testament to skin's durability, properly tanned animal hides can function for centuries. If skin is well cared for and protected from sunlight it can be healthy for over 100 years.

Throughout lifetime, skin experiences exposure to a hostile environment presenting a large target to a variety of injurious agents such as trauma, infection, cancer and allergies. Skin like the eyes reflect events taking place within the body. In respiratory collapse, lips and skin become bluish (cyanosis) from lack of oxygen. Hepatitis turns first the eyes yellow (jaundice), and later in the skin as unprocessed pigment, bilirubin spills from vessels, staining the skin. Jaundice is from the build-up of excess bilirubin, a waste product a sick liver cannot process. Anxiety, shock, chronic illnesses and anemia result in pale skin. In shock and heart attack, skin may be damp, cool and pale. Excessive bruising without trauma implies a bleeding disorder, while chronic diseases such as diabetes and alcoholism are manifested by skin changes. The skin of the face, hands and genitalia contain the highest concentration of nerve bundles known as receptors and account for the excessive pain levels from wounds, especially burns to these areas.

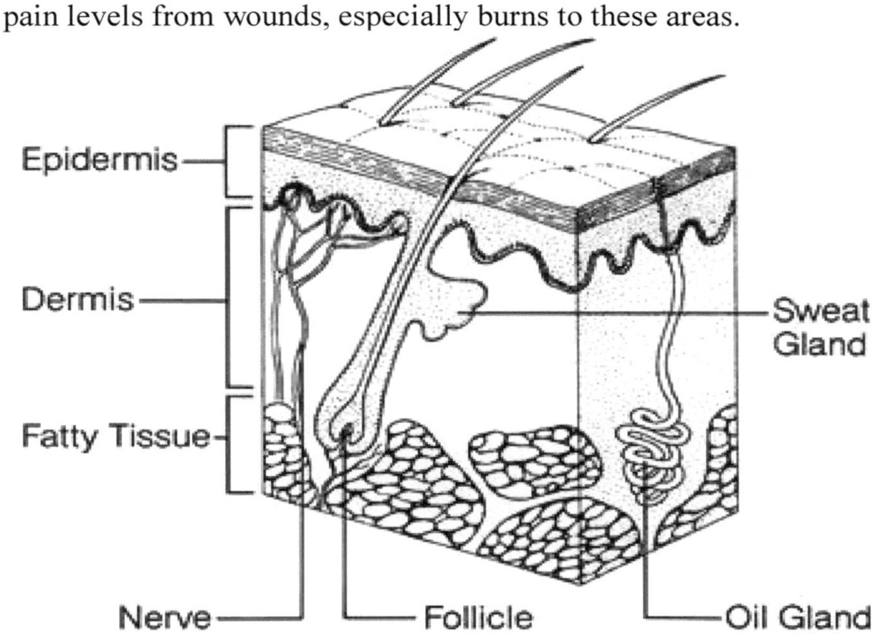

Puncturing the dead upper layer of skin are hairs, narrow necks of sweat and oil glands. NLM

Skin Glands

There are three primary glands found within the skin. Oil (sebaceous), sweat and cerumen (ear wax) glands residing deep in the living skin with their narrow necks reaching the surface, any of which can serve an infection site. Sebaceous glands are associated with fur or hair follicles, where they secrete an oily mixture of fats, cholesterol, proteins and salts to protect and groom hair. They occur in large numbers in the genitalia, eyelids, neck and upper chest. Sweat glands are simple structures when compared to the more complex oil and wax glands. Concentrated in the underarms, pubic region and chest, they secrete a complex mixture of water, salts, urea, ammonia, sugar, vitamins (C) and contain blood components such as drugs and infectious viruses. A special type of oil gland found in the axilla and pubic areas secrete an oil that has no use in the human, however the oil serves as food for the bacteria expected to be there. Everything in circulation may be found in sweat. Wax glands are best known in the ear canal, where they produce cerumen, a heavy oil that provides protection for the fragile ear canal. Ear wax should be left alone unless it has blocked the opening, removed by lavage and not with a Q-tip. Soap removes natural oils from hair strands, requiring conditioner after shampoo to separate and control longer hair.

Wound care is covered more completely elsewhere to prevent small wounds from becoming serious field medical problems. Infected wounds with their local swelling and redness may slowly spread towards the interior body without proper care. The red streak leaving the wound and migrating up the extremity must have appeared as a poison in the past. Infected wounds in late stages of sepsis, result in coma. In the fairy tale of "Sleeping Beauty", she is awakened by a kiss from a prince after a small wound put her to sleep. Cleaning, dressing and antibiotics have replaced the "kiss" for wound infections. The story of "Sleeping Beauty" is to warn the danger of small wounds, where a foreign body is left in place. Earliest versions emerged in mid fourteenth century, on the eve of Black Death. In three different versions, Sleeping Beauty's wound and embedded foreign object was a rose thorn, splinter from a spindle and in the earliest version, a sliver of flax. There must have been thousands of grieving family and friends gathering at the bedside of a dying loved one, struck down by a simple wound aggravated by an embedded foreign body. Splinters flung from projectiles into wood ships maimed and killed more sailors than the direct effects of cannon balls.

Skin Color

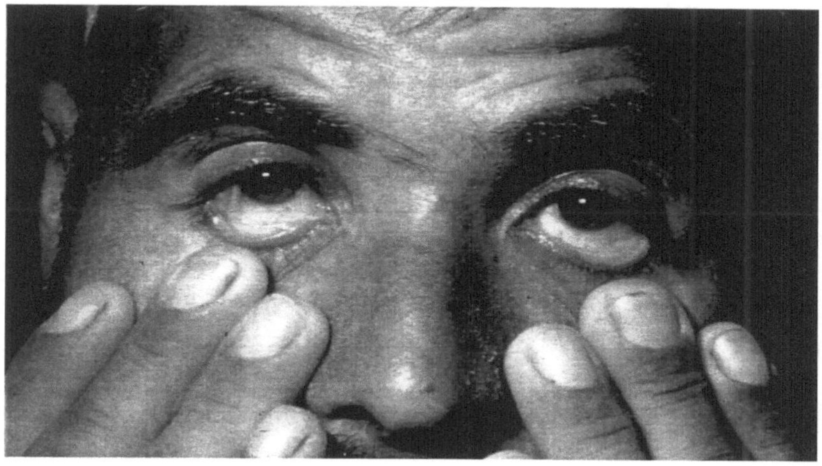

Pale skin in the lower inner eyelids and fingernail beds are classic skin findings of low blood count. Anemia is common in the third world where intestinal parasites roam free in the gut and urinary tract consuming nutrients the bone marrow and immune system needs for blood cells and protection. They also lower blood levels further by causing bleeding. There is a common urinary parasite (*Schistosoma haematobium*) in Egyptian farmers who wade in their Nile-soaked fields, in their early adolescence begin to have bloody urine. 19th century English medical officers referred to this teenage onset of hematuria as "male menopause". Photo by author

Solar Injury

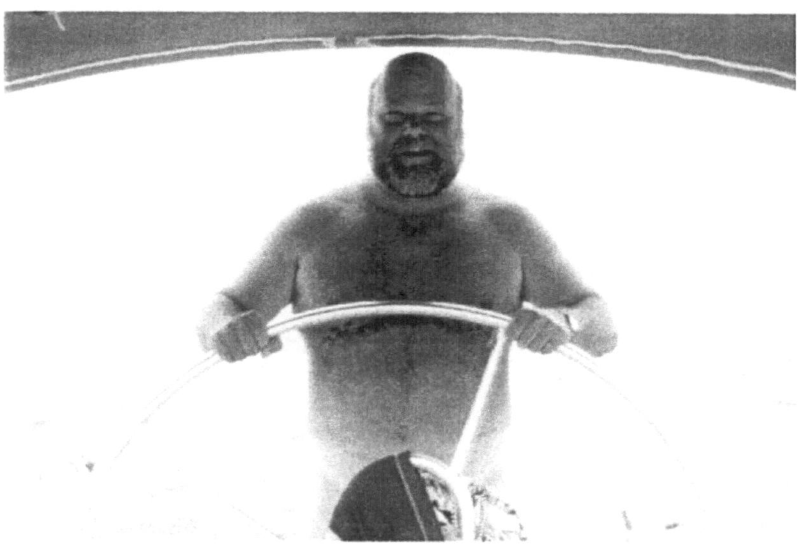

Even though this person is in the shade of a dodger cover he is still receiving reflected cancer-causing radiation to a large area of exposed flesh. Some of this skin has seen little

sun before and is more likely to burn in reflected sunlight. Cover up with clothes or sunscreen, even in the shade. Photo by author

Skin color is reflected light from subterranean streams of blood, just underneath the skin's transparent surface, the capillaries. This color varies with skin thickness and pigmentation. Pigmentation is due to melanin, brown granules of protein produced and packaged by the melanocyte. These cells sense increased sun exposure which encourages deeper skin color as melanocytes respond by transporting pigment from its production sites in the dermis to the skin's surface in long hollow tubes (dendrites). Exposure to sunlight or tanning increases pigment formation and therefore increases tolerance (protection) to solar energy. However, excessive tanning reverses this beneficial effect and increases risk of early skin destruction and skin cancer. The variety of skin pigmentation found among the world's people is due to their ancestor's level of sun exposure since sunlight is necessary to convert vitamin D into bone. The lower latitudes receiving daily direct sunlight, produced darkly pigmented people, whereas in the relatively sun-starved northern latitudes with long dark winters and only a few hours of sunlight produced a blonder lightly pigmented population. People with dark skin have the same number of melanocyte (pigment producing cells) as people with fair skin, but they are larger and contain more pigment and therefore block more solar radiation than light skin people. The risk of skin cancer is related to the amount of sunlight filtered, thus light skin and light eye-colored people are more susceptible to sun injury. Australia leads the world in skin cancer as many people living are descendants of Northern Europeans whose ancestors did not evolve skin color for lower latitudes.

Skin color varies widely among animals depending upon the climate they inhabit. The white polar bear has black skin, its ivory color comes from refracted sunlight in its long hollow guard hairs. Guard hairs stay erect and will not mat when wet, allowing the bear to quickly shake off water, reducing the risk of water freezing in the fur. The hollow hairs also work like "light pipes', funneling ultraviolet sunlight from the sun to the bear's dark underlying skin.

It is important to realize that more than skin is being exposed to solar radiation. The sun is a giant fusion nuclear reactor, and its radiation passes through the skin's semitransparent membrane. Cells and chemicals transiting the spidery network of vessels in the skin are bombarded by tiny units of the sun's discharge. Blood components absorb solar radiation and carry it to deeper organs, playing an active role in the internal environment. Exposure to sunlight activates some drugs causing adverse reactions such as itching, rash and extreme redness. Antihistamines, antibiotics (especially, tetracyclines), diuretics, anti-inflammatory drugs and even sunscreens can cause skin problems when exposed to ultraviolet radiation. If solar radiations can cause cancer in an organ as durable as the skin, it is not hard to imagine that it could also trigger the development of cancer in less durable internal organs. Melanoma, which can spread widely, can occur in places never exposed to sunlight. Circulating immune cells are known to be quite sensitive to radiation, may be adversely affected by an overindulgence of sunlight, increasing the risk of leukemia, lymphomas and malignancies other than skin cancer.

Temperature Regulation

In all warm blooded (homothermic) animals, the skin serves to prevent overheating or, when confronted with cold, becomes an effective insulator keeping heat in the body. Deep within the primitive layers of the brain lies a group of nerve cells known as the temperature regulating center. Slight variations in the temperature of the blood flowing by these cells triggers the center's activity which will then either radiate heat away or trap it within the body. Evaporation or sweating is initiated by overheated blood bathing the central nervous system. As the body's temperature rises, this center becomes more active, stimulating nerves and chemical messengers to direct more blood to the skin's surface wile opening sweat glands. If temperature continues to rise, more vessels open, routing additional blood to the skin. Tiny sweat glands stimulated by this increased flow, begin to secrete a mixture like diluted urine onto the skin's surface, where its evaporation cools the body. This sweat contains many substances like salts, antibodies, infectious agents such as hepatitis or AIDS, proteins and drugs, all of which reflect the contents found in the circulating blood. Sweat on the skin evaporates taking heat away from the body through radiation, since to evaporate the sweat away, heat must also leave the body.

Sweating is paramount to temperature regulation in hot environments and should not be hindered. The former practice of using salt tablets to conserve water loss and reduce thirst is poor medical practice. Salt tablets have no place in the field medicine. If the body's ability to sweat is impaired, overheated blood within the brain cause the symptoms of heat stroke: distorted judgement, physical collapse, coma, brain damage or even death. If delicate brain tissue is heated above 105 F, serious irreversible damage may occur in adults. Children's brains can tolerate high temperatures, and seizures are not uncommon in high fevers. Heat injury is preventable with adequate water intake, intake which may reach two to three gallons per day in the tropics or in the heat of an engine room. With fevers, fluids are paramount in protecting the person, whether elevated temperature is from infection or heat stroke. Former students lost a boat in the Tuamotus's Islands (the Dangerous Archipelago) when they struck a reef due an error in navigation. They believed the heat induced confusion had distorted their judgement. Probably not the only boat lost due to heat-related injury.

Dermatology-
The Study of Skin Disease

Perhaps to a greater degree than the other medical specialties, dermatology has developed its own vocabulary. It helps to be familiar with the more common terms used in the description of skin disorders.

Dermatology Definitions

Macule: a small area of altered skin color without elevation (age spot)
Plaque: a raised "plateau" of skin (flat mole)
Nodule: a solid small "bump" (mosquito bite)
Papule: a solid tiny "bump" (chill bumps)
Vesicle: a fluid filled cavity (blister)
Bullae: a larger filled cavity (larger blister)
Ulcer: a localized area of skin loss
Fissure: a crack in skin (athlete's foot, cracked lips)
Wheal: Raised fluid filled streak of swelling, a "welt", hives or urticaria

Crust: raised platform of dead skin and debris (impetigo, healing chickenpox)
Ecchymosis: area of blood under skin (bruise), usually associated with trauma
Petechiae: tiny dark spots of bleeding, looks like "buckshot", associated with fevers that cause hemolysis (bleeding under skin) known as hemorrhagic fevers.

Contact Dermatitis

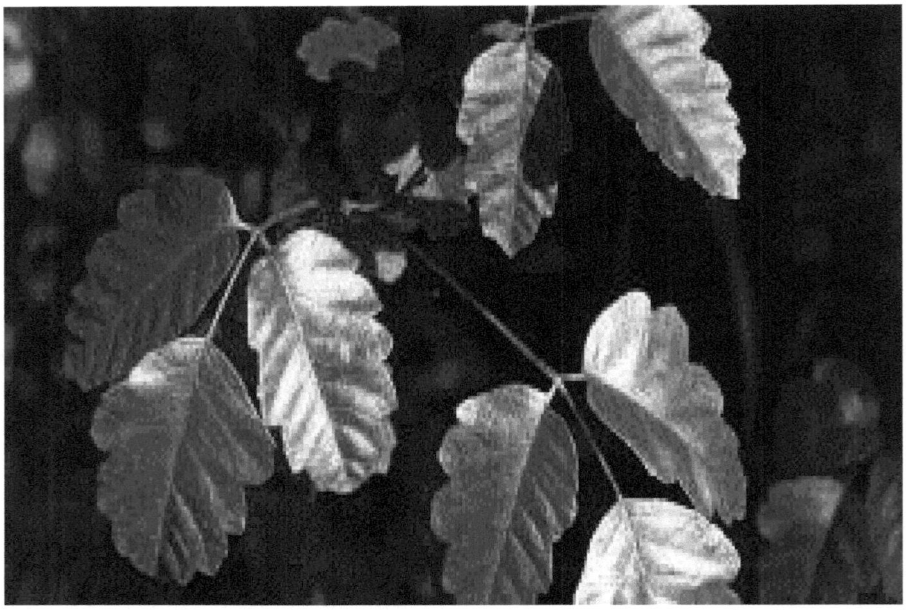

"Leaflets, three, let it be!" Both poison oak and ivy leaves occur in threes and this poison oak (*Toxicodendron diversilobum*) is common on the author's Pacific coast farm and one of the most toxic plants found anywhere.

This common acute rash is caused by direct contact with a toxic chemical or one that triggers allergic reactions. The results of this chemical reaction are redness, itching and in some cases blisters and ulcerations. Poison oak and poison ivy in the plant class Anacardiaceous, produce some of the strongest known plant toxins among many other toxic plants. Other causes of contact dermatitis include hydrocarbons such as diesel fuel, paints, cleaners, metals (especially, nickel), rubber products, sea animals (fire coral, sea cucumbers, starfish, etc.), new clothing, make-up, sunscreens or in many cases of unknown causes.

Contact dermatitis is a common who visit outdoors, where some plants contain toxic oils or resins, and when warmer temperatures reduce protective clothing. The Cocobolo tree and wood products in central America, in the West Indies a type of manzanita, the manchineel tree, along with most tropical gourds and cucumbers, tulips and mango leaves, contain irritating resins. All the "stinging" plants such as nettles, prickly pear and the Spanish dagger cause skin penetration along with a chemical injury when the plant releases histamine and acetylcholine (two active chemicals found in the body). Whatever the cause, emergence of redness, swelling, vesicles or the larger bullae (blisters) strongly suggest contact dermatitis, especially if the site itches. These eruptions are generally well defined but can become continuous over a large area. When contact dermatitis affects thin skin such as the eyelids or genital area, swelling can become severe enough to close eyes and inhibit urination, or when rash is widespread, consider the use of oral steroids (Prednisone).

Contact dermatitis usually clears without treatment, however, there is the risk of infection if itching is not controlled. It is important to minimize the action of scratching, which may open and contaminate already injured skin from the abrasive action of bacteria-laden fingernails. Wet soaks with Epsom salts, Dome Burroughs, or any soap will lift remaining plant residue while soothing the injured skin and reducing bacteria. The area of inflammation should be lightly coated with a topical steroid or astringent (calamine) and covered with dressing of cloth or Saran wrap which keeps the medicine from being rubbed off while reducing scratching during sleep. Nails should be kept clean and short, especially in children. Benadryl (diphenhydramine) capsules are helpful in reducing itching. Itching can be done with ice cubes whose smooth icy surface will numb as it soothes.

Topical steroids are the commonly used agents in treatment. They are more effective in the milder form of contact dermatitis or when the rash is limited to one area. In more severe cases where itching has led to early skin infection or when the rash is widespread, oral antibiotics and oral steroid should be considered. A steroid dose such as Prednisone or Solu-Cortef of 60 mg each day for two days, 40 mg each day for two days, and 20 mg for two days, will be helpful in reducing the more severe inflammatory responses. If the rash begins to show signs of infection (increased redness, pain, swelling and red streaks), a wide spectrum antibiotic such as erythromycins or cephalosporins should be used for 7-10 days. Clothing, including shoes, should be thoroughly cleaned after contact with poisonous plants. It is possible for a person to get another case of contact dermatitis months later from contaminated boots.

Eczema

In this common allergic skin condition of chronic dry itchy skin with "scaly rashes" over the elbows, knees, hands, face, and in some cases, large blocks of skin. These areas can crack, fissure deeply and become infected, especially in children from nighttime scratching. People with eczema should avoid exposure to irritating harsh soaps, wool, and oils such as lanolin and petroleum products. Treatment includes moisturizing creams and bath oils, intermittent use of topical steroids and antibiotics if the area becomes infected from itching. Keeping the skin clean and dry is important. The habit of frequent bathing, which is a recent (last century) innovation has greatly reduced chronic skin irritation from the grit of dirt abrading the skin with friction. The constant dampness to parts of the body, such as the groin, promotes fungal growth. Until recently, skin infestations such as scabies, lice and fleas were a constant source of skin irritation. Bathing, laundry cleaned with soap in hot water and sanitation has greatly improved skin health.

Psoriasis

A common life-long incurable disease marked by irregular patches of raised red skin, covered by silvery-white scales. New biological drugs are effective in controlling the disease; however, it appears to be a life-long condition and in an unfortunate, few has affects internal organs. The first areas affected are elbows, knees and scalp while in some more severe forms, psoriasis is associated with severe disfiguring arthritis, is one of the most destructive disease of joints. Symptoms may come and go early in the disease and the condition can be improved by exposing the affected skin to sunlight. In some respects, psoriasis behaved like a malignancy and anti-cancer drugs have been used to control.

Leprosy is mentioned several times in the Old Testament and once in the Gospel of Luke. However, most people labelled as "unclean" lepers were likely suffering chronic skin lesions from other causes. At the time Leviticus (the Hebrew Book of Laws) was written describing leprosy, Greek medical literature makes no mention of leprosy but describes other chronic skin disorders. By the time of the Crusades there was leprosy in the Middle East, but the author believes leprosy mentioned in the Old Testament was more likely chronic forms of dermatitis which could cause losing digits, skin deformities and the foul odor of chronic wound infections. Certainly, they would appear unclean.

Fungal Infections

With a vast number of fungi in the world, only a few cause skin problems and those are normal skin inhabitants (dermophytes). In most cases dermophytes are microscopic scavengers, cleaning up debris on skin that accounts for a tiny part of the hordes of microscopic inhabitants of our skin. So hardy are fungal creatures that they can feed on keratin found in the outermost layers of dead skin, hair and nails. If the protective layer of keratin is breached through dampness and cracking, fungus colonies will invade and increase, provoking an inflammatory response of redness, itching and scaling. In the scalp and beard, tinea capitis, on the trunk causing "classic ringworm", tinea corporis, not a worm, but clusters of tiny colonies growing outward over the skin, like lichen on a rock. On the feet, tinea pedis causes "athletes' feet". Another common skin fungus, tinea versicolor is characterized by slowly spreading white spots that will not tan.

All common tinea infections can be treated with a variety of topical agents. Older preparations including Whitfield's ointment, Castellellani's Paint and Gentian violet solutions, some are still used in some parts of the world where they are effective although irritating and messy. Undecylenic acid was introduced during World War II and is still today in most over-the-counter preparations. Most common topical anti-fungal is clotrimazole and other similar drugs will end in "zole".

A shampoo containing selenium (Selsun Blue) is useful in treating chronic fungal dermatitis afflicting the scalp and beard. Selenium shampoo is also effective in treating tinea versicolor when used most days for several weeks. Miconazole and clotrimazole are of the most common fungicides, and when combined with a topical steroid cream relieves the inflammatory response as the fungicide eliminates the dermatophyte infection, reducing itching. On the feet and body, these creams should be used intermittently for several weeks after the skin appears clear. Allylamines such as Lamisil are currently the most effective.

There are several oral agents used in treating fungal infections. The first is nystatin, which has enjoyed a long, safe, and successful battle against oral and vaginal yeast infections. Thrush is a common problem in infants causing a white membrane developing over the tongue and inner cheek, treated by placing nystatin on a finger or swab and wiping the area two to three times each day for several days after clearing. Thrush also appears in the immunosuppressed. Diaper rash is usually caused by candida, a fungus producing an angry red rash with surrounding red patches and satellite colonies. This rash is best treated with clotrimazole and mild steroid cream. Ketoconazole is a recent arrival on the scene of fungicides and useful for yeast infections such as chronic candida vaginitis. It is effective against more severe or aggressive forms of skin fungal infections that may be encountered. Oral Ketoconazole is available worldwide and although generally safe, can have serious side effects if taken with other drugs. Do not take oral antifungals if you do not have a list of all medications it may react with.

Sun Burn - Solar Radiation

Redness, tenderness, pain and in severe cases, blisters are signs of excessive sun overexposure. Treatment is limited, prevention is paramount. After the injury, cold compresses, fluids and pain relief with aspirin, acetaminophen or other analgesic. If blisters form, they should be left intact (do not deliberately puncture) and managed like a second-degree burn. Repeated sunburns or deep tanning results in the life-long accumulation of radiation leading to destruction of the skin connective tissue (wrinkling) and several types of skin cancer. The desire to tan increases in all types of skin cancers including basal cell and melanoma now occurring in younger victims.

The sun radiates a wide spectrum of light energy, fortunately, the most destructive never reach the Earth's surface, but are reflected back into space or absorbed by the atmosphere. The most significant wavelength for skin cancer is the ultraviolet B wavelength emitted in the midrange of the solar spectrum around 300nm. Sunlight of this wavelength has several possible mechanisms that can damage or cause mutation of fragile, unprotected DNA inside the cell's nucleus. Blood cells are bombarded by solar energy with every passage through skin in sunlight. It is theorized that ultraviolet light damage is usually repaired over time, however solar-injured cells may experience faulty repair with continued exposure. An example of faulty repair is the scaly, wrinkled skin of solar-caused actinic keratosis (sailor's skin in old med texts) causing irregular red thickening or thinning over sun exposed skin. If untreated and continued sun exposure, it slowly becomes malignant. Solar radiation can trigger herpes outbreak and leads directly to cataract formation and is partially blocked by covering clothing and sunglasses. Actinic keratosis is treated with liquid nitrogen or Retin A. cream, preventing premalignant skin lesions from becoming malignant.

Blocking the Sun

The most effective way to block solar energy is not with sunscreen, but sunblock, such as reflective clothing covering the entire body or an occlusive dressing such as zinc oxide (can be manufactured from diaper powder and petrolatum). Shade, although reducing sun exposure, allows a substantial amount of radiation to strike the skin as reflected light. Surfaces such as water, sand, decks, etc., reflect 25 to 40% of the cancer-causing wavelength. Snow intensifies the effects of sun. Clouds reflect only one-half of solar radiation back into space, permitting sunlight access to cloud-shaded skin.

Sunscreens lying over the skin's surface absorb UVB sunlight before it penetrates skin. These include PABA, padiate 0, benzophenones (oxybenzone), cinnamate, and salicylates. Sun blocks, such as zinc oxide, are much more effective since they reflect light as opposed to absorbing it.

Sunscreens are labelled with a sun protecting factor which relates to the length of time of safe exposure to the UVB. The higher the number, the more time one can safely stay exposed. Even at the higher sunscreens, there is still solar radiation reaching the living skin and is not as effective as clothing. Swimming, sweating, contact with sand or towel decreases the effectiveness of the sunscreens and therefore repeated applications are required. Staying in water is no protection since 96% of UVB will penetrate several feet of clear water.

Skin Cancer

People who work and play outdoors are recipients of the most common malignancy, skin cancer. Fair complexion, light eye color, easily sunburned people are at the highest risk, especially with a history of repeated sunburns. The closer to the equator and the higher the altitude (thinner air and less absorption), the greater the risk. The irritation of wind friction passing over skin increase risk of skin cancer significantly when added to sunlight (at least experimentally in rats). Common sites include the face, back of hands and neck, top of ears and back. Basal cell skin cancers, the most common, first appear as small mounds of pearly pink, scaly, flaky skin known as actinic keratosis. Later, these areas become raised with a central cavity or crater which ulcerates and bleeds becoming a sore that will not heal.

The signs of early skin cancer are subtle. Any mole that changes in size, color, or shape should be removed and examined by pathologist. A mole that begins to itch or one that develops multiple colors should be removed. Some recommend any pigmented (dark) mole as large as an eraser head should be removed. It is not always wise to be suspicious and wait for other changes that may herald cancer such as surrounding redness or the development of a nodule at the site. Early removal of any unusual, localized skin change is paramount to diagnosis and treatment of skin cancer. It is important to examine the skin in its entirety, using a magnifying glass and bright light to carefully examine moles for color, loss or disruption of skin lines at the margins of moles (Lines of Langerhans's) and irregular margins with the color spreading out just under the skin. Redness surrounding a mole and itching increase suspicion, as these mild symptoms may be the body's immune system paying attention to a problem.

Malignant Melanoma

The incidence of melanomas has been increasing, especially among younger Caucasians in the USA. Until recently there was no effective treatment for this aggressive cancer. Keytruda and other Sulphur-containing anti-tumor medications in this class have been a breakthrough saving many lives. In the past, the cure was only effective with early diagnosis and surgical removal, sometimes removing large sections of tissue containing lymph nodes. People who sunburn or freckle easily and those with multiple moles, are at an increased risk to develop melanoma. A family history of melanoma increases a person's risk 100-fold.

The signs of melanoma include the ABCD warning. A is for the asymmetry of a mole's borders, appearing to "leak" out into the surrounding skin as ink will do when wet. B is for border irregularity instead of being smooth, the border reveals an irregular coastline of tiny bays and peninsulas (east coast of Newfoundland). Another border change is the loss of tiny skin lines that crisscross the skin. In normal moles these lines appear unmolested across the mole, whereas, with skin cancer the lines often stop at the irregular border as skin architecture is being disrupted. C is for color variation. Common moles are usually one or two colors. In melanoma, there are often three or more colors with blue, red, and white found within the same lesion. D is for diameter. Moles the size of eraser heads (6 mm) or larger are more likely to become malignant.

During the yearly physical exam, all skin should be viewed in people with risks of skin cancer since melanoma may occur in skin that has received little to no sun exposure. Suspect moles should be removed at the earliest opportunity. If possible, have a pathologist examine the mole to make sure that if it is malignant and that the cancer has been removed in total. In some cases, cancer cells will have penetrated deeper into the skin and escaped to other parts of the body through the lymphatic system.

Burns

There are several mechanisms whereby the skin can be injured by a burn. Injury from the sun occurs over hours whereas superheated metal or steam will severely and deeply damage skin in less than a second. Burns have been classically described as first, second and third degree depending on the depth of skin involved. A newer classification is based on an exam to determine the full or partial thickness of the skin injured. In any case, all burns should be cooled as soon as possible to reduce further injury.

All burns are hazardous to the entire person, not just the skin. First degree burns such as sunburn are accumulative over one's lifetime and may lead to the development of skin cancer. Second and third-degree burns breach the skins protective barrier increasing the risk of deeper infections. Burns are often avoidable with protective clothing, sunscreens and healthy respect for all things hot. It is a good habit to wear a long apron in the galley, with hot pads and a fire extinguisher close at hand.

Burn Dressing

Over the ages, many substances have been employed to reduce the pain and suffering of burns. These have included poultices containing plant products, animal oils, petrolatum even manure, and some have been effective. Aloe dressing made of fresh plants (cacti) has been efficacious for centuries. The right combinations are effective, and the ideal burn dressing would be soothing, non-stick, have some anesthetic as well as antibiotic properties and work as a wick to draw fluid out of the wound. Keeping burn wounds free from discharge may require frequent changes. The author's recommended dressing is prepared with the following: Silvadene cream (Silver sulfadiazine 1%) liberally spread over the wound after cleaning. On top of the cream, non-stick Telfa or Adaptic pads placed and covered with 4" x 4" sponges held in place by rolled gauze or tape placed away from the burn edge. This dressing, if kept dry, will "wick" fluid from the wound, decreasing contamination. If the dressing becomes damp with either wound discharge or water, the dressing will act like a wick in the other direction. Wicking fluid into the wound allows skin bacteria along the wound margins to be pulled into living tissue. Dressings must be kept dry and changed as soon as they become soiled. The presence of damp soiling of the dressing means that the dressing is now a hindrance to wound healing and should be replaced. Most burn wounds be better off without a dressing than a one damp soiled covering.

With each dressing change, dead tissue is removed gently and completely as tolerated by the burn victim. Dead tissue is identified by its color of black, brown, green or yellow. The presence of tiny bleeding spots at the bottom of the wound means viable tissue has been reached. Prior to debridement the wound can be soaking under a gauze damp with the local anesthetic, lidocaine. In addition to local anesthetic, an oral narcotic given fifteen minutes before may reduce the discomfort associated with wound debridement. The area should first be gently scrubbed with warm soapy water to remove the surface debris that forms over the burn. Using small forceps (tweezers) and scissors, the dead tissue should be gently cut away. Replace the burn dressing and change once a day, more often if it becomes damp. Debridement should be carried out at least every other dressing change, while wound margins are carefully monitored for signs of infection.

Insect Bites

Insect-borne diseases constitute some of the worst afflictions that plague mankind causing sudden and slow deaths. Throughout history and today, they account for the greatest numbers of deaths and much of the world's misery. Typhus, malaria, plague, yellow fever, sleeping sickness, typhoid fever and others are carried within the arthropod's body and transmitted to humans through the wound of the bite. The damage to humans by the Tsetse Fly and the sleeping sickness, kept mankind and livestock out of the Serengeti, allowing large native animal herds to exist there and nowhere else in the world. The microbe carried by Tsetse flies unknowingly preserved the plains of the Serengeti from human domestication. Arthropod-borne diseases occur when the pregnant female mosquito, tick, louse, flea or fly takes a blood meal from tiny vessels just under the skin. The virus, bacteria or parasite is injected or regurgitated into the victim's blood stream during the feeding process. This type of infection is referred to as the anterior approach, while an even more unsavory infection can be delivered in the posterior manner.

Insects such as the Ridivid bug of Central and South America (now in southern USA), to make room for a blood meal, expel a bowel movement at the time of feeding. The Ridivid's stool is irritating to the skin around the wound site triggering itching. The unknowing victim during sleep, mindlessly scratches the site, rubbing infected stool into the bite wound, allowing the parasite access to vessels just beneath the skin. This bite may lead to a serious and often deadly Chagas' disease. This insect is common in thatched roof huts in moist hot climates where hundreds of beetles reside in each hut and drop onto sleeping victims in the dark. Although rustic and romantic, avoid sleeping under thatch in the tropics and have a thorough appreciation of the parasites and other infectious agents common in tropical travel.

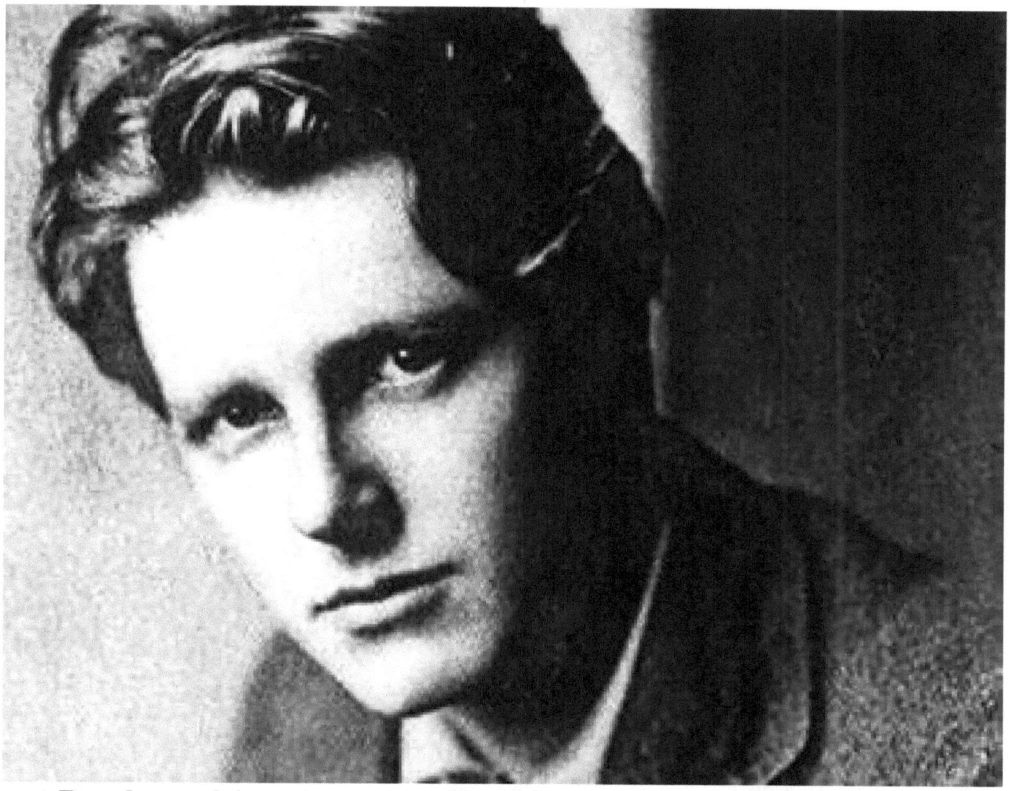

Rubert Brooke, a rising star among English poets was a scholar and an athlete at Cambridge, who after graduating travelled and studied in Germany, Italy, Canada, United States, and the South Seas. The Irish poet W. B. Yeats described him as "the handsomest young man in England". At the beginning of World War, he obtained a commission as an officer in the Royal Navy, saw combat in the retreat from Belgium, contracted dysentery in Egypt and died on a hospital ship off a Greek island of an insect bite while awaiting landing at Gallipoli. The wound became infected and spread causing blood poisoning. National Portrait Gallery, London

If I should die, think only this of me:
That there's some corner of a foreign field
That is forever England

Rubert Brooke died before the age of antibiotic and like thousands of other soldiers, a small wound became fatal. If there is any doubt about a wound becoming infected, clean, dress and give antibiotics. Even if the insect bite carries no harmful agents, they should be avoided. Itching and subsequent scratching may damage skin, allowing surface bacteria access to the deeper tissue, created by insect wound. Insect bites are best prevented by protective clothing and repellent. Bite sites should be cleaned and left open to the air to reduce irritation and local itching. Swelling can be controlled with ice (using an ice cube to scratch). Should itching become a problem, the application of mild steroid cream or oral antihistamines (Benadry) may be useful. The development of swelling, redness, heat and a red streak moving away from the wound signal an infection, and antibiotics and hot soaks should all be employed

Scabies

Scabere is Latin for scratch

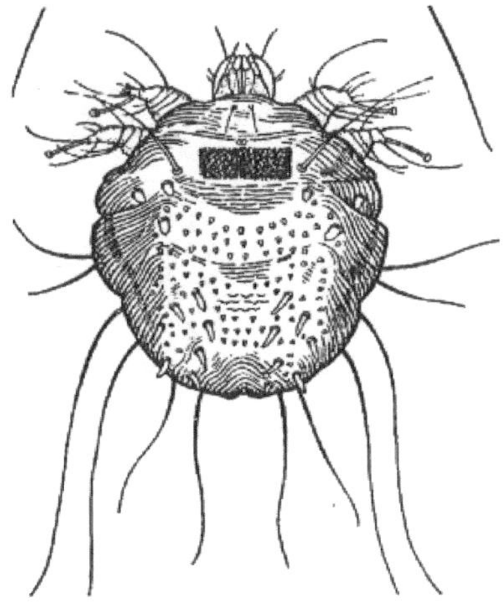

The female scabies has been described as an armored excavator. Textbook of Clinical Parasitology 1932 by David Belding

Scabies (mites) have been around as human companions well before recorded history. It is especially common when bathing is rare. Mite infestations of the scalp and skin have afflicted humans throughout history and are still common throughout the world. Outbreaks continue in the USA occurring even among the affluent. The tiny, submicroscopic insects causing scabies are impressive in their attack on the human skin. The pregnant, *Sarcoptes scabiei*, that digs her way into skin is a true Alien-like horror. Electron microscopy reveals a female animal that is armed with multiple tooth-filled jaws, covered by armored plates and sprouts digging claws capable of quickly excavating a tunnel many times her length. After copulation on the skin, most males die of exposure while the pregnant female excavates a 3mm burrow within 2-3 minutes. The female may lay eggs for up to four to five weeks after fertilization, depositing eggs in different burrows. A few fortunate males enter these burrows where they may live the bachelor life for two to three weeks. The female deposits a catch of eggs and fecal pellets (sayballa) providing her newborn mites their first meal. Some 4-5 days after hatching and having consumed their mother's leavings and possibly their father, emerge from the burrow and scatter to surrounding hair follicles. In ten days, they are adults, fertile, reproducing and soon digging new bungalows.

Their burrows appear as tiny winding threadlike elevated channels ending in a grayish speck. The most common sites for these creatures are the finger and toe webs, wrist, elbow, nipples, genitalia and underarms. Vigorous scratching at these lesions often leads to a skin infection of impetigo making it important to manage the itching of scabies along with killing the mites and their hibernating offspring. Scabies likely attributed to many labelled as "lepers" in ancient history. Lindane (named for James Lind, Royal Navy), a preparation of 1% hexachlorobenzene (the benzene ring kills the animals) is available world-wide, effective, and reasonably safe. Before application, the entire body should be washed, dried and then covered completely with Lindane cream and rinsed in 24 hours. If mites continue to appear, repeat the process in one week. Itching will continue for as long as one month after the mites and eggs are killed because the skin still retains the body parts while the immune system continues to remove them. Do not apply more than two treatments, even if itching continues, as the benzene ring of Lindane is also toxic to humans. Crotamiton 10% (Eurax) can also be used to kill scabies, but it is less effective in the scalp. The cream is massaged into the entire skin surface from chin to toe following a routine bath or shower and left on for 48 hours. A second application is recommended 24 hours after rinsing the first application. This is more effective in scabies infestations of the body and is not as effective in scalp scabies. In most cases, head and body hair is removed.

All this activity in the skin leads to a great deal of irritation and therefore scratching. It is easy to imagine our forefathers, with no adequate bathing facilities and no effective drugs, sitting first around campfires and later around conference tables scratching. Meeting first as tribal leaders and later as leaders of nations, making historical decisions while digging at itchy sites. Early European sailors to Japan and China were called barbarians by the Orientals because of their filth, stink and infestations. Sailors spent months at sea without bathing, living in the same unwashed clothes and bedding. Ships with the wind astern could be smelled before being seen. James Lind a 17th century English ship's surgeon routinely "baked" clothing and bedding of sailors combined with frequent bathing to reduce vermin and the diseases they brought. Scabies come through contact with contaminated bedding, animals and sleeping partners. The intense itching of this disease is mechanical due to burrowing tunnels under the skin.

Flea Bites

These wounds are common throughout the world in both temperate and tropical climates. The diseases they carry are spread by close human contact with an infested dog, cat, rat, mouse or other humans. Blood-fed fleas can survive for weeks and months in bedding after the meals provided by animals or guests have departed. Some fleas can produce thousands of offspring if provided enough blood meals. Designed like flattened stickers and burrs of plants seeds, anchored between hair follicles where they survive claws, nails and teeth trying to remove them. Their bites begin as small papules with a tiny central puncture wound and may evolve to vesicles or pustules with surrounding redness. These bites tend to be clustered in groups of three and lead to intense itching and secondary bacterial infections such as impetigo.

The common treatment is lindane cream or shampoo. Management includes killing the fleas (by thorough washing of bodies, clothes and bedding), reducing itching and responding to a possible wound infection, coupled with Benadryl to control itching. All bedding and clothing should be cleaned in hot soapy water with vigorous rinsing. Fleas in many parts of the third world may carry tropical fevers and should be suspected in multiple bites. It was the flea and louse that brought Black Death to 14th century Europe, and they can transmit serious disease today. An engorged flea may go one year before needing to feed again. They can even survive freezing for several months, revived by a warm blood meal. They have a sensory component of their nervous system that can detect heat and carbon dioxide of a near possible host.

During blood meals, fleas and lice have spread diseases that changed the very fabric of human history such as the destruction wrought by the Bubonic Plague during the mid-14th century. Millions of humans and untold animals died an agonizing death during a few short years beginning in 1346. The disease came in two forms, the first and the more deadly attacked the lungs, causing severe sudden pneumonia and death, the less severe form though survivable still killed in great numbers. The early 1340's were the last good years in Europe for a very long time. Weather changes produced by volcanic activity in the East Indies on the other side of the world brought several years without a summer and began the "little ice age" that lasted until mid-19th century. Almost all plagues are preceded by climate induced famine which reduces human immune systems. Volcanic activity and extraterrestrial impacts (Justinian's Comet) from space brought catastrophic climate changes precipitating the Plague of Justinian in Mid-6th century AD, begetting the Dark Ages. The Dark Ages lasted five hundred years and depopulated much of Northern Europe. Climate change, wrought by events well outside any human activity led to wet cold summers and even colder, dark winters combined with shipping are the perfect storm for great pandemics in human history. Following several seasons without summer and the Justinian plague, the legend of the Holy Grail emerged from the darkness as a hope for mankind.

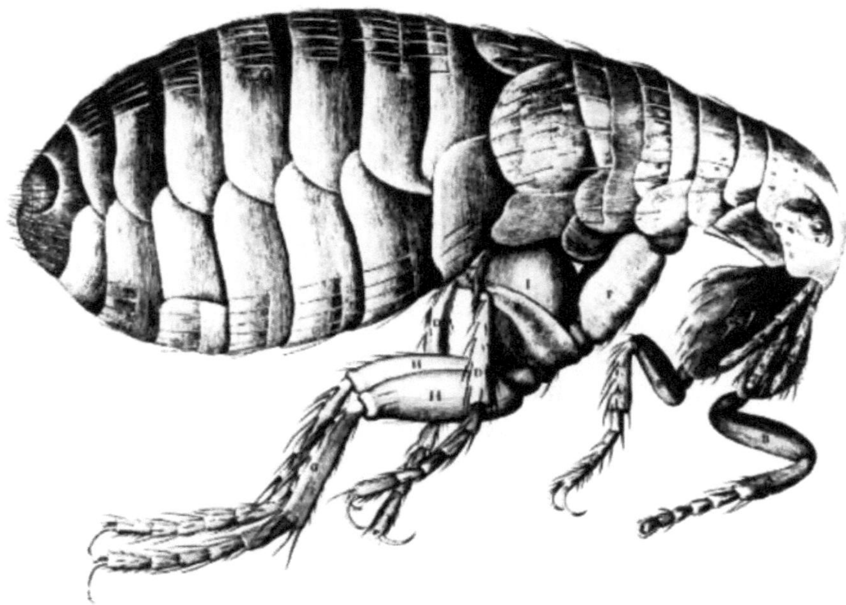

Robert Hooke published "Micrographia' including his drawing of a flea in 1665. This flea, like other tiny animals that appear in his book, were found on and in him. "Justinian's Flea" is a good read for the plague that damaged 6th Century Byzantine.

The Black Death

According to the historian Haester, around twenty-five to 40% percent of the entire European population died in a brief five-year period. The pneumonic form was the more merciful, killing within hours. So devastating to the body, physicians who arrived healthy sometimes died before the patient. It was the deadly pneumonia that brought about the childish jingle "Ring around the rosary, a pocket full of posies, a-choo! a-choo! And we all fall down". The rosary was the Catholic beaded necklace for God's protection, the posies were a common folk cure-all and the person that begin to cough or sneeze would surely fall down and die. In non-pneumonic form, there was some chance of survival depending on the number and size of the large tender nodules, buboes arising under arms and groin. These huge lymph nodes soon would break through the skin and ooze the foul stench of deep infection, an odor that was soon extruded by the breath, bowel and even skin.

Death in Bubonic Plague was so horrible that children would desert parents and parents would desert children, while priest would refuse Sacrament in fear of the contracting Black Death.

The medical world was helpless to explain or treat the disease. Philip VI, the French King implored the medical University at Paris for a report on the disease that was rapidly decimating his population and wealth. His ministers reported village after village being deserted and the cities filling with dead bodies all over his empire. After seven months of study, the premiere medical faculty in Europe reported to the king, "The cause is a triple conjunction of Saturn, Mars and Jupiter in the 40th degree of Aquarius". As to the treatment, they admitted that the knowledge was hidden from even the most highly trained physicians. Medicine during this period even at the Universities was based more in astrology and theology than the medical science of Aristotle and Galen. Greek and Roman knowledge was lost from much of Christian Europe. Most blame the Church for the low quality of medical education in Europe and what competent medicine that was practiced was by Hebrews and Arabs, rarely by Christians.

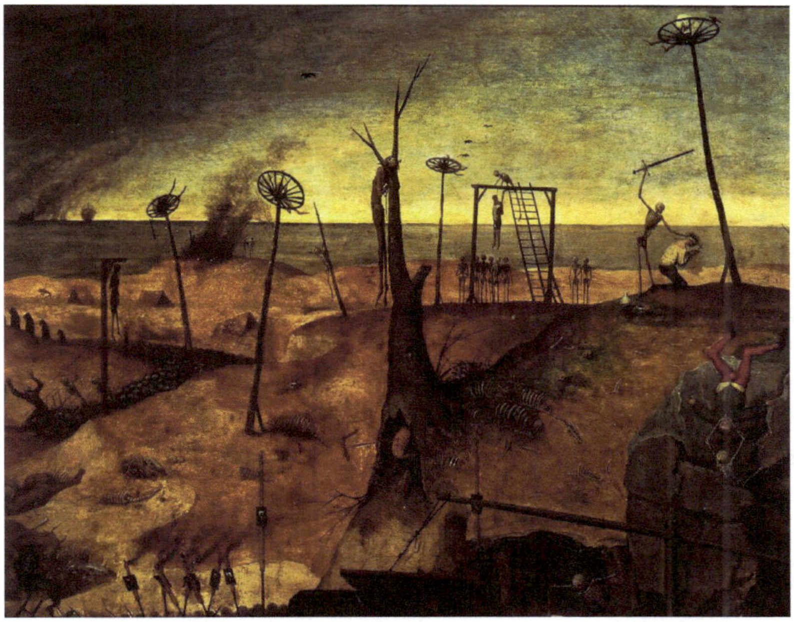

A portion of the "Triumph of Death" by Pieter Bruegell. A painting depicting a world doomed with death, famine and warfare because of a deadly and easily spread bacteria. After entering history in the 14th century, it remained dangerous and fear for nearly a millennium. The Allies in England believed Germany was going to parachute plaque-infected rats and paid a bounty on rats brought for exam for Bubonic Plague.

The death rate in Black Death was highly variable as in some isolated villages, the disease was barely felt while in coastal and river ports over half were killed. Death was highest where there was direct contact with shipping since incoming ships brought rats and their accompanying fleas with plague. The historian Haeser reported mortalities were the lowest where there was a shortage of doctors. In plague as in other infectious diseases, children were the hardest hit. In many coastal hamlets and cities of the 14th century children became a rare but joyful site. This paucity of children coupled with normal high infant mortality rates produced a labor shortage for several generations which helped shape the early industrial revolution where machines replaced people.

The disease continued to ravage Europe in populations living in crowded cities, along with garbage, human waste and rats for centuries. Those who have on lived on the water know how rats thrive in these habitats. Sailors and their ships continued to deliver new strains of Bubonic Plague throughout the 14th and 15th centuries. Sporadic episodes were still reported early in the 19th century, occurring in dock workers and sailors. Rats in some of the world's busiest and most heavily polluted harbors carry this formidable disease today. Five hundred years after Bubonic plague descended on Europe in coastal Viet Nam, the cause was discovered to be *Yersinia pestis* living alternately within the gut of the flea and the bloodstream of the rat. Man became an accidental host to the bacteria when bitten by either the rat or the infected flea. Pestilences have rendered profound effects on civilizations. In the panic and fear of infectious diseases, people have abandoned farms often fleeing to crowded conditions. Because of insect-borne infections, there have been food shortages creating famine, causing displacement of populations, revolutions and civil wars, all combined to encourage fanatical religious movements and political upheavals.

As ill a wind as the plague was, Black Death did have some positive effects on Europe. At the time of the plague there were around 17,000 lepersoriums throughout Europe. Every city or rural area had a leper colony, its occupants were shunned and reduced to begging. Leprosy disappeared after the plague, only persisting in small numbers in northern Europe, especially Scandinavia. Some believed the plague bacteria had somehow eradicated the TB-like bacteria that causes leprosy. And it did so indirectly. The sudden decrease in population, necessitated a rise in mechanization; windmills and water wheels for the felting of wool into clothing and blankets, grinding grain, powering forges. Wages for the first time were paid to common people as now their labor had value. Now with money, wool clothing and blankets could be purchased, decreasing the previous need for entire families and sometimes villagers to huddle around a single fire sharing blankets and animal skins for warmth. Leprosy requires prolonged skin to skin contact with friction as in shivering next to infected skin. People were no longer huddling so much, except in the colder parts of northern Europe.

Fire Ant envenomation

Envenomation from this aggressive insect is more common than stings from other insects of the Hymenoptera class insects (bees, wasps, yellow jackets and hornets) in Central and South America, Southeast United States and the Caribbean. Reaction ranges from local redness to intense pain, and possibly death of anaphylactic shock. The fire ant causes an unusually large local reaction at the bite site that causes enough damage to develop into an infection. To some people, the venom may produce a severe allergenic reaction as insect venoms contain large foreign proteins and a high concentration of toxic alkaloids. These chemicals may cause significant local destruction of skin and underlying connective tissue, forming puddles of pus and dead tissue (necrosis). This event is often preceded by formation of a clear bubble (vesicle).

Little can be done to prevent necrosis from insect and spider envenomation, since the tissue destruction is difficult to halt. Hyperbaric oxygen in decompression chambers is used throughout the Southern USA for spider bites primarily for the Fiddleback and Black Widow spiders. Moist heat, frequent gentle cleaning with medicated soap and water, removal of dead tissue and wound covered with a clean dry dressing will decrease the risk of infection. If infection develops then an oral antibiotic such azithromax would be recommended. In most cases the spider bite occurs undetected until pain, redness and swelling develops.

Ticks
Arachnoid-eight legs

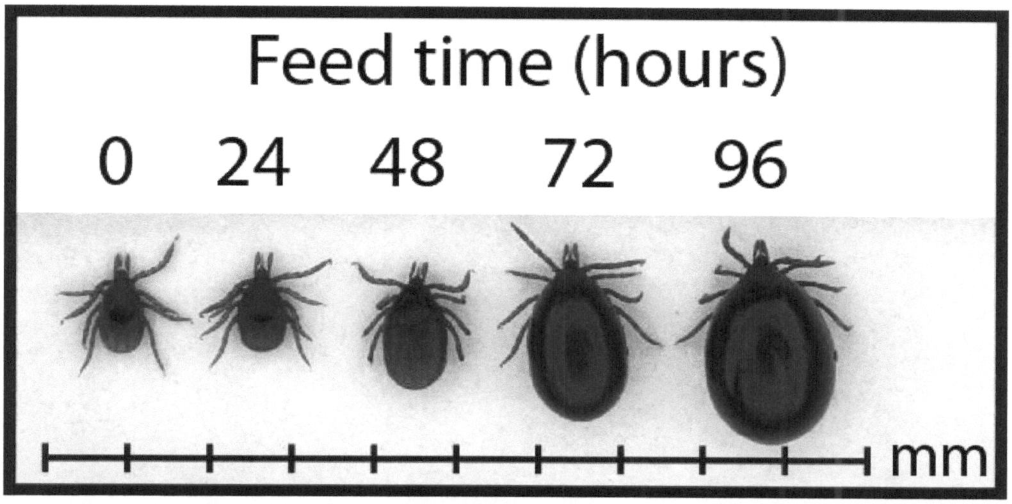

The pregnant female needs blood to feed fertilized eggs and during the blood meal inject a variety of microscopic pathogens and with large numbers of ticks can bleed mammals to death. CDC

Ticks, one of the author's least favorite creations have caused human suffering throughout history and continues today. They can harbor bacteria, rickettsia and viral infections passed to humans when the pregnant female takes a blood meal. Lyme's Disease, Rocky Mountain Spotted Fever, Tick Fever and Typhus are tick-borne rickettsia infections causing fevers and rashes. Some are fatal while others may become life-long diseases. Generally, the smaller the tick, the more likely to have disease. The author, his family and pets endure year around tick bites in Northern California requiring frequent removal and treatment. The tick should be carefully removed in total. A small, curved hemostat is a good tool or fine pointed forceps. Grasp the tick's head as close to skin as possible, careful to not to puncture the blood-filled bag or compress contents of bag back into the host. Larger ticks are less likely to be infected verse the smaller ticks as Lyme's disease and other infections also kills the tick. The author recommends cleaning the wound after tick removed followed by antibiotic, in most cases only a single dose. Most antibiotics will reduce risk of tick-borne diseases with doxycycline favored, however with sun exposure, it is more likely to cause a skin reaction. Bruising and swelling at wound site, fever and generalized body-wide complaints require more than a single dose. In these cases, treat for 7-10 days. Spider bites can be treated in similar fashion.

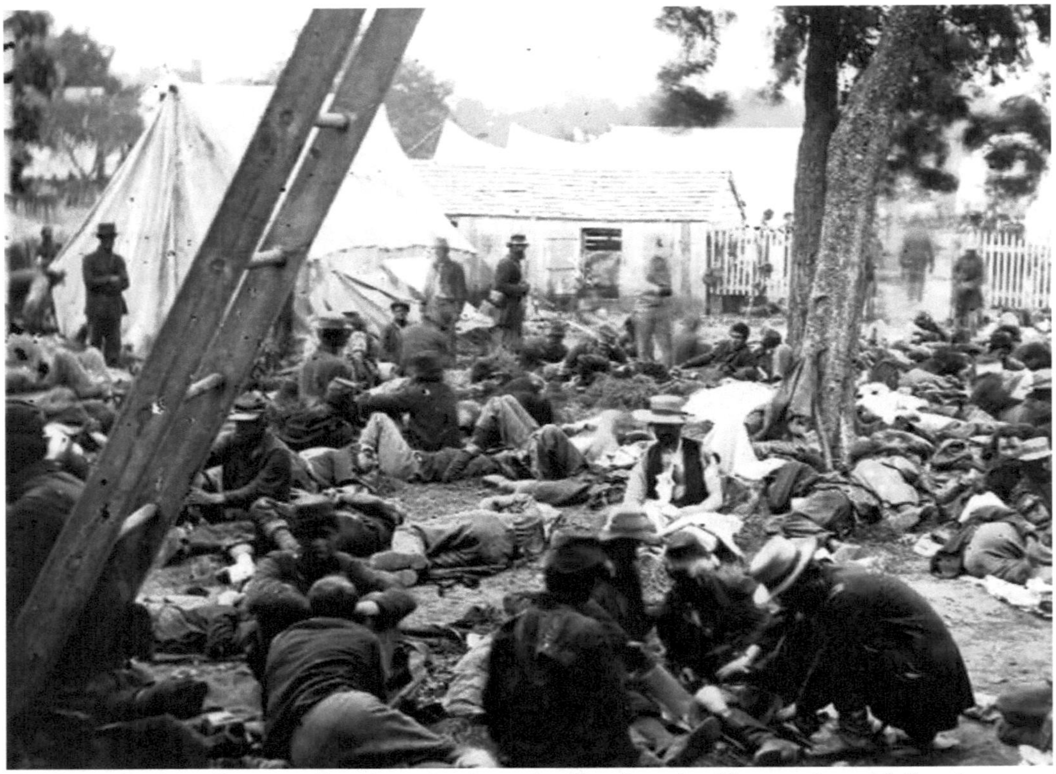

The field hospital at Savage Station during the Peninsula Campaign of the Army of the Potomac attacking Richmond. McClellan built a mighty army, an army he was afraid to risk. Unlike US Grant, who believed his job was to destroy the enemy army, not capture its capitol, McClellan based his strategy on capturing Richmond. Napoleon had already proved that capturing Moscow, Russia's capital is not winning a war. The Union landed on March 17, and slowly and cautiously moved inland without contacting the enemy until April 5. McClellan, with any sense of battlefield command, would have moved quickly and attacked before the Confederates could concentrate, instead he dragged huge siege guns through swamps. The real fighting did not start until June 1, when both armies began fighting on a wide front. Also engaged was an army of ticks. Soldiers in the field, without bathing and clothing changes, begin to experience hundreds of tick bites, while the wounded become infested with blood-filled arachnoids. The swamps of the peninsula had a reputation for fevers in the summer and having two armies of thousands on this ground provided an abundance of blood meals for pregnant female insects and ticks, some leaving disease in their wake. National Archives

Animal Bites

Bites from animals with jaws and teeth are a combination of crush and penetrating injuries, carry a high degree of infection. Animal bites are considered contaminated and should be cleaned with attentive carefulness. Soaking and scrubbing is not useful in puncturing wounds, so a large syringe connected to a soft needle cover of an IV catheter is used to deliver bactericidal soap and warm water to the deeper tissue. Insert the tip well into the wound while holding the wound open. Dilute povidone-iodine 1% (betadine) solution repeatedly into the wound with syringes full of soapy warm water is good management. After cleaning, cover with an antibiotic ointment like Silvadene and keep a dry dressing with frequent changing. Ice to the wound may reduce swelling and pain while lessening deeper soft tissue damage associated with a crush injury. Reducing swelling in crush injury reduces the risk of hydraulic pressures damaging cells (compartment syndrome). Infections such as rabies and hepatitis can be imparted in a mammal bite. All bites should be meticulously examined for the possibility of fracture, nerve, or tendon damage and cleaned as thoroughly as possible. The author recommends antibiotics in animal bites soon after the injury, with addition of a second stronger antibiotic if the wound shows early signs of infection. Erythromycin, amoxicillin, cephalosporins are recommended. A tetanus vaccine should have been given if 5-10 years has lapsed since the last tetanus.

Bites over joints are high-risk wounds as tendon sheaths are shallow and easily injured and infected, leading to scar tissue and reduced range of motion. Some scarring can permanently impair the joint's function and bites with fractures carry even a higher risk of infection and disability. Animal bites are usually left open and not sutured closed since closing the wound may prevent healing by sealing infectious material in the wound. However, for cosmetic reasons, wounds on the face, after thorough cleansing, can be closed with small loose sutures. Use antibiotics, warm soaks, and careful wound care in bites that penetrate the skin. The most serious domestic animal bites are delivered by cats, five times more infectious than dogs, especially over hands. Most instances of rabies are rare and seen in wild animal bites. In the United States, skunks, raccoons and bats occasionally carry rabies. The rabies virus is quite fragile and early good wound cleaning will go a long way towards preventing rabies. Human bites can transmit hepatitis, AIDS, and one or two cases a year of rabies.

Of all bites, the human bite is considered the most likely to get infected and the most common human "bite" occurs when the closed fist forcibly meets a hard object. The skin over the knuckles and the underlying bone is broken. When contact with teeth punctures skin, the trauma Imparts millions of oral bacteria into normally sealed compartments. This wound should be treated with antibiotics within 6-12 hours, to prevent a serious infection. "Boxer's Fractures" often occur under the effects of alcohol, increasing the risk of infection, since the injured person does not seek medical care until the next day. Immediately remove any rings, soak the wound in medicated soap followed by lavage into puncture sites, begin antibiotics (consider an antibiotic injection) and splint the hand with bulky dressing. Keep hand in elevated position.

Rats

Although rat bites are uncommon in the United States, these mammals have caused a huge amount of human disease. Even though it is a late addition to human activity, the rat has been a major player occupying a special woeful place in maritime medical history. There is no mention of rats in the Old Testament nor by the Greeks or Romans, although they described mice and considered them a pest. There is no evidence that rats were present in the Western World before European shipping reached the Far East, although some historians believe the Plague of Justinian was Bubonic, yet there is no mention of rats in 6th century Byzantine. Prior to the 1400s there is no written description of an animal that resembles the large aggressive omnivorous rodent that appeared suddenly in the mid-14th century. The first rats arrived at a Mediterranean habitat filled with places to nest and breed with no natural predators, surrounded by human activity and abundant food. It would not be hard to imagine sailors carrying these intelligent playful animals in cages and on their shoulders as pets. The author believes the Ship Rat was likely confined to a few islands in the East Indies where they "hitchhiked" on passing vessels. Some escaped captivity to live and breed in the bilges of ships and later the filthy harbors of Mediterranean port cities began to grow in great numbers as the humans around them were doing. Soon they begin to compete with people for grain, bedding and space.

Shipping delivered and serviced the Crusades which resulted in trading in the eastern Mediterranean at some point became colonized by *Mus rattus*. Known to history as the ship rat or black rat it came, scattered and entrenched in all of Europe. This rat has also been called the Alexandrine rat and Arab rat since the Islamic port of Alexandria was probably the first Mediterranean port where the rat entered written history. Its size, intelligence and reproductive capacity enabled it to become quickly established in Alexandria, and from there, the ship rat spread over all of Europe and into the Near East, Africa, the Americas and later to Polynesia. A large population of rats were already living among humans when rats from the east brought the infected fleas carrying *Yersinia pestis*.

Even before the rat brought Black Death to Europe, rats had become a major cause of human misery. So destructive were rats, Medieval European taxes could be paid in rat tails. The rats that overran Europe were much like humans, it that they were omnivorous, able to breed in all seasons, adaptable to many types of environments and have the social skills to organize into hunting groups, even making war on rival groups. The earlier black rats were soon displaced by the more ferocious and cunning rat, *Mus decumanus*, the Asiatic or brown rat. "Rat Wars" were documented by legitimate historians (Hans Zinsser in "Rats, Lice and History") as the brown Asian rat outbred, outfought, and destroyed the black rat in most of Europe. By the end of the 18th century the brown rat had conquered the black rat and colonized all of Europe including the British Isles. It spread across the continent after arriving in European ports abroad vessels returning from the Far eastern ports of Cathay, Ceylon and Batavia. These same brown rats now are found on every continent except possibly Antarctica. Today, only scattered colonies of the black rat have survived in the far north of Scandinavia.

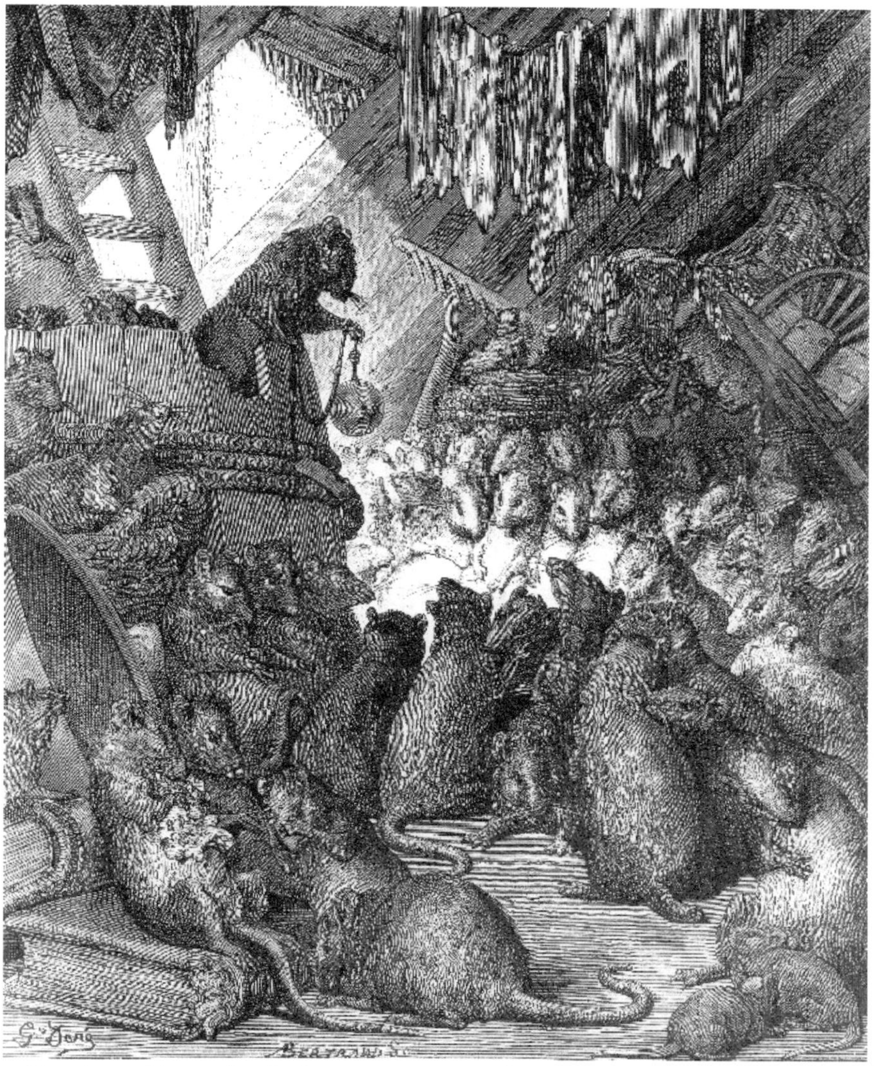

Drawing by Gustave Dore depicting concentration of rat population combined with concepts of social engineering, leadership and command

The story of the Pied Piper (Rattenfanger von Hamelin legend) who piped the children away from their parents when the town refused to pay for his disposal of the rats into the river Weser around 1300. Rats not only inflicts humans but other animals by carrying diseases such as plague and typhus to wild and domestic mammals. Rats eat the young of others, especially birds and their eggs, in some places wiping out entire species of bird life. Children have been attacked by the brown rat, causing injuries and deaths. Dr. Kane of the Artic ship *Advance* returned the favor by eating the numerous rats within his ship through a winter trapped in ice after consuming all fruit and vegetable sources of vitamin C. Rat meat prevented scurvy in the crew that expanded their culinary limits, while the pickier shipmates suffered. Rats can be an excellent source of vitamin C, proteins and nourishment in times of need. Many besieged cities in the past centuries from Paris to Vicksburg have gladly seen rats on the dinner table.

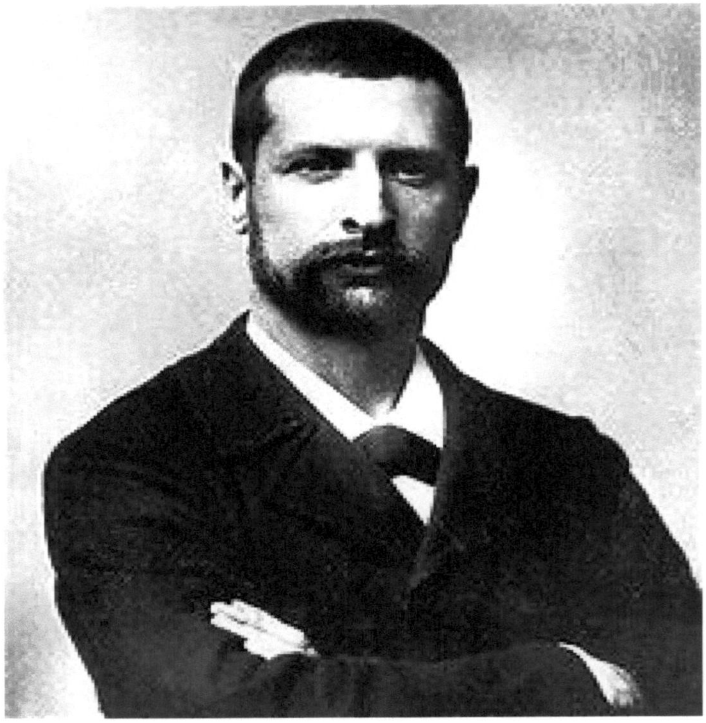

Alexandre Yersin (1863-1943), a French-Swiss physician discriminated for his Huguenot beliefs, left France after medical school and spent several years at sea as a Ships Surgeon, finally settling in the village of Nha Trang the south-central coast of France's colony of Viet Nam. There he studied and discovered the bacterial cause of Bubonic plague and by giving the infection to cows developed the first successful treatment of plague by giving retrieved bovine serum to patients. The bacteria, *Yersinia pestis* is named for him and his gamma globulin injections became useful for other infections and is being used in COVID-19. He had the first private airplane in Viet Nam and is responsible for developing civil aviation in that country. Photo at Yersin Museum, Nha Trang

Incision and Draining Abscesses

Abscesses have been treated by incision and drainage for thousands of years and is still the treatment of choice. Antibiotics will not effectively treat an abscess, only suppress the infection, often leaving a small hard knot under the skin. Abscesses should be opened with a sharp knife, drained completely as possible, and a wick placed to keep the wound open and draining. The premature closure of an incised abscess will lead to continued infection. The step-by-step plan for abscesses treatment is simple, requiring a few surgical tools, an absorbent dressing and wick, good lighting and the ability to render the surgical site painless.

Equipment required for incision and drainage

Q-tip or Forceps Hemostat
4" x 4" gauze pad
Iodoform gauze tape
Scalpel, #11 blade

Local Anesthesia
Hydrogen peroxide or clean water for irrigation

Position the patient comfortably with good exposure of the site and good light. Gently scrub the area overlying and surrounding the abscess for one minute. Vigorous scrubbing is unnecessary when using a medicated soap. Shave the site if needed for exposure and anesthetize the skin over and around the abscess. For a superficial lesion with obvious fluctuance (softness just under a thin layer of skin), one could use ethyl glycol spray or even ice for anesthesia. The first contact of the spray on an abscess site is uncomfortable, so lead up to it by demonstrating the cooling effect on your own hand, on the patient's hand, then over the abscess. Maintain a steady spray until a white "frost" appears, then proceed immediately to open the abscess with a single blade thrust. For an abscess that is too deep or large for a single brief incision, infiltrate the overlying skin with lidocaine. Injection may be painful and adds to swelling, so limit injection sites and the amount of lidocaine to the minimum necessary for anesthesia. Locate "softness" (pocket of pus) by two-finger gentle pressure or, if necessary, use the 22-gauge needle to aspirate the site to demonstrate pus.

Note: If you do not demonstrate the soft pocket of pus underlying the area of redness and swelling, do not proceed with incision because it may open tissue compartments and spread infection. Instead, continue intermittent moist heat and elevation for 24 hours, treat any cellulitis with oral and/ or injectable antibiotics and re-examine every eight hours.

After anesthesia achieved, make a single quick incision parallel to skin lines (Lines of Langerhans) from edge to edge across the softness. Expect spontaneous drainage of some pus, often mixed with blood (it may appear more blood than pus). If no spontaneous discharge occurs, try light pressure on the surrounding skin or deeper incision. Avoid this step if the site is on the face or around the ear since it might infect the sinuses by pushing the infection deeper.

Gently probe the opened abscess with a sterile swab (Q-tip) or curved hemostat to break up and clean out locations. An abscess is seldom smoothly spherical but more likely to be irregular in shape, with finger-like extensions that spread into tissue planes or partially sectioned by fibrous and necrotic debris. Gently opening and closing a small, curved hemostat is helpful in breaking down the abscess's interior walls (bulkheads). After probing, lavage the abscess with saline or hydrogen peroxide, using the lidocaine syringe and a blunt needle if painful. When probing and lavage no longer yield pus, examine for bleeding. If the abscess is relatively large, packing will stop a slight oozing of blood. Insert a gauze wick or, if the abscess is relatively large, pack the abscess site with 1/4" or 1/2" strip of Iodoform gauze tap, Betadine-soaked gauze, or plain gauze. Cover with sterile 4" x 4" gauze pads, and expect some oozing of pus (exudate), and a little bleeding. Change the dressing and wick at least every 24 hours if wound is still draining, more often if the dressing becomes soiled. Oral antibiotics are not necessary unless there is evidence of surrounding redness or cellulitis, however giving a single dose of antibiotic could be contemplated.

Ingrown Nails

A common affliction of people who wear shoes, especially if too short, is the ingrown toenail caused by injury to the nail bed deep within the nail base. This injury occurs with repeated big toenail trauma such as new tight shoes, "stubbing" the toe, etc. This in turn causes the nail to form a spur that juts out into the surrounding, tissue creating infection as if a foreign body was present under skin. Although hot soaks and antibiotics will help, it will only be resolved with surgical removal of the nail spur. This is done by removing the entire nail or just a vertical sliver from the offending side. The toe must be anesthetized with lidocaine on both sides and ample time to lapse before surgery, since anesthesia is often slow getting to the nail bed. Proper anesthesia is achieved when the patient cannot feel a needle prick to the area along the infected nail. If pain is encountered during the procedure wait for several more minutes or administer more lidocaine. After removal of the sliver of nail, the site is dressed with a layer of Silvadene and lightly covered with non-stick gauze. Some bleeding is expected as is some pain. However, by the next day the toe should feel well enough to resume normal activities.

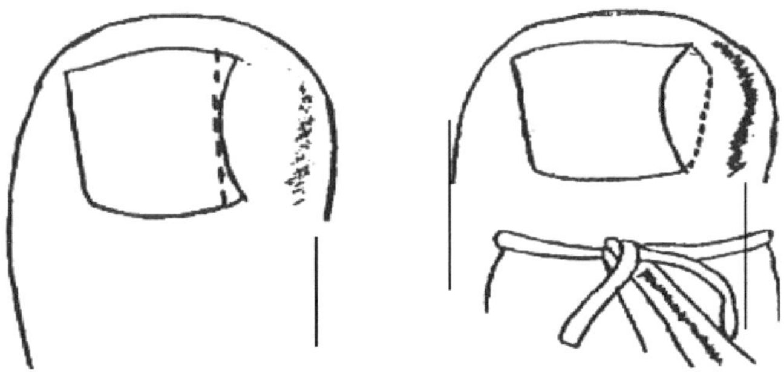

A small rubber band held in place by a hemostat will reduce bleeding when the offensive part of the toenail is removed.

Skin Infections

Impetigo and cellulitis deserve special mention since they can develop rapidly from a small wound to a spreading infection. Impetigo is common around the nose and mouth where small sores are easily infected by the abundant bacteria found around these two orifices. A common cause is insect bites that have been aggressively scratched and has spread, not only to other parts of the skin but also to others who contact infected skin through touch, shared towels and bedding. Treatment consists of scrubbing the wound with a medicated soap and brush. Topical antibiotics such as Silvadene or Bactroban (mupirocin) are helpful in reducing wound bacteria. However, if distant sites develop similar infections, oral antibiotics are indicated.

Cellulitis is a serious infection that is spreading under the skin, uncontained and has gained access to the skin's circulation system. It is manifested by a large area of tender, red, warm, swollen skin sometimes around a seemingly tiny wound. Without treatment, red streaks radiate from wound and begin spreading through the lymph channels that drain infected area. Hot moist towels placed over the wound and the area elevated, will discourage congestion at the site. Oral antibiotics should be started at the first suspicion of wound infection, using erythromycin, amoxicillin or azihtromax to prevent cellulitis. The presence of fever with the skin signs of infection requires stronger second antibiotics in addition to the first. Cellulitis around a major joint such as the knee, in a diabetic person or in the head and neck, should be treated aggressively. These infections may need antibiotic injections along with oral antibiotics, long hot soaks, elevation, good nutrition and rest to prevent a deeper joint infection.

Local Anesthesia

The use of injectable anesthesia to block pain during minor surgery is surely one of the more comfortable advances medicines has made in field surgery. Commonly used agents are lidocaine (Xylocaine), mepivacaine (Carbocaine) and bupivacaine (Marcaine). In the past, cocaine was frequently used, especially in trauma to the head and neck, but due to its potential for abuse, is currently out of favor. For the rare person allergic to all "caines" of local anesthesia, Benadryl (diphenhydramine) can be injected producing moderate anesthesia. These agents block pain nerves radiating away from the wound or expectant surgery site. They are also effective in blocking pain when injected into a fracture site, placing the injection into the hematoma or swelling forming around the broken bones. Do not use more than 8-10 cc of local anesthesia since it may slow the heart or cause an allergic reaction. The site to be injected should first be scrubbed with a bacteria-killing soap.

Using a small 25-30-gauge needle, inject a small amount just under the skin, raising a tiny white mound. In a few seconds, this anesthesia will numb tissue at that site and afterward, another 2-4cc can be injected in 1/2cc amounts in different directions away from the wound. Most local anesthesia drugs are combined with epinephrine, which decrease bleeding by vessel constriction and keep the anesthesia in place longer. Bottles of lidocaine with epinephrine will have a red label, those without epinephrine a blue label. Wait at least 20-30 seconds, then probe the skin around the wound with a sharp point to determine the level of anesthesia. If one area still feels pain, give 1/2 cc more anesthesia over that site. Normally anesthesia will keep an area pain free for thirty minutes or more, especially if epinephrine is present. Infiltration of local anesthesia is often needed for placing sutures and draining abscesses. In a laceration repair, small amounts are injected into each side of the wound and at both ends, usually 1/2 cc in each area. With the abscess it is somewhat more complex but proper anesthesia will make the procedure much more comfortable.

The Gut

Abbreviation for the alimentary canal from the Latin word *alere*, meaning to nourish

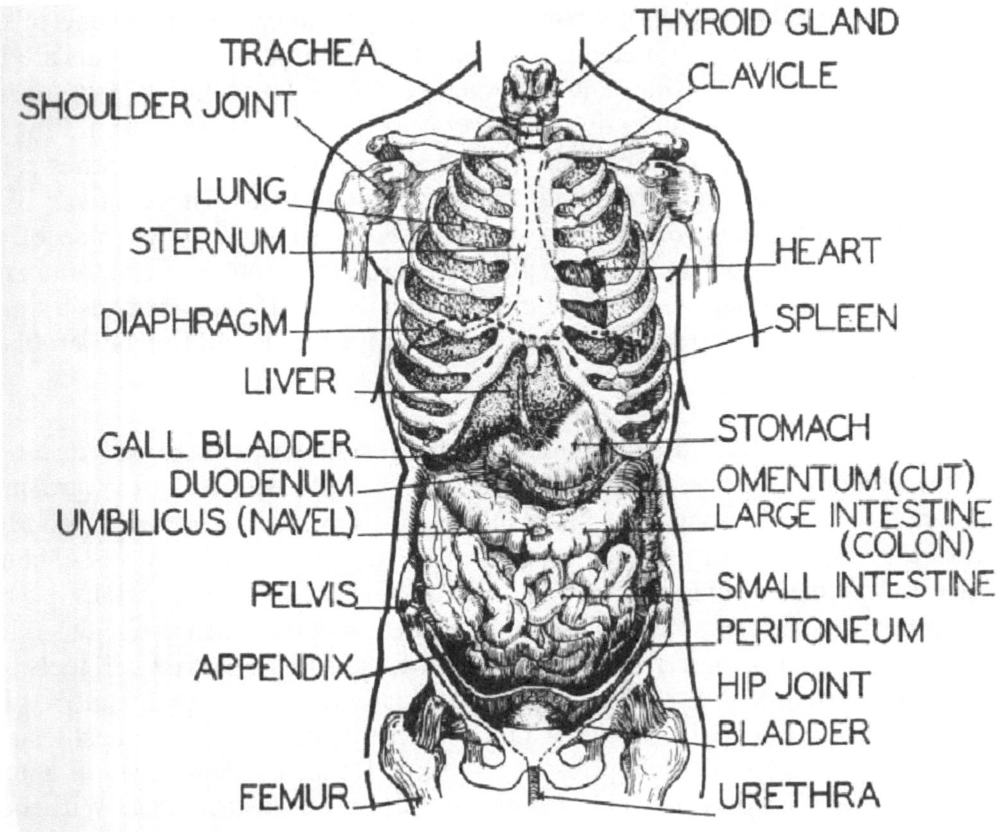

21. General view of the internal arrangement of the trunk (chest and abdomen).—Adapted from Cole and Puestow.

This illustrates the relationship of the abdominal contents to its neighbors

Beginning with the mouth and ending at the anus, is a hollow living tube, with the primary purpose to break down, digest and absorb nutrients. There is one creature, *Demodex foliculorum* that has a gut containing mouth but no outlet. This nearly transparent microorganism eats dead skin and oils from eye skin glands, slowly filling with feces as it has no anus for discharge. As it will eventually succumb from having no outlet for its digestive waste, the creature rots quietly among the eyelashes. Fortunately, humans possess an anus, although if the gut becomes obstructed and unable to move fluids and materials through its tube, death can occur.

In the following pages, the reader will learn that the gut is much more than a place for food processing. Beginning life as a simple microscopic canal in the forming embryo, and ends up in the adult, as a complex system over seven meters (21 feet) long, punctured along the way by canals, valves and side passages to other organs. Its total surface area is an amazing 300 square meters, about the size of a large room, producing 200-2000 ml (2 quarts) of vapor each day, the dreaded bowel gas. On average there are around 10-15 dispersements each day and each is a sign of life.

Bowel gas is noxious due to its components, a heady mixture of nitrogen, oxygen, carbon dioxide, Sulphur, hydrogen and methane (CH_4). These last two are produced by bacterial fermentation of bowel contents are flammable, and severe burns have occurred from explosions within the colon during surgery with electrocautery and by the juvenile prank of lighting farts.

The gut welcomes food and drink to its flow of enzymes, organic soaps and de-greasers, hormones, acids, bicarbonates and body fluids as it courses down its winding stream through the chest, abdomen and pelvis. Stools are brown because bile from the gall bladder has been added, and its absence in hepatitis results in stool becoming pale, almost white. Stools normally are firm because water is removed in the final stages of the lower bowel. If stool passage is too rapid, as in diarrhea, stools will be watery and loose. Too slow, and constipation can occur.

Mouth
(*stoma*-Latin for opening)

The mouth, forming the funnel-shaped opening to the gastrointestinal tract, is primarily for chewing and mixing the food with saliva. There are some enzymes added by oral secretions, but they are few compared to the ones that will be added later by the pancreas. This oral process, however, is important to an omnivorous animal-like a human that consume all forms of food. Humans and carnivores tend to have smaller mouths requiring meals to be taken in bites, as opposed to animals that swallow the meal whole. It allows humans to break food into smaller pieces, eating all or only part of the meats, vegetables and fruit that may be present. We share this trait with few other large mammals as most have a metabolism designed as either a meat-eating hunter (carnivore) or grass eater (herbivore). Being able to chew food allows humans the luxury of swallowing only a portion of the meal at one time. Compare this to a snake that swallows its food whole and often alive. Without the aid of teeth or saliva, the snake's digestive juices must break down the entire animal, including hard tissues such as bones, shell, hide, and hair. It is no wonder that the digestive enzymes of snakes are the most potent in the animal world. Viper venom, whether the nerve type of cobras or the blood poisoning variety of rattlesnakes, are modifications of digestive enzymes.

Esophagus
Greek-*oisophagos* for passage of food, gullet

Joining the mouth (proximal) to the stomach (distal) is the esophagus, a smooth 25-35 cm (10-16 inches) tube, collapsed in the resting state but capable of great distention. Like a snake, the esophagus moves by rhythmically contracting muscles wrapped around a hollow tube. Like the snake, humans can swallow large objects, passing down the expanding esophagus in waves of movement (peristalsis). Food and liquids sometimes return to the mouth in reverse peristalsis, vomiting (emesis). The esophagus can be a site of great discomfort when acid from the stomach escapes through a normally closed valve system (lower esophageal sphincters) at its base. Even without noticeable belching or discomfort, stomach acid can splash onto the sensitive lining of the esophagus, which is rich in pain nerves. The old term for this condition was hiatal hernia is now called reflux. This can be diagnosed when barium is swallowed, and in reflux, barium on X-ray is flushed back through the upper stomach into the lower esophagus. Endoscopy is now the gold standard for diagnosis by inserting a flexible scope through the mouth and into the stomach, visualizing the lower esophagus.

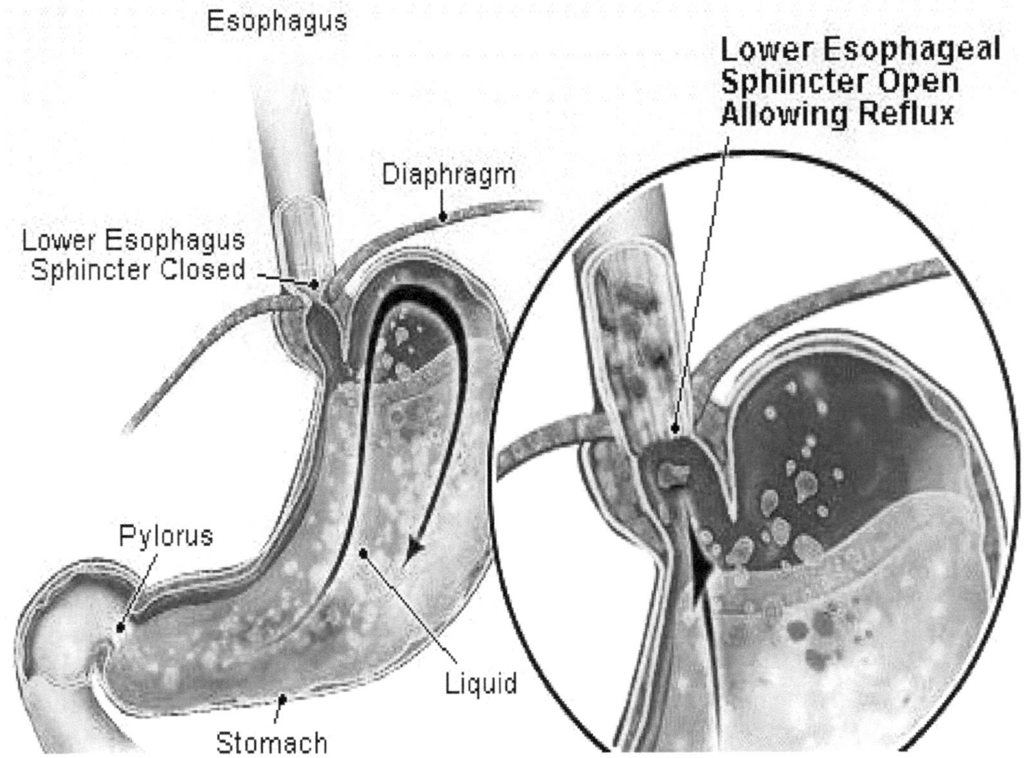

The esophagus perforates the diaphragm, muscular sheaths separating the chest from abdominal contents. In a "hiatal hernia", the upper stomach is pushed up into the chest through the perforation created by esophagus. NIH

To protect the esophagus from stomach acid, avoid overeating which can stretch the lower esophageal sphincters (valve-like structures), rendering the distal esophagus partially ajar. Reflux-induced heartburn at times will generate chest pain that is as severe or more severe as chest pain caused by a heart attack. Long-term treatment of reflux is aimed at reducing stomach acid production with drugs, such as cimetidine (Tagamet), the first true drug to reduce heartburn, has been replaced by the more effective proton-pump inhibitors. These inhibit a cellular pump which allows stomach cells to produce high concentration of hydrogen. In addition to medications, reducing chemicals that increase acid, such as caffeine and tobacco should be avoided. Staying upright for at least two hours after eating enables gravity to keep stomach acid from the esophagus. Eating a large meal and then reclining to digest is a common history in reflux complaints. Remember that aspirin-like drugs (the non-steroidal anti-inflammatory drugs, NSAIDs such as ibuprofen, Naprosyn, etc.) will all increase the risk of heartburn, especially with a history of similar attacks. Chronic reflux is more than an aggravation, since a history of chronic reflux is common in esophageal cancer, a very bad actor. Three men in the very first "Medicine at Sea" class were constantly eating Rolaids and other over-the-counter antacids, later died of esophageal cancer.

The Stomach

Greek-*stomachos* meaning gullet

Lying behind the heart along the mid to lower chest and upper abdomen is an S-shaped, thickly muscled widening of the gut tube. Measuring approximately 10-12" by 4-5", the stomach represents the most dilated portion of the digestive tract where it stores, mixes and delivers food to the small intestine. In most primates, rodents, bears and other carnivores, the stomach is a single chamber of circular muscles covered by longitudinal muscles, running the stomach's length. In humans, it can hold about one liter of volume when fully loaded as the meal is mixed with acid and other stomach excretions by gentle contractions. Normally, the stomach contracts in an orderly fashion towards the small bowel. However, it can reverse its course and do so with violent vomiting (emesis). The stomach responds to different types and amounts of meals, changing digestive secretion production. Stress and shock damage the stomach lining from reduced blood flow. Probably the most common cause of acid disturbances encountered by the author was from aspirin-like anti-inflammatory drugs (pain meds such as ibuprofen) which are potentially dangerous and may be responsible for thousands of deaths each year from gut bleeding. NSAIDs also cause hypertension and heart disease.

The stomach has two major microscopic glands, one secreting hydrochloric acid, while the other provides a thick protective mucus coat, keeping acid from contacting the cells of the stomach's lining. When too much acid is secreted for prolonged periods of time, this mucus coat breaks down. Acid then spills directly onto the stomach's living membrane of tissue, blood vessels and nerves, where a process of inflammation begins that may lead to bleeding and ulcer formation. The stomach's lining is deeply furrowed with multiple valleys and ridges allowing for possible acid pools to form. It is important to protect the stomach's lining from agents that either increase acid formation or promote the destruction of the mucus membrane. Stress, caffeine, alcohol and especially nicotine increase the deleterious effects on the stomach and small bowel. The high calcium content of dairy products has also been shown to increase acid production. Therefore, the former treatment of drinking milk for ulcer pain has been discarded since it may aggravate the condition.

It now appears that an infectious agent, the bacteria, (*H. pylori*), may play a major role in ulcer formation and multiple antibiotics are needed to treat ulcers infected with this durable creature. Chronic infections, cigarette abuse, the elderly and starvation increase the possibility of an ulcer infected with *H pylori*. Imagine how tough a creature must be to survive immersed in an acid bath that would quickly destroy most cells. Under normal conditions, the stomach and small bowel are sterile. Ulcers in the elderly or with weight loss increase the risk of stomach cancer. Stomach pain is often described as a "hot" pain, boring through the upper abdomen or lower chest to the back. Ulcer-caused pain usually is accompanied by bleeding into the gut resulting in black and "tarry" stools. Blood appears dark after it has been mixed with stomach acid and passes through bowel. Less than one teaspoon of blood in a bowel movement will be occult (hidden), requiring a simple test (guiac or Cologuard) to discover.

Cancer of the stomach is a dismal painful disease (it has a low cure rate) and is often presented with bleeding, producing melena, and almost black stools. In the past, stomach cancer was the most common form of gastrointestinal cancer. Refrigeration greatly reduced the consumption of smoked meats and stomach cancer is now much less common. Charcoal or smoke-prepared food eaten regularly, over long periods of time, exposes the stomach's lining to a known cancer-causing agent. Weight loss, upper abdominal pain and persistent blood in the stools indicate possible cancer somewhere in the gut or chronic ulcer.

Another more rare but interesting cause of stomach pain is a ball of hair, the bezoar, that slowly grows in the stomach of grazing mammals. The English word derives its source from several Oriental languages. The word for antidote or anti-poison in Turkish is "panzehir," in Persian, "padzahr" and in Arabic, "badzehr". Evidently, poisoning was common in these Islamic countries and their harems of multiple consorts producing multiple offspring. Few medical conditions are steeped in more mystical and fraudulent medical lore than the bezoar. It was believed that by swallowing a thick stomach-shaped wad of indigestible hair and fur (most coming from goat stomachs), protection from poisons was imparted. These would be swallowed prior to the consumption of possible poison-laden food and later retched up for future use. So valuable were bezoars, they were handed down through generations, some were gold plated, becoming heirlooms to kings and queens in medieval Europe as well as sultans and vizors of the Ottoman Empire. They still occur today in people who pull and swallow hair along with cats. The ultimate Serengeti scavenger, the hyena, has no problem eating hair, for it possesses a digestive tract that can not only break down hair and hide but also derive nourishment from it. A feat normally reserved for fungi.

Ulcer Formation

At the narrow end of the stomach is a sphincter-like area formed by constrictive firm muscle tissue. Through this portal, in multiple movements, a meal is passed into the waiting first component of the small bowel, duodenum. It is here that most ulcers occur, not in the stomach, because the duodenum produces a thinner mucus membrane less protective than stomach mucus. The actual site of ulcer formation is confirmed by diagnostic imaging or with a scope inserted down into the stomach (endoscope). The pain of stomach versus duodenal ulcer (or inflammation) is similar enough to be indistinguishable at sea and in the field, but this is not important since treatment is the same. Suspected inflammation and bleeding in the stomach or small bowel is treated with the same drugs for reflux by reducing stomach acid, such as Tagamet, Zantac, Carafate, Axid, along with the newer proton-pump inhibitors Dexilant, Nexium, Prilosec and others. These medications are available worldwide and highly effective.

From the time the meal arrived, the stomach has been in communication with the bowel, pancreas and gall bladder through blood-borne chemical messengers. Messengers informing downstream organs of digestion, information about the type and amount of meal on its trip down the gut. By working in concert, the gastrointestinal tract ensures that as much of the meal as possible will be absorbed. A meal laden with red meat and fat will increase both bile release from gall bladder and pancreatic enzymes. A particularly large meal will signal the colon to empty in preparation of incoming bulk. This stimulation can be overplayed, causing the "dumping reflex," creating a sudden need to evacuate the bowels, sometimes during a meal. In some older people, the dumping reflex is so sensitive, they must be close to a toilet when sitting down for a meal.

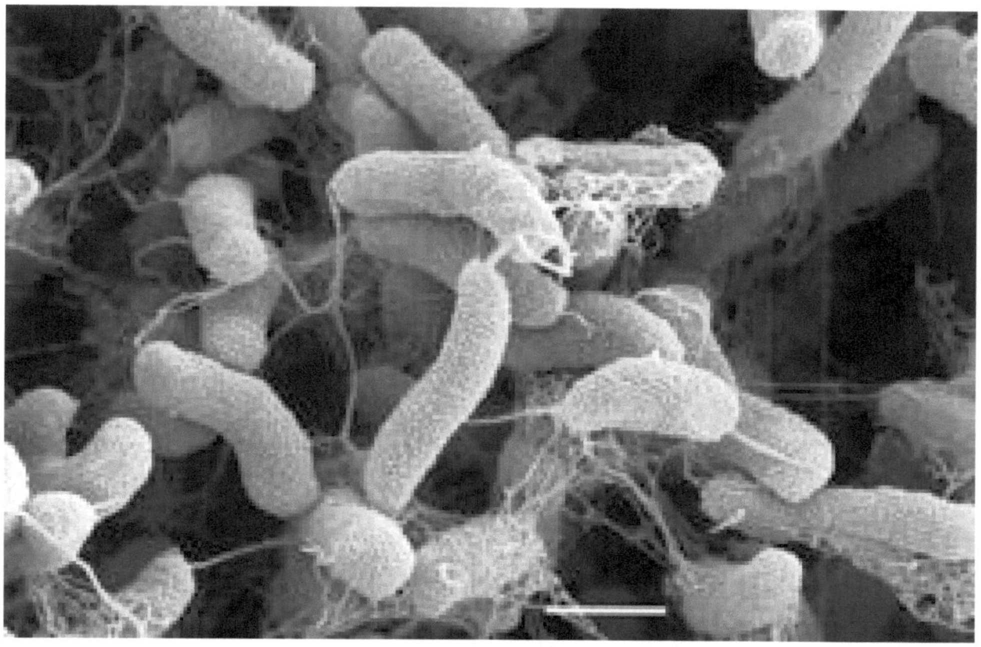

Electron microscopy of the rod-shaped bacteria that is a top human killer, *vibrio cholerae*. Here with a single tentacle. Under electron microscopy in real life, they have multiple tentacles used to attach to the small bowel wall, releasing a toxin that results in continuous fluid loss from the gut. Another vibrio bacteria produces the bio phosphoresce in plankton on dark nights at sea. Muhsin Ozel

The Small Bowel

(intestine)-Latin word *intest i num* meaning inside

Most of the digestive action in the gut takes place within the dark, airless confines of the small bowel. It is here that the bulk of nutrients is absorbed, and here that most of the symptoms associated with disorders of poor absorption (malabsorption) take place. The small bowel is hardly small when its surface is considered. It is divided into three segments: the duodenum, the jejunum and the ileum, the latter empties into the colon. The small bowel is smaller in caliber than either the stomach or the large bowel, thus early anatomists labelled it, small. The large surface area of the small bowel is designed for the optimal absorption of sugars, proteins, and fat. The complex compounds found it food are broken down by organic soaps and enzymes so the smaller units can be transported across the lining of the gut into waiting blood. Digestion is a simple word for an extraordinary chain of events whereby raw materials brought into the mouth are coupled and converted into streamlined molecules that plucked from a steamy effluvium stream into the swirling currents of circulation.

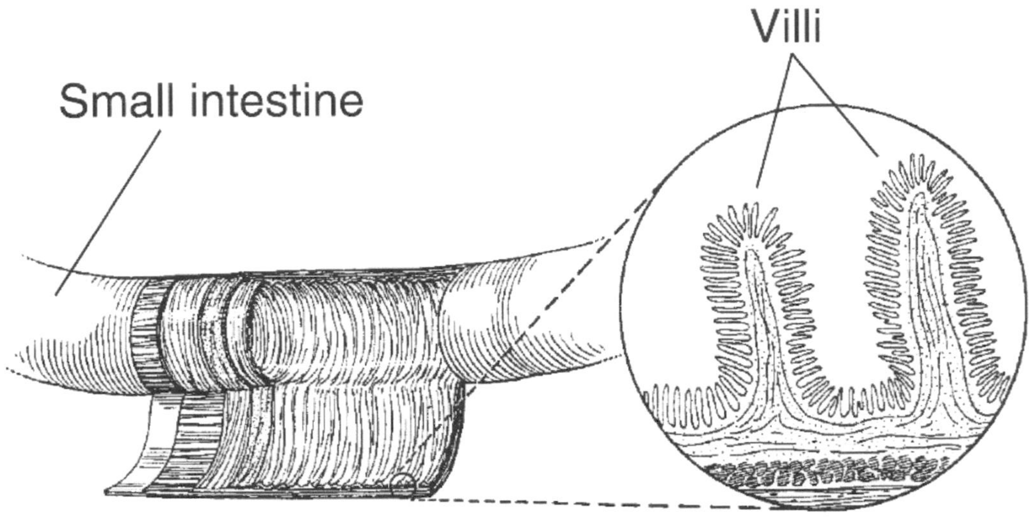

Among the microscopic ridges and valleys (villi) of the small bowel where digestion primarily takes place. It is also a site for immune activity and new research points to its effects on the central nervous system. Although most gastrointestinal bacteria reside in the colon, microbes are being discovered in the previously believed to be sterile small bowel. NIH

The small bowel does more than digest food. Lymph tissue spread about in the small bowel contains the bursa component of the immune system where B-lymphocytes are activated and trained to secrete their antibodies. The nervous system has its solar plexus here while the circulatory system has vast beds of vessels in and around the small bowel for the storage of blood. This long (8-12 feet) hollow, coiled, serpentine organ moves constantly within the abdomen, as gas and the slurry mix of ingested food is squirted wetly along its length. This movement creates most bowel sounds, the rumblings that can sometimes be heard from across the room. Bowel sounds are always present under normal conditions, even though heard only with a stethoscope. The loss of bowel sounds indicates bowel obstruction, a serious sign of abdominal distress.

Within the interior of the small bowel there are more convolutions and not just a simple hollow tube in appearance, but one filled with ridges and deep valleys, greatly increasing the interior surface area of this part of the gut. On the surface of these folds are tiny finger-like projections (villi) which further increase the surface area for absorption of nutrients. Covering the villi are even smaller projections, the microvilli (2,000,000,000 per cubic centimeter of bowel surface). This surface is very fragile and is easily washed away in diarrhea. Diarrhea has many causes, but they all cause malabsorption. When fluid is rushed through the small bowel as it is in diarrhea, there is little time for absorption. A serious life-threatening form of diarrhea is dysentery, cholera being the most common etiology throughout history and in the world today. There is a big difference between diarrhea and dysentery, the latter combines the frequent watery "rice-water" stools with fever, abdominal pain and discomfort with each passing of stools. The Vibrio bacteria that produce cholera releases a toxin that traumatizes the bowel lining, destroys the absorptive membrane resulting in the small bowel's inability to retain fluid. Because of this destruction, much of the body's water is lost by frequent painful water stools. Sudden severe diarrhea without fluid replacement can quickly lead to dehydration and shock, especially in children. Replace fluid losses with oral electrolyte fluids and IV fluids, if possible. Cholera has possibly killed more humans and altered the courses of history, especially wars, than other single agent. Certainly, it played a greater role than any general. In the Swedish Russian wars between Sweden's Charles XII and Peter the Great in the 18th century, entire armies melted in their trenches. During the so-called Reconquista as the Spanish Catholics pushed the Spanish Muslims out of the Iberian Peninsula, armies just disappeared under the onslaught of cholera. There are cases where entire ships crews died leaving ghost ships at sea. A single human could spread cholera to thousands through contaminated bowel discharges. Even today after earthquakes, hurricanes, wars and famines, cholera emerges. The development of oral electrolyte solutions has saved countless lives.

Under the microscope, microvilli form a microscopic "brush border" covering the valleys and peaks of the small bowel's wall. Each microvillus is unique, differing from the billions around it. Imagine a tropical rain forest, a jungle carpeted in foliage of different sizes, shapes and species. This microscopic jungle can harbor parasites just as the jungle is inhabited by dangerous, carnivorous animals and disease carrying insects. Most gut parasites are microscopic while some are the size of pencils, a few even larger. The small human bowel, a maze within a maze creates a large surface area where liquids and semisolids are moved along through a labyrinth of bends and convolutions by progressive contractions in one direction, peristalsis. As part of the intestinal wall is stretched by food contents, the segment directly behind it contracts, pushing the food ahead. This can be intense at times creating almost explosive movements (peristaltic rushes), which cause cramping and diarrhea.

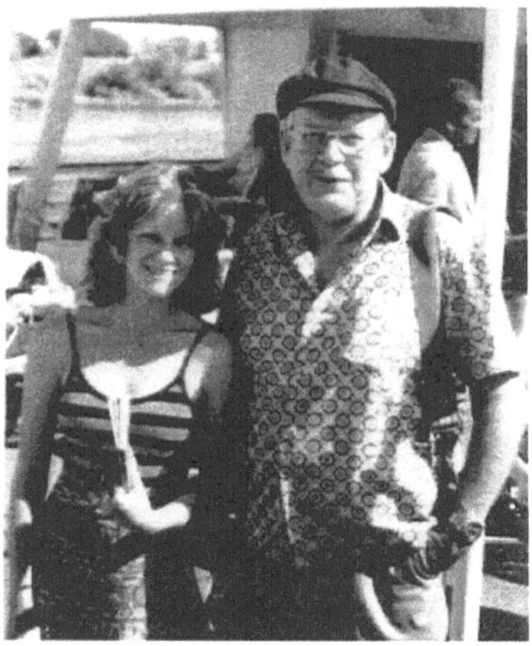

Captain Ray Watton USN, MC pictured with the author's wife on the Nile River, was one of the WHO researchers that developed the powdered electrolyte solution that has been so successful in replacing lost fluids. He was not one of the scientists to make any money from research that led to Gatorade. Dr. Watten was a seasoned traveler while visiting China, fell ill with a flu-illness requiring IV fluids. Although he was assured the needle used on him and his wife had no previous use, there was doubt. There is legitimate concern in the third world of receiving previously used needles. Therefore, carry your syringes and needles!

The Pancreas

Dubious word root for this organ, *kreas* is Greek for flesh, Jerimiah 51:34, the Hebrew word *KaRaiSH* means belly, in culinary history this tissue was considered trash and seldom consumed.

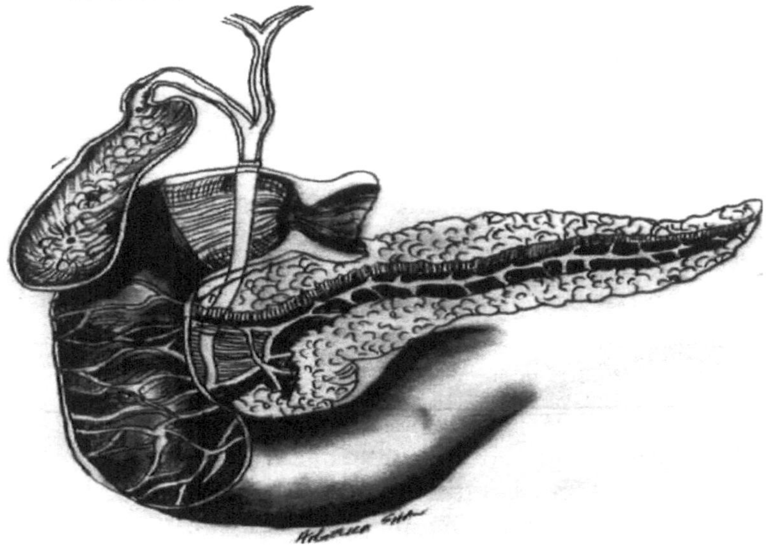

Lots of things happen in this drawing where food, bile, stomach fluid and pancreatic enzymes come together quietly in health but loudly in disease.

This soft tube-shaped organ lies in the upper left abdomen just under the stomach and across from the liver and gall bladder. The pancreas was known as the "finger of the liver" in the Jewish Talmud. It was the last organ of digestion whose function was defined. In most mammals, the head of the pancreas fits into the "C" of the duodenum, its body and tail nestled along the underside of the stomach. Just as people vary in skin color and face shape, so do their digestive systems vary. The human pancreas is an example of how the gut is often different in function in different groups of humans. Ancestors' dietary habits affect the way food is digested today and because of this, they have tendencies to gain weight. What developed as a defense mechanism to store fat for lean times has turned into an increased likelihood of diabetes.

Previously nomadic people such as the American Indian now experience an extremely high rate of diabetes because their pancreas has been unable to adjust to today's diet. The gut of the Plains Indians was designed for a "feast or famine" type of existence where large amounts of meat were consumed at a single feeding. While at the same time, their diet was low in carbohydrates. The nomadic gut could eat eight to ten pounds of meat in one sitting and digest most of the protein if allowed to rest for days. The American Plains Indians were magnificent looking people, according to the early explorers. In the journal of Lewis and Clark, they described the Mandan, Shoshoni, Sioux and Arapaho Indians as lean, muscular people with good teeth, perfectly formed bodies and disease free. Perhaps the most famous American Indian was the Shawnee chief, Tecumseh. He could read and write English and was described by many as the most handsome man in the Ohio River Valley. This was in sharp contrast to the often weakened, disease-scared and wasted bodies of those living in congested large European cities. Nomadic people also ate the entire animal, not just the muscle, and games have much less fat than today's meat products. American Indians lived on marginal diets, their guts able to digest every scrap of protein to ensure survival and poorly designed for large amounts of carbohydrates daily. Although a few tribes, especially those of central and eastern America developed some form of agriculture, most American Indians existed by hunting and gathering edible roots, berries, seeds and nuts. Oak acorns, poison when raw, made up a large part of the diet of west American coast Indians after the tannic acids "leeched" by immersion in clean water, pounded into a paste and consumed like flour.

Meriwether Lewis described an episode of Shoshoni Indians feasting on a freshly killed animal. The tribe had been fasting for several days with no meat available and were famished. When Lewis shot a deer, the tribe descended upon the fresh meat and devoured the deer in total, eating guts, drinking the blood and tearing at the scraps of meat stuck to bone and skin. Lewis wrote "Indians would snatch up a piece of liver, kidney or spleen, and tear at it with his teeth, the blood running down the corners of mouths." Every scrap of animal protein consumed was turned into the effort of survival. The Plains Indian gastrointestinal tract could pour out large amounts of bile, pancreatic enzymes and insulin to process all that meat and organ. Few Americans could eat a meal such as this unless they were truly starving, and fewer still could digest it completely because diets are used to smaller, more frequent feedings.

The American Plains Indian's pancreas evolved to function in response to a large protein-rich meal and then to rest for days. It is unsuited to today's diet of daily meals high in carbohydrates (sugars) and fats. Therefore, a high rate of diabetes in overweight American Indians are the result of their gut's design. It takes a long time for the gut to modify a pancreas capable of secreting insulin continuously, processing incoming food and maintaining fat stores. The pancreas well suited to the feast or famine existence becomes a detriment in modern society. Alcohol is another example of a digestive system limited by evolutionary differences in people. Europeans had a long history of exposure to ethyl alcohol, especially sailors, soldiers and frontiersmen. They consumed large amounts of low-grade alcohol, often daily. The Old West was full of alcoholics, and alcohol was one of history's most common trade goods. It was the "money" of the American west as soldiers in western forts were not paid in money, as there was no use for it, instead they were paid in whiskey. As a consumable, whiskey could be consumed or traded for other items, such as dry goods, female company, game foods, and exotic Indian-made items and in rare cases, books. European livers had developed enzyme systems to break down alcohol after generations of exposures. The American Indian had no such exposure and alcohol quickly intoxicated them breaking their spirit and health. This lack of enzymes allows alcohol levels to rise and stay elevated, creating a very intoxicated Indian. Continued drinking damages liver and pancreas, accelerating the severity of diabetes.

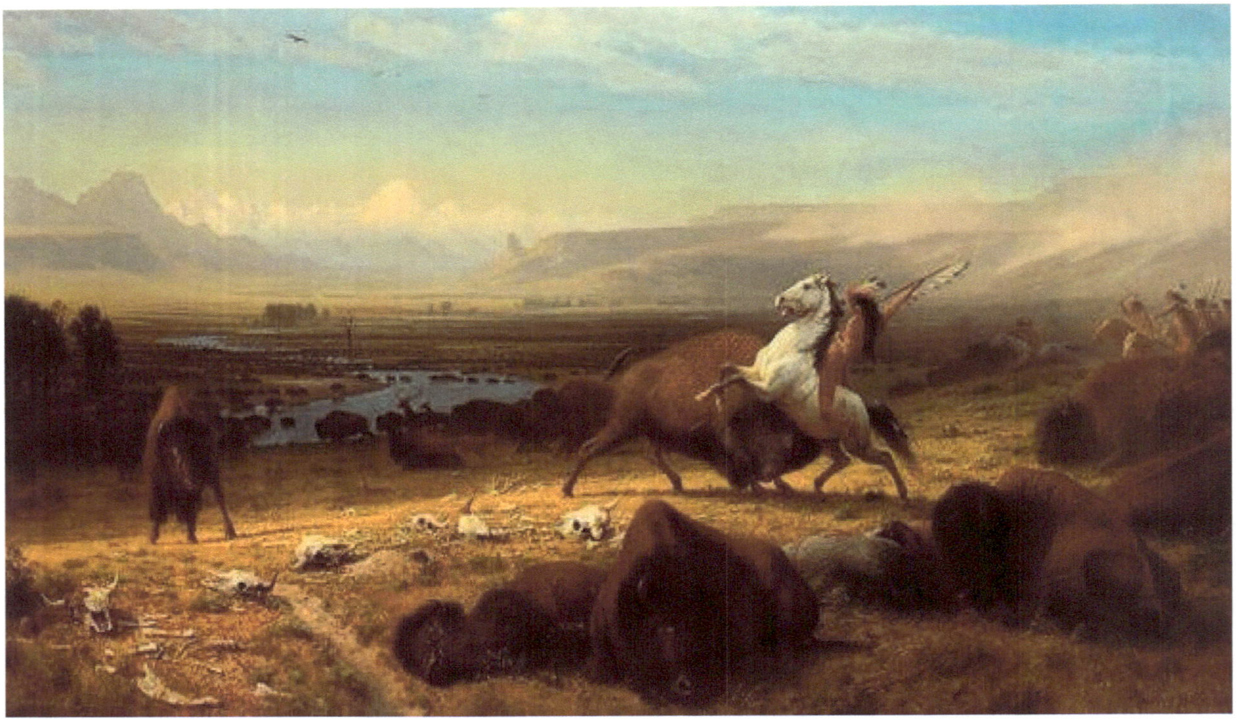

"The Last Buffalo Hunt" by George Catlin. The plains Indians relied on this animal for much of their food, clothing, housing, tools and the dried manure burned for cooking. The horse, introduced by the Spanish in Mexico, was extremely helpful in hunting the buffalo and forever changed the Plains Indians. Coronado's expedition searching for the Seven Cities of Gold brought them to the southern edge of the Grand Canyon, seen first by Europeans in the mid-16th century. The expedition continued northeast into the pueblo cities and finally terminated in the great plains of the present-day Oklahoma panhandle and western Kansas, where for 10 days the explorers were in a continuous buffalo herd. Travelling at 20 miles a day, this meant that the herd was probably over 200 miles wide.

The pancreas contains tissue capable of producing a hellish mixture of enzymes intent on destroying proteins. These enzymes are mindless, and if they somehow escape the confines of the gut, they will digest any protein encountered, attacking the body's own tissue and causing a form of self-digestion. When the pancreas "leaks" its secretions, they become deadly to tissue surrounding the gut. Fortunately, the pancreas is not likely to leak, which is good since pancreatitis can produce profoundly serious causes of abdominal pain. Pancreatitis causes upper left abdominal pain that steadily increases relentlessly with no intermittent relief as seen in other abdominal pain. It also causes severe nausea and vomiting; nausea is not relieved by vomiting. The pain often follows a large meal, heavy in protein and fat, combined with the consumption of alcohol. This combination of protein, fat and alcohol produces a strong response from both gall bladder and pancreas, a response that can unfortunately become obstructed by a gall stone or swelling near the ampulla of Vater. Obstruction and stagnation of this site is not fortunate for the affected. Fortunately, under normal conditions pancreatic juices are activated only when exposed to bile, hopefully exposure only occurs within the confines of the small bowel. However, if this exposure and activation takes place prior to the enzymes passing through the ampulla and into the lumen of the small bowel, the obstruction causes swelling of the tissue at the head of the pancreas.

This swelling if not resolved will worsen the obstruction leading to pressure, pain, severe nausea and vomiting as the now activated pancreatic enzymes begin a destructive rampage.

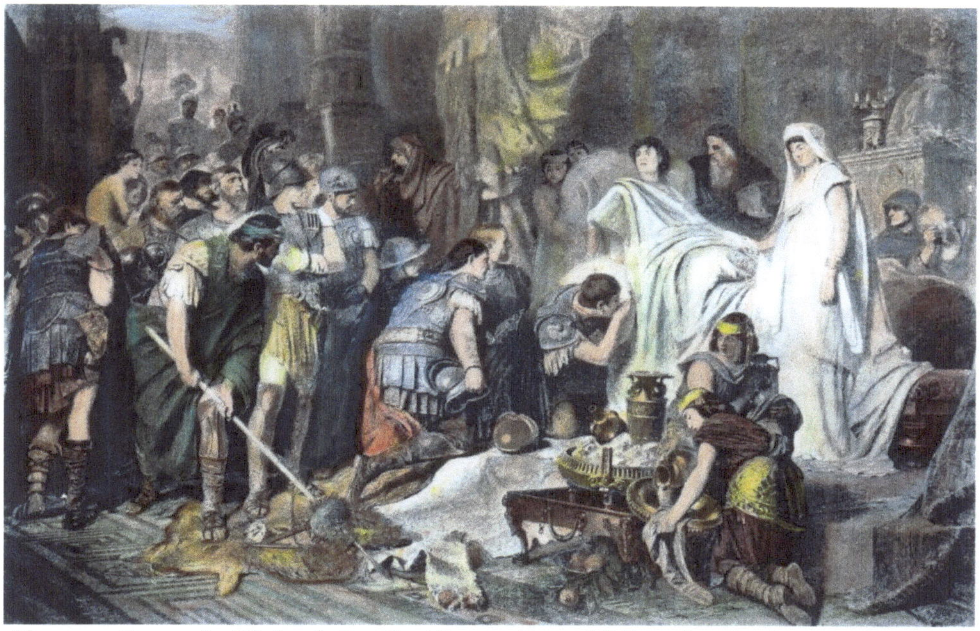

Posterazzi's greatly embellished death Alexander of Macedonia, known as Alexander the Great on his horse, on his deathbed.

The upper left abdominal pain that persists and increases in discomfort without intermittent relief, is strongly suggestive of pancreatitis, especially when accompanied by vomiting without relief of nausea. Alexander the Great, at the young age of 29, was stricken with abdominal pain following a victory celebration in Bagdad after his armies were turned back by the fevers of the Indian subcontinent. In June of 323 BC, after just thirteen years of leadership he had conquered the former Greek world, Egypt, the Middle Eastern kingdoms of Syria, Mesopotamia and Babylon, Bactria (Afghanistan), Persia and had penetrated the Khyber Pass into India. After his army refused to march further into the Indian subcontinent because of the deadly tropical diseases, tigers, snakes and seemingly endless battles, he returned to Baghdad where he entered a period of banquets and drinking bouts with his victorious soldiers.

Baghdad was an area known for bad water, and one of Alexander's priority engineering projects was to provide safe drinking water and irrigation canals in the Euphrates River basin. The lack of drinking water in this desert capital in the summer led to restricted water intake. Banquet meals tended to be large portions of pigs and other rich animal flesh, consumed with wine and not water. Unfortunately for the young warrior-emperor, one of these banquets was his last meal. The following morning, he awoke with abdominal pain, which over a few days developed into severe abdominal pain, symptoms suggestive of peritonitis and increasing fever. He lived for ten agonizing days after the onset of abdominal pain, dying with a high fever and delirious. There was time enough for each of his soldiers to pass by for his review and blessing. The author believes Alexander's death caused by pancreatitis while others have listed typhoid fever, malaria and deliberate poisoning. The upper left abdominal pain that persists and increases in discomfort without intermittent relief, is strongly suggestive of pancreatitis, especially when accompanied by vomiting without relief of nausea. Pancreatitis fits the location, circumstances and description of Alexander's demise. It also serves to warn about the risk of large fatty protein-rich meals taken with alcohol in the face of dehydration.

Treatment of pancreatitis, even in modern hospitals, is limited to bowel rest, pain relief and antibiotics if fever is present. Bowel rest in the hospital is complete bowel rest with IV fluids and a nasogastric tube inserted to continually remove stomach fluids. This can hardly be done in the field where management is limited to clear fluids by mouth in small amounts to lightly stimulate the gut, while giving enough fluids to ensure hydration and urine flow. Pancreatitis is a serious cause of abdominal pain and should not be managed at sea or in the field if the person can be delivered to a modern health care facility. The symptoms can persist for weeks, sometimes for life, requiring the addition of pig or beef pancreatic enzymes with each meal. Chronic pancreatitis leads to weight loss and chronic intermittent abdominal pain, loose frequent stools and early death. The best test to detect pancreatitis is the serum amylase level.

Alexander was wounded by sword, spear and arrow more than twenty times. After death, his generals divided up the empire with Ptolemy going to Egypt, where he continued Alexander's work in building a powerful merchant marine base at Alexandria and founding medical school while building the great library. It was supposed to be the world's most complete library of Greek medical texts and continued to serve as the major center for maritime medicine for more than 1000 years.

The Gall Bladder

two Greek words, *khole +kystis* meaning gall containing bladder

The gall bladder is another component of the gastrointestinal tract normally silent unless provoked. It lies under the liver and behind (posterior) where it serves as a contractible reservoir of bile, a yellow-green soap-like fluid that aids in digestion, especially meats and fats. The golden-green substance appears in later stages of retching, as the stomach has emptied its contents, and now fluids from the proximal small bowel are being ejected, causing a very bitter taste. Bile is a waste product of the breakdown of old red blood cells and recycled in the gut as an emulsifier, an organic soap. Bile is derived from bilirubin, a yellow pigment found in the hemoglobin of mammals. After the liver has extracted iron from old red blood cells, iron is returned to the bone marrow, a yellow chemical, bilirubin remains. After further degradation, bilirubin is rendered into bile and stored in the gall bladder. Diseases affecting the liver's ability to breakdown bilirubin into bile, will turn a person yellow in hepatitis, pancreatic cancer and Yellow Fever. Yellow Fever was known as Yellow Jack in sea-going terms and flying the Yellow Jack flag as a warning often prevented pirates from taking a ship as the disease was so deadly to sailors. A gall bladder is not necessary for survival, and many live every day simply fine after having the gall bladder removed. Mammals need the organic soap of bile to more fully digest the fat found in the animals and plants eaten.

As the bile is discharged via the gall bladder it serves the body on its outbound passage from the digestive tract by breaking fatty substances into smaller pieces. Removing grease from hands and dishes, even with repeated rinsing with water does little, yet by adding soap, the film of grease disappears down drain. "Degreasing" foods by emulsifying fat is the primary function of bile in the gut. The gall bladder's neck collapses between meals, opening when food enters the stomach and contraction of the bladder as the meal enters the small intestine, opens the long slender neck. Hopefully, just before entering the small bowel, bile meets and activates the pancreatic enzymes. This is all done on the command of hormones released by the stomach. When the liver is unable to convert bilirubin into bile, first the whites of the eyes and later the skin become stained with this yellow pigment (jaundice).

The most common problem of the gall bladder are stones that form in the stagnant pool of bile and accumulate over time in the bladder. Stones that can later squirt into the narrow neck of the gall bladder as it joins the pancreatic duct just before the Ampulla of Vater. It is within this narrow passage that stones block the outflow of a contracting gall bladder leading to intermittent sharp (colicky) pain in the right upper quadrant of abdomen, nausea, vomiting and diarrhea. The pain often radiates to the right shoulder blade and this history is diagnostic of gallstone disease. Gallstones can remain dormant for years, especially if meat and fat are avoided. Typical gallstone attacks follow a meal heavy in fatty meat and the ingestion of alcohol (like a pizza and six-pack of beer). Treatment includes bowel rest (clear liquids), control of nausea and pain, antispasmodic drug (Donnatal), encouraging fluids and antibiotics if fever appears. After the attack has passed, the person should avoid fats, meats, gravies, fried foods and alcohol until consulting a physician.

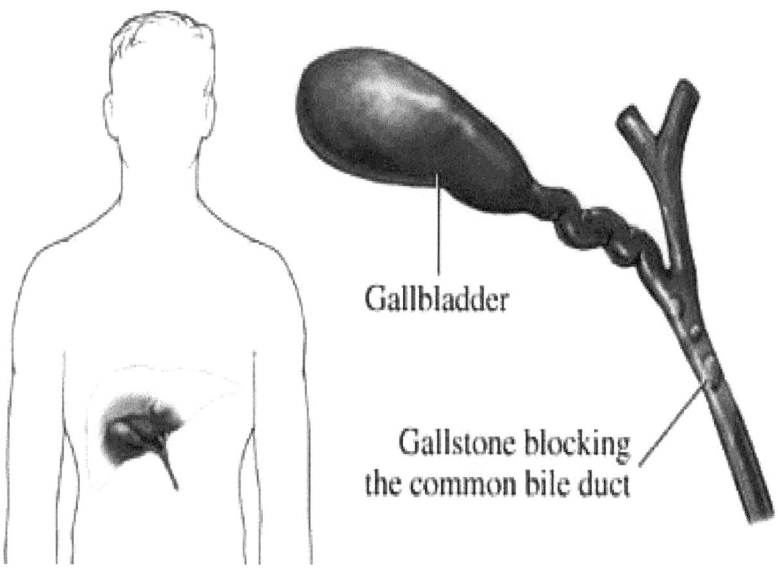

In this picture a gallstone has obstructed the bile outlet, causing the cystic duct to swell. This swelling will result in considerable abdominal pain and gas-passing that come and go, usually relieved by bowel rest and gut tranquilizers. Stones are formed when thick salty solutions congregate in a stagnant gall bladder. NIH

Not that ago, gallstone attacks resulted in painful surgery followed by 5-7 days in the hospital, the first 2-3 days, with a tube down the nose and into the stomach. The surgery now is done with a fiberoptic scope through several small incisions, the patient often goes home the next day. Another recent treatment is the use of drugs that dissolve gallstones while reducing the risk of attacks. This drug, Actigall, is made of cow gall bladder contents, exactly like the oxgall carried on Egyptian vessels 4000 years ago. It has been used for the management of abdominal pain for many centuries.

The Liver

Greek *liparos* meaning fat, Old English *lifer*, Dutch lever, German *leber*

The largest internal organ in mammal, fish, fowl or reptile is the liver. In the human, it is not only the largest but one of the busiest organs in the body. Twenty-four hours a day, the liver is detoxifying chemicals, activating hormones such as the sex steroids, regulating carbohydrate (glucose) metabolism, producing much of the proteins needed for repair of tissue, removing old cells from circulation, manufacturing antibodies for infection control and sending bile to the gall bladder for storage.

Infection of the liver, viral hepatitis is a common disease. There are several types, none of which are pleasant, while some are fatal. The most common form (outside the tropics) are hepatitis A, B and C. Hepatitis A is commonly contracted via food contamination and can make a person very ill for weeks or months, but usually has no long-term side effects. However, hepatitis B and C can become a chronic life-long disease requiring liver transplant, killing thousands of people every day throughout the world. For every health care worker dying of AIDS or Ebola, thousands die from hepatitis B. Fortunately, there is an immunization for hepatitis B in the form of three injections given over a six-month period, but these must be boosted every 10 years. Hepatitis A is two injections over 6 months and requires a booster every 10 years. Since hepatitis is much easier to prevent than treating, immunizations are the preferred course. Gamma globulin is safe but used less now and may offer some protection from hepatitis A for several months after injection. Hepatitis C until recently was difficult to treat and was a life-long illness with grave consequences. However newer medications offer many a cure with limited side effects outside of high costs. Some medical officers recommend travelers to developing countries with questionable sewage control, receive gamma globulin for hepatitis A (if available), along with immunization for hepatitis B and A.

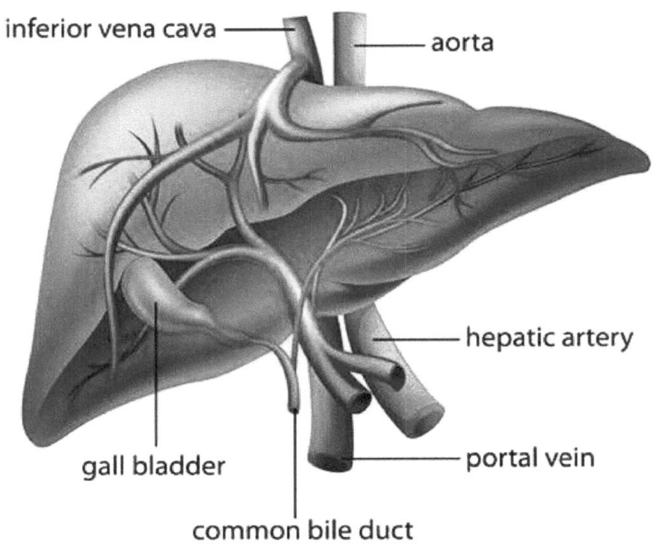

The liver is blood vessel rich and can easily bleeds with abdominal. It serves not only the gut, but the endocrine, vascular, lymphatic and nervous system. One can only be healthy with a healthy liver. NIH

Liver function is indirectly measured by detection of the amounts of two liver enzymes, SGOT and AST coupled with serum bilirubin which elevate prior to jaundice. Loss of sense of taste and smell are sometimes early symptoms of hepatic dysfunction. The liver plays hosts to many tropical infections including schistosomiasis, amoebas, liver flukes, malaria, intestinal nematodes and others. Abdominal pain that is persistent with or without fever in the tropics should increase suspicion of liver parasites. Fortunately, the medical communities in the tropics are well equipped to diagnosis and treat these diseases. Unfortunately, treatment is often prolonged and uncomfortable.

The Small Bowel

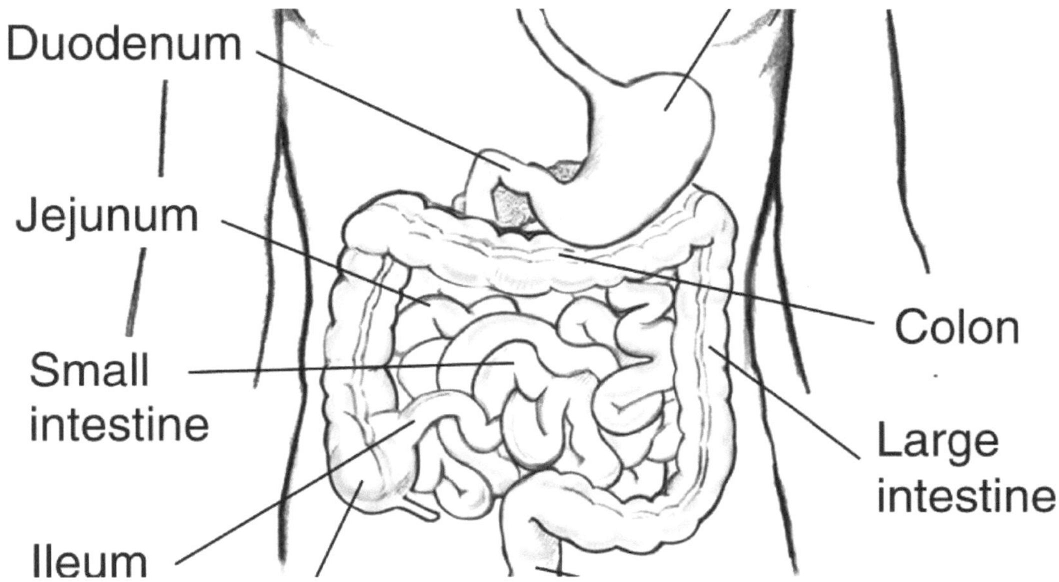

The small bowel has three components, duodenum, ilium and jejunum. Its combined surface in the adult is the size of a tennis court. NLM

The Duodenum

Complicated Latin word *intest I duod num digit o rum*, meaning intestine of 12 fingerbreadths

The beginning (proximal) of the small bowel, duodenum is a C-shaped piece of small bowel measures about ten inches (25 cm) in length and is responsible for receiving secretions from the stomach, gall bladder and pancreas. It is a very active place and can be the site of a great deal of pain and misery since problems with any of the above organs can impact on the duodenum. If too much acid is received from the stomach, it inflames the duodenum's lining, causing pain and bleeding. Both the gall bladder and pancreas gain access to the bowel's interior through a shared valve-like structure, the ampulla of Vater, embedded in the duodenum's wall. Here, bile and pancreatic juices containing bicarbonate to neutralize the stomach acid and powerful enzymes destined to break down proteins, find their way into the hollow gut. The content and amounts of secretions from the gall bladder and pancreas are customized for the type of meal discharged by the stomach. Large meals high in fat and protein are the most difficult to digest. These types of meals strongly stimulate bile and pancreatic release, as large amounts are needed to emulsify (de-grease), break up and absorb such a feeding. In the duodenum, digestion begins in earnest. This is the first site of absorption for most nutrients as well as water and most drugs, although glucose, alcohol and some water taken up in the stomach. Beginning in the duodenum, proteins are rendered into smaller chains of amino acids which can be absorbed by the brush border in the following jejunum and ileum. At the same time, the soap action of bile mixes and begins to emulsify and break up the fat found in many foods.

Ileum/Jejunum

Latin word for Troy, easily confused with the ilium, which is bone in pelvis, jejunum is Latin for fasting.

This is the final component of the small intestine and is the longest in length and varies widely in humans from 7 to 14 feet. Here any remaining nutrients the body needs are absorbed, especially B12. In dysentery, especially cholera, it is the site of major fluid loss. The jejunum terminates in several valve-like constrictions (jejunum-cecal valves) before emptying its slurry-like contents into colon

The Colon

Greek word *kolon* meaning large bowel (also family name for Christopher Columbus)

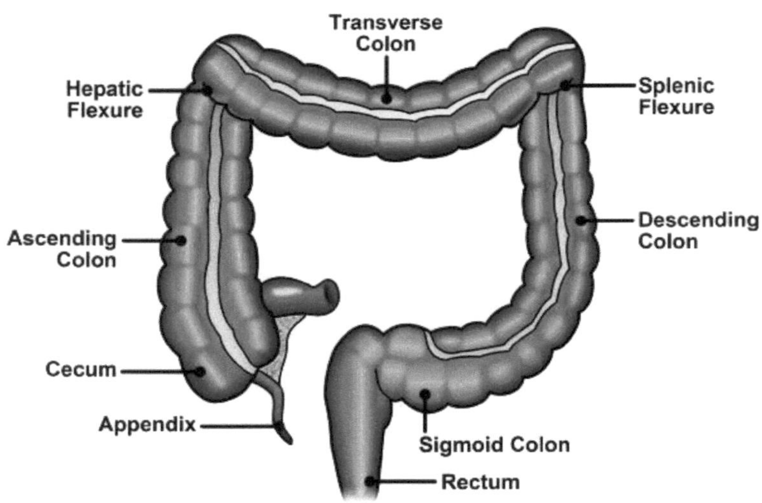

The large bowel is much more than the final passage for food and water. It has a large self-controlled nervous system, and it provides a home to billions of microbes, some necessary for health. Colonic bacteria have been discovered to affect personality, body size and intelligence. NLM

Storage and fluid removal from the feces are of the primary gastrointestinal function of the colon as there are still many useful chemicals in feces, some of which the colon attempts to absorb. The brown color of passed stools is caused by colon bacteria fermenting bile. Some animals, including rodents under conditions of need, will eat their own feces to recover even small amounts of nutrients. Elephants routinely eat other elephants' feces to capture useful bacteria and the most expensive coffee in the world is recovered coffee beans from elephant feces. Surprisingly, humans are now sharing stool materials in a procedure called fecal transplants, where another person's feces transferred to a receptive colon. There appears to be no precedent in the history of medicine for this procedure and is being used for weight loss, inflammatory bowel diseases, irritable bowel syndrome and some auto immune diseases. Drugs such as aspirin, caffeine and anti-nausea medications are absorbed in the colon along with as much water as time will allow. Bacteria are absent or found in low numbers in most of the gut but play a huge role in the colon. Here they begin the breakdown of feces by fermentation, a process that continues after the feces has left the body. Colon bacteria produce vitamin K, which is absorbed into the body and is needed for normal blood clotting. As much as one-half of the material in a bowel movement is bacteria, amounting to several pounds of teeming organisms within normal colons. The total number of bacteria living peacefully in a human colon is estimated to be 10 to the 23rd power, a number so large as to be incomprehensible.

Colon bacteria for the most part, enjoy a relationship which benefits themselves and their host. That is unless they escape the GI tract and invade the sterile confines of the peritoneal cavity. When this happens, the very serious condition of peritonitis develops, requiring the best medical care available to avoid death. Prior to the advent of abdominal surgery and antibiotics, any leakage of bacteria from the colon into the abdominal cavity was almost universally fatal. Punctures of the colon from swords, spear, projectiles, blunt trauma, rupture of the appendix and ectopic pregnancy had few if any survivors in the pre-antibiotic and modern surgery era.

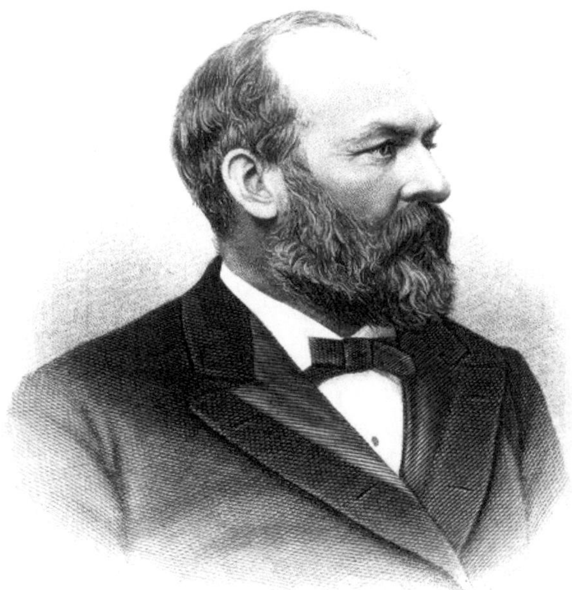

James Garfield, the 20th president, congressman, Union Major General, led troops at Shiloh and Chickamauga, only served for six and one-half months, yet instituted

agriculture reform, strongly supported civil rights for African Americans and believed in state-sponsored primary education. National Archives

People with possible peritonitis must be watched carefully at sea and in the field, while treated early with antibiotics. It can last for days and even weeks, depending on the cause, severity and quality of care. President Garfield was gut-shot by a small-caliber pistol at close range and spent long, painful weeks dying. It is not known if the bullet ultimately killed him or the multiple physicians that put unclean fingers into his wound probing for the bullet. Even Thomas Edison tried to find the bullet using a machine he had invented but did not account for the metal in the bedsprings the dying president was laying on. When President Garfield realized that his abdomen had been penetrated by the bullet, he said "I am a dead man." He had seen many comrades die similar wounds in the Civil War.

The length of the colon is approximately the person's body height. It has two sharp turns and contains muscle fibers that run around (circular) and along its structure (longitudinal), allowing the hollow organ to constrict and push material and gas forward. Many problems inflict this part of the gut, especially if colon contents become stagnant. Adequate water intake, dietary fiber, such as psyllium (Metamucil) and physical activity all increase colon flow. In the lower descending colon before its termination into the rectum often contain diverticula (Latin for byway), especially as the colon ages. They appear as pouches protruding away from the lining of the colon almost like small fingers when filled with barium on X-ray. They are usually silent but can become infected (diverticulitis) if stagnation occurs. These pouches can be blocked by dietary seeds or small pieces of hard stool. Like hemorrhoids, diverticula are often inherited, seen with chronic constipation and are more likely with long periods spent sitting on toilet. In some cases, they slowly enlarge like a tree root and find a way to penetrate the surrounding tissue and come to the skin's surface around the rectum forming pilonidal cysts. Left lower abdominal pain, especially cramp-like painful spasms, rectal bleeding and in more severe forms, fever requiring treatment including antibiotic (especially with fever), stool bulking agents (fiber) and increased fluids.

Diverticulitis

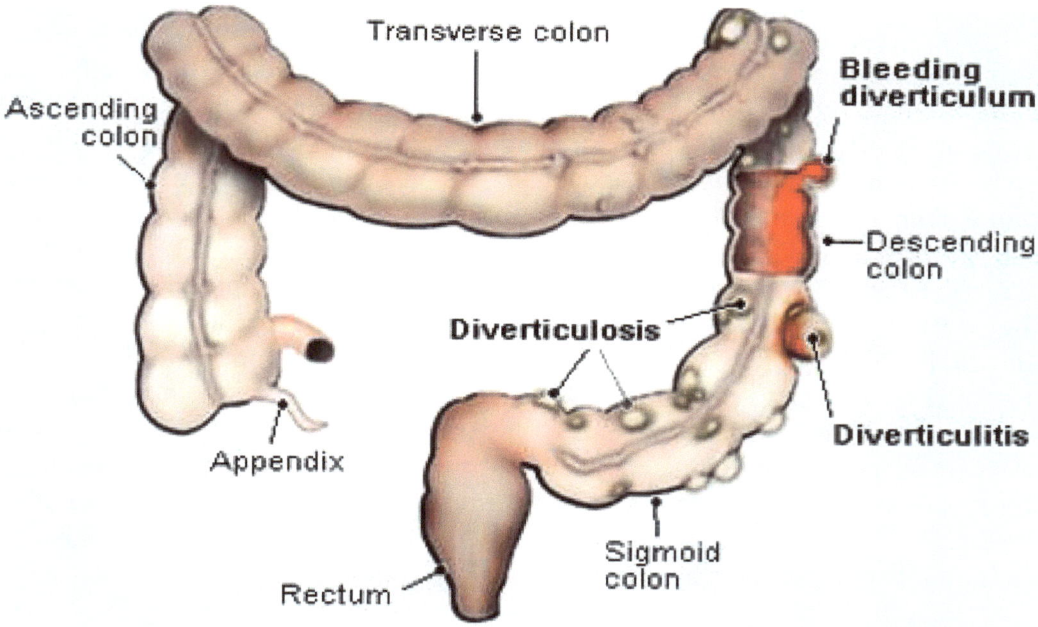

Images from CDC of common sites of diverticulitis, many people will have the pouch-like diverticula but only a few will develop disease, and some will rupture creating a surgical emergency. NLM

A common malady in the lower colon where tiny pouches form in the soft mucosa usually causes no symptoms and are only found on barium enemas and colonoscopy exams. These blind finger-like projections can become inflamed and infected resulting in lower abdominal pain, fever and bowel movement changes. Clear liquids and antibiotics usually resolve these problems but in severe cases and in chronic complaints result in colon resection to remove these sites of obstruction.

The **rectal fissure** is another common cause of rectal bleeding. It can be painless and sudden, producing blood-tinged discharge at the time of a bowel movement or bright red blood on the tissue paper. It may be difficult to tell the difference between hemorrhoids and fissure as both cause bleeding, fissure tends to be painless while hemorrhoids cause discomfort. Treatment is usually the same, with laxatives, extra fiber, sitting in baths of hot soapy water, no straining, shorter bowel movements time, mild steroid cream or better, steroid ointment, suppository at bedtime and after bowel movements, gentle wiping techniques using moisturizing cream on toilet paper (if rectum very irritated) and increased fluids to thin stools. Most of the over-the-counter hemorrhoid preparations are fish oil and when combined with mild, topical steroids are effective in reducing irritation and promoting healing of inflamed rectal tissue. Simple care of the rectum requires keeping the area clean and dry, sometimes several times through the day, especially in hot moist climates. Keep hydrated, avoid spicy hot foods, eat extra fiber, and avoid prolonged bowel movements and straining.

The Rectum

Latin *rectus* meaning straight as compared to preceding coiling bowel

This nearly vertical segment of bowel in the upright position is composed of complicated musculo-neuro connections to both involuntary and voluntary series of valves. The location and function of this structure is different in every person, both in anatomy and function. The rectum is blood vessel rich, as is the oral cavity and esophagus where bundles of large venous blood vessels (hemorrhoidal) are found, their function is to reduce and dilute concentrations of bacteria. Rectal length is 6-8 inches and like the nose and ears tends to get larger with age. Its muscular coats are thicker than the rest of colon, composed in circular (inner) and longitudinal (outer) layers. Its absorbing power is remarkable (thus making it a good pathway for fluids used in resuscitation). This is due to the thick submucosa layer rich in blood vessels and lymphatic channels; finally, the innermost layer is the mucus membrane rich in vessels. Just prior to exiting the body is a thin transitional layer, where the gut meets skin. This tiny strip of flesh is rich in blood vessels and a common site of irritation and itching known commonly as puritis ani (inflamed rectum). Muscles are voluntary and involuntary in action, the most important is the levator ani (lifter of anus) when the sphincter relaxes to defecate, compressing the urethra. External sphincter is usually voluntary, while the internal sphincter is generally involuntary (dumping reflex).

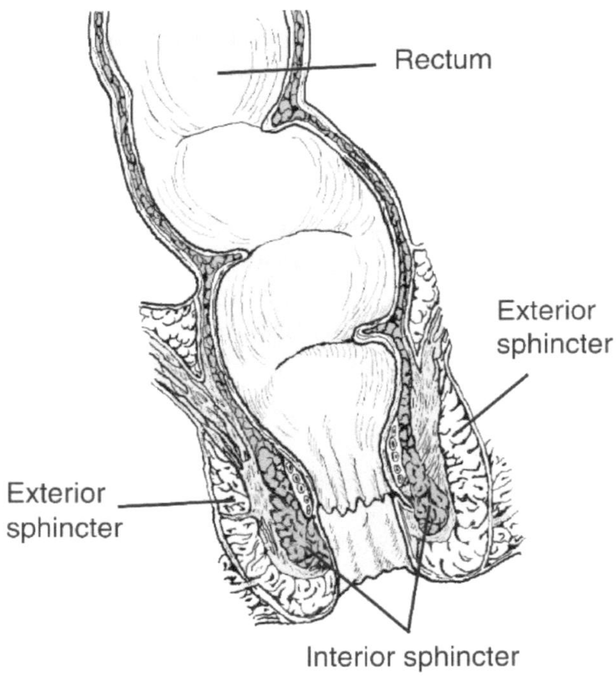

The gastrointestinal tract terminates through a series of valves that allow for voluntary discharge of bowel wastes. The rectum lies within a thin-layered muscular wall of blood-rich tissue. NLM

The anus is the termination of gut and filled with sebaceous follicular glands producing lubrication and usually an unpleasant odor. In many mammals, discharges from these glands are used as a scent to attract and discourage other animals (in some breeds of dogs need to be cleared manually).

The anus can be stretched in all directions without injury if done slowly, while easily can be torn with sudden violent opening. Itching is common and is seldom due to worms (as is often feared) but usually caused by poor hygiene, i.e. areas not kept and dry. Even though there is a small part of the gut, it accounts for many medical complaints. It is a common site for gastrointestinal cancers, rectal bleeding from hemorrhoids and fissures, constipation, "dumping reflex" (uncontrolled rectal discharge with little warning, especially with meals), abscesses, cysts, venereal diseases and prolapse.

One of the most common rectal complaints, hemorrhoids, occurs when large venous blood vessels encompassing the rectal area become engorged with stagnant blood flow. These heavily laden vessels over time can "breakthrough" the thin muscle walls leading to bulges inside and outside the rectum. External hemorrhoids form soft and sometimes hard "knots" around the anus, while internal hemorrhoids form within the rectum. As a rule, external hemorrhoids cause pain, internal hemorrhoids leak causing peri-anal itching. Both bleeds, resulting in bright red blood in stool and on toilet paper. Sudden gushes of bright blood are often due a tear in the fragile mucosa of rectum, this is usually painless and the result of hard firm stools that "tear" their way out of rectum.

Hemorrhoids and History

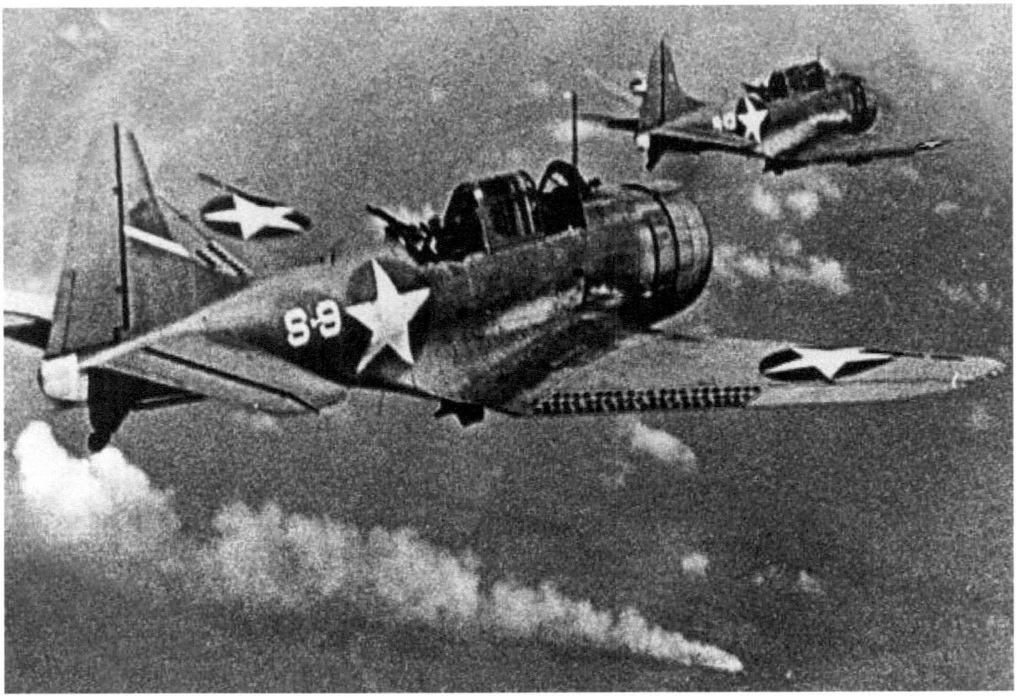

The Battle of Midway was possible affected by hemorrhoids. National Archives

Rectal pathology is widely dispersed in history, occurring frequently and managed by many treatment modalities, some highly effective. Napoleon received some relief with the application of blood-sucking leeches in draining the emperor's hemorrhoids. Salves of heavy oils, vegetable poultices, hot soaks and at last resort, painful excision in the less fortunate have all been effective in the past. Stool softeners increased oral fluids and topical mild steroid ointment are the current conservative treatments, but a large external hemorrhoid may require drainage. Often a blood clot gets trapped in the ballooning hemorrhoidal tissue requiring it to be opened and drained. The procedure is not difficult since anesthesia has followed by opening draining the hemorrhoid is not to be attempted unless necessary. The excision and drainage of a large external mass of blood extending from a sailor's rectum prompting him to comment upon completion, "I hope you enjoyed that Dr Hill, because you will never do that again to me"! The injection of local anesthesia was the primary cause of transient discomfort, and once lidocaine took effect, the surgery was nearly painless. Hemorrhoids are common today and have been a persistent human affliction throughout history playing a possible role in human events as the following story recounts.

No battle in human history compares to the significance and brevity of the Battle of Midway on June 4, 1942. Within minutes, three of the Imperial Japanese Navy's finest aircraft carriers were destroyed, leaving its surviving pilots, no place to land. In a "blink of the eye", much of the offensive power of the Imperial Japanese Navy was on the bottom of the Pacific Ocean. Winston Churchill in the early 20th century feared that a single naval battle could lose a war. Midway did not lose the war for Japan, but it destroyed a large part of Japan's offensive abilities and inhibited its plans for isolating Australia. Before the US fleet left Pearl Harbor for its ambush the Japanese,

Admiral Bill Halsey was replaced for medical reasons by a non-aviator, Admiral Jack Fletcher. In the first Hollywood movie, "Midway" Halsey was replaced due to severe hives, while in the 2019 movie, it was shingles. The real reason is a piece of medical lore that has come through the "scuttlebutt" within the US Navy Medicine that Halsey's hemorrhoids had become severe enough to render him unfit to command. His removal may have changed the battle in America's favor.

Halsey was replaced by the next senior naval officer, "Jack" Fletcher who had primarily commanded heavy cruisers but had led the two previous carrier battles, the Battle of Coral Sea and the Eastern Solaman Islands. These were the first naval battles in history where the opposing fleets were not in visual contact, fighting with aircraft instead of shipboard guns. Like many medical officers, he was learning carrier fighting "in the field". After sinking three Japanese fleet carriers, the Americans lost the carrier *Yorktown* and Admiral Fletcher aboard the sinking *Yorktown*, transferred command to Admiral Raymond Spruance aboard the *Enterprise* when the fourth Japanese carrier was found and destroyed. The aviators with their blood up wanted to pursue and finish off the retreating enemy ships, but the more cautious Spruance demurred and withdrew. Halsey with an offensive personality such as Robert E. Lee and Horatio tral would have likely sent his remaining ships in pursuit. However, a few hundred miles away Yamamoto was waiting with dozens of heavy battleships and cruisers that would have made short work of the smaller United States Pacific Fleet including the last two American carriers.

Rectal hygiene may be difficult in the field, especially in hot moist climates because of sweating and inadequate cleaning after bowel movements which can irritate the rectum and surrounding skin. Water hoses, cleaning towelettes, and gentle wiping with defecation will reduce the need to scratch, which worsens the complaint of pruitis ani (chronic itchy anus). Sometimes it may be necessary to clean and dry the rectal area several times a day even without defecation to reduce irritation while application of petroleum base ointments with or without topical steroids can be very useful.

The rectum is not the dirtiest spot on the body when compared to the types of bacteria found in the oral cavity, however it is highly contaminated and rich in bacteria. The rectum is another site on the body where bacteria-laden contents interact with skin and the outside world. Remember this when you are shaking hands with strangers, since you have no idea where that person's hand has been since its last washing. Fingers that are likely to have been in nose, mouth and rectal area. The rectum is known for common medical complaints, such as bleeding, itching and pain from hemorrhoids, cysts and fissures. The termination of the colon is surrounded by tissue containing large veins which easily become distended into varicose veins. The Western-style toilet offers an excellent opportunity for these vessels to over-fill, stretching venous tissue into hemorrhoids. While sitting atop the typical western toilet, the entire weight of the abdominal contents suspended over the outlet of lower colon, the surrounding skin stretched taut. All the while, the toilet rim acting like a tourniquet, further enhancing stagnation. Here a person sits comfortably, daydreaming or perhaps reading several chapters of Tolstoy's *War and Peace*. During which, rectal veins are swelling with pooling blood. These toilet habits over time risk the formation of hemorrhoids. It is not uncommon for an exposed hemorrhoid to form a blood clot, causing a tender hard knot at the rectum which is best resolved with opening and drainage. Straining to pass hard firm stools is a common etiology of hemorrhoid formation.

Since any rectal bleeding could be the result of cancer, all should be investigated even if likely caused by hemorrhoids. The author recommends colonoscopy exam as soon as is prudent. Colon cancer is the number one cancer in the American population, and although it is primarily a cancer over the age of 55, it is striking younger and younger people. Checking the stool for blood with an occult blood test is warranted every year, more often if there is a family history of colon cancer.

In addition to rectal pathology, psychology played a role at Midway and later in the battle for the Philippines when considering the "mind set" of naval aviators and giving command of fleets to fliers. At the Battle of Midway the only carrier USS *Hornet* commanded by aviator Marc Mitscher played no role in the battle. Believing he alone knew the position of the Japanese fleet, he sent planes to "the flight to nowhere" in disobedience of orders from his non-aviator superior. Added to this mistake was Mitscher's after-battle report included untruths to "cover his ass". Later in the war, William Halsey in command of a huge American, with the aggressive behavior so common among fliers, abandoned Douglas MacArthur's landings at Leyte Gulf chasing a Japanese decoy of carriers devoid of airplanes that represented no threat to the invasion. Just as the Japanese hoped he would do. Halsey not only took all the fleet carriers with him but also the battleships and heavy cruisers supporting the invading army. When the Imperial Japanese Fleet appeared off the Gulf of Leyte, one of their ships, the world's largest battleship *Yamato* weighed more than all the American ships Halsey left behind! Some believe his abandonment of the invasion beach invasion was the largest single mistake in US Navy history costing the lives of hundreds of sailors, several warships and the near destruction of the landing forces transport ships.

Cancer in the Gut

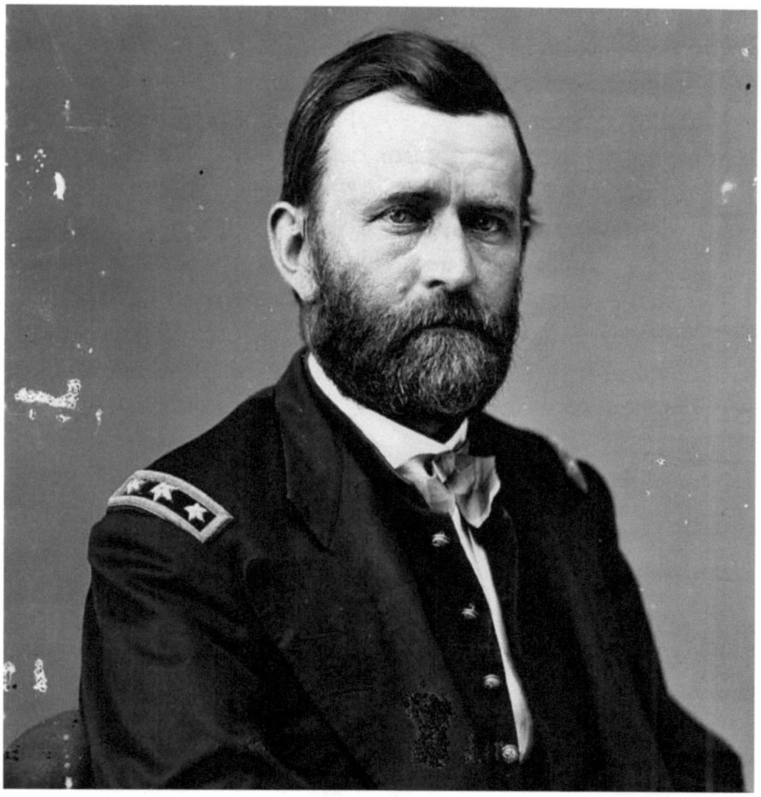

Grant only ate charred meat, never eating any meat with red or pink showing, and he smoked twenty cigars each day. He was known to be one of the best horsemen in the army and personally collected more maps than any other individual. US Grant, the 18th president, sometime called "Unconditional Surrender" Grant. At Yalta, the dying President Roosevelt surprised his generals and Churchill with using Grant's term for Germany's unconditional surrender. Whether it was a slip or planned, some blame this demand for unconditional surrender for Germany's suicidal fighting in until May 1945. If not for a single bullet that struck down the commanding Confederate General Albert Sidney Johnston at the Battle of Shiloh, he and his lieutenant, William Tecumseh Sherman would have been disgraced and cashiered for gross incompetence. They did survive and they learned from their mistakes, going on to win the American Civil War. National Library of Congress

There has always been cancer in the gastrointestinal tract. Until the mid-20th century, the esophagus and stomach continued to be the primary sites. In the 1960's it faded away except in the elderly. However, Japan continued to experience high rates. Refrigeration greatly reduced stomach and esophageal cancer, first in the US and later in Japan, reduced cancer by converting high carbon smoked meat to fresh meat. Carbon has been identified as the causative agent for much of esophageal cancer along with tobacco. Dysphagia, or painful swallowing is the hallmark complaint along with weight loss and anemia. Ulysses S Grant died a slow painful death from esophageal cancer but fortunately Samuel Clemmons (Mark Twain) prompted him to dictate his life story. Grant's memoir is good reading. All gastrointestinal cancers are usually associated with low blood counts (anemia).

Monitoring the stool for blood is an excellent first line of diagnosis. The blood is often occult (unseen) in the stool and detected by simple stool sample for blood which should be done yearly. Colon cancer is the # 1 cause of cancer in the United States when men and women are lumped together and require vigilance to detect with stool for occult blood, abdominal CAT scans and colonoscopy. The lower colon is the primary site, but colon cancer can occur in the more proximal (closer to the ileum). The author recommends a full colonoscopy, not just a sigmoidoscopy. Colon cancer tends to spread to the liver first and then beyond. Lymphoma cancer is found in the colon but will not cause bleeding. Pancreatic cancer is often silent until too late. Symptoms include pain in the left upper abdominal quadrant and early diagnosis requires either an ultrasound or CAT scan of abdomen. This author obtains a CAT scan of abdomen and pelvis every 3-5 years to detect early cancer and evaluate other internal organs such as liver, prostate, and colon. Liver cancer is associated with colon cancer, lymphoma and chronic viral hepatitis of B and C.

The Urinary Tract

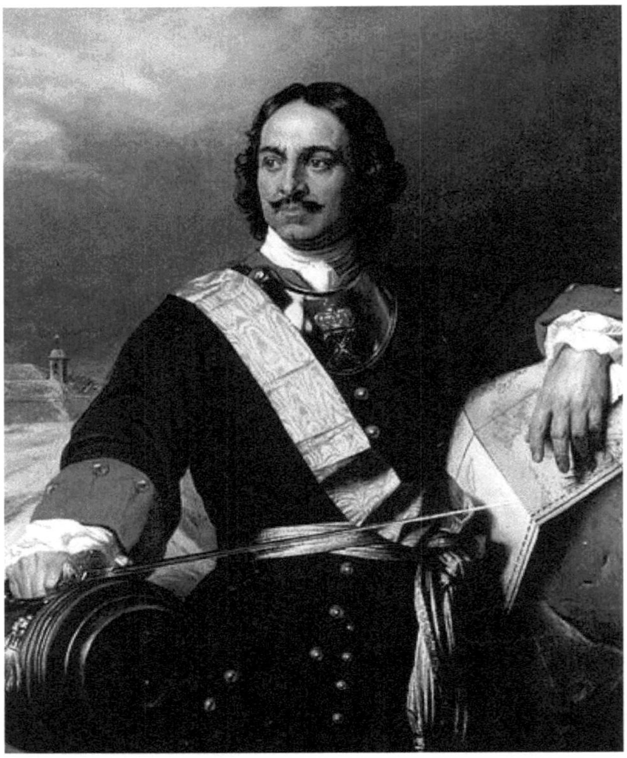

Peter the Great, 1672-1725 at six foot eight inches was a giant in size and ambitions. He enlarged Russia in successful wars, built two world-class fleets and forced his subjects to become more European while starving millions of serfs to pay for his projects. Just as Stalin did to the Ukrainians in 1930s. When Peter's only son fled Russia and his future throne, Peter violated Austrian sovereignty, had him captured and put him on trial. His father, serving as prosecutor and judge, found him guilty and he was found murdered in prison, saving him from being broken on the wheel. Peter suffered much of his adult life

with chronic urinary tract disease and died from complications of kidney failure. Painting by Paul Delacoche, Hermitage Museum

As an experiment of one's urinary system, measure the input and output of fluids in a 24-hour period. In addition to measuring amounts of urine produced, note that colored fluids enter the body, and depigmented (except with beets) urine comes out of a complicated filtering system. Normally, there will be less output compared to intake because with each exhaled breath, water leaves circulation. Sweating and bowel movements also remove fluid. An exception where output may be greater than input is when a diuretic is deployed, changing the kidney's ability to retain fluid. Alcohol and diuretics such as furosemide (Lasix) may result in urine formation greater than intake. There is a great deal of information in urine, information easy to retrieve with urine test strips. Test strips detect glucose (diabetes), white blood cells (infection), blood (stone), bilirubin (hepatitis), protein (kidney disease), ketones (fasting) and concentration of urine compared to water. Urine is composed of excess water, dissolved waste products, dead cells sloughed off from the interior of the urinary tract, occasional bacteria, a few white blood cells and drugs. Drugs not only detectable in urine but are still active in many cases.

While visiting South Africa, the author met a professor of ichthyology (*ikhthys*-Greek for fish) who was studying catfish in water systems connected to city discharges. They were finding significant levels of fluoxetine (Prozac) in fish that should have never met a human antidepressant in the wild. In municipal waters systems where wastewater is recycled, the same would be true since antibiotics, hormones, psychotropic drugs are not currently removed. Many excreted unchanged, active and with the baggage of side effects possibly most of the body's cells. Are these unknowingly consumed drugs, affecting human behavior?

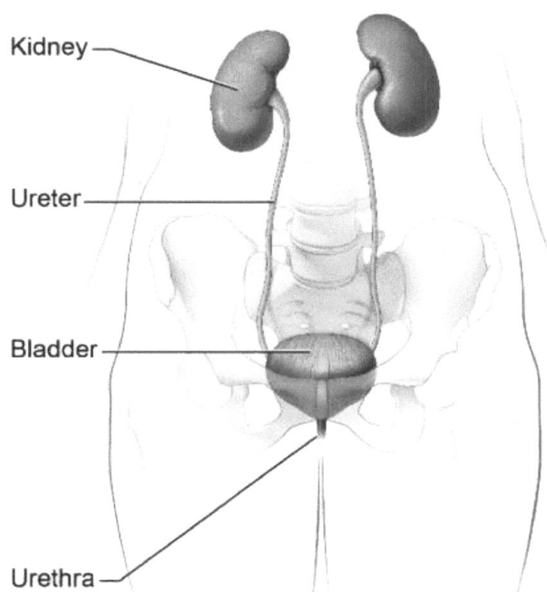

Large amounts of arterial blood are delivered to the headwaters of the urinary tract in the kidney where it is filtered by the hydraulic pressure generated by the heart's left ventricle. Much of the filtered fluid is reabsorbed along gracefully curved nephron tubes which form

most of the kidney tissue. Fluid in the bladder contains chemicals unwanted nor needed dissolved in excess water. NIH

During periods of exertion, especially in hot and humid conditions, more water is lost through perspiration and increased respiration. Exercise increases the need for water to support demands of cells in the musculoskeletal system, kidneys, heart and central nervous system. Even with exertion, urine should flow at regular intervals. Dark urine indicates inadequate fluid intake. The author believes urine should not be darker than light beer. The light color indicates that even with perspiration and breathing loses, the kidneys have excess water to dilute waste.

As the body burns sugar, manufactures proteins and repairs tissue, chemical waste products are generated. Accumulation of these products of metabolic activity would soon become harmful and must be eliminated. The kidneys' primary responsibility is to filter blood, selectively removing toxic materials while recycling others the body can still use. Along with the liver, the kidneys are the most active recycling center within the body, removing toxins and discharging them before they become a problem.

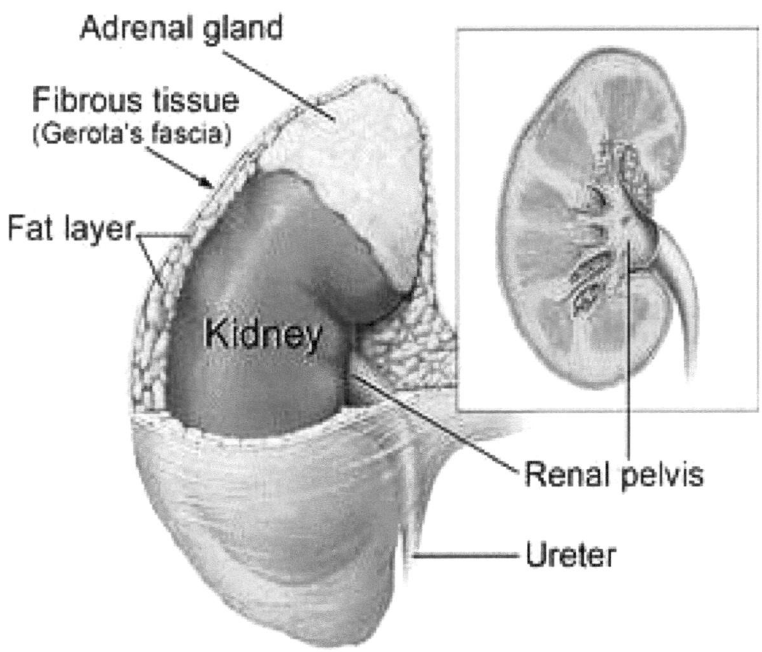

Normal kidney anatomy in most people, however the urinary tract contains more abnormalities than any other human system. Extra kidneys, extras ureters and malformations are common. The adrenal glands release adrenalin, aldosterone and cortisol. NIH

The kidneys normally occur as a pair of two fist-size bean-shaped organs found under the muscles of the lower posterior chest, in the flanks. Each kidney is enclosed in a tough fibrous capsule and layers of densely packed fat for protection. So well protected are the kidneys that they are rarely injured during trauma. The ancient Egyptians, during the mummifying process, removed all the internal organs of the royal family members, placing them in jars with the mummies. The kidneys were so well hidden in the body that it was generations into this process, before they were first discovered and placed in jars, even though thousands of bodies had been opened and examined by these early undertakers. The kidneys contain the "headwaters" of the urinary tract, a complex system of small streams, cisterns and canals connected to an expandable reservoir (the bladder). Blood from the heart reaches the kidneys through the large renal arteries, receiving 25% of all blood pumped, seconds after it exits the left ventricle. Over one liter of blood passes through the kidneys and its millions of tiny filtration units, the nephron, every sixty seconds at rest. The kidneys will experience damage if blood flow is interrupted even briefly. Shock victims may recover initially, only to develop kidney failure because shock deprived the nephrons of the blood flow needed to keep them living.

Nephrons resemble a ball connected by a long curved semipermeable tube where fluids and salts pass in and out until the final product of urine is discharged at the end of the nephron. Each nephron is like a tiny spring that along with one million other nephrons, drain into a central area (calyx), where urine awaits entry into the ureter which transports it down to the bladder. The calyx is a cistern draining region of the kidney which in turn opens into the larger kidney pelvis. The calyx and pelvis are the sites of kidney stone formation in the salt-rich fluid created by the nephrons. The brinier and more concentrated the urine, the more likely is stone formation. Initially, the nephron removes fluids, salts, drugs and other compounds from the passing blood, most of which is returned to circulation after "scrutiny" by the kidney tissue. Under normal conditions, urine is composed of items the kidneys consider waste and mixed with excess water.

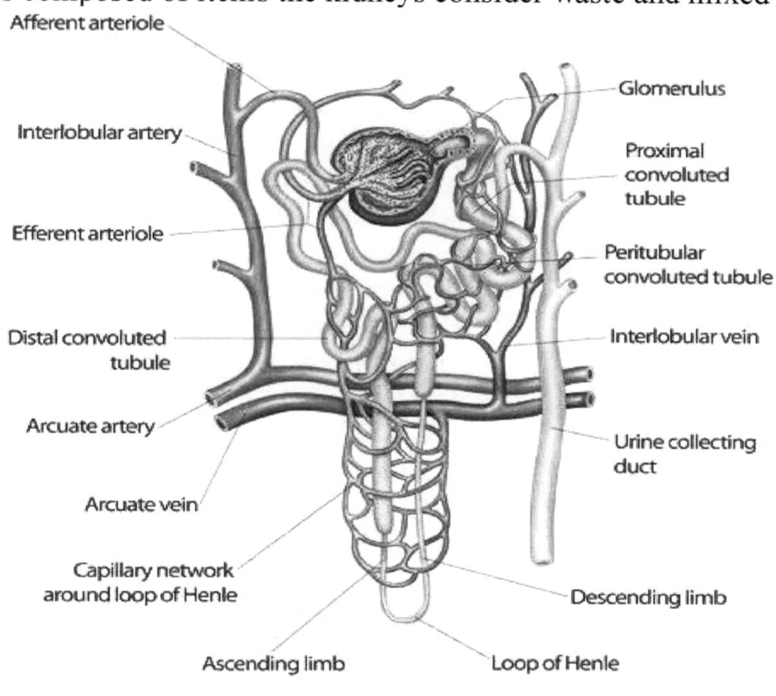

STRUCTURE OF A NEPHRON

A National Institute of Health illustration of the complicated functional unit of the kidney. Arterial blood comes in from the left, is filtered in the ball of vessels of the glomerulus, chemicals are useful and returned to circulation through the venous system while

unwanted chemicals and excess water expelled. There are useful chemicals in urine, and Mohandas Gandhi drank his first morning voiding every day.

Nephrons like people, come in different sizes and types. In periods of low cardiac output such as dehydration, blood is diverted to nephrons that specialize in retaining water, while in times of plenty, other nephrons are utilized to increase urine formation. In heart failure the kidney may increase the problem, by retaining fluid. As the left ventricle fails, there is reduced cardiac output which the kidney perceives and by shunting flow to fluid-retaining nephrons, retains more fluid. This increased fluid retention further aggravates heart failure. The author has seen the results of this several times around the holidays, where congestive heart failure patients are "drowning" in excess fluid. Holiday meals are large and often contain excess salt which also promotes fluid retention. In these cases, a heart already compromised, is confronted with increased fluid to pump. Unable to increase output, output drops, signaling the kidneys increase fluid retention. These patients are literally drowning in their own fluids. In the emergency room, the author inserted a large IV needle, and one to two units of excess fluid is withdrawn, reducing circulating fluid and reducing workload on the left ventricle. Holiday meals are notorious for increasing cardiac deaths.

The young Peter visited the Dutch shipyards observing how they built and launched 1000 ships each year allowing a small nation to dominate hipping and become the richest country in Europe. He had assets in Russian timber and pitch, large numbers of people coupled with the breadbasket of Ukraine. He later spent time in France which had Europe's most powerful army learning how to organize his manpower into a military force. Peter brought these concepts back to his backward people and attempted to drag them into the modern 17th century, but the effort ultimately failed. And Peter the Great died at the peak of his productive life, due to chronic kidney failure because of his lifestyle. He drank little water while consuming a diet high in protein and alcohol. Adding to the insult of little water intake, he spent much of his adult life bouncing around in carriages and sleds. He traveled almost constantly between his growing fleets in the Baltic and Black Seas, covering the distance between Vancouver and Los Angeles many times in a country with few roads. Bouncing along in vehicles without suspensions, it is little wonder that even organs as well protected as the kidneys would suffer under such abuse. Peter's greatest moment in his quest for sea power was off Cape Gangut in 1714 where the modern Russian warships so painfully and expensively built by the Russian people, defeated a much smaller Swedish fleet, giving Russia its first naval victory.

By the end of Peter's reign, Russia had become the world's largest producer of iron, and he had thirty-four warships as good as England's best along with fifteen frigates and 800 galleys. A fleet completely built during a single lifetime by brutalizing its population to pay for it. Unfortunately, almost all the officers and builders of his fleets were Greek, Venetians, Danes, English and Dutchmen who melted away after Peter's death. Peter's greatest failure as a sea lord was that he could not convince his people to embrace sea power, modern economics and even the western health care he brought with imported Europeans. Had he practiced better health habits, lived another decade and left a competent heir, Russia could have joined Europe much earlier in a less confrontational relationship. A German princess who became known as Catherine the Great in the 18th century embraced much of Peter's program and Russia under her control emerged as a world power.

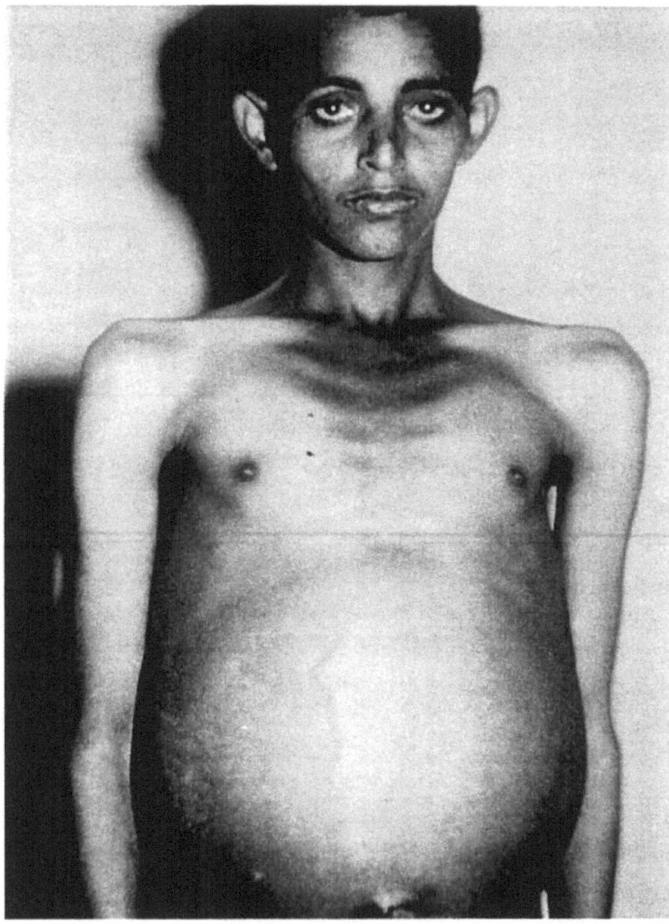

This is a young Egyptian farmer admitted for study at the in the US Naval Medical Research Unit #3 where the authored studied tropical medicine. Note the large abdomen filled containing fluid and loss of soft tissue in arms and face, hidden in the image is his kidneys and liver writhing in parasites. Photo by Author

The young man pictured has a belly full of fluid (ascites) that has left circulation caused by thousands of reproducing creatures. Ascites occurs in a variety of maladies including kidney failure, liver failure and congestive heart disease. As the kidneys reduce the amount of fluid expelled from the body, excess fluids pool in the abdominal cavity, ankles and sometime in the face. It may occur in starvation as well as in urinary tract disease. If the body does not ingest enough protein, the liver will strip protein from the muscles. Thin arms and legs in big-bellied starving children shown in famine news clips is due to kwashiorkor, protein starvation. Weight gain, swelling and decreased urine output, and urine positive for protein, consider kidney failure.

Urine is 95% water, with the remaining 5% a mixture of many substances, some of which can be detected with urine testing. Examination of urine reveals much about the state of the body. The presence of sugar, proteins, white blood cells, red blood cells, nitrite, bilirubin, and ketones can quickly and easily diagnose a wide variety of conditions. Early physicians often had an assistant taste the urine to detect sweetness (sugar diabetes) and sourness indicated infection. Fortunately, this technique is no longer necessary.

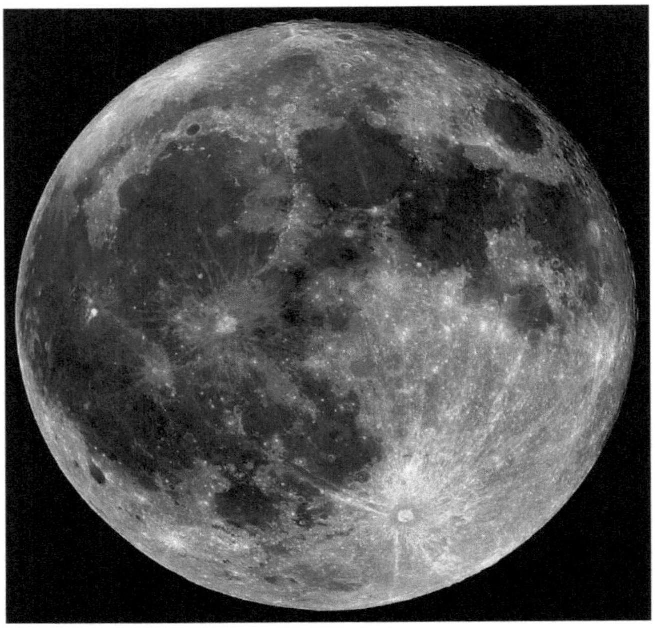

The large crater at the bottom of a full moon with impact rays is named for Tycho Brahe, the 16th century night observer that collected thousands of records of planet and moon positions. He died from complications of a ruptured overfilled bladder after refusing to heed the desire to urinate. A dinner party in his honor with frequent toasts to his health delayed his urination, resulting in bladder rupture followed by peritonitis and death. NASA

The author cared for a similar lethal urinary rupture in a retired sailor. In this case, the injuries resulted from a failed bosun chair while some 25 feet above his deck. In the fall, both femurs and the pelvic bones fractured. These are serious injuries, however, what killed him was his ruptured full bladder, flooding the peritoneum with urine, resulting in peritonitis. Therefore, empty the bladder before climbing mast as the Russian astronauts do before entering their launch spacecraft. Driving an auto at high speeds with a full bladder can be fatal.

Under normal conditions, only a small portion of kidney tissue is necessary (25% of one kidney) for kidney function. This extra or redundant kidney tissue in today's world of safe drinking water and effective medications appears to be an example of how "overbuilt" some of the body's systems are. Until recently, survival often depended upon this redundancy in the pre-antibiotic era, when recurrent kidney infections reduced the number of nephrons with each assault. Many humans died of kidney failure caused by successive losses of tissue leaving the kidneys pitted with scar tissue or pockets of pus, blocked by stones and connected to the bladder by dilated stagnant ureters. Reduced renal function is a major killer of pet dogs, if not encouraged to drink water.

Today, most infections do not ascend the urinary tract to assault the kidney but are eradicated while still in the bladder. However, under adverse conditions, especially dehydration, bacteria can gain access to sterile kidney tissue, producing a kidney infection, pyelonephritis. Symptoms include fever, back pain, vomiting and are one of the few causes of hard shaking chills outside the tropics. Kidney infections are potentially life-threatening and therefore treated aggressively with oral and injectable antibiotics and fluids. Amoxicillins, sulfas, quinones (Levaquin) are good choices coupled with injectable antibiotics.

Stagnation is the enemy of all body systems with the kidneys most dependent on fluids. Pushing fluids keeps urine flowing while delivering blood-born antibiotics. Stagnation in the kidneys leads to infection, stones and perhaps cancer, problems prevented with adequate fluids. Drinking water is a mainstay in preventive health by providing the kidneys with enough fluid to continuously flush the body of waste.

Kidney Stones

Within the funnel shaped collecting pools (calices), fluid gathers, rich in dissolved salts. Under certain conditions, tiny crystals begin to aggregate one to the other until a large and too often ragged, razor-sharp calculus emerges from the urine pool. There are several theories for stone formation, but all are enhanced by low urine flow. These include dehydration, fever, infrequent urination and poor fluid intake habits. Some stones may form in a few hours in hot dry weather if the person does not keep well hydrated. The most common symptoms associated with kidney stone are back pain and blood in the urine (hematuria).

As urine forms, it passes down the collapsible ureters collecting in the bladder. When these outlets become blocked by stones, pressure builds within the kidney causing a deep severe flank pain, sometimes accompanied by fever, and perhaps vomiting. Stones block the flow of urine, creating stagnation and increased pressure. In the field, when a kidney stone is suspected, it gives fluids, pain medications and antibiotics, especially if fever present.

Microscopically, some stones have an irregular surface of sharp pointed edges and spikes. As they transverse the urinary tract, the stone periodically embeds and tears the urinary lining, causing bleeding and pain, although most of the discomfort stems from the pressure. Encouraging water or other fluids will help wash the stone out along a corridor dilated by increased urine flow. Opiates will also dilate the smooth muscle found in the urinary tract as well as reduce pain.

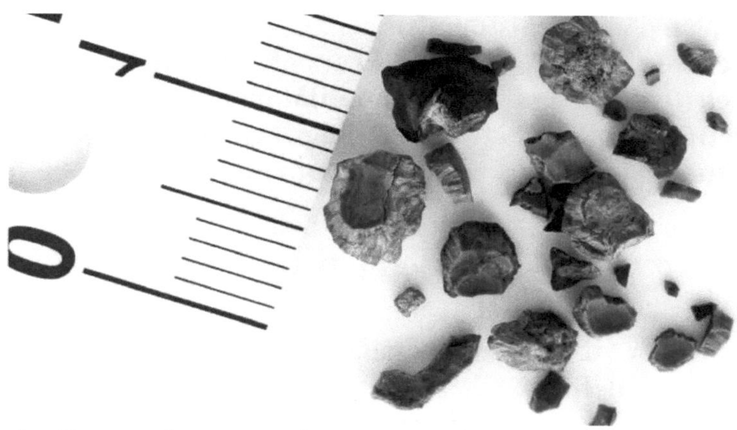

Kidney calculi come in many shapes and sizes. Note the sharp edges. NIH

Urinalysis

The following items are not found normally in urine, and their presence may indicate a diagnosis for the following conditions:

Glucose- diabetes
Protein-kidney disease
Blood-kidney stone, infection, trauma, cancer
Bilirubin-hepatitis
Ketones-fasting
White Blood Cells-infection
Nitrites-infection

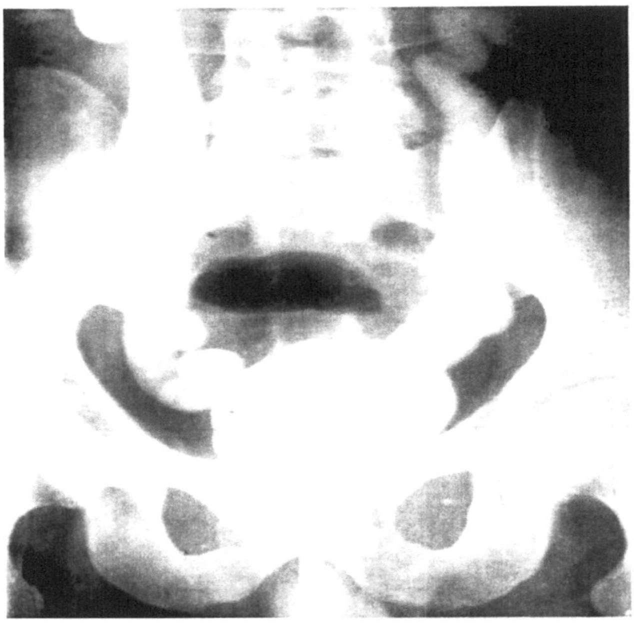

An intravenous pyelogram revealing the results of chronic parasitic urinary infection. This Egyptian farmer is infected with schistomaisis, a parasite capable of penetrating intact skin while wading in waters of the Nile. Great numbers of the creature inhabiting the urinary tract have caused obstruction and subsequent dilation of normally threadlike ureters. These ureters, connecting the kidneys to the bladder look more like highways than threads. Chronic kidney infections have been a constant companion for humans throughout history.

Urinary Tract Infections

Under normal conditions, urine is sterile, containing no bacteria. Good urine flow is essential in maintaining this sterility, as it flushes the urinary tract continuously. If urine flow becomes sluggish or stagnant, bacteria may gain access to the bladder or even the kidneys, and cause infection. Low back pain, painful urination, fever, foul smelling or cloudy urine, blood in urine and fatigue are all signs of a urinary tract infection. Dipstick urine examination may reveal the presence of leukocytes (white blood cells, infection), nitrites (infection), blood (infection, kidney stone), and protein (kidney disease, inflammation).

Simple bladder infections are more common in women, due to the short distance from the vagina to the bladder. Sexual intercourse often precedes a female bladder infection and can be reduced with post-coital urination, flushing the short urethra. Early bladder infections can sometimes be managed in one dose of nine 500 mg amoxicillin tabs or five double strength sulfa tabs. Otherwise treat for 7-10 days with either antibiotic. Good urine flow is important to a healthy urinary tract and a healthy body. Drinking enough fluid to produce a clear stream of urine several times a day will prevent many bad things from happening. Hydration not only helps prevent urinary disease, but it may also prevent heart attack and stroke as both are states of stagnation.

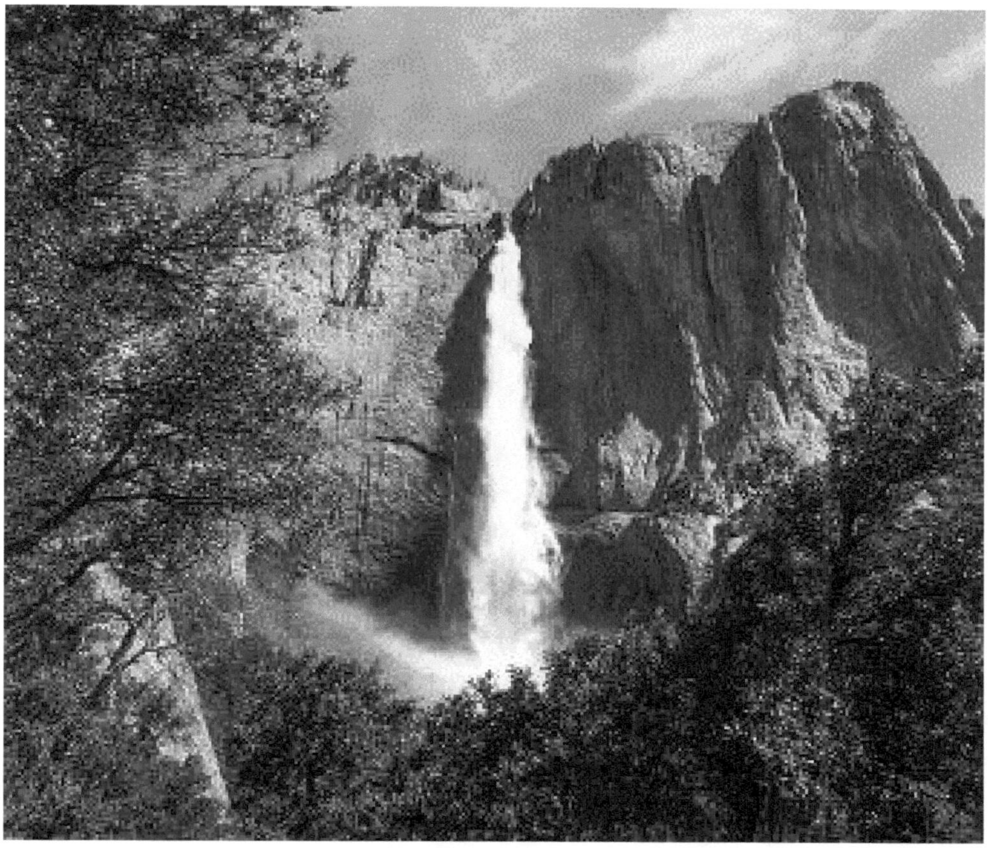

Yosemite falls is an example of good flow. If both the upper and lower falls are added together, Yosemite Falls are the tallest in the world. National Park Service

The Female Reproductive System

"What is a woman? A woman is the vehicle of life. Life has overtaken her. Woman is what it is all about -the giving of birth and the giving of nourishment". Joseph Campbell

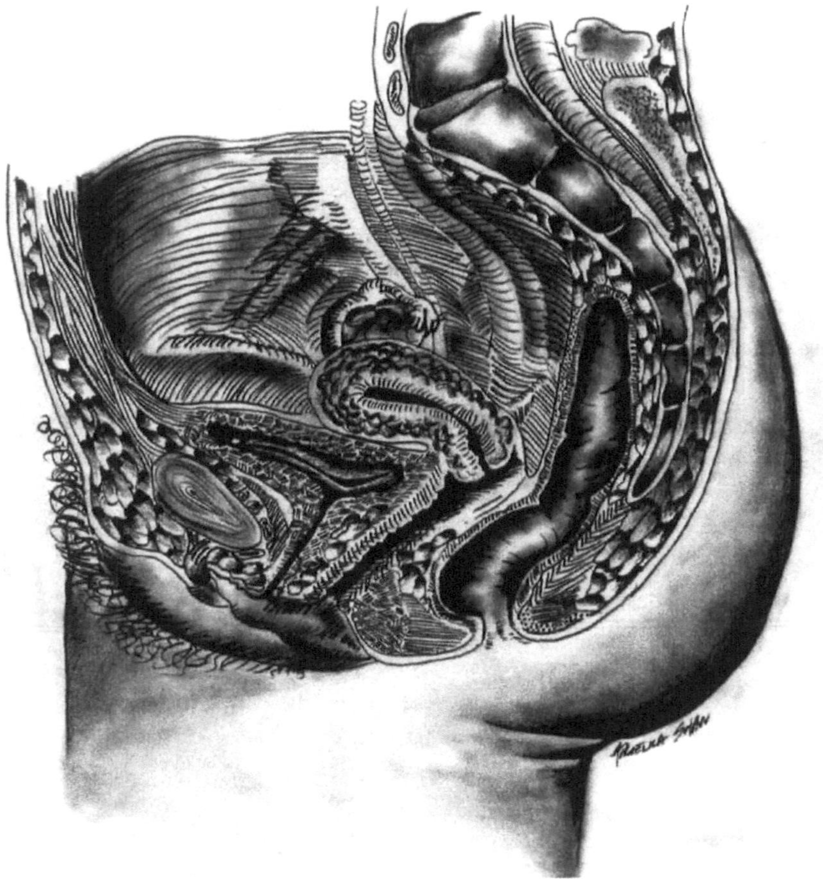

Whether you believe in the simultaneous evolution of man and woman or whether you believe that Adam was created first followed closely by Eve makes little difference. Male and female are similar in humans (they even have the same number of ribs), as they are in other animals and plants. Men and women primarily differ in reproduction, the more obvious differences in appearance and function are due to the synthesis, release and effects of sex hormones from special organs. This process is much simpler in the male when compared to the complex orchestration necessary for the female to maintain fertility. The cycle of menses, the development and release of eggs from the ovary and the competent way the female reproductive organs sustain and deliver a living human being is perhaps the most miraculous system in all of nature.

Reproductive System of Human Female

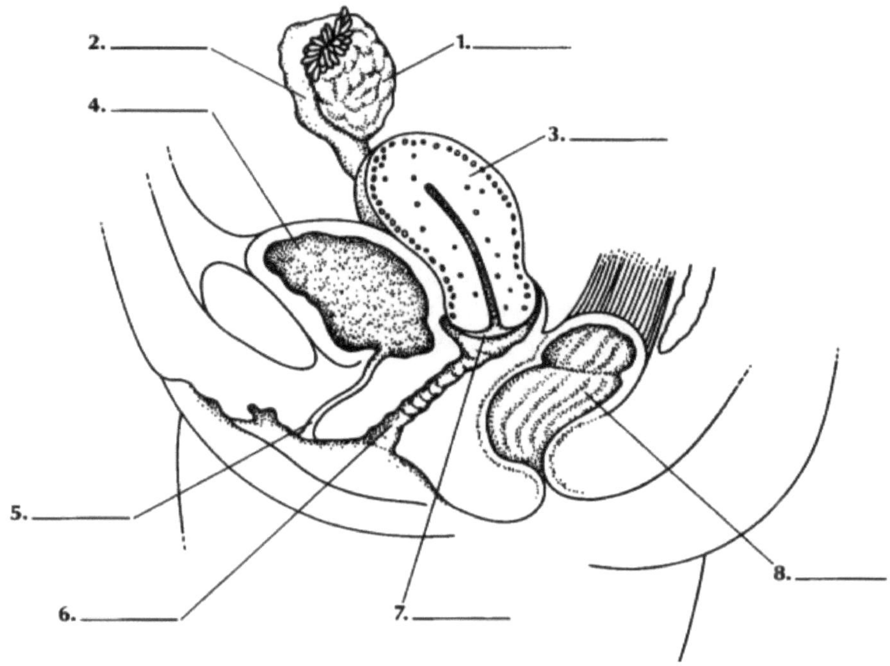

1. Ovary 2. Fallopian tube 3. Uterus 4. Bladder 5. Urethra 6. Vagina 7. Cervix 8. rectum

With the first menses (Latin-month) a young woman begins to be stimulated and influenced by a group of closely related substances formed from cholesterol molecules. These sex steroids and hormones prepare the woman's body so that it can reproduce. Body changes such as breast development, hip widening and the laying down of fat stores are brought about by chemicals released by the ovaries, adrenals, hypothalamus, pituitary and others. Chemically, the differences between the male and female hormones are quite small, especially when compared with the differences in their effects. Both sexes produce male and female hormones in vastly different amounts. Some animals can undergo a sex change from male to female, and back again, such as the common reef parrot fish, by changing the ratio of these hormones.

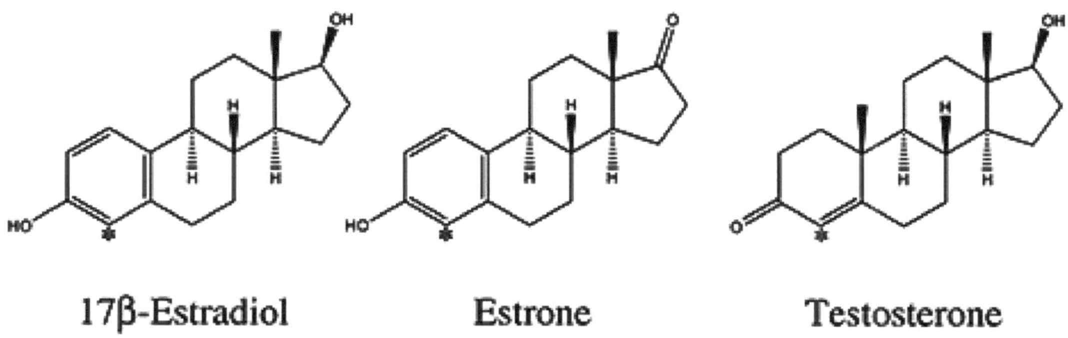

The sex steroids begin life as a cholesterol molecule. Note how similar in structure are male and female sex steroid, yet they function in the human much differently. Usgs.gov

Women with an excess of male hormones will develop features such as muscular body shape, facial hair, early heart disease. Some men on the other hand, produce higher than normal levels of the female hormone, estrogen, giving them a more female-shaped lithe body and a higher pitched voice. The Catholic Church of the Middle Ages castrated pre-puberty choir boys to prevent sexual development and deepening voice associated with fertility. The *Castrati*, a child's voice in a grown man body, were featured in plays, operas and choirs of Europe's great cathedrals. Castrated males (eunuchs) obtained positions of high power in the Byzantine and Ottoman Empires as medical officers, generals and advisors. In the male, cholesterol is converted to testosterone by the testicles, while in the female, estrogen is manufactured in the ovaries (estrogen is released in small amounts from body fat in the female and the male). It is the periodic build-up and withdrawal of estrogen that causes the menstrual cycle of vaginal bleeding. Menstruation derived from Greek word for moon, as menstrual cycle tends to mimic the moon cycle. As young females pass into adulthood, they begin to have vaginal bleeding (menarche), sporadic at first and then becoming more regularly cyclic, indicating fertility. The later sputtering menses, hot flashes and mood swings indicate the passing of fertility (menopause). The menstrual cycle begins with the ovaries being stimulated to release increasing amounts of estrogen which cause the womb's lining (uterus) to swell, while an egg or eggs develop and then are released. This spongy uterine tissue is richly supported by a network of tiny blood vessels in preparation for receiving and nurturing a fertilized egg. If fertilization does not take place, the lining is sloughed off through the cervix and into the vagina, causing the only visual sign of the events around menstruation. Pliny considered the foremost scientific mind in first century Rome described mensuration as "Wild indeed are the stories of the mysterious and awful menstrual discharge". Oral contraceptives artificially cycle the bleeding with synthetic estrogen, while preventing the ovaries from releasing eggs. Oral contraceptives "trick" the reproductive system, preventing fertility.

Pregnancy

Most pregnancies are uncomplicated, presenting little danger to the sea-going or travelling expectant mother. This was not true in the past, as pregnancy accounted for great numbers of deaths in women and their newborns. Skeletons with a baby wedged tightly in the pelvis are not uncommon and is a grim testimony to the hazards of childbirth. It is also not uncommon to find graves with the remains of a woman nestling a newborn infant, both succumbing to the travails of childbirth. A testament to the danger of delivering a human being.

Even after a successful birth, bleeding and infection took many lives in the past and continue as a concern today. Even with good prenatal care and healthy mother, pregnancy exposes added risks to a female. An understanding of the physiology and possible complications in the delivery of an infant should be helpful in the field. A complex group of chemicals released from the brain involving the hypothalamus and pituitary glands combined with the adrenal glands and the ovary itself, an egg is released from a Graafian follicle (named for the Dutch anatomist who described it in 1677). The egg is then captured by the tiny tentacles of the fallopian tube and transported into the tube's interior, where in confined quarters, it is easier prey for swarms of sperm. It is in the fallopian tube where most fertilizations occur, not in the womb. Sperm cells must be hugely numerous and healthy, since a protective barrier must be eaten away by enzymes carried in the sperm's head. Usually only a single sperm enters the egg and is then closed to other penetrations.

Under normal conditions, the fertilized egg is then gently swept into the waiting uterus where it buries itself in the soft network of blood vessels and begins to grow along with the placenta. Unfortunately, this normal scenario of fertilization sometimes goes awry, and a deadly risk of a tubal pregnancy occurs. Because this condition is possibly fatal and must be surgically corrected, it should be understood by sea going personnel.

In the tubal or ectopic pregnancy, a fertilized egg has become implanted not in the uterus, but in the wall of the fallopian tube. Previous infections in the woman's reproductive tract increase the risk of tubal pregnancy since scar tissue is often the cause of blocked tubes. As the embryo grows, it begins to stretch the thin muscular wall of the fallopian tube causing pain in the lower abdomen. Pain intermittent at first, but soon does not come and go, but steadily worsens until the growing fetus and placenta ruptures, causing internal bleeding, peritonitis and finally shock. It is a problem that can only be cured by abdominal surgery. No amount of pain medication will relieve the pernicious pain and ultimate fatal outcome.

As the egg implants, it burrows into the tissue lining the tube causing erosion and often bleeding, blood that appears in the vagina. This "spotting" of blood is soon followed by pelvic pain, especially during intercourse. Physical activity such as running, climbing stairs or even prolonged standing will aggravate the pain as the heavy embryo-filled tube applies traction to the pelvic organs. Sexual intercourse becomes more painful as the tube enlarges. Rupture in the ectopic pregnancy can occur throughout the first trimester (as early as three weeks from conception), depending on where along the length of the fallopian tube the egg implants and how fast it grows.

The Deadly Pregnancy

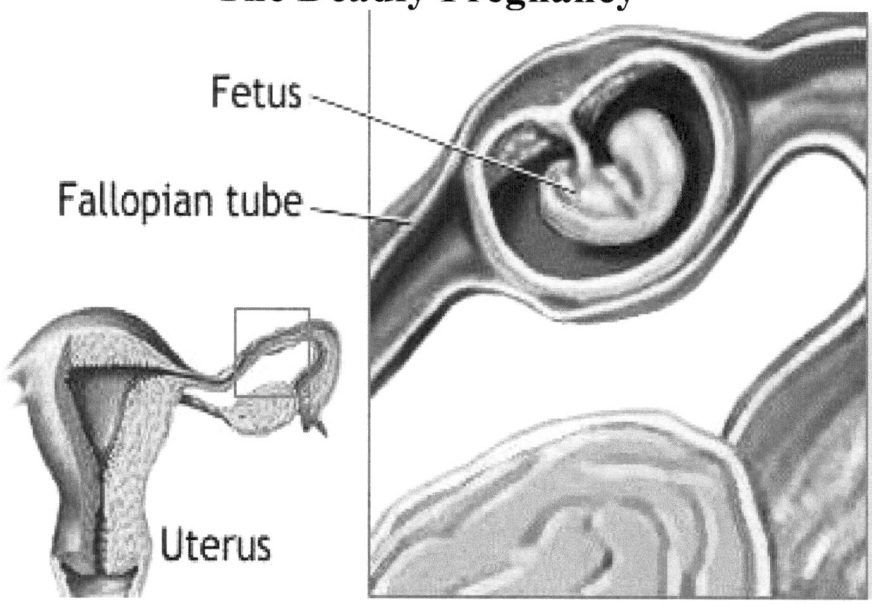

Illustration of pregnancy outside the womb, entrapped and developing with the too small fallopian tube. National Library of Medicine

It is especially important to determine if pregnancy present with complains of abdominal pain in sexually active females. Modern urine pregnancy tests are positive within days of conception although the test will not discern a pregnancy in the womb verses an ectopic. Still, it should be employed in evaluating any abdominal pain, even when the female denies sexual activity. If the test is positive and the pain continues to increase, plans for evacuation should begin. Management in the interim consists of clear liquids, pain relief and antibiotics if fever develops. Remember that some women may complain of spotting and abdominal pain even in normal pregnancies, however, if the pain continues, appears to be centered on one side, and any signs of rebound develop, a diagnosis of tubal or ectopic pregnancy must be considered. This is a surgical emergency requiring early transfer to surgical care.

Delivery of an infant

It is not within the scope of this text to teach the art and science of labor and delivery, but instead, an overview of general information and the possible need for field delivery. Most labor and deliveries require only minimal assistance for mothers and child. However, many people today do not know even the simple rules for labor and delivery that were common knowledge in the days of home delivery. Labor begins with the continuous rhythmic contractions of the uterus, the softening and stretching of the cervix and ends with the delivery of both baby and afterbirth. The time for these events varies from minute to days in some cases. Most labor and deliveries last around 8-12 hours, usually decreasing with subsequent children, since bones and soft tissue around the birth canal have been pre-stretched.

.

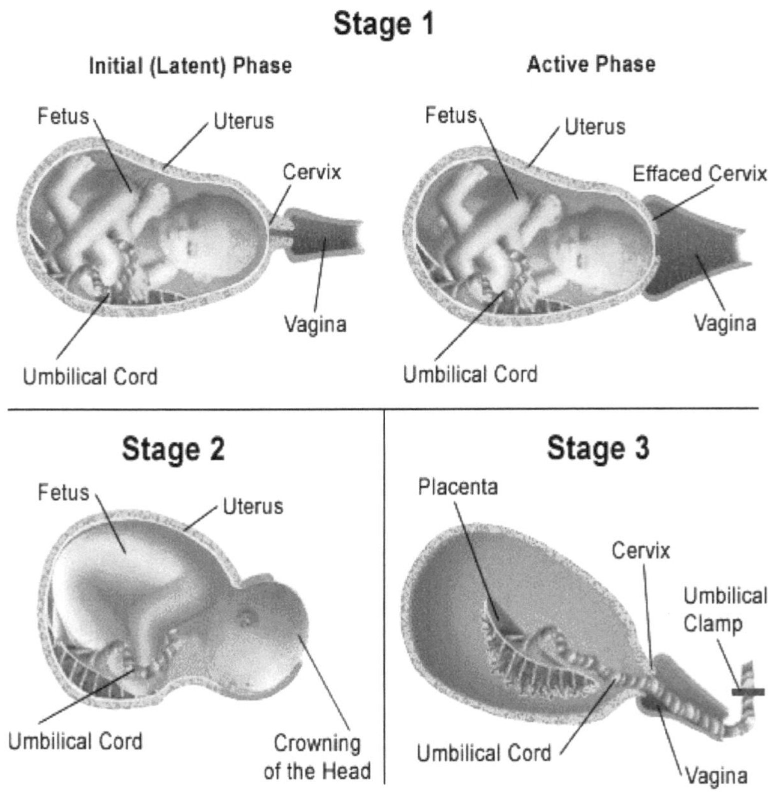

The 3 stages of delivery normally take 8-12 hours, longer with the first delivery, usually less with subsequent births. NIH

Near the beginning of labor there is usually a bloody show, which represents a plug of protective mucus that has sealed the cervix from the interior of the womb during pregnancy. This is usually followed by a "rush of fluids" as the bag of water surrounding the infant has burst or torn (the bag sometimes is deliberately opened to induce labor). If not a rush of fluid, then a new sense of dampness from the vagina indicates that membranes are releasing amniotic fluid in anticipation of labor. As the power of the contractions increases, the baby is ever so slowly pushed into and through the birth canal. The cervix is remarkable structure, beginning as firm thick tissue, perforated by a tiny canal. Tissue combing strength with flexibility enabling it to stretch first over the baby's head and later the shoulders in a normal delivery. Until the cervix has fully dilated (10 cm) the infant cannot be safely pushed through the canal, and the desire to push by the mother should be restrained. Any medications given to the mother for pain will reach the baby, therefore, administer as little as possible. However, if the mother begins to fray (or threatens the life of the father), pain relief is important to allow some respite from the discomfort of contractions. Buprenorphine, a synthetic narcotic developed to reverse opiate overdoses is an excellent pain medicine allows the mother some relaxation between contractions and unlike opiates, will not suppress baby. The dose is 1-2 mg every 2-4 hours dissolved in the mouth for pain control.

As soon as the cervix is wide enough to allow the head to pass, delivery assumes a much faster pace. It is during this time that the baby deserves special attention. As the head appears outside the vagina, the mother should stop pushing so that the newborn's upper airway is cleared of secretions prior to the child's first breath. The baby is often moving but is unable breath since the chest is held tightly within the mother's bony pelvis. There is time to place a bulb syringe or regular large syringe in the mouth first and then each side of the nose until all fluid appears to be suctioned away. A brown stain (meconium) indicates the possibility that the child was overstressed during delivery and may cause breathing problems for the new infant. Meconium, the dark plug of stool formed in the later part of fetal development (looks like moist tobacco) is normally passed out the infant's rectum within the first 24 hours of life outside the womb. If this first bowel movement occurs while in the uterus, it can contaminate newborn's fragile lungs with the first few breaths. The presence of meconium increases the need for clearing the airway before allowing the child to breath, followed by close observation, some low flow oxygen if available, and medical help if possible.

After the child has been suctioned, gentle traction along with mother's-controlled push will usually remove the rest of the child from the birth canal. The newborn should not be waved triumphantly around in the air but warmed immediately by drying, placement on the mother's bare warm abdomen, usually with the umbilical cord still attached, and covered with a dry, warm blanket. After several minutes, the afterbirth (placenta) should also be expelled. Do not attempt to pull the placenta out since the cord could part and increase the risk of a retained placenta, only rarely must the placenta be removed gently by hand if not delivered spontaneously. Sometimes, gentle traction may be necessary to coax the placenta out of womb.

Bleeding after delivery is common, and to the lay person and a new mother, the amount may appear frightening. Just prior to the baby's delivery, the mother's cardio-vascular system is delivering large amounts of blood to the uterus and this blood flow must cease. The anatomy of the uterus combined with chemicals released directly into the blood stream by the pituitary, hypothalamus and adrenal glands should slow as the uterus continues to forcibly contract after delivery. The failure of the uterus to shrink to a much smaller size can result in shock. Throughout history, post-partum bleeding has taken the lives of females in great numbers. The presence of midwife, medical officer or competent attendant (historically the father) reduced this risk.

Gentle massage to the top of the uterus, while somewhat uncomfortable to the new mother, is helpful in encouraging the womb to clamp down. Stimulation of the nipples, via breast feeding or by hand, also causes increased uterine contractions. The mother depends heavily on the strong muscular contractions that spewed forth the child to seal off bleeding. Aspirin should be avoided in and around childbirth.

Delivery of the Baby (step-by-step)

As the baby's head is born, it normally faces down, and as labor progresses, the head turns sideways, the nose pointing to the mother's left thigh. As soon as the baby's head appears, support the head with one hand and stop delivery (even if the mother has a strong desire to push and finish delivery). Delivery must be halted here to allow the infant's upper airway to be cleared before the first breath. At all times support the head with one hand.

With one hand, compress the bulb syringe before bringing it to the infant's face. Place the syringe 1 to 1.5 inches into the newborn's mouth and gently into both sides of the nose, removing all secretions. This is usually done several times until the syringe sounds dry with successive aspirations. As the head is gently pushed through the birth canal, the hand supporting the head continues to control the speed of delivery. When the head is delivered outside the vagina, use the other hand to check the neck for possible umbilical cord coiled around the infant's neck (nuchal cord). If a nuchal cord is present, use two fingers to gently lift it over the shoulders, back into the birth canal. In the unlikely case the cord is too entangled to remove, it should be clamped, cut, and unwrapped from the infant.

Delivery of the shoulders (the widest and sometimes the most difficult part) is best accomplished by continuing to support the head as it is gentle elevated. Upward traction allows the lower shoulder to slide more easily through the birth canal. As the shoulders appear, be prepared for a rather rapid delivery of the rest of the baby and continue to apply gentle continuous traction. As the abdomen and hips appear, place the other hand under the buttocks, holding the moving baby in both hands for the first time. Expect the baby to have a bluish tint for the first few minutes of life. Hold firmly since a newborn is naturally slippery, covered with a heavy lubricant (vernix). Immediately warm the newborn by placing it on the mother's abdomen and covering it with a warm cloth. There is no hurry to cut the cord, it can wait for the delivery of the placenta.

Delivery of the Placenta

Place one hand on the mother's abdomen, feeling for the hard, contracting uterus. It should feel like a large hard grapefruit just under the abdominal muscles. These contractions should deliver the placenta in about ten to twenty minutes. Do not pull on the cord to hurry along with the placenta's delivery. Gentle firm pressure over the top of the contracting uterus will help the mother expel the placenta and membranes.

Expect some bleeding as the placenta passes through the cervix and into the vagina. Gently guide the placenta through the vagina and if the placenta is still uncut, lay it alongside the infant, to help keep the baby warm. The placenta and newborn have been constant companions for many weeks, there is no hurry to sever this relationship.

Cutting the Cord

Place two clamps (hemostats) on the cord about three inches (10 cm) apart, six inches from the baby. Using umbilical tape (or other thin cloth ribbon), tie one inch from the clamp closest to the baby, compressing the cord firmly, but slowly to avoid cutting through the cord (do not use string or thread as it may cut the cord). Tie the tape with a square knot. Cut the cord between the newly tied tape and the clamp furthest from the baby and check the end for bleeding. Treat bleeding with direct pressure to the vagina.

Post Delivery Bleeding

It is normal for there to be bleeding after delivery, around 500 cc, one to two cups. If bleeding appears to be coming from a vaginal tear, apply firm pressure with gauze and hand. Treat vaginal tears with daily cleaning, leaving open to air and light. After the author's first delivery in Western Oklahoma with a long-time general medical officer told me about post-partum blood loss, "its half as much as the mother thinks she has lost and twice what the physician thought". Place dressings of sanitary napkins or fluffy gauze over the vagina and rectum (after completely removing any stool also delivered with the baby). Having the mother keep her legs pressed together will increase the effect of a pressure dressing.

Apply gentle, firm pressure to the mother's abdomen to further encourage the uterus to contract. Even though it may be uncomfortable, the uterus must fully contract or expose the mother to the risk of bleeding to death. Breast feeding and other breast stimulation such as pinching the nipples will also enhance uterine contracture. If the uterus did not contract quickly, blood loss can be catastrophic. Just before delivery, liters of blood are flowing thorough the placenta every minute into the infant. As soon as the placenta separates from the uterus, stopping this blood flow is paramount. Fortunately, the uterus is designed to contract forcefully, staunching this flow. Give the uterus all the help available which is mainly "laying on hands" with nipple stimulation and deep firm massage over the collapsing womb.

Note: the author and wife elected a home delivery for 2nd child with midwife in attendance, however the midwife was unable to attend (same thing happened for the third child). During both deliveries, the experience was enhanced by having these steps read aloud. This book works.

Pelvic Inflammatory Disease

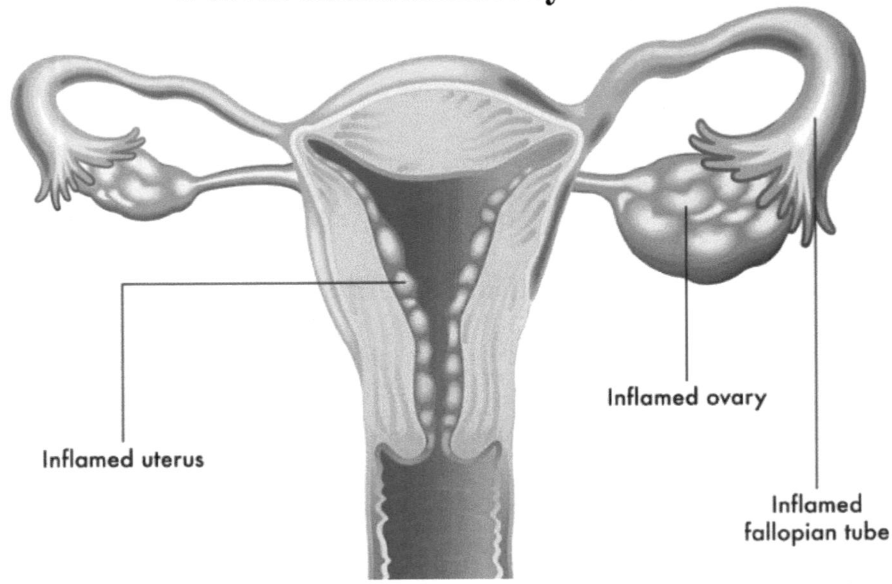

NIH illustration of the inflamed ovary and its connected fallopian tube of pelvic inflammatory disease. Like most infections the complaint of lower abdominal pain is accompanied by fever.

Pelvic pain, fever, backache, painful intercourse, are signs of infection in the female reproductive organs. The symptoms come on suddenly with gonorrhea, more slowly with the more common Chlamydia. In the era before antibiotics, this was often fatal. In the field, antibiotics greatly reduce risks of peritonitis and fallopian tube scaring found in ectopic pregnancy

Pelvic inflammatory disease (PID) may present with vague, longstanding complaints of low- grade fever, pelvic discomfort and low back pain with sex, physical activity or prolonged standing. Complaints that may have been presented for several days to weeks. Doxycycline is the drug of choice for pelvic inflammatory disease as it is effective in bacterial and chlamydial causes of PID, and unless the person develops signs of worsening, is used alone. A pregnancy test is recommended since doxycycline is not recommended in pregnancy. Metronidazole is effective but alcohol must be avoided. Antibiotic injections should begin if the person develops any symptoms of peritonitis (rebound). In all cases of female venereal disease, the partner should receive the same therapy, even with no complaints. Syphilis, gonorrhea and Chlamydia are all effectively treated with doxycycline, 100 mg every 12 hours for ten days. No other single antibiotic is likely to kill all three of the leading causes of venereal disease, but even doxycycline will not hamper herpes or the AIDS virus.

Vaginitis

There are several things capable of causing injury and subsequent inflammation of the vaginal wall. These include trauma and infectious agents of bacteria, fungus, viruses and parasites. Generally, the vagina can protect itself from infection, unless normal vaginal mucosa has been altered, or highly infectious agents such as herpes or gonorrhea are introduced. Mucus glands in vaginal walls produce fluid which continuously flushes the vaginal vault, keeping the vagina swept clean. Vaginal walls are thin muscular rings, covered with soft, moist, exquisite contractile tissue that is sometimes injured with rough intercourse. Excessive friction, either from inadequate lubrication, lengthy intercourse or violent activity, breaks down the protective mucus coating over the delicate vaginal walls. It is not uncommon to see vaginal pain, discharge and itching after prolonged or too frequent intercourse.

Antibiotic use increases the risk of yeast vaginitis because the drug disrupts the balance between bacteria and fungus, both often found in the vagina. As bacterial numbers decrease with antibiotic use, it allows candida fungus, which is normal flora in the vagina, to greatly increase the number of colonies and overgrow the vaginal wall. Candida causes a thick itchy discharge from the vagina. It responds to nightly applications of clotrimazole cream with a mild steroid for 5-10 days. Oral medications (ketoconazole) are highly effective and quicker acting. If this fails to clear vaginitis, the cause could be either from a parasite (trichomonas) or bacteria. In these cases, the discharge is heavy, almost cheese-like, and will have a foul odor. There is pain with intercourse, implying the vaginal wall irritation.

In trichomonas, both female and her partner/partners must be treated with metronidazole (Flagyl), even though the male feels no symptoms. The dose is 250-500 mg (lower dose for smaller patients) three times a day for 5-7 days or a more recent recommended treatment is 2 grams (200 mg) in a single dose. Metronidazole is closely related to the drug Antabuse and may cause nausea if combined with alcohol.

If pain and swelling are the major symptoms of vaginitis, it is probably herpes or another venereal disease. Herpes causes very tender blisters, surrounded by redness, sometimes so painful, it may be difficult for the woman to urinate, leading to urine retention and the need for catheter placement. Zovirax (acyclovir) or other antivirals, if available, are given in large doses. If vaginal pain is associated with deep pelvic pain and fever, suspect pelvic inflammatory disease, and treat with doxycycline 100 mg every 12 hours for 10 days. If signs of a more severe peritonitis appear (rebound, increasing fever, decreasing bowel sounds, increasing pain), add injections of strong antibiotic every 12 hours, in addition to giving doxycycline. In some women, mild symptoms of discharge, pain during or after intercourse, pain with urination and itching can persist for weeks after treatment.

Male Reproductive Organs

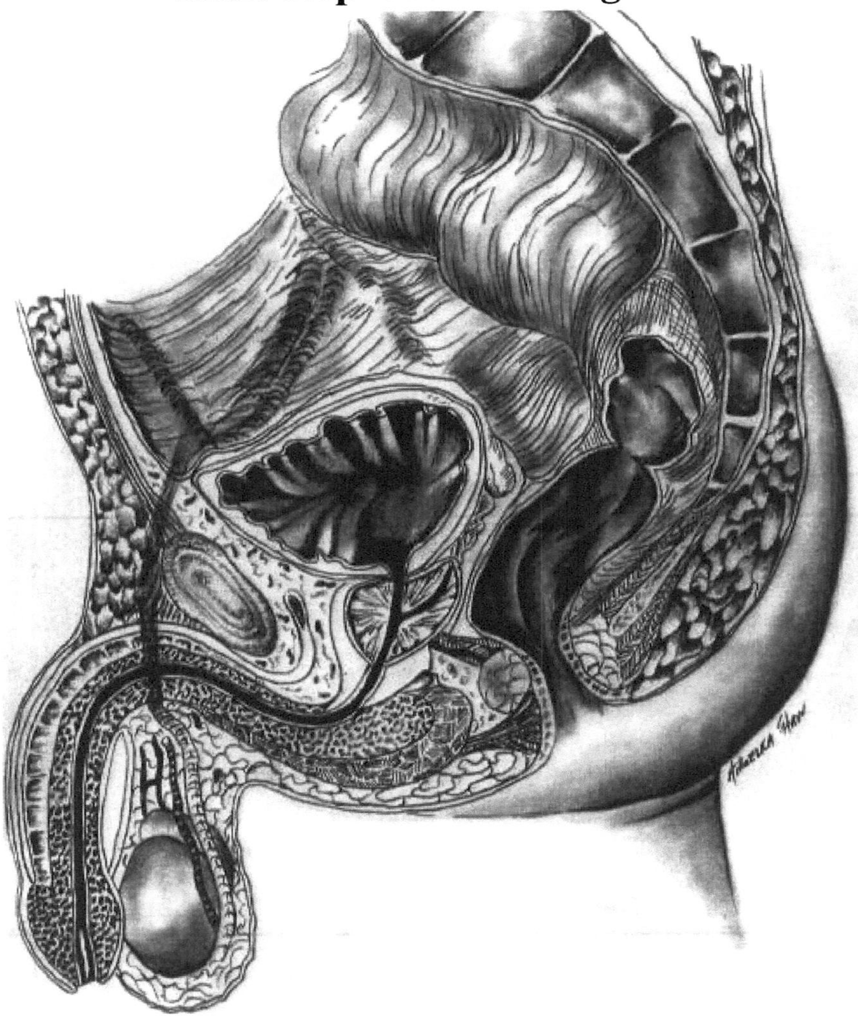

Most of the male reproductive system is outside the body and exposed. For sperm to become "infective", they must mature at temperatures below body temperature. The scrotum is corrugated the same way a radiator functions by radiating heat. AM

Compared to the female, male reproductive function is simple. The primary organs are found clustered around the base of the penis, the testicles, epididymis and prostate gland. The penis is composed of erectile sponge-like tissue, when filled with blood, becomes enlarged and erect. Testicles, the site of sperm production is the central organ, suspended within the insulating scrotum, where sperm cells mature at an ideal temperature, several degrees below the rest of the body. Testicular tissue is perforated by thousands of tiny canals, estimated to be over 250 meters long in man.

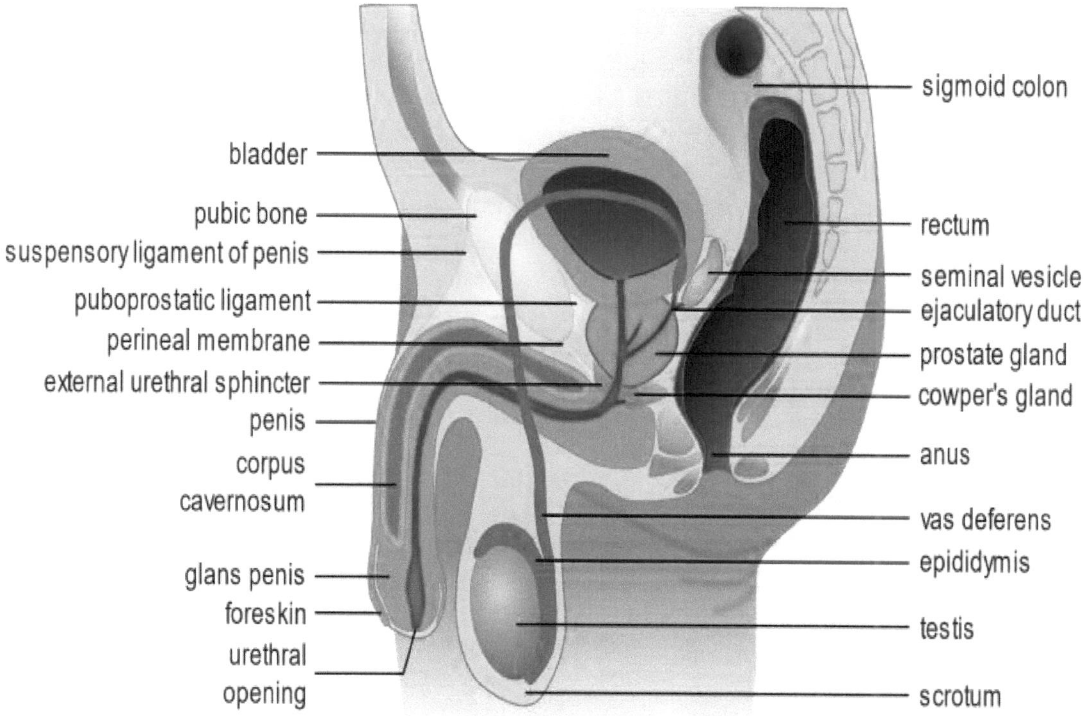

Anatomically, the male reproductive system appears more complicated than the female, however, physiologically the male systems pale when compared to the female. NIH

Sperm cells consist of three parts; head, connecting middle piece and tail, each manufactured and assembled in this labyrinth of streams and microscopic lakes connecting testicles to epididymis. Sperm cells are different than any other cell found in the male, having only twenty-three chromosomes in a community all other cells having forty-six. Sperm deploy a contractile tail for locomotion driven by a tiny manufacturing component using fructose sugar providing energy, and the acrosome containing enzymes that "eat" a passage through the female egg's surface. As a former member of the submarine navy, the author visualizes sperm cells as torpedoes. Self-powered, mission oriented, carrying the charge to penetrate the target at its tip and a similar shape.

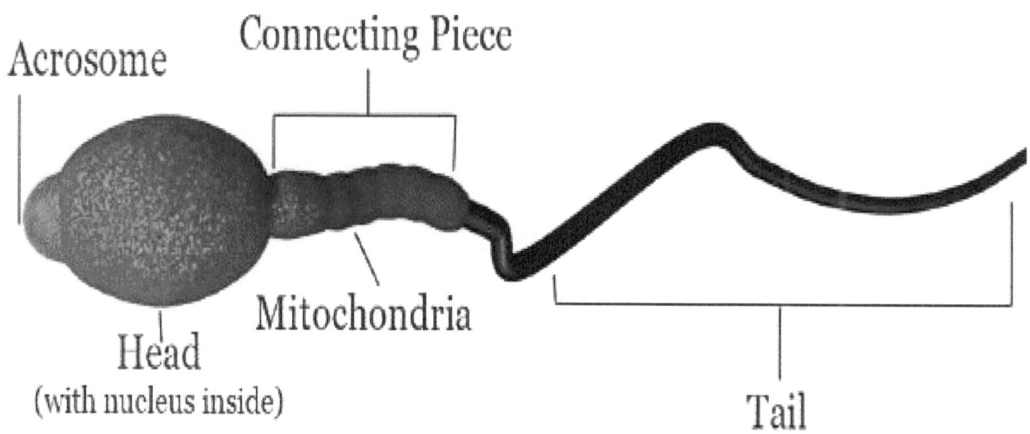

NIH illustration of mature sperm cell with all pieces in place. NLM

Sperm is a Greek word for seed and several hundred million sperm are found in a single ejaculate, creating lottery-like numbers for the chances of a single sperm fertilizing an egg. In humans the sperm cell is the smallest cell, attacking the largest human cell, the egg. Human sperm cells are the most motile of all human cells, powered by a powerful tail, moving like a tadpole or crocodile. Not all animal sperm cells are as diminutive as the tiny 0.06mm human sperm. One species of fruit fly discharges a sperm cell that is longer than the male fly! The head of a human sperm contains 23 chromosomes from the father, half are males (y) while half are females (x) and hydrolytic enzymes used to dissolve the protective coat of the receptive (victim) egg. The mid segment contains the power unit of packed mitochondria needed to make the energy to "whip" the tail vigorously back and forth. It takes hundreds if not thousands of sperm to dissolve the egg's coat but once the lucky one (rarely 2 or 3 may simultaneously enter, giving rise to paternal twins or triplets) enters the egg, the others were only there for augmentation.

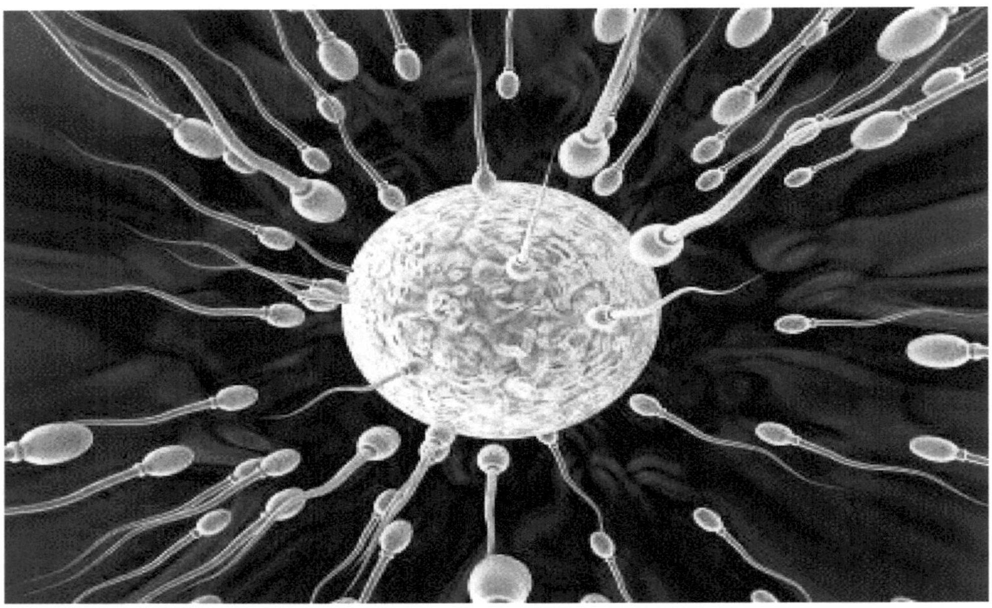

An artist's image of sperm "attacking" the egg. NIH

Sperm produced in the testicles, must traverse the epididymis, a 4–6-meter trip, taking 4-6 weeks, as they mature. With ejaculation, the most mature sperm are swept out of the epididymis, passing quickly through the prostate in waves of prostate muscle contractions, where sperm is mixed with its nurturing semen. In the developing fetus, tissue that becomes the womb in a female, become the prostate in the man, the contractions of the male orgasm, reflect on a tiny scale, those of uterine contraction during labor. The healthy prostate is believed to be drained frequently, and drainage occurs with the male orgasm or nocturnal emissions (wet dream). Some of the pleasure of the male orgasm is the rhythmic contraction of the orgasmic prostate gland, as semen is ejaculated with the sperm from the epididymis. Semen contains vitamin C, which is necessary for sperm to activate the rapid contractile cells of the sperms' tails, allowing them to whip back and forth, propelling sperm over the uncharted course of the female reproductive system. Semen also contains fructose (fruit sugar), as there is nothing to eat in the female reproductive tract. The vagina, and to a greater degree, the interior of the uterus are hostile environments for sperm, requiring them to bring their own provisions.

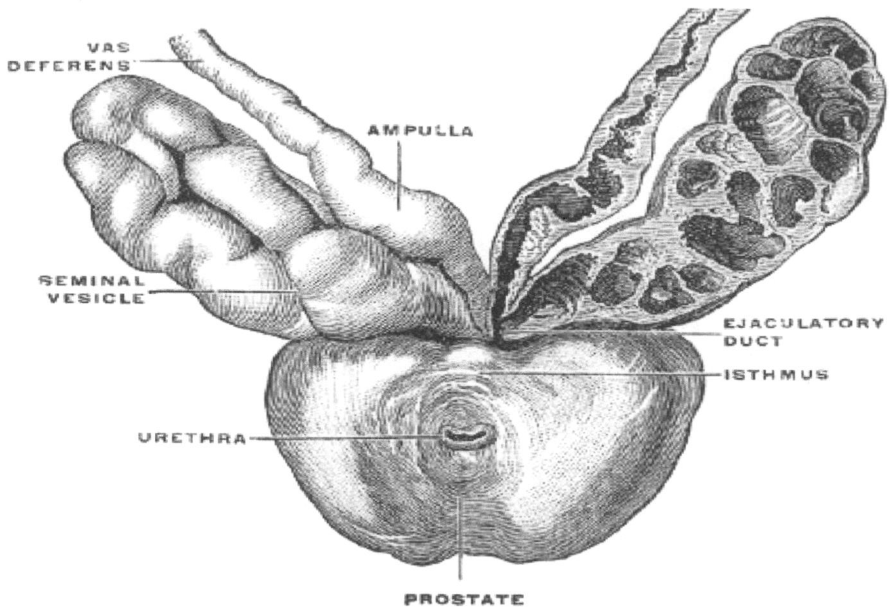

Prostate from the Greek prostates word for guardian, as it is front of bladder Epididymis from two Greek words, *epi* meaning upon, *didymis* testicle. Urethra is Greek for passage of urine, *ouron* is Greek for urine, Testicle is Latin for witness, as presence of testicles bears witness to man

Not only does the prostate in the male fetus develops from the same tissue as the uterus, it occupies the same essential body space also. As the boy turns into the man, the voice deepens, pubic hair sprouts and the prostate enlarges and becomes functional under the effects of testosterone secretion by the testicles. Later in life the prostate enlarges as part of aging. A large prostate in the older male is to be expected and often accompanied by constricted urine flow. This leads to more frequent urination and a weaker urine stream.

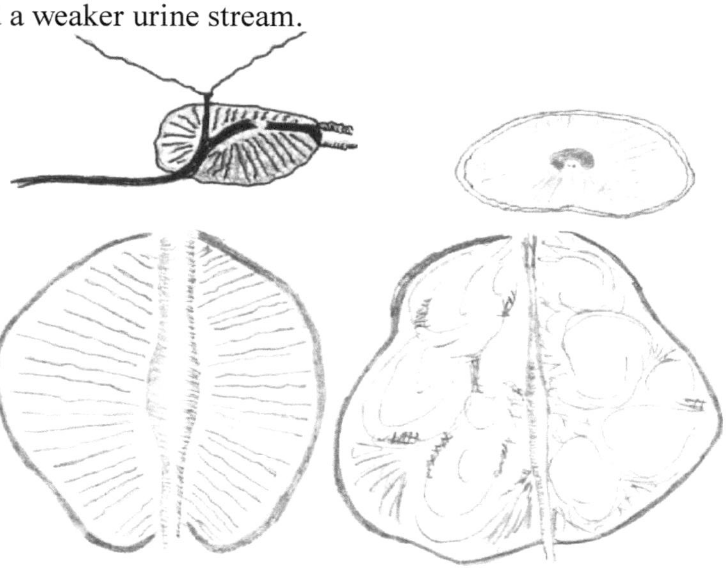

The aged prostate on the right is larger and firmer compared to a normal youthful prostrate on left with wide open passages surrounded by smooth soft tissue. The prostates above show the normal architecture in three views and the older congested and swollen

prostate at the lower right. In this prostate the ureter passing through the body of the prostate is constricted causing decreased urinary flow, multiple small urinations, especially at night and increased risk of cancer. A common procedure in the aged prostate is TURP- transurethral resection of prostate, where the channel through prostate is "dredged" as would a shipping channel would be deepened and widened.

Prostatitis is common, as the prostate gland is a "dead end organ", increasing risk of stagnation. Prostate infections manifest deep pelvic pain, fever, painful urination especially at end of urine flow, milky discharge, low back pain, with these complaints becoming chronic and intermittent. It is commonly caused by agents who are not associated with sexually transmitted diseases (STDs). Epididymitis may present with similar symptoms, primarily on one side of groin, usually more acute and seen often in younger males. Pain is more severe, settling in testicles and may involve swelling of the testicles. Often caused by other than STDs. Urethritis (pain deep in penis with discharge) can be acute in gonorrhea or more chronic in chlamydia and almost always caused by STDs in males. Infections in the reproductive tract are best treated with doxycycline. Prostate cancer is one of the costs of aging for men, becoming more common each year after age 50. The cancer is quiet until it has spread beyond the prostate and is more aggressive once outside the gland.

During digital rectal exam, only the posterior portion of the prostate can be felt, however, it is site where most tumors are found. Lumps, nodules or irregularities palpated on the digital exam require further evaluation. Follow-up with a urologist and CT scan and a blood test, PSA-prostate specific antigen is sometimes helpful but alone is not adequate. There are many cases of prostate cancer with normal PSA and elevated PSA does not always indicate prostate cancer. The prostate gland is small before adolescence, enlarging and becoming active in semen production when testosterone arrives. Stagnation within the male reproductive tract can lead to infection in two primary sites, the prostate and epididymis. The prostate has only one exit with no continuous flow, dependent upon ejaculations for cleansing. Because of this, it is the most often afflicted organ of the male reproductive tract.

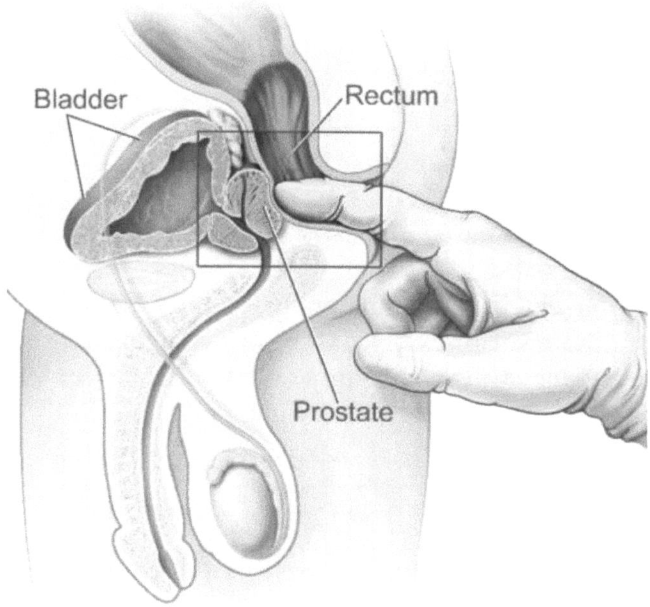

Even though only a small part of the prostate can be palpated, most cancer is found in that portion. NLM

Stagnation in the prostate is prevented by using the organ as celibacy appears to increase rate of dysfunction. In the act of orgasm, the prostate contracts several times, discharging its contents in a flushing motion. Contractions of the prostate is sensed by the "waves" of orgasms. Infection, inflammation and cancer of the prostate are all reduced by exercise, low fat diet and regular prostatic discharges (orgasms). Almost all prostates, if old enough, become malignant. Rectal exams once a year in men over the age of thirty-five are important in early detection of prostate cancer and over fifty, a blood test (prostatic specific antigen- PSA) is recommended. Men who live alone or are sexually inactive (celibate) have the highest rates of prostate cancer.

Inflammation or infection of the prostate (prostatitis) causes rectal or low abdominal pain, pain on urination, especially at the end of urination, a light creamy discharge from the penis, and chronic low-grade fever. The symptoms can come on suddenly or over weeks. Excessive alcohol intake is known to aggravate the chronic condition. Treatment can be difficult, requiring antibiotics for 2-3 weeks or longer. Doxycycline, Cipro and some penicillins are all used to treat prostatitis, sometimes in combination in resistant cases.

Bloody ejaculate is not rare in men and extensive lab and exam seldom identify a cause. Considered a normal aberration, the author has seen several cases, and none proved to be pathological. However, painless blood from the male urinary or reproductive tract should be evaluated for cancer

The epididymis when infected causes pain, swelling and redness on one side, known as "blue balls," to lay people. The pain is severe, sometimes ice to the area and opiates may be necessary. Antibiotics have limited success, with doxycycline being the most used, even though it may not prove helpful. Epididymitis does not appear related to venereal disease. Herpes is a skin infection of the penis that is a sexually transmitted disease that appear as tender blisters with surrounding redness. It is treated with acyclovir or other antivirals.

Gonorrhea causes redness and swelling at head of penis and heavy yellow-green discharge oozing from urethra and extremely painful urination. It is treated with ampicillin or amoxicillin 500 mg capsules given as one large dose of 4.5 grams (nine capsules). Injectable cephalosporins (Rocephin-cephtriaxone) is painful but very effective as single shot. Doxycycline will also treat gonorrhea when given over ten days, and is the only antibiotic that will kill gonorrhea, chlamydia, and syphilis. Chlamydia is currently the most common sexually transmitted disease in men. Unlike gonorrhea it does not cause dramatic thick discharge nor is it extremely painful. Instead, it causes mild discomfort at the end of urination and a light creamy discharge. Syphilis, formerly rare, is once again on the rise. It causes a painless ulcer on the penis or mouth.

Syphilis

The word is believed to originate from a poem by Italian medical officer Girolamo. Fracastoro about a shepherd named Syphilis. The word appears to be a Latinized version of the Greek word for pig-lover? It has been known as the French disease, the Great pox, Lues

"One moment with Venus, a lifetime with Mercury"
17th century sailor's lament

"If one knows syphilis, one knows medicine" William Osler

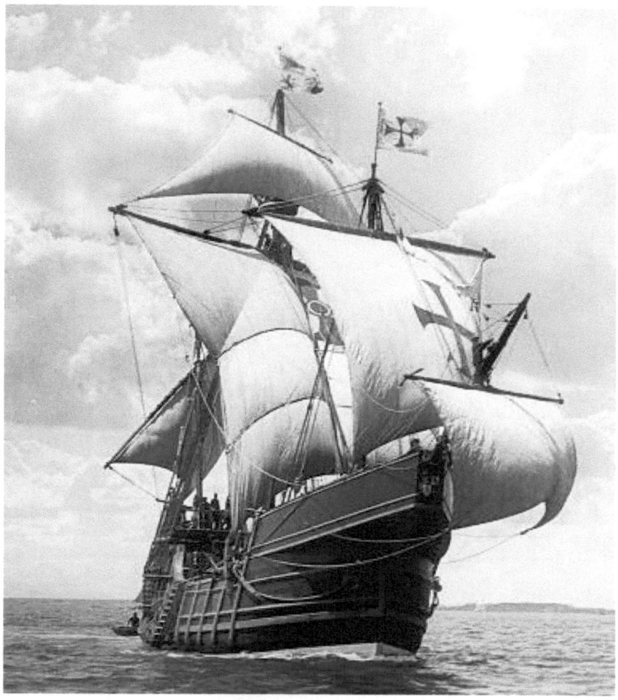

An artist illustration of the largest of Columbus' three ship fleet, the Santa Maria. A small fleet harboring diseases in both directions that would profoundly affect the world. National Archives

In August of 1492 Christopher Columbus departed Seville with three small ships (Nina, Pinta and Santa Maria), 90 men (some carrying infectious diseases) and assorted livestock, sailing west to find the shores of Cathay. Instead, he found the Caribbean coast of the Americas. Unknown to him at the time, he and his crew also found a new scourge that was soon to ravage Europe, the Middle East, North Africa and later the paradise islands of the Pacific. After landing and allowing his crew to mingle with natives in the island of Hispaniola he returned to Spain in March of 1493 with only one ship, a smaller crew (64), six "Indians", assorted artifacts and a microscopic corkscrew-shaped bacteria (spirochete) that "syphilized" Europe. Some historians believe syphilis was already present in Europe; however, this author believes it was a new infectious agent in the Western World as there is no mention of any disease resembling syphilis in Hebrew, Greek, Roman or Byzantine historical texts.

The people of late 15th century Europe were no strangers to terrible diseases. The increased shipping activity of the Crusades had brought leprosy, smallpox, Black Death, typhus, cholera and other infectious diseases in wave after wave of misery to the populations of Western Europe. However, the emergence in the late 15th century of syphilis was perhaps the most hideous. It was a devastating illness that within a few days ravaged and disfigured the victim as skin became covered first with blisters that later turned into angry red swollen ulcers, reeking with foul odors. If they survived for more than a few days, gummas (syphilitic abscesses) developed deep within the body or limbs, later erupting with a foul odorous white sticky mucus. So bad was their appearance that even lepers shunned them, mothers deserted children, priests refused to give communion, sailors threw the still-living sick overboard and villagers drove the afflicted out of town, to die unattended, lonely and unburied.

Within one year of the arrival of syphilis it was being spread in the wake of a French army marauding across Europe. The disease first appears in print in 1494 as the "French Disease" because of a large outbreak that followed in the wake of the French Army of Charles VIII during a military campaign in northern Italy. The spirochete harbored by a component of Spanish mercenaries containing some of Columbus' sailors. Syphilis was so infectious that within three years of Columbus' return, it had penetrated all of Europe, even the remote northern Shetland Islands far north of Scotland. A single ship was enough to plant the seed of syphilis in the many small coastal ports, where even under the prudish ways of medieval Europe, the disease was spread rapidly inland from the waterfront.

Dutch and German physicians labelled syphilis as *Bosen Blattern*, the evil pox, in French *la gross verole*, the great pox. Perhaps its earliest medical observer was Rodrigo Ruy de Isla, a Spanish naval surgeon that not only documented the disease in Columbus' crew but also traced its origin to the Caribbean Island of Hispaniola. Ruy de Isla was the first to recognize the beneficial effect of fever on the course of the disease and the first to deploy mercury as effective treatment. Sailors whose immune system could generate a high fever suffered less deleterious effects of syphilis. In the beginning, it was a lethal infection with high death rates. Fortunately, or perhaps unfortunately, it became a chronic almost hidden life-long infection, still ultimately fatal as this disease affects every organ system in the body. Syphilis has adversely affected human history since its introduction to the world by Christopher Columbus and is currently under appreciated and nearly forgotten but not dead. Until recently, hospital admissions, pre-marital blood tests and military physicals all required a VDRL blood test to detect the presence of syphilis. Testing for syphilis is no longer routine, and unfortunately it is on the rise again worldwide, and in fact a major site of syphilis infection is among the elderly in nursing homes per the author's daughter-in-law who manages the blood bank in Oklahoma City.

Within 1-2 generations after its introduction to Europe, either syphilis underwent a change, or the human immune system adapted, rendering it a chronic smoldering infection. It appeared to weaken as a virulent infection and though still fatal, now slowly kills over years and decades. The bacteria were somehow modified by the human immune system into a weaker form, or the offspring of the original spirochetes selectively chose the less aggressive traits. Did the bacteria engineer its own natural selection to a less aggressive more effective parasite? However, it was achieved, syphilis became a contagious infection for life, affecting human history for centuries. Some historians estimate that by the late 19th century, twenty-five percent of the Western World was infected.

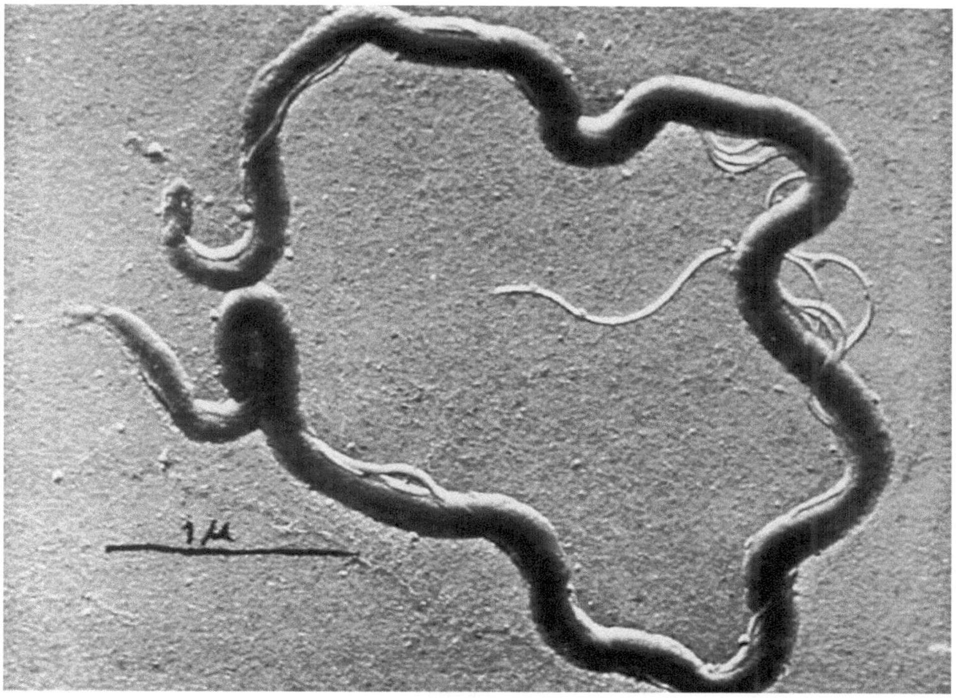

Note the cork-screw shape which makes this creature difficult to treat, as does the similar spirochete that causes Lyme's disease which can also become life-long. CDC

Hundreds of treatments were tried on syphilis but until the mid-20th century, the only effective treatment was the highly toxic heavy metals, arsenic and mercury. Mercury treatment remained unchanged for over 400 years and though often effective, was a poisoning almost as bad as the disease. Arsenic became the base metal in Nobel Prize winner Paul Erhich's discovery of Salvarsan for treating syphilis in 1909. Arsenic at low doses proved to have antibiotic activity and improved the patient's stamina. In the beginning and today, syphilis is treated easily in its infancy, soon after exposure, when a painless sore or ulcer appears on genitalia. Almost any antibiotic will destroy the spirochete if treated immediately after exposure, however if untreated initially, treatment is difficult and lengthy.

Mercury was found to be effective within the first few years of the emergence of syphilis and continued in use well into the 1930's. It is the oldest effective antibiotic but a very toxic agent. Even before Columbus, mercury had been used for centuries by Greek, Arab and Hebrew medical officers to treat leprosy and yaws (another disease caused by a spirochete) as well as fevers in small doses. It was being used as early as 1497 by a French naval surgeon Julien for syphilis and who noted the disease later in coastal natives of Hispaniola.

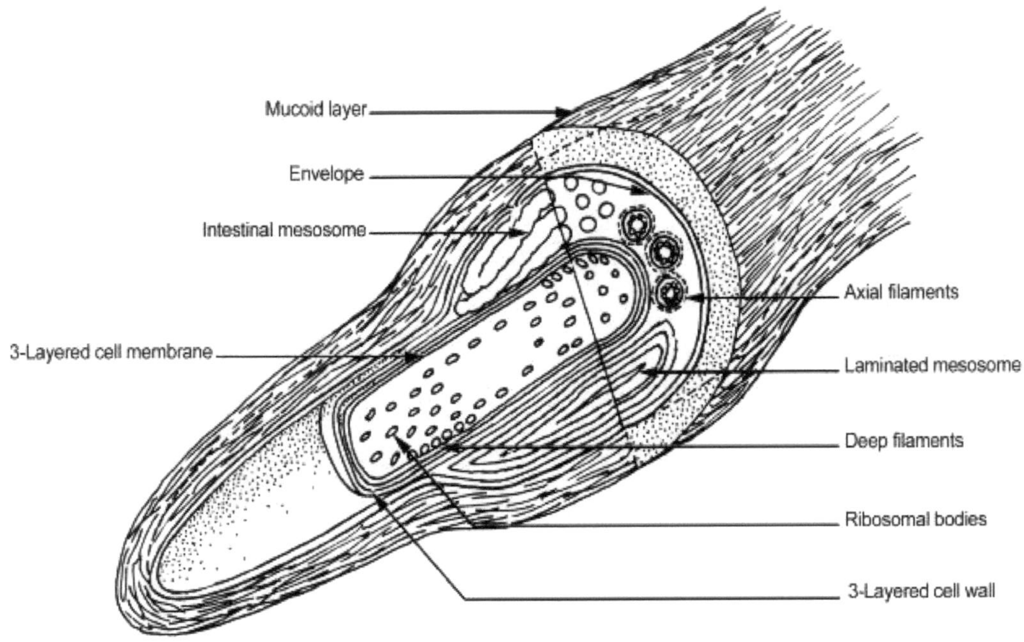

Just the head of a "simple" single-cell pathogen, CDC

Although Mercury-containing solutions produced favorable results on the disease, it was hard on the patient. Syphilis and mercury treatment became so common that early European druggists were called Mercers. An early form of syphilis treatment was named for a Dutch ship's surgeon, Van Swieten, whose solution found its way into all well-equipped shipboard and army apothecaries of the 17th, 18th and 19th centuries. Sailors were frequently "dosed" with Van Swieten's Solution when returning from ports known for the disease. Not unlike sailors during the Second World War reported jugs of penicillin at the gangway when returning from certain shore leave.

The island of Hispaniola played an important role in another sexually transmitted disease five hundred years after Columbus when the western half, the nation of Haiti served as a conduit for the spread of AIDS from Africa to the Americas. There are several differing theories about the origin and spread of AIDs including the human creation of the virus. The author finds the most likely and interesting story in the following. The virus that became known as AIDS may have begun as a primate (monkey) virus found in the green monkeys in the jungle around Kinshasa, the capital of Zaire (now renamed as the Congo). Kinshasa along the Congo River and surrounding jungle has long been known to harbor dangerous diseases. Joseph Conrad's "Heart of Darkness" is a fictional account of the river's dangers, especially the fevers. It was not unusual for Europeans to become ill and die within days after they stepped ashore. Many were never to be seen again after heading upriver, while others left the Congo area with broken health.

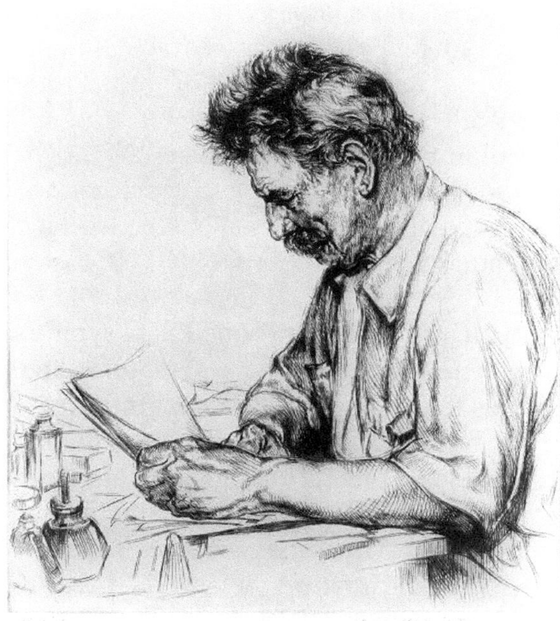

Sketch of Dr. Sweitzer by Arthur W. Heintzelman. As a German citizen, he was treated badly by the British and French during the World War II.
National Library of Congress

It was in this area of West Africa where Albert Sweitzer practiced medicine and surgery during and between both World Wars. As a young man he was an internationally known pianist, published composer and a professor in theology. His two books, "The Quest of historical Christ" and "The Mysticism of Paul the Apostle" were highly regarded and widely read. At age thirty he experienced an "epiphany" from God to become a missionary physician and after finishing a three-year medical program was sent to West Africa north of the Congo River. Along the Ogooue River which drains the Congo's Bateke Plateau, Dr. Sweitzer and his anesthesiologist wife did thousands of surgeries, most inguinal hernia repairs. Many patients walked for weeks holding their hernias in place with the promise of having it repaired in his clinic. The fevers and long hours under minimal living conditions eventually broke their health requiring return to Europe. After seven years he returned without his wife and worked until the end of World War II.

West Africa's central coasts are rich with infectious agents, so it is no surprise that AIDs could have been harbored here (as is Ebola), just waiting for human hosts. There are widely held beliefs about the origin of AIDs, some even claim it was man-made; however, it is not new disease, and serum specimens from a Dutch merchant sailor in the mid 1950's and a British seaman in 1968, both serving ports in West Africa were found to contain evidence of the AIDs virus. The following account is this author's story about the recent rise of this deadly disease. When a new garbage dump was needed for the growing population of Congo's capital, Kinshasa, it was carved from jungle displacing green monkeys that lived in the trees. Like many animals, the monkeys quickly adapted to foraging among human waste and contact between humans and monkeys became common. As people came to the dump to discard or gather refuse, they were sometimes attacked and bitten by monkeys who became more accustomed and therefore less fearful of humans. This contact might have resulted in the transfer of the virus from monkey spittle to the human blood stream. Beginning in the 1970's, there was a large cultural exchange between the Congo and Haiti, with thousands of sexually active young people crossing the Atlantic, spreading the virus through sexual intercourse. The AIDS virus was carried to Haiti by the returning young people, who in turn visited the brothels and bars of Haiti where they coupled with vacationing Americans. As the natives of this island did with Columbus's men. Haiti had for years been a popular destination for male homosexuals, especially those from New York and Montreal where the disease first appeared in numbers AIDs would have arrived in the United States even without the homosexual connection, just as syphilis would have eventually reached Europe without Columbus.

Until well into the 20th century, it was true that if one knew syphilis, one knew medicine, since syphilis affects every organ system and causes more symptoms and physical findings than any other single disease. Syphilis was the known as the "Great Imitator" in medical studies as almost any complaint could possibly be attributed to it. One of the author's pathology professors and a historian remind his students that today's lecture could be related to syphilis. Towards the end of each lecture, doing a good imitation of Maurice Chevalier, he recited with a French accent "and every little breeze whispered Louise", (Lues being another name for syphilis) and why it is included in today's lesson. A medical text of the late 19th and early 20th century would be dominated by syphilis with some tuberculosis thrown in. The serum test to diagnosis syphilis was developed by a German bacteriologist August von Wassermann in 1909 and was used throughout the 20th century. In the same year, another German scientist, Paul Ehrich on the 606th trial of an arsenic (heavy metal like mercury) discovered Salvarsan which although still toxic, was safer than mercury. Syphilis was not safely and successfully treated with antibiotics beginning with penicillin until the 1950s but in its chronic form is still difficult to manage. Medical officers should be aware of its possible presence and be prepared to treat early with doxycycline in STDS.

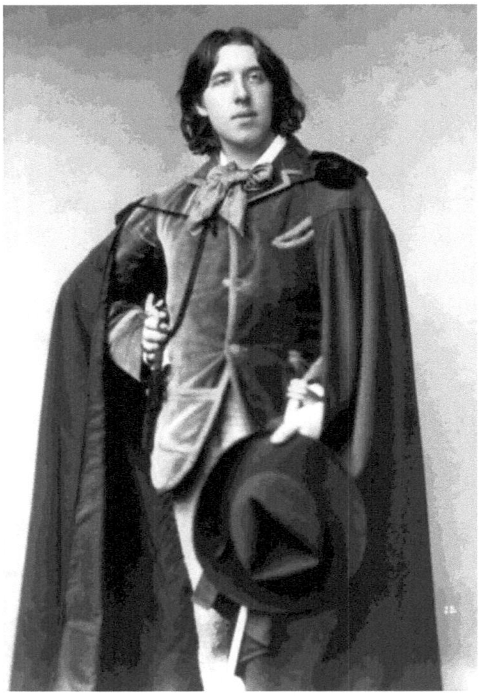

Oscar Wilde, "History is merely gossip" supposedly contracted syphilis as a young student at Oxford where activities with prostitutes were common. His promiscuous sexual activity brought the legal system against him and in the face of British hypocrisy, dared the

courts to punish him which they did, sentencing him to two years in prison for "commission of acts of gross indecency with another male person". One of his novels, "The Portrait of Dorian Gray" depicted perhaps his own life of early sins and later consequences. He died a painful death at the age of 46 from complications of cerebral syphilis. NPR

Syphilis has not played a small role in the history of the Western World since its introduction in the late 15th century. The following are examples of historical major figures probably infected. Beethoven's deafness was a condition commonly associated with the central nervous destruction by syphilis, and it was well known fact that he hung out with prostitutes. Vincent van Gogh was another artist who was known to associate freely with prostitutes and reported he was treated with mercury and urethral strictures with painful dilation. Strictures in the urethra were common in sexually transmitted infections.

Syphilis is classical described into three stages, the first, a painless ulcer-like lesion on the genitalia or within the oral cavity. It may not even be noticed, especially within the vaginal vault. The lesion resolves with seemingly no other symptoms until later, when a red rash appears, and unlike most rashes involves the palms of hands and soles of feet. The rash resolves and once again no symptoms appear for years, even decades for some. In the late third stage of syphilis, bacteria have crossed the blood brain barrier in great numbers and begins its slow destruction of the central nervous system. An image of Mongrel hordes relentlessly conquering Persia, Turkey and the Middle East on its path to meeting Europe on the east bank of the Danube, comes to the author's mind. This slow pernicious destruction leads to serious chronic and progressive symptoms, headaches, loss of sensation in extremities and increasing weakness, tremors, imbalance with walking, a shuffling gait (tabes dorsalis) caused by brain and spinal cord ravages. Seizures, wasting, personality changes, insanity, coma and death appear late in the disease.

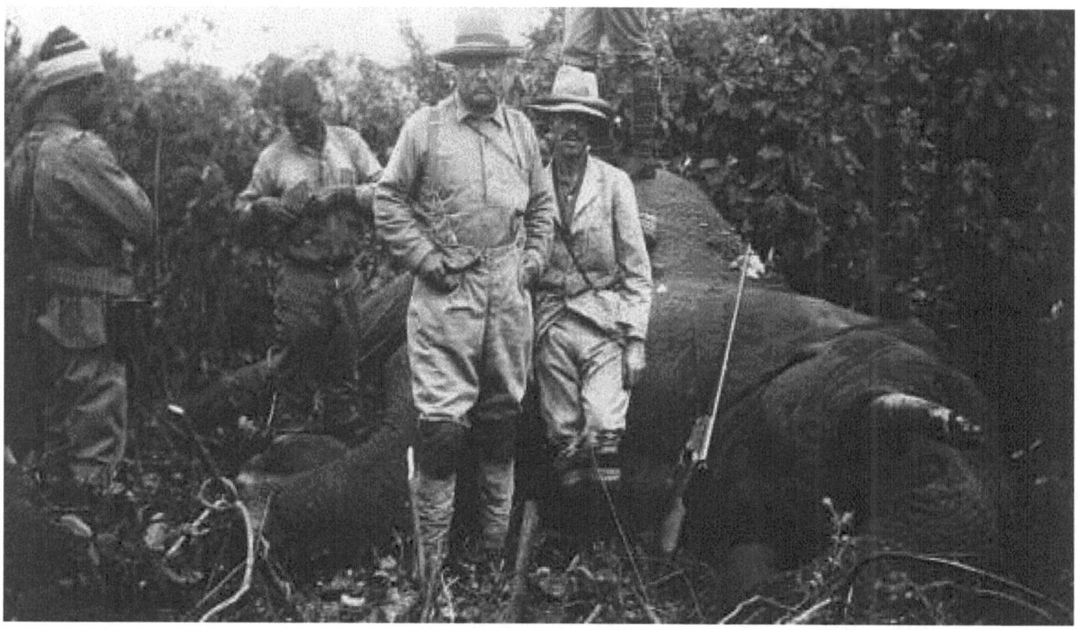

Teddy Roosevelt in East Africa, hunted with the big game hunter, Baron Blixen
National Archives

"Out of Africa" the book and movie were based on the true-life story of Karen Blixen (pen name Isak Dinesen) who contracted syphilis from her cousin and husband Baron von Blixen-Fineke. In the early 20th century, Holland was not only a center for world shipping but also a center for syphilis treatment since the spirochete invaded Europe four hundred years ago. After contracting the disease from her husband, she went to Amsterdam for mercury and probable arsenic treatment, unfortunately it was only partially effective, slowing the infection, not curing it. By 1930 the disease had damaged her central nervous system causing problems with balance and walking requiring her to be carried by her secretary later in life. She lived until age of 77, dying of emaciation, looking like a concentration camp victim. "I myself was the lightest thing of all, for fate to get rid of". Her husband infected wives of European hunters and Masai women who in turn infected their husbands. The syphilitic Baron probably indirectly infected thousands of victims. One of history's truly bad men.

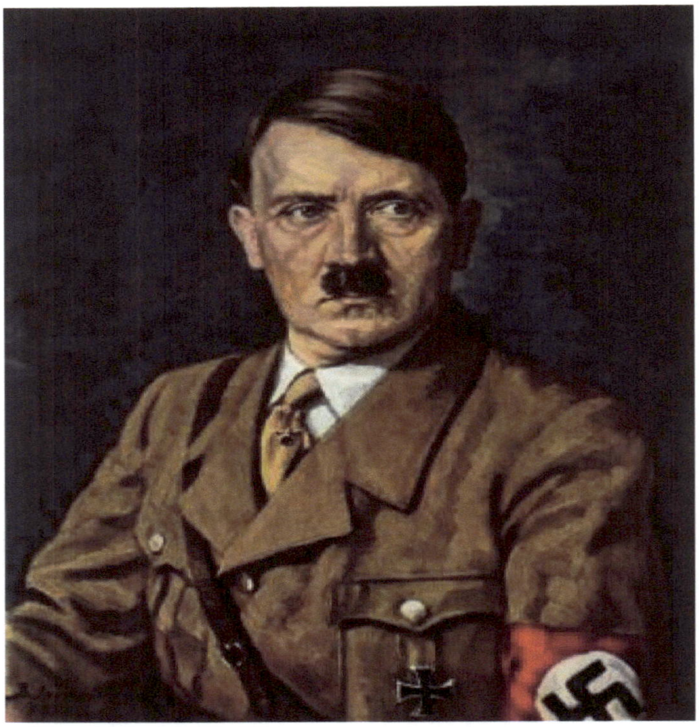

"Combating syphilis should have been made to appear as the task of the nation. Not just one more task. Everything — future or ruin — depended upon the solution to this question." Adolf Hitler, 1933. He was a strict non-smoker and had wanted to make tobacco illegal (the military said that was impossible, as smoking was paramount to the soldier's morale). He was a vegetarian and non-drinker, always dressed plainly wearing a simple Iron Cross metal he earned in the Great War, often surrounded by generals wearing uniforms adorned with decorations. He owned almost nothing, as he did not acquire the art, precious metals and jewels, estates, castles and even libraries that some of his lieutenants pillaged throughout Europe. He loved Wagner's music, Charlie Chaplin movies and his dog, Blondi. As a young man, it is believed that he contracted syphilis in Vienna and blamed it on an encounter with a Jewish prostitute. Adolf Hitler painting by Bruno Jacob 1933

By 1945, Hitler looked much different, the effects of third stage syphilis, years of heavy metal treatments and drug abuse were evident in his appearance, behavior, body movements, tremors, personality changes and heart disease. In addition to chronic syphilis attacking every part of his body, he had received hundreds of doses of mercury and arsenic over several decades. In the mid 1930's chose the care of Dr. Theo Morell, a well-known syphilologist as his primary medical officer. It was not unusual for leaders to choose a medical officer that specialized in their medical needs. President John Kennedy chose a well-known chronic back pain specialist, Janet Travail, becoming the first female medical officer to the President of the United States private medical officer.

Few medical officers have played a greater supporting role in human history than Theodore Gilbert Morell. Dr. Morell was responsible indirectly, for aspects of the Second World War by medically manipulating his patient, Adolf Hitler. Although being recognized as one of Europe's experts in syphilis, he was suspiciously regarded by Germany's military physicians as most believed he was a danger to the Fuhrer. Why did Hitler, who was meticulously clean, changing his shirts twice daily, choose a physician that seldom if ever, washed his hands? With dirty fingernails, he gave thousands of injections over the years to Hitler. His injections included a bizarre list of drugs and materials, a mixture of modern and tropical folk remedies. Dr. Morell was well travelled after serving as a combat medical officer in the Great War near the front. After the war he worked as a Ships Surgeon visiting ports in the tropics, where he interacted with local medical practitioners developing a poly-pharmaceutical type of medicine. This approach was controversial, leading to constant accusations by the German medical establishment, criticism Hitler chose to ignore. His injections included belladonna, human placenta, bull semen, methamphetamine, opium (later when opium became unavailable, methadone) and preparations made from Romanian peasant's feces! Morrel occasionally used leeches on Hitler's temples for headache, which Hitler believed was effective (as they were for Napoleon's hemorrhoids). Morell's role vaguely resembles that of the mad monk Rasputin, whose bizarre activities helped bring down the Russian Tsar and the Bolshevik takeover of Russia.

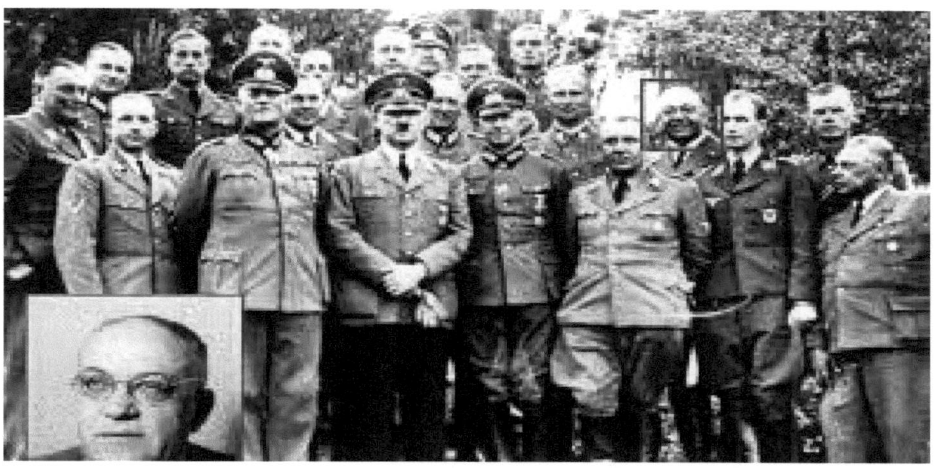

Hitler looks healthy in this photo while Dr. Morell seems to be one of the few grinning. Morrel's "fragrance" of poor body hygiene was the butt of many offhand comments and even though most Nazi physicians considered him a quack, much of his controversial treatments continue today. He became rich establishing his own pharmaceutical manufacturing which later suppled the German Army with his products. elespanol.com

During episodes of his congestive heart disease, Morell injected Hitler with iodine potassium and IV digitalis. At the time, intravenous digitalis (a plant toxin) treatment was considered radical by the medical establishments of the mid-20th century, however later it was used in millions of patients for heart failure. The treatment of Hitler's syphilis by Dr. Morell played a huge role in Germany's supreme leader's decisions, judgements tainted by disease and toxic drugs. His decline was noted by those around him beginning in 1942 when he decided against his military advisors to attack across southern Russia towards the Caucasus oil fields and the city named for his enemy, Stalingrad. The city had little strategic value and the German 6th Army, Germany's most powerful and most mechanized army was leading the attack. In was like a powerful spearhead attached to a weak shaft. Behind the German 6th Army were thousands of flat featureless miles of the Russian plains, intersected by bridgeless rivers, connecting the army to its supply base 2000 kilometers to the rear. A supply line protected by poorly equipped and led armies of Italy, Hungary, Bulgaria, Romania and assorted small groups of Spanish, French, Dutch, Finnish and other regiments that had fallen in with the German Army. In late 1942, while the German 6th Army was engaged in the ruins of Stalingrad where their tanks were as useless as their airplanes, their supply line was shattered, and the survivors surrendered. Tens of thousands of men in a Russian winter, no food, little if any medical care and no hope of returning home. This terrible strategical disaster begins a long line of similar battles, all decided under the influence of Hitler's disease and his medical officer. Of the 250,000 German troops that left for Stalingrad, only 6,000 returned decades later, some becoming officers in the Soviet dominated East German secret police.

In the early 20th century, it was estimated that one-in-four of the western world was infected with active syphilis. Some nations experienced much higher rates. During the Great War 1914-1918, there was such a high syphilis rate among the French civilians and French army, that blood transfusions were not accepted from the French population. "Defeated Flesh" by Bertrand Taithe traces much of France's high rates of syphilis to the siege of Paris during the Franco-Prussian War of 1869-71. Women and children were ordered to evacuate as the Prussians drew near. However, reluctant to leave were several thousand prostitutes, becoming trapped with thousands of soldiers and the remaining male population, resulting in an extremely high concentration of the spirochetes. Since many soldiers, politicians, writers, painters and other artists stayed in the city and endured the siege, this group experienced an especially high rate of infection. Taihe believes the syphilis incubated during the siege of Paris, spread throughout France, adversely affecting the French leadership in the late 19th and early 20th century, leading to France's decline as a world power. The Dreyfuss Affair, financial disaster of the failed Sea-to-Sea Panama Canal and weak military leadership early in World War I were at least in part, due to neurosyphilis.

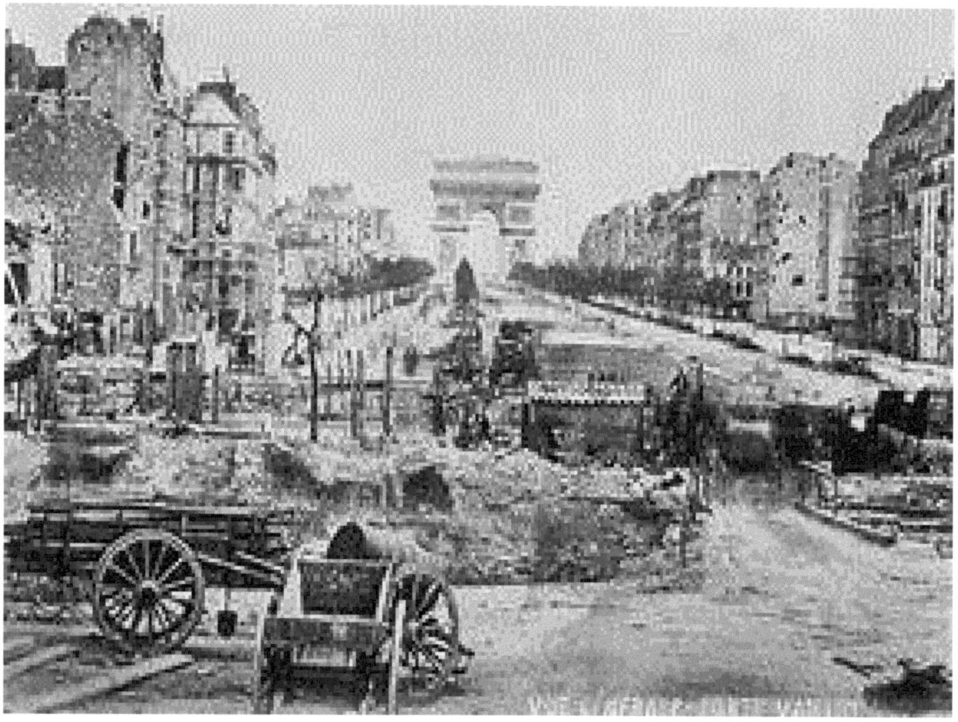

The Siege of Paris, September 1870-January 1871 led to starvation of the condensed population. After exhausting food stores, they ate most of the animals in the Paris Zoo, followed by their pets and finally the rats of the sewers. It was the only time in Paris, there were no rats.

In the late third stage of syphilis the bacteria have entered and begin destroying the central nervous system, causing serious chronic and progressive symptoms. No place in the body is safe from this clever parasite syphilis that developed the ability to survive and thrive in every human organ system; cardiovascular, especially the aorta, gastrointestinal, lung, kidneys, liver, skin, central nervous system and immune system. Antibiotics for decades had the ability to destroy spirochetes in all the above systems, but they could not cure syphilis. Without chronic use, the infection returned after antibiotics withdrawn. The patient's infections were thought to be from exposure to new hosts, however it proved to be the same infection that somehow was avoiding the antibiotics. Due to its unique spiral corkscrew shape, the *Treponema* allows it to screw its body into spaces no other shaped cell could enter, retreating a place in the body unknown to the human immune circulating cells. When exposed to attack, the bacteria screw itself into the anterior chamber of the eye, where it slowly waits and "hibernates" as resources scarce in that part of the eye. Physicians used special lights to examine the eye for the presence of spirochetes in the anterior chamber where no antibiotic could enter.

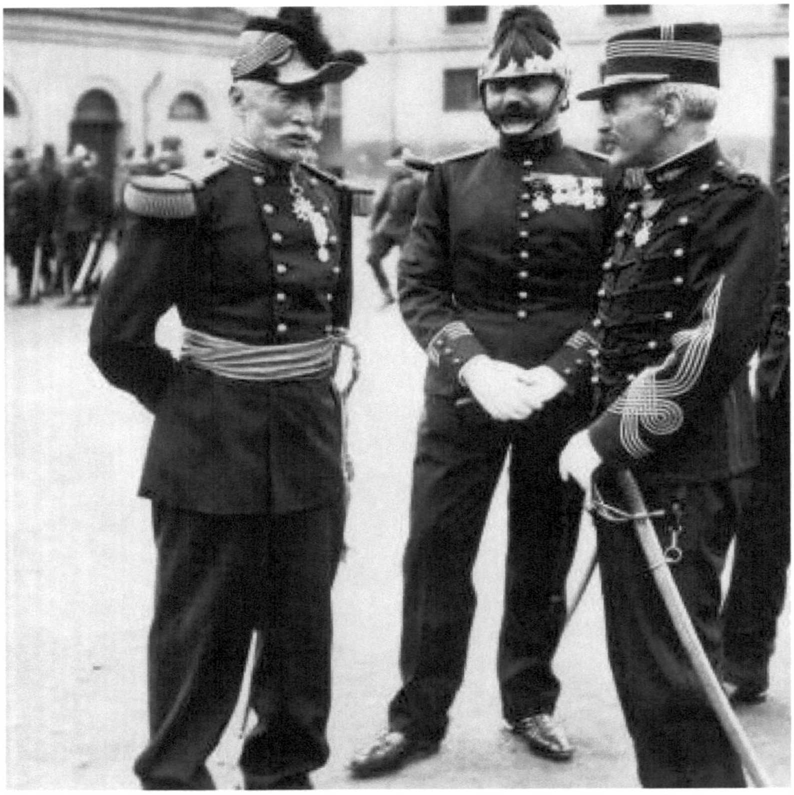

Captain Dreyfus on the right after reinstatement in the French Army. Dreyfus was a wealthy Jewish dedicated artillery officer falsely accused of passing military secrets to the Germans. Information of minimal use to the enemy, yet on a few scraps of forged material, Dreyfus was convicted of treason, public humiliated in front of the Army and imprisoned on the formally closed French penal colony on Devil's Island off NE coast of South America. The prison was reopened and staffed for him alone for years under extremely harsh conditions. The cover-up of The Dreyfus Affair exposed antisemitism and corruption within the highest levels of the French Army, bringing down the government and the Army. The Dreyfus Affair in the late 19th century badly wounded France in the years before the First World War. Neurosyphilis played a role in this affair that divided France, created more anti-Semitism, and severely damaged the leadership of the French Army and its morale. The microscopic spiral-shaped treponema bacteria had penetrated and damaged France on the eve of Germany's invasion in August 1914. Alfred Dreyfus returned to the Army and with the Germans bearing down on Paris in the summer of 1914, a small contingent of French officers and men sallied forth from Paris and attacked the west flank of the Alexaner von Kluck's First Army. In the van of this French attack was Major Alfred Dreyfus, risking his life for the French Nation he loved. A recent book, "An Officer and Spy" by Robert Harris is a good read on the Dreyfus Affair. On the other side of Europe, a medical condition, hemophilia in a single person, was preparing to wreck France's primary ally against Germany, Imperial Russia. National Archives

Rulers from Russia's Ivan the Terrible in the 15th century to the 20th century's Uganda's Idi Amin. Napoleon, Stalin, Churchill's father Lord Randolph Churchill, Friedrich Nietzsche, Franz Schubert, and thousands of others of historical significance were suspected or proven to harbor these bacteria.

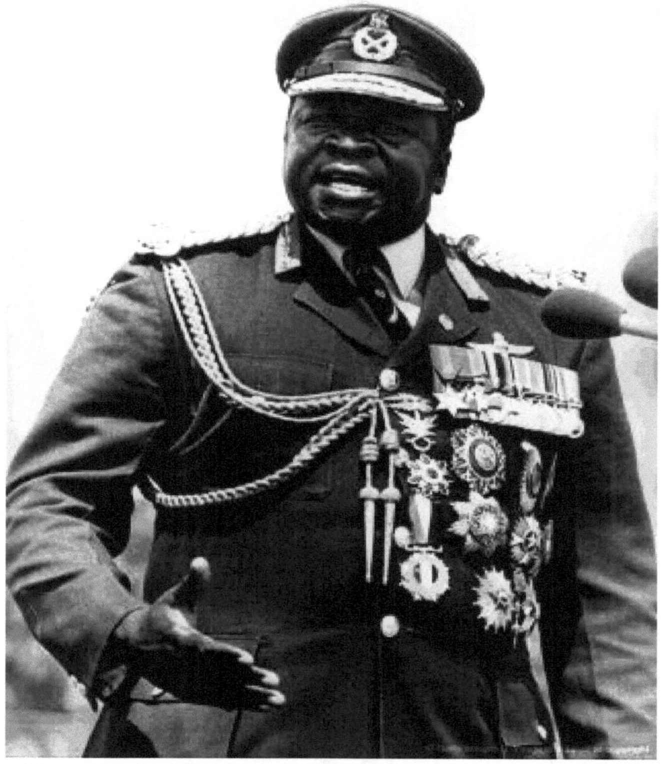

The heavily "heroically metaled" Idi Amin, dictator of Uganda was an effective leader early in his country's independence, even impressed Queen Elisabeth of England. Syphilis, the spirochete turned him into an angry vicious man, with bouts of personalities changes, incredible acts of cruelty, finally killed him. "The Last King of Scotland" is an excellent movie depicting this tyrant. National Archives

In the beginning, if syphilis is diagnosed and treated while in its first stage, its infancy, it is easily resolved with simple antibiotics. However, if the bacteria gain a foothold, allowing numbers to multiply in the internal organs, it may become a life-long disease without aggressive treatment. Doxycycline is the drug of choice in suspected sexually transmitted disease (STD) as it will treat syphilis, gonorrhea and chlamydia, making it the best choice for sexually acquired bacterial infections, but must be given early.

References for some of the author's assertions in this chapter:

"Pox" Deborah Hayden
"The Bunker" James P. O'Donnell
"The Fall of Berlin 1945" Anthony Beevor
"The Last One Hundred Days of the German Reich" John Toland
"Defeated Flesh" Bertrand Taithe, "Blitzed" Norman Ohle

The Basic Sciences

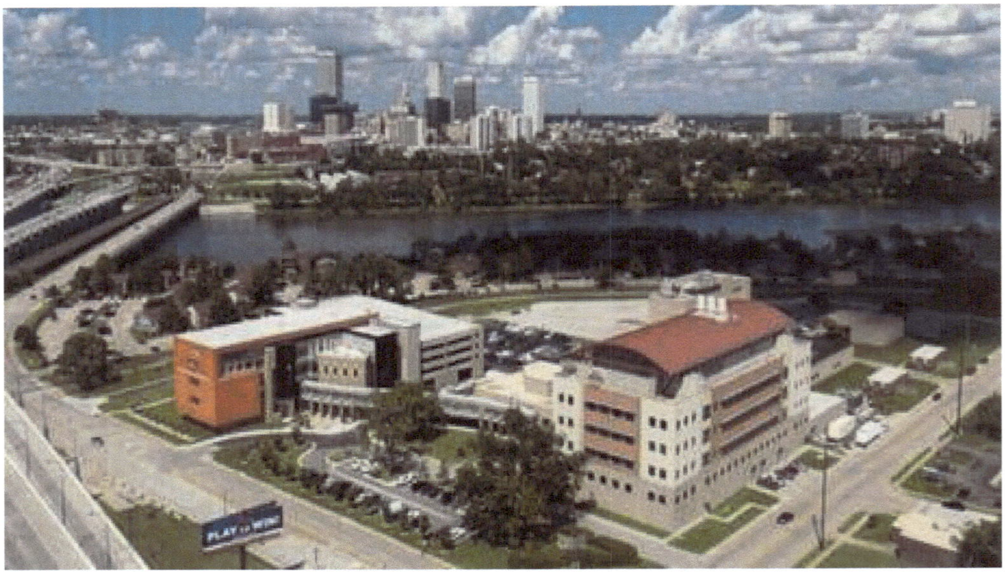

Oklahoma State University College of Osteopathic Medicine, Tulsa, Oklahoma. The site where the author studied much of the basic sciences that went into this text.

Medical education in the past was primarily founded on apprenticeship training, not unlike the way a blacksmith, soldier, cook or mechanic was trained. Medical schools were few in numbers when compared to the needs of physicians and surgeons in a violent and diseased world, requiring most training to be on-the-job in villages, cities, ships and on battlefields. Currently physicians are required to complete many hours in undergraduate and later graduate basic sciences course in medical schools. The basic sciences include biochemistry, microbiology, physiology, immunology, pathology, anatomy and medical terminology (heavily Latin based). Most of these subjects are spread among in the discussions of diseases and injuries. The sciences of biochemistry and microbiology have their own sections here. Although not necessary in the field, a good foundation makes for a stronger structure.

Biochemistry

Bio, Greek for life, chemistry an uncertain word root, likely from the Arabic word *al-kimia*, Latinized to alchemy in the Middle Ages. Some believe the word originates from ancient Egypt since *"Kema"* is a word for the Land of the Nile. In this text, biochemistry is defined as what happens inside a cell when chemicals meet life leading to controlled chemical behavior.

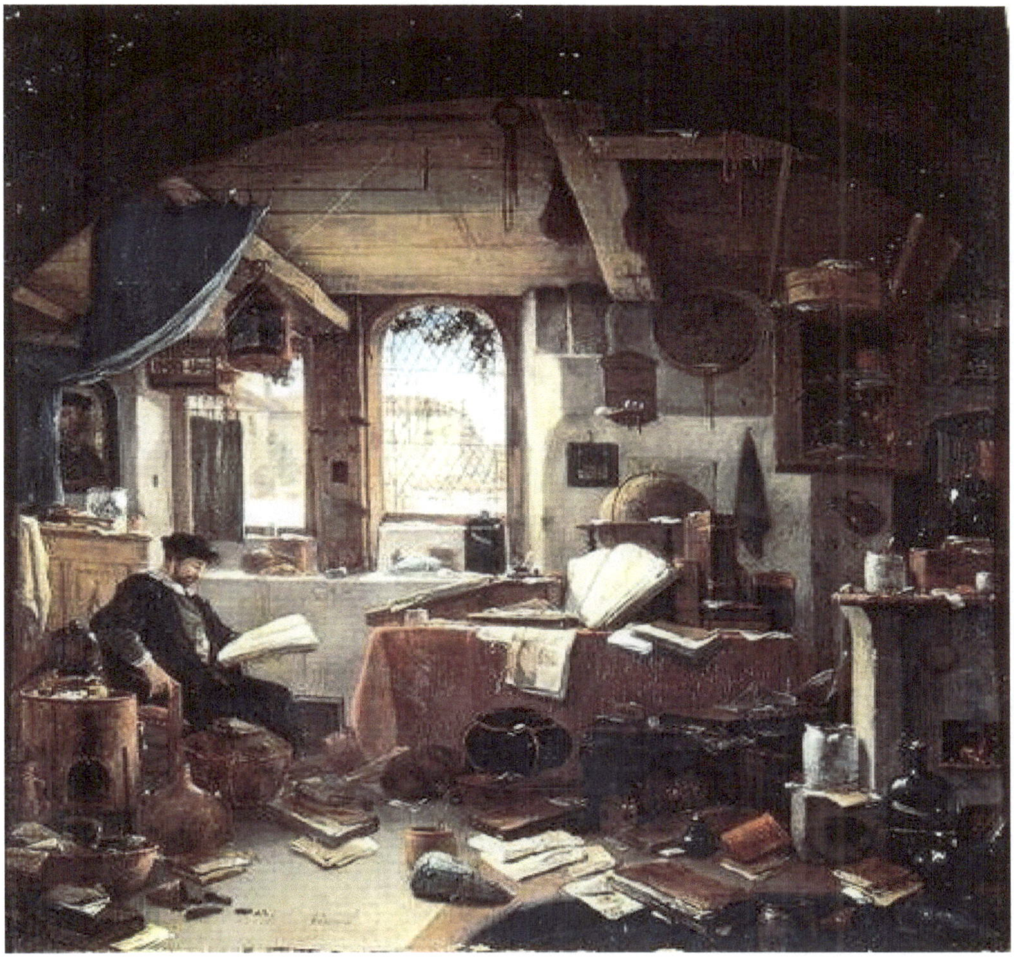

"The Alchemist" by Thomas Wijck, 1616-1677. He lived and worked in 17th century Venice, London and Holland. His paintings favored people found around ships and seaports. Note the confusion in this office, as alchemists were not yet engineers. The Dutch became the premier maritime nation in the 17th and 18th centuries, in no small part due to their embrace of alchemists.

The alchemist and biochemistry were extremely valuable to the maritime world in the late Middle Ages, especially the Netherlands. They were a source of literacy, books, maps, scientific instruments, informed fellowship along with medicines of the chemical type. Alchemists were an important reliable source of mercury, the only effective cure for syphilis, and due to its toxicity, exact dosing reduced its disabling side effects.

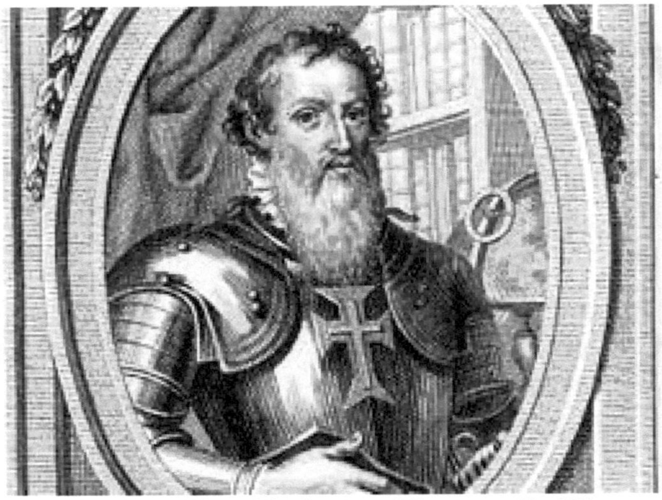

Henry the Navigator, 1394-1460, the third son of Portugal's King was more of a soldier than a sailor and yet earned the title of navigator as he was the force behind pushing Portuguese shipping out of the Mediterranean and into the Atlantic pursuing valuable spice and pepper trade. Pepper was so valuable it was sold by each single berry.

After many attempts and lost lives, the Portuguese opened the sea route between Western Europe and the Spice Islands of the Far East by sailing around the tip of southern Africa. Where, with the innovation of long-range sailing ships and shipborne cannon, they raped and pillaged their way up the eastern coast of Africa. After arriving in Zanzibar and bribing an Arab pilot, Ahmed Ibn Majid, crossed the Indian Ocean to the rich Indian subcontinent. The name of Ahmed Ibn Ahmed is still reviled by Moslems. The Portuguese had an accidental biochemical advantage over other northern European maritime powers in citric fruits brought to the Iberian Peninsula by invading Moors from the oasis of North Africa. The key to preventing scurvy, ascorbic acid (vitamin C) was fortunately part of the Portuguese ship's stores. The "spices" brought back from the Far East were so valuable and the risks so high, that if only one ship in five returned, the voyage was a huge financial success. These spices were valued as medicines, not as food enhancers. One of the four spices only found on a handful of islands, nutmeg, contains myristicin, a precursor of MMDA (ecstasy) a monoamine oxidase inhibitor that enhances its effect. Along with nutmeg, cloves, cinnamon, mace and pepper largely drove the spice trade due to their high value per weight. The book "The Scents of Eden" by Charles Corn is a highly readable account of the Spice Trade but will lower one's view of the Dutch.

The Dutch, scenting profit followed the trail blazed by the Portuguese down the west African coast and across the Indian Ocean with many more ships and men. Without the benefit of citric fruits, the Dutch used an inferior source of vitamin C, cabbage pickled in vinegar, sauerkraut. Within two generations the Dutch, now armed with citric fruits from their colony in South Africa, overwhelmed the hegemony of the Portuguese. The government of Portugal and the repressive Catholic Church required all crew to be Portuguese, kept secret logs of voyages, currents, weather and landmarks. Information strictly guarded in a nation under the shadow of the Spanish Inquisition and limited trade to Portuguese and Spanish ports. At its peak, the Portuguese had perhaps 4000 merchant marines and a few hundred ships. By the late 17th century, the Dutch overwhelmed the Portuguese with 10,000 ships crewed with men and women, regardless of religion, race or creed. The Dutch freely provided ships with logs and charts, while encouraging trade with all countries.

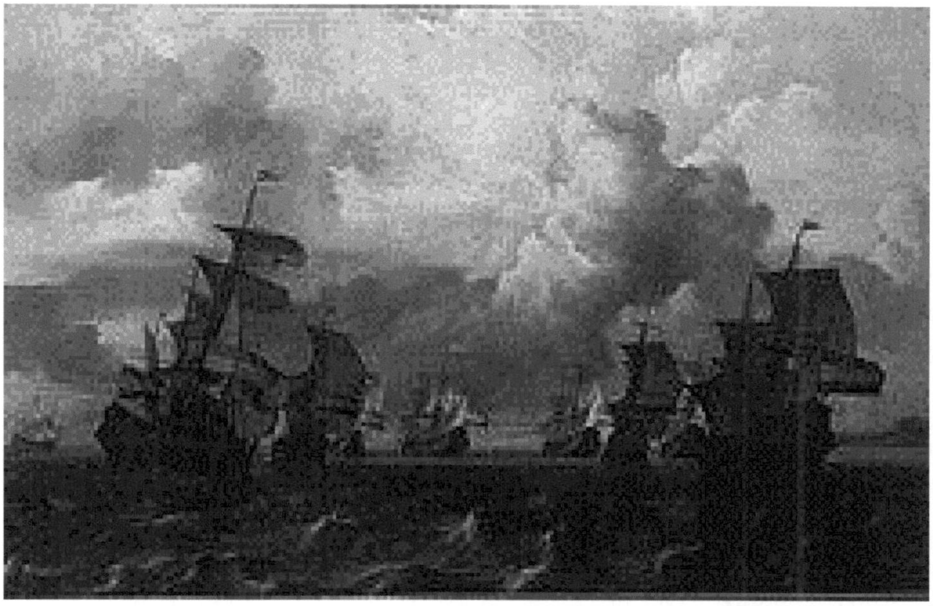

The Dutch East Indies Fleet by Ludolf Bakhuizen 1630-1708. The Dutch developed a new type of ship, lightly armed, wide bodied to increase storage, designed more for trade than warfare and at their peak were launching 1,000 new ships each year. The invention of the windmill allowed the Dutch to mill trees into lumber much more efficiently than hand sawing.

Chemistry is a history-rich component of medicine and has contributed significantly to seafaring and exploration. The combination of elements into specific structures and their chemical interactions within the cell have changed human history. Alchemists in the Netherlands served as a "nidus" for development of other sciences, i.e. the microscope (microbiology), the telescope (astronomy), accurate navigational instruments, training and medicine chests. Developments stymied by the Spanish Catholic Church in the Iberian Peninsula. Just like oil and water will not mix, alchemists and the Inquisition were not compatible. The repressive nature of Spanish Catholicism played a major role in the demise of Iberian maritime power and the rise of Protestant maritime nations. The English were late to worldwide shipping as they were dealing with removal of the Scottish Stuarts and deciding on monarchy vs citizen leadership while the Dutch were devouring the East Indies, shoving out the Portuguese and initially blocking the later-arriving English. The Netherlands became the richest nation in Europe due the spice trade, enhanced manufacturing and in a large part due to the Protestant separation from the Catholic nations of Spain and France. The Netherlands controlled the island nation of Indonesia for over three centuries until December 27, 1949.

The early sailors of the Iberian Peninsula had two advantages over their northern brethren with their Atlantic Ocean ports and citric fruit brought by the invading Arabs of North Africa. Biochemistry in the form of oranges and lemons provided to the crew, quite by accident, reduced the incidence of scurvy. This enabled them to sail further and longer than other European ships of the 15th and 16th centuries. The Dutch medical officers, knowing the ravages of scurvy, forced crew to eat sour pickled cabbage and were happy to replace it with citric fruits. Not until the 18th century did the British medical officer James Lind prove that citric fruits contained a substance that prevented and treated scurvy. The British eventually solved their domestic quarrels and rapidly built its maritime strength. After a century of conflicts in Europe and abroad, a united Great Britain subdued both the Dutch merchant and military navies, establishing British naval supremacy until the 20th century.

The "Spice Islands" were four tiny volcanic tufts of land between New Guinea and Celebes, that fueled the European conquest of Indonesia. So valuable were nutmeg, mace and cloves, that men and ships were willing to risk years at sea to collect the few chemicals found here and no other place on earth. The Arabs were first to exploit them in the 14th century, naming them the Maluka Island (Islands of Kings in Arabic) and creating a huge market in Europe through merchants in Venice. Like the Opium Wars two and one-half centuries later, the Spice Wars between the European sea powers were about money. The value of spices was not for enhancing food dishes as they are today, but were believed to be powerful medicines, making riches worth the enormous risks (50-80% loss in ships and crew). The Portuguese arrived in the early 16th century followed by the Dutch in the early 1700's and eventually the Maluka Islands' natives were murdered and replaced by slaves working the plantations.

Almost everything that happens in the cell appears to follow rules and paths of strongly supposed biochemical theory. It is important to remember that biochemistry uses science to explain what the cell does; however, the cell may not be aware of what we think it is doing. No one has seen what happens at the molecular level and there is still much unknown about intracellular events when chemicals meet life. The "blueprints" of cellular activity are believed to be contained in the coils of DNA and RNA, blueprints that can be altered by chemicals (toxins), trauma (radiation), alien organisms and by chance encounters with particles passing through cells. An example of chance encounters are neutrinos, minute particles that pass through each cell at rates of hundreds of millions during the cell's life. Travelling at 7 million miles per hour, these tiny subatomic (much smaller than an atom) objects rarely strike any intracellular molecules, since most of the cell is empty space, however, when impact occurs, change is possible. This could be the mechanism for change within a cell, an organ and an organism, accounting for adaptations seen by Charles Darwin in the Galapagos Islands. Changes could lead to "improvements" or in some cases diseases such as cancer.

Cancer cells become more aggressive than the normal cells around them, growing and reproducing at a higher rate. To sustain this increase in growth, cancer cells "steal" resources from normal cells, soon displacing the less aggressive native cells, as the European Americans displaced the Native Americans. The Europeans were aided by germs and steel, the germs working at the cellular level while steel represented technology. Jared Diamond's "Guns, Germs, and Steel" describes how technology and infection allowed the European conquest of much of the Western world. Cortez landed 600 men a few horses and some big fighting dogs. Imported fevers and large numbers of death deaths preceded Cortez and continued to aid this tiny force in the destruction of an enormous civilization that in size and sophistication rivaled any European Nation.

Even larger effects aided Pizarro in South America where in a single generation populations and cultures collapsed. So destructive was the power of imported fevers, the population of the Amazon

Basin crashed to near extinction. Suddenly cities, millions of acres of agriculture and the total collapse of a culture reduced atmospheric CO_2 when millions of square miles of jungle replaced cultivation "overnight" in geological time. The Amazon Jungle is recent, appearing in the 16th century after Europeans introduced Smallpox and other infectious diseases that ravaged a population of tens of millions. Huge numbers of plants appeared on the vacant native agriculture, forming the world's largest jungle, requiring huge amounts of CO_2 to be sucked from the atmosphere. The sudden appearance of the Amazon jungle removed so much CO_2, it lowered global temperatures, reduced food supply and played a large role in "The Little Ice Age". This period saw glaciers growing, in some cases engulfing settlements in Europe, shortening summers, leading to poor harvest, famine and social disruption. The Little Ice Age preceded Black Death and increased its intensity after the depopulation of the Americas lasting into the 19th century.

In 1541a small part of Pizarro's invading force detached itself in the eastern Andes Mountains, and began an unexpected two-year boat voyage down the Amazon River. Here they encountered thousands of huge cities, large tracts of cultivation and an advanced civilization. Francisco Orellana's description of that trip had been disbelieved for centuries until recently because no one believed that a civilization of that enormous size could have been present. Cities and tens of millions of people disappeared under the rise of the massive Amazon jungle; their existence is being uncovered slowly as the jungle removed by clearing the great river basin. "River of Darkness" by Buddy Levy is an almost unbelievable description of Orellana's journey, a trip collaborated by a literate priest on the trip. For centuries these accounts were not believed because the "experts" of academia discounted the presence of an advanced extensive culture in the Amazon basin. The diseases Orellana spread on his trip down the Amazon depopulated an entire civilization and significantly enhanced The Little Ice Age.

The Kreps' Cycle

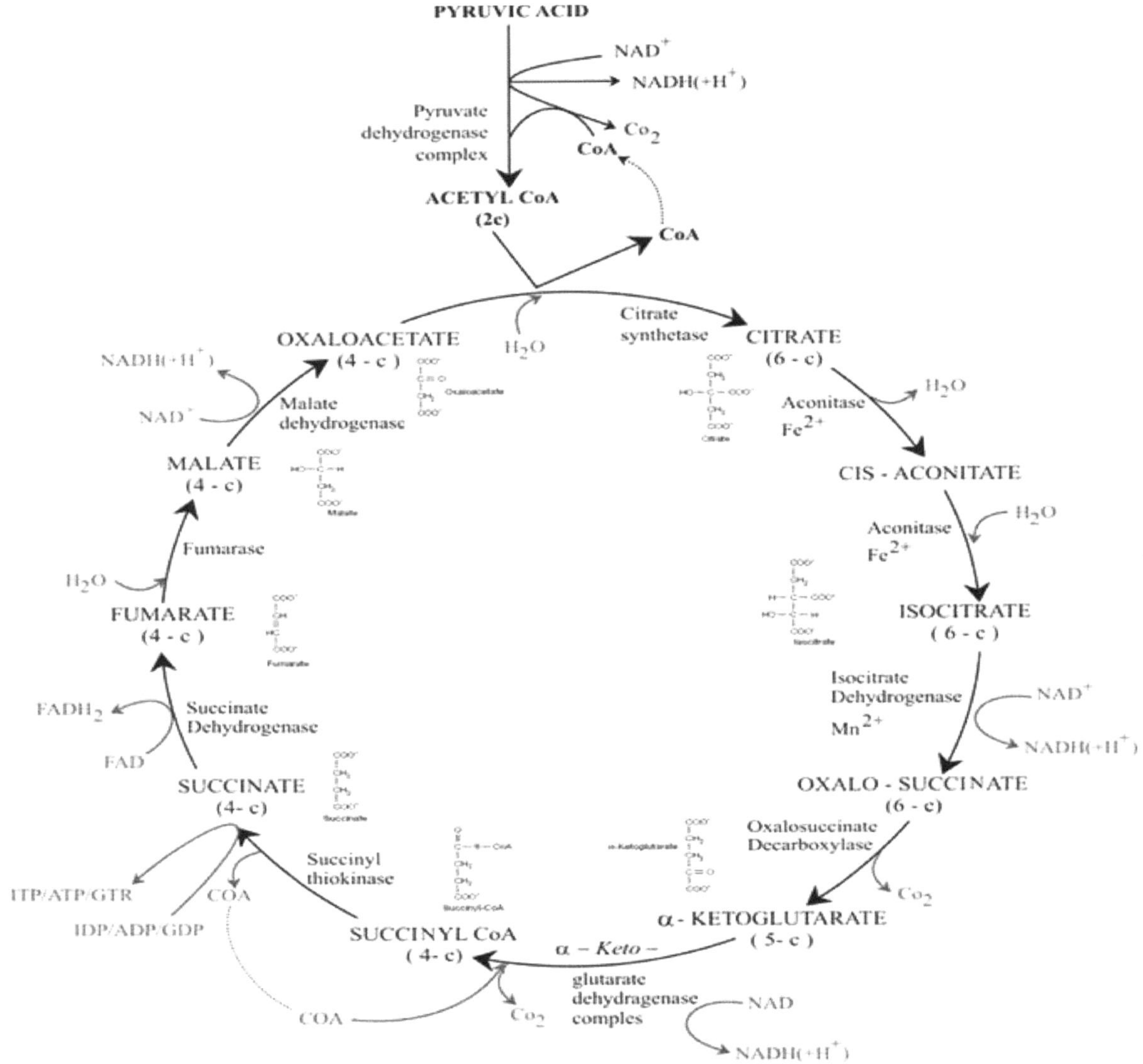

Complicated looking, isn't it? No one truly understands every reaction in the cycle at the molecular level, so do not feel bad if it looks complicated, because it is! In this two-dimensional picture, a larger "wheel" of chemical reactions is connected by smaller "wheels" of chemical reactions known as electron transfer systems. It starts with pyruvic acid which is formed when glucose is cleaved into two molecules. Once started, it follows a predictable series of chemical reactions, each reaction requires CoA, coenzymes (vitamins) such as NAD (vitamin B3), FAD (vitamin B2), H_2O and energy. NIH

The Elements

Chemistry study begins with the concept of elements, each unique structure with unique activity based on that structure. It is important to realize that these structures have never been seen; only strongly theorized and everything in the universe is made from the 92 known elements. These are represented on the periodic table discussed later. It is called The Periodic Table because the structures of elements on the table are repeated periodically, one atomic number at a time. The vertical columns are elements that have similar properties, and the horizontal columns are arranged in ascending order by the number of protons representing their atomic number. The first table was published in 1869 by the Russian scientist Demitri Mendeleev and even though his original table was incomplete, so predictable was his work; he predicted the presence and properties of undiscovered elements.

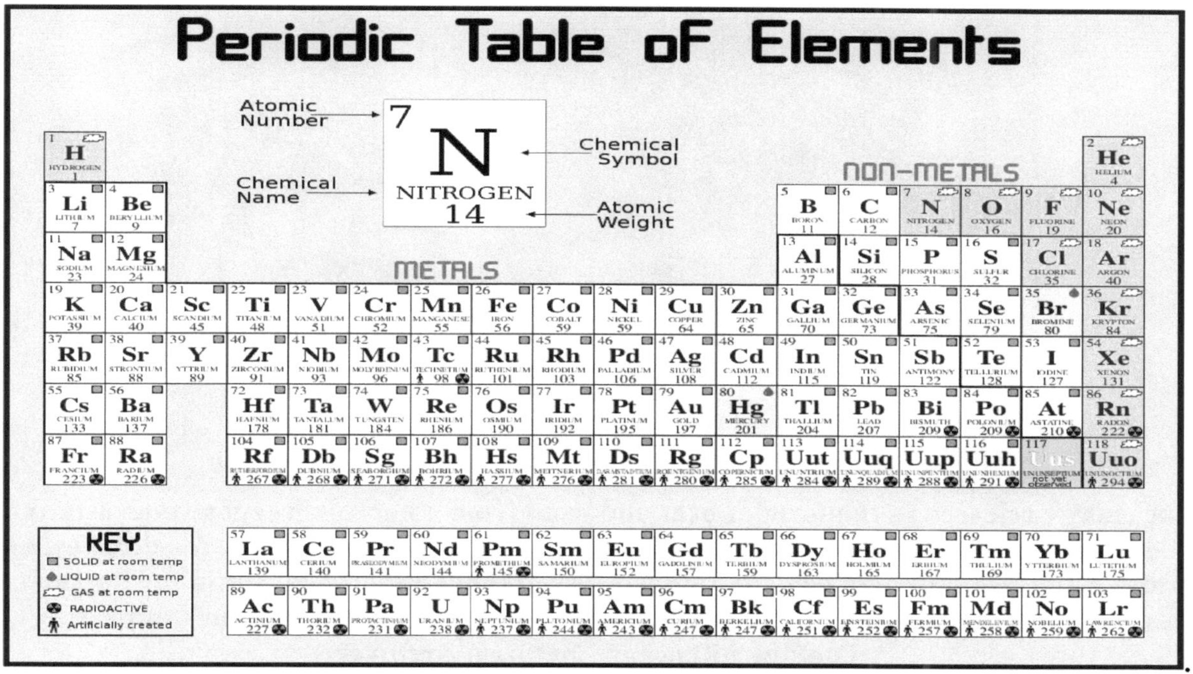

Periodic Table of elements contains the elements that make up everything in the known Universe. Only a minority of these elements are used in human cells under normal conditions. Some elements are essential to human cells while others are toxic. There are ninety-two natural elements found on earth, the heaviest being uranium with an atomic number of 92. The others following uranium are created in the lab, some lasting for only a few moments. The most famous man-made element is plutonium, the material used in the 2nd atomic bomb dropped on Nagasaki August 1945. NIST

There is a predictable order to the vertical and horizontal columns and the elements sharing similar properties are found together. In simple terms, chemical reactions occur because most elements have particles and/or units of energy to give up or to accept. In both cases, giving or accepting achieves a more stable, perhaps more comfortable existence. Giving and taking is the basis of biochemistry in the living cell, and in that respect, is not unlike human history. The tendency to transfer from one group of elements to another is reflected in the geography of the Periodic Table, as elements of the left side are more likely to interact with elements on the right side. Generally, the further apart from each other, the more likely the interaction, i.e., sodium (Na) on the extreme left side reacts eagerly with chlorine (Cl) on the extreme right side, both highly reactive elements by themselves. However, when combined, produce one of nature's most stable compounds, sodium chloride (table salt). The transfer of energy from one molecule to the other is the basis of the Krebs' Cycle and all reactions within the cell.

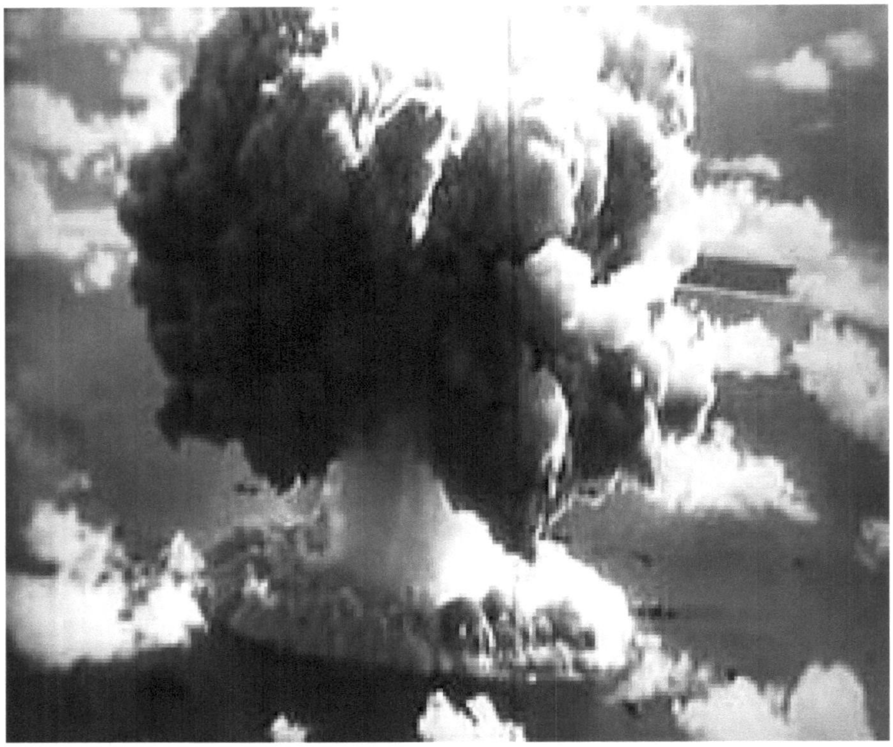

The energy released in the form of heat and wind from a nuclear weapon is devastating, while the delayed radiation effects of subatomic particles release continue for decades, even centuries, the result of high velocity impacts. Even though the atom within the human cell is overwhelmingly empty space, if bombarded by overwhelming numbers of particles, damage will occur. National Archives

Chemical reactions begin at the molecular level when atoms interact in a "dance" generally between two willing partners. However, the nuclear reaction in the image is too violent to be consensual. Atoms are composed of a dense nucleus of positively charged (+) charged protons clinging to neutrally charged neutrons, surrounded by clouds of negatively (-) charged electrons. If the nucleus of an atom were the size of a basketball, the first orbiting electron would be 2 miles away! This space between the nucleus and electrons is believed to be essentially empty, void of particles. Thus, almost all the space occupied by each atom is empty, allowing subatomic particles to pass through the atoms and cells in the tens of millions every moment without impact. Electrons migrate across these empty spaces as do people, seeking more stable environments. Migration to the molecular level is explained by valance.

Valance describes the number of electrons in the outer shell of an atom. Atoms are composed of a dense + charge nucleus with – charged electrons circling, traveling at a speed estimated at 36 million mph. Imagine the solar system, with the sun as the nucleus and the orbiting planets as electrons, however planets are much closer to sun and much larger than electrons. Electrons are moving so fast; they form a weaved shell (protective?) of energy around the nucleus. Piercing electron shells allows atoms to be split, thus nuclear power. Splitting extremely large atoms like uranium with its dense nucleus of 92 protons releases huge amounts of energy (nuclear fission), however nuclear fusion of atoms releases even more. The bombs used at Hiroshima and Nagasaki where fission bombs, later more destruction nuclear weapons were fusion bombs.

The closest shell to the nucleus has room for only two electrons, with successive shells holding 8, 18, 32 and 50. The sun is a huge mass of hydrogen atoms composed of a single proton and single neutron nucleus with a single orbiting electron. With intense heat and pressure in the forge of the Sun, hydrogen atoms are fused together forming Helium with two electrons circling its two protons and two neutrons. This fusion of hydrogen releases massive amounts of energy, energy that has been flooding the earth for billions of years. Much of the sun's energy is damaging and the earth's atmosphere and magnetic field protects living things from harmful radiation of nuclear fusion. The sun, like other stars will eventually run out of fuel but not before finishing this text.

When the outer shell of an atom is full, the atom feels no need to accept or donate electrons, rendering it less likely to react with other elements and compounds. Some elements contentedly contain full outer shells such as the "noble" gases. These elements are inert and chemically snobbish, refusing to react with others from the far-right side of the Periodic table. The closer the outer shell is to being full, i.e. needing electrons to fill, the more aggressive the atom is in attracting electrons from other atoms. On the other hand, atoms that have isolated electrons in their outer shell are electrons readily given up.

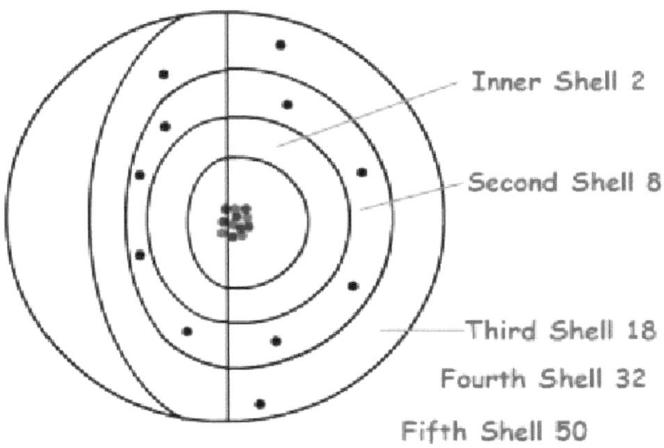

The more the electrons, the more the shells, the more the potential energy. The higher the placement on the periodic table the denser the atom.

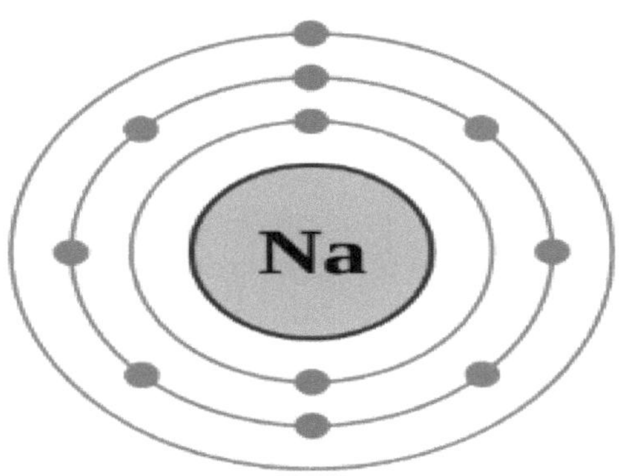

Note sodium's single electron, all alone in its outer orbit, eager to migrate, leaving behind a more stable atom with its outer shell filled. After electron release, sodium now has positive charge, Na+

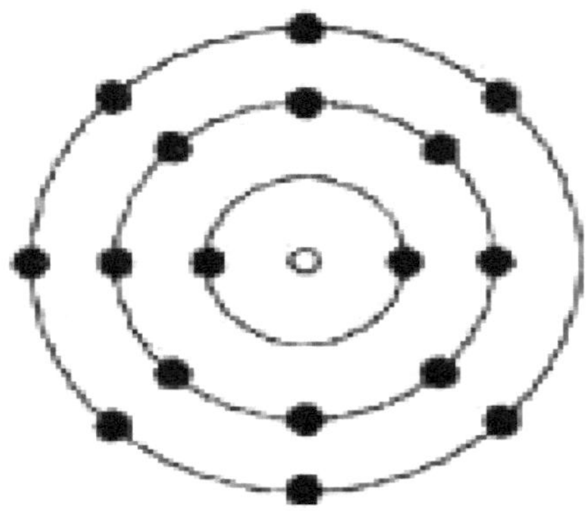

Chlorine has 7 electrons in its outer shell, needing a single electron to obtain a more stable atom. Acquiring that electron gives it a negative charge Cl-. The electron transfer from sodium to chlorine satisfies both, creating one of nature's most stable molecules, table salt. However, when combined with water, they eagerly separate into charged particles. Chloride, like the other halogens, need electrons to fill outer shells, making them highly reactive, therefore, useful in purifying water. Iodine is a halogen vital to human health. The thyroid gland captures dietary iodine to produce thyroxine, a hormone that affects all cells. It is also used in the event of a nuclear accident or nuclear warfare to prevent thyroid cancer when exposed to ionizing radiation.

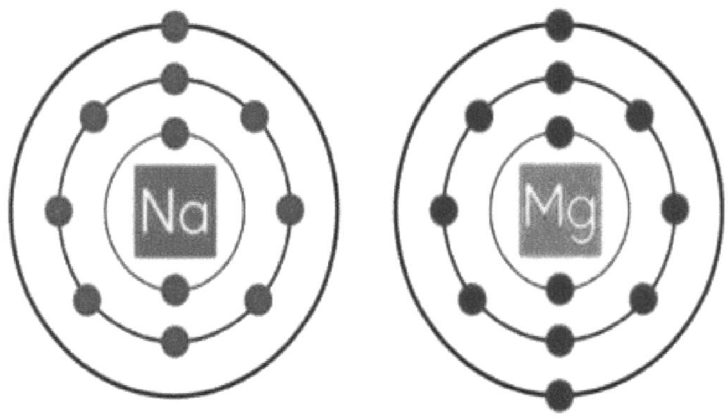

Compared to sodium, magnesium has 2 electrons to donate, becoming Mg++. Magnesium is commonly found bound to calcium which needs 2 electrons to fill its outer shell.

All chemicals have a structure, and the shape of a molecule dictates its function. Just as the hand is formed a certain way allowing it to grip, stroke, illustrate, perform surgery and a host of other functions, combining strength and finesse. A molecule is a single element, or a single group of elements bound together. A single atom is a molecule while insulin, also a single molecule, contains 257 carbon atoms, 383 hydrogens, 65 nitrogens, 77 oxygens and 6 sulphurs.

The periodic table begins with hydrogen, the simplest element with a single proton giving it an atomic number of 1. As the number of protons increases one at a time going from left to right, the elements become larger, heavier and more complex. The atomic number is the number of protons in the atom, the atomic weight is the summation of protons and neutrons. After hydrogen, helium has 2, lithium with 3 and so on until uranium with 92 protons is reached as the last of the known natural elements. Currently 18 synthetic (manmade) elements have been added beyond uranium.

The most notorious of these, plutonium, atomic number 94, is the explosive material that was "split" in the second atomic bomb dropped on Nagasaki august 1945. So powerful is plutonium that the amount of explosives in that bomb was the size of a 25-cent piece containing enough energy to destroy a large modern city. It did require several billion dollars, the creation of three new cities (Oak Ridge, Tennessee Los Alamos, New Mexico and Hanford, Washington) complete with schools, hospitals, shopping centers along with thousands of scientists to produce enough atomic material to build three atomic bombs.

Elements active in the human cell are found in scattered clusters on the Periodic Table, some are interchangeable in the biochemistry of the cell. On the left side, the four metals of sodium (Na), magnesium (Mg), calcium (Ca) and potassium (K), all with electrons to donate and critical to the human cell. While on the opposite right side, the cluster, carbon (C), nitrogen (N), oxygen (O), phosphorous (P) and sulfur (S) are found together in both vertical and horizontal orientation. These nine elements along with chlorine compose most of the chemicals necessary for life. The "alkali" metals on the left side have electrons to donate and are highly attracted to the halogens and other select elements opposite them on the right side. The halogens, fluorine, chlorine, bromine and iodine are considered the most likely to enter relationships with other elements, as they need electrons to fill their outer shells. Halogens are the only group of related elements that are found in all three states on earth, chlorine as a gas, bromine as a liquid and iodine as a solid. Halogens are found in teeth, hair, ivory, blood cells, thyroid gland, and in trace amounts in all animal cells. Florine is 2nd only to Sulphur in its ability to acquire electrons.

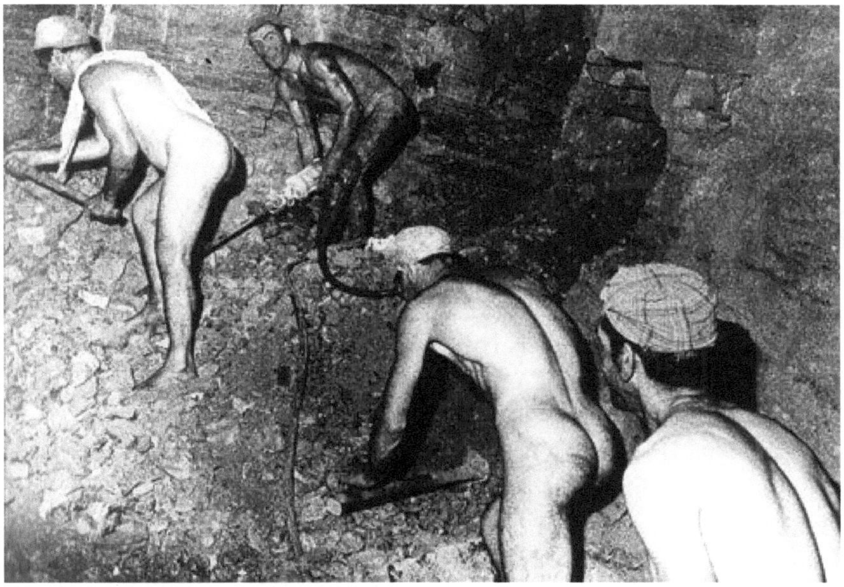

Little had changed in three millennia of sulfur mining in Sicily. National Library of Congress

Sulfur, atomic number 16, is especially interesting to the author for both medical and historical reasons. It is the most active element, reacting with every other element except gold, platinum and noble gases. Sulfur is the 10th most abundant element on earth and a common component of oil refining (important for the history of Sicily). It was used in ancient Egypt for eyelid infection (trachoma) and by the Greeks to fumigate rooms to kill insects. Alchemist of the Middle Ages compounded topical ointments of sulfur and tar for skin ailments, a treatment still commonly used in scalp and skin disorders. Even before Greece and Rome, the mines of the volcanic island of Sicily provided the bulk of sulfur in the Mediterranean world and the mines were notorious man-killers. The largest volcano in Europe, Mt Etna, the world's most dangerous volcano, dominates an island of other volcanoes filled with sulfur-laden rock. Generations of slaves spent their short lives, providing this element to the world.

For thousands of years, Sicily's slave mines were notorious man-killers. Working in dark underground caverns where temperatures of 113 degrees were common and air filled with sulfuric acid, made for a short, painful life. By the 19th century, boys entered the mines at 6-8 years of life and each year in the mines, suffered repeated respiratory ailments. Poorly fed, only a few grew over 5 feet, and fewer were alive at 40. Silicosis, chronic lung disease from inhaling minerals, was first described in Sicily's miners and later seen in coal miners and the asbestos industry. It is a disease still commonly seen today. As oil refining came into use in the early 20th century, removing sulfur from crude oil replaced mines. Mining in Sicily collapsed suddenly, leaving a population of unnecessary workers and their families, sending a large wave of immigrants to the United States as the Irish potato blight did sixty years earlier. Booker T Washington, born in slavery, rose to be a respected scholar, advisor to Presidents and world traveler. He visited Sicily after the mining collapse and wrote about it in his manifesto, "The Man Farthest Down". His description of poverty, disease and oppression on the island was dismal when compared to oppressed African Americans living in the South in the early 1900s. Dr Washington wrote that the American negro has greater access to education, property, a higher standard of living, longer life and greater religious freedom than the natives of Sicily. He compared the sulfur mines "to the nearest thing to hell I expect to see in this life". Not surprisingly, people are left in great numbers and currently 5 million Sicilians live in Sicily while 17 million live in the US alone.

Sulfur was essential to the rise of the industrial world, and Sicily was the primary source. Many nations' economies depended on its supply, causing conflict over its control. The "Sulfuric Crisis" was a near war between France and England over control of Sicily's valuable sulfur in the 1830's. The resource had been controlled by the British, who had ruthlessly exploited both the mines and the people of Sicily, acquiring a monopoly on the mining, processing and transport of the world's most abundant supply. The French recovering from Napoleon's defeat demanded a share of this abuse, almost leading to a shooting war. It was Sicily's sulfur that helped power 19th century's Industrial Revolution as almost every industrial enterprise required large amounts of sulfur. There are other smaller deposits of sulfur in the form of cinnabar, a blood red ore found in much of world. After extracting the sulfur, the vermillion pigment is used as dye for textile and wool, body paint in Native Americans, to color pottery and for the red color of art on caves and canvas. Brimstone in the Bible and other ancient texts is Sulphur, essential for human cell function, and at the same time extremely toxic. It is found on the Periodic Table among a cluster of elements representing some of the most active in life: Oxygen, Phosphorus, Nitrogen, Selenium and in some animals, Arsenic.

The term arsenic, atomic number 34 comes from the Greek word *arsenikon* meaning male and virile, as low dose dietary arsenic appeared to improve vitality. Later in the Bronze Age it was added to tin and copper to produce a stronger metal. Teamsters in mountainous terrain knew to add small amounts of arsenic to their horse's fodder as it increased their stamina pulling loads uphill. Dr Hahnemann, known as the father of Homeopathy, recognized that arsenic, even though a poison, at low doses has positive effects on cells. Small doses of arsenic are essential for rats, hamsters, goats and chickens. Animal husbandry used arsenic for centuries to increase size and weight of chickens, hogs, cows and other meat animals. Today, some commercial feed contains small amounts of arsenic for the same reason. Herds of herbivores also require salt supplement to reproduce.

Arsenic was used by the ancients as an antibiotic and penicillin replaced it and mercury for treatment of syphilis. It was applied to wigs as a powder to discourage lice. An arsenic containing chemical was Paul Ehrlich's agent #606, named because it was the 606th drug studied to treat syphilis with less harm than mercury. In the First World War, arsenic combined with organophosphate produced a blister agent poison gas and later as a defoliate (agent blue) in Viet Nam. In high doses, arsenic uncouples oxidative phosphorylation due to its close association with phosphorus on the Periodic Table. Inside the cell, arsenic can replace the phosphorus molecule in essential reactions. It has been used as a pesticide, herbicide, insecticide and as a preservative in wood for centuries. Arsenic is still being used in medicine as a radioactive molecule in a PET scan. Arsenic is also the 2nd most common semiconductor in electronics and has contaminated much of the world's drinking water.

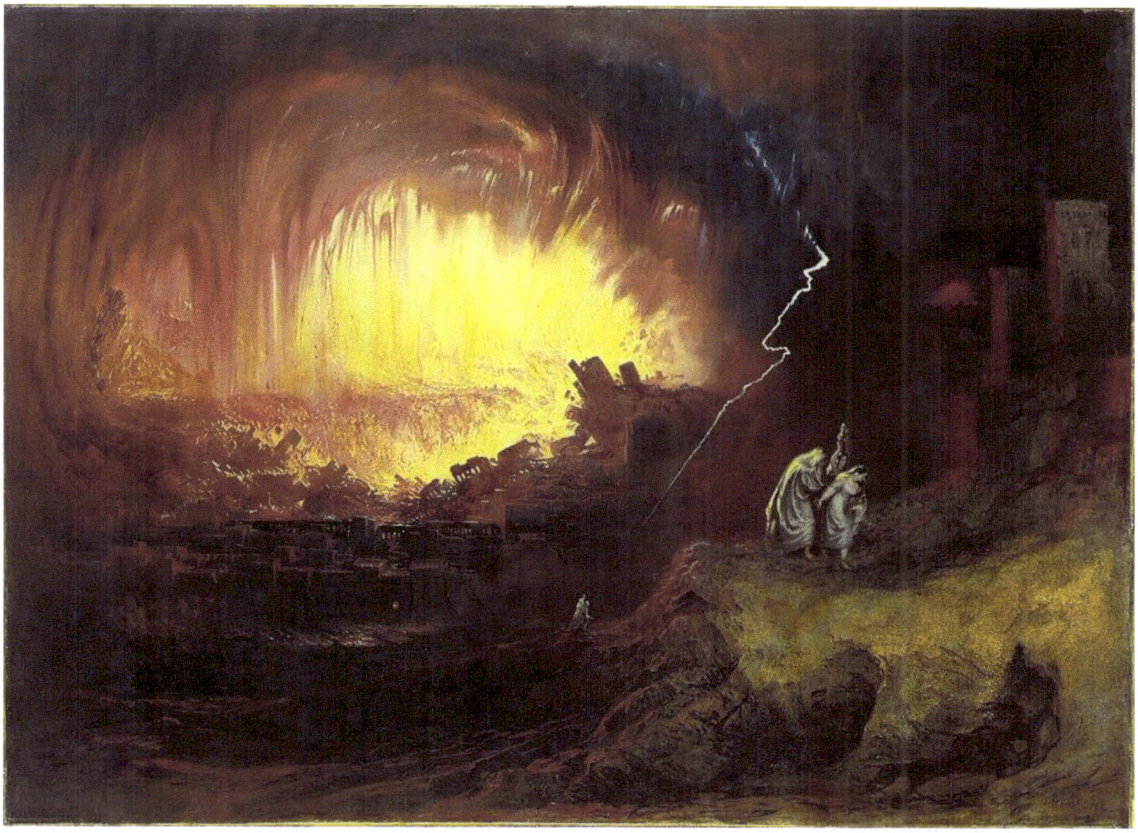

"The Destruction of Sodom and Gomorrah" by John Martin, 1852. The story of God's destruction by a rain of fire found in Torah, Christian Bible and the Quran.

Phosphorous, atomic number 15 is too reactive to be found alone in nature since it freely attaches to other molecules, especially oxygen forming phosphate, PO_4. Phosphorous is one of the "party animals" on the periodic table. The word phosphorus is Greek for "light-bearer" while the Latin word is Lucifer, and phosphorus was called "The Devil's Element" by the Catholic Church because of its incendiary use in munitions. Phosphorus was the 13th element discovered by Hamburg chemist, Hennig Brand in 1669. Hamburg was the first city to receive phosphorous-incendiary bombs July 1943, code name Operation Gomorrah which created one of the largest human-generated fire storms of World War II, killing and wounding 80,000 civilians and destroying the city. The book "The 13th Element" by John Emsley is a good read about the history and chemistry of phosphorous. Organic phosphates are used in detergents, pesticides, fertilizers and nerve gas. When mixed with sulfuric acid it creates a superphosphate fertilizer. In humans, 90% of phosphate is found in bones and teeth. It is essential for most chemical reactions and structures in the cell.

Another cluster of elements essential to the biochemistry of life are three metals in the mid part of Periodic Table. Mn (manganese), Fe (iron) and Co (cobalt) each with a higher atomic number going left to right. These are "inorganic" (term means not associated with living things) metals with similar structure and behavior, becoming "organic" within the cell. Chlorophyll contains manganese, hemoglobin contains iron and B12 contains cobalt, all three closely related metals found enclosed in similar phosphate-rich ring structures (pyrimidines) in widely different cells performing similar functions.

At the molecular level, human cells take incoming molecules and transform them from one structure to another, depending on the function needed by the cell. Why is the study of chemistry a large part of medicine since few medical officers use chemistry in practice? Because even if unseen, chemistry plays a role in every medical condition, including those encountered in the field. An understanding of chemicals and their interactions within the cell, although not required to be a good medical officer, makes more sense. At any moment within trillions of every human cell, thousands of interconnected chemical reactions are all following specific pathways. The cell never rests. Visible findings of diseases known throughout history, i.e. fever, rash, eyes and skin staining yellow in hepatitis, bleeding in hemorrhagic fevers, shortness of breath and pain in heart attack are symptoms and signs of manifestations of chemical events inside the affected cells and tissues.

Great events in human history have been shaped by biochemistry when human cells are deprived of essential chemicals or exposed to toxic chemicals, the human story has been affected. For all to go well, a healthy cell needs circulating fluid, oxygen and a constant supply of "the right stuff", while protected from "the bad stuff". The absence of essential chemicals has begun a chain of historical events like a chain of chemical reactions in the cell. Biochemistry has been an often silent yet important player in historical events, in some cases due to the lack of "the right stuff". One such story is about a simple missing chemical; its absence came close to changing world history.

Thiamine

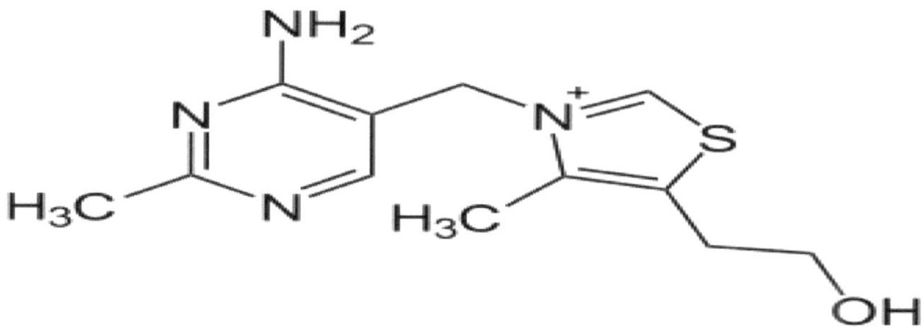

The lack of this chemical structure has affected armies, navies and explorers

Thiamine is a vital essential component of the human diet lost from certain foods in their preparation and storage. A loss that can lead to deficiencies and serious disease. A diet dependent on polished rice where the unattractive husks (stores longer without its water-retaining husk) are removed, will not sustain the human cell. A diet inadequate in thiamine occurred during the Russian Japanese War 1904-5, with almost disastrous results for the Imperial Japanese Navy. Once again in Napoleon supposed words, "an army moves on its stomach", however in the following story, it was a navy.

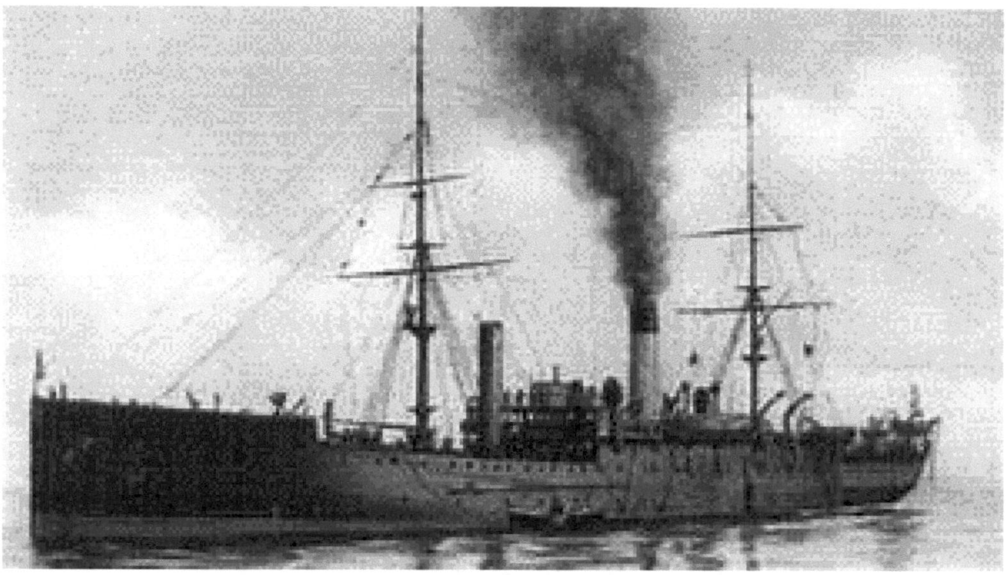

The Imperial Russian repair ship *Kamchatka*, the most infamous repair vessel to ever sail

Thiamine, vitamin B_1, C_{12} $H_{17}N_4$ O S (note the sulfur molecule) contains five of the six most common elements in a human cell and is essential for cell survival. Early summer 1905 found two modern steam-driven steel fleets fighting with rifled cannons and self-propelled torpedoes for the first time, in one of the most important sea battles of the 20th century. The absence of thiamine could have led to the destruction of the Imperial Japanese Navy, only saved by the ineptitude of the Imperial Russian Navy. A vitamin deficiency (beriberi) that should have been prevented by competent Japanese medical officers almost rendered their navy dysfunctional. The diet of the Japanese Navy was primarily based on polished rice, as it has a longer shelf life once the husks are removed. The advantages in storage were the cost of nutrition. The Imperial Japanese Navy (IJN) had essentially been a coastal fleet fed a diet dominated by polished rice augmented by frequent stops at local ports where unpolished rice, fresh vegetables and meats were obtained. However, in the war between Russia and Japan, the Japanese Navy was forced to attack and blockade the Russian fleet anchored in Port Arthur on the Asian mainland. This required the Japanese fleet to be at sea for months with no supply vessels to replenish stores. The ships and their medical officers were not prepared for a preventable disease caused by living on stored rations without fresh supplements. The Russian fleet was also suffering from widespread disease and medically disability that even competent medical care could not overcome.

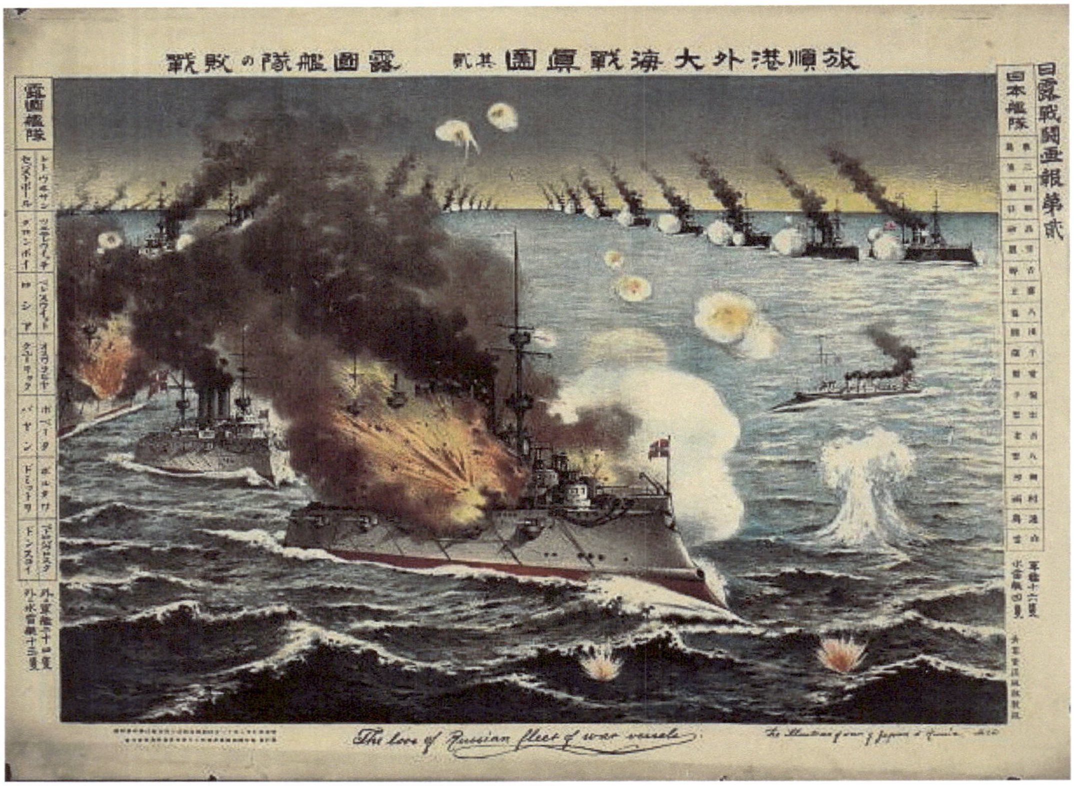
旅順港外大海戦圖 其弐 露國艦隊の敗戦
日露戦闘画報第弐
The loss of Russian fleet of war vessels

Battle of Tsushima Straits May 27-28, 1905, was the most important sea battle since Trafalgar a century earlier, and a battle that would have profound effects in the first half of the 20th century. Drawing was done by art student at Kyoto University and turned into mass produced post card. In forty-five minutes of the first shot, the battle and ultimately the war was lost by Russia. National Library of Congress

The world expected Imperial Russia to defeat Japan on land and sea. Unfortunately for the Russians, they were successful at neither. The mighty Imperial Russian fleet was so soundly defeated in a single battle, it ultimately lost the war. However, Russia refused to realize it until tens of thousands Russia soldiers were lost. The Russia Fleet leaving the Baltic Sea started with the flagship running aground minutes after lifting its anchor. A common Russian saying "and then things got worst" rang true when the *Kamchatka* mistaking British fishing trawlers for Japanese gunships (18,000 miles from Japan?) opened fire almost resulting the Russian fleet being attacked by the British Royal Navy. The Russian fleet's speed was dictated by the slowest ships, took months to reach the Far East in an effort that has been compared to Hannibal crossing the Alps with elephants. After sailing and steaming from the Baltic and Black Sea around South Africa (the French and English refused them passage through Suez Canal and the Russian Admiral feared a Japanese attack in the closed space of the canal?), across the Indian Ocean, up the South China Sea. After 18,000 miles of steaming, the Imperial Russian fleet was worn out, the men and ships fatigued. There were forty-two warships in the fleet, some were crudely converted large pleasure yachts from the Black Sea with deck guns fitted. The Russian officers knew there was no Pacific Fleet left to aid them because earlier in the war, Japan attacked Port Arthur without declaring war (as Japan did at Pearl Harbor in December 1941), leaving much of Russia's Pacific Fleet on the bottom of its harbor. The Second Pacific Squadron was on its own, hoping to defeat a waiting fleet after steaming thousands of ocean miles with many of the crews ill and the ships worn out from steaming with flammable coal dust on decks and in corners. Taking on coal often at sea (the first time in history) from other ships and dock had scattered coal dust throughout the ships. Russian Medical officers reported increased respiratory complaints in the fleet likely from coal dust inhalation.

Deprived of the Port Arthur Fleet and its deep protected anchorage to rest and refit before battle, a decision was made to dash through the Straits of Tashima instead of sailing around the east side of Japan, the longer and safer route. Admiral Razhdestvensky and his command decided to sail between the Korean Peninsula and the Japanese islands in the confined space of the Tashima Straits in part for medical reasons. Illness had overwhelmed the medical services (after refueling in Madagascar, much of the crew came away infected with STDS) and upon entering the straits, the Russian fleet was ill-prepared to fight in storm-torn open sea. The author could find no accounts of the "Voyage of the Damned" by the fleet's medical officers, but it must have been a grim experience for those entrusted in providing medical care. Dozens of ships, thousands of men, some too exhausted or ill to leave their bunks, faced high winds, waves breaking over decks and an enemy fleet armed with rifled artillery and fast-moving torpedoes. A few hours destroyed Russia's vaunted sea power, a power that Peter the Great begin building 200 years before.

The Russian sailors were in poor shape for an ocean battle; however, the Japanese sailors may have been in worse condition due to a serious medical condition, thiamine deficiency (beriberi). After months at sea, thiamine was absent from the Japanese sailor's diet, exclusively fed on polished rice, rendering most too weak to stand duty. Since cells have no way to store thiamine, the Japanese sailors needed a steady supply to maintain function. A cell must have "the right stuff", otherwise it cannot maintain its health and without the right stuff, performance suffers. The Battle of Tsushima Straits established Japan as a Pacific Ocean Sea power, setting the stage for later conflict with United States. Fought over two days, May 27-28, 1905, in rough seas with fleets filled with tired and ill sailors. Dozens of ships and thousands of men perished in weather and seas too severe for survivors to be rescued.

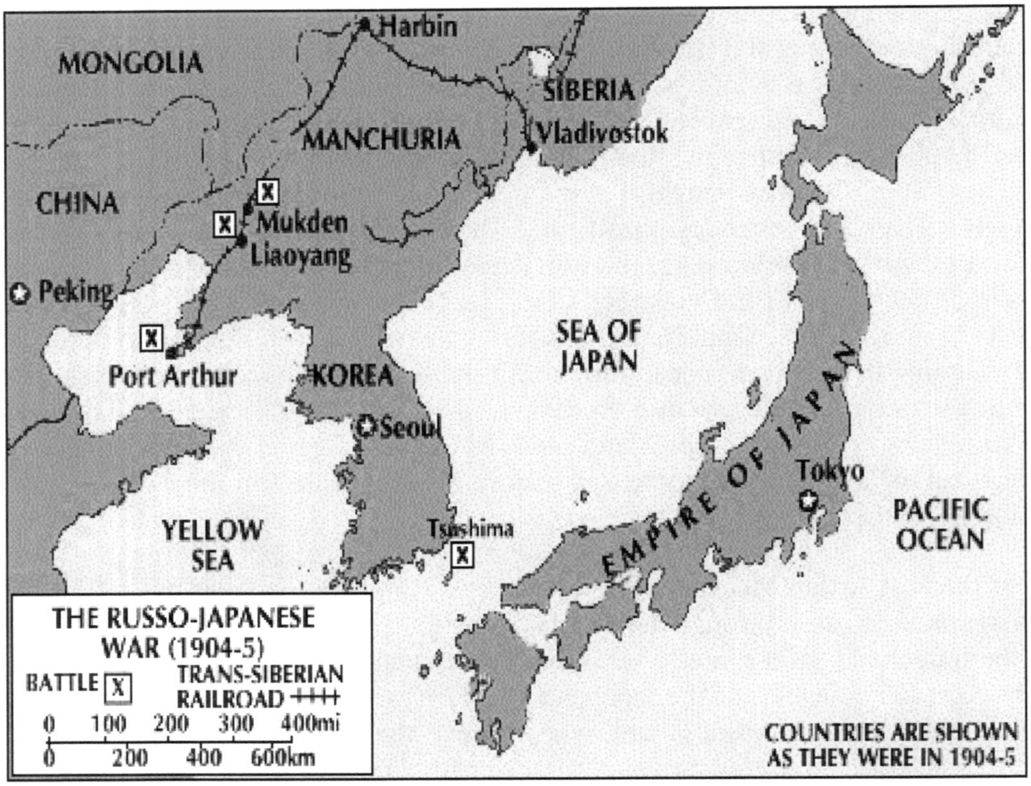

Port Arthur was closer than Vladivostok and better protected from weather, but the Japanese blockade of Port Arthur forced a passage through narrow enemy controlled waters. Note the battles at Mukden and Liaoyang that isolated Port Arthur from land. Machine guns were used in large numbers for the first time in warfare, accounting for the high numbers of infantry dead. The battle of Mukden had military observers from several European nations but the lesson of the machine gun effects on infantry must not have been appreciated.

Most of Japan's ships contained enlisted men so lethargic, few were able to man their battle stations. Fortunately for the Japanese, officers had access to small amounts of dried fish and vegetables providing just enough men to fire guns and launch torpedoes while keeping the ship's engines and steerage functional. At the time of battle, the Russian fleet arrived with thirty-eight warships including eight battleships, four of which were modern with assorted armed escorts. Since the Russian fleet left with minimal ammunition, little to no gunnery practice had been employed on the outbound voyage and due to at-sea coaling, the ships' deck had a layer of flammable coal dust reducing the enthusiasm for gunnery practice. The Imperial Japanese Navy had only four modern battleships (all built in Europe), with smaller guns and fewer supporting cruisers and destroyers but was fighting in its home waters with adequate gunnery practice.

The Russian Fleet might have escaped ambush had not Admiral Rozhestvensky obeyed international maritime law requiring his trailing full-to-capacity hospital ships (some converted yachts) to display running lights. The lights of hospital ships alerted the waiting Japanese fleet to the long-exposed line of Russian ships in the van of the hospitals. Imitating Horatio Nelson at Trafalgar one hundred years earlier, Admiral Togo with fewer ships and with most men in sick beds "crossed the T" of the line of Russian ships and all but annihilated the enemy fleet. Russia lost 30 ships with most hands, leaving only a small portion of the fleet still floating, never to challenge Japan again at sea in the war. Rumor has it that the sailors cheered *Kamchatka's* sinking.

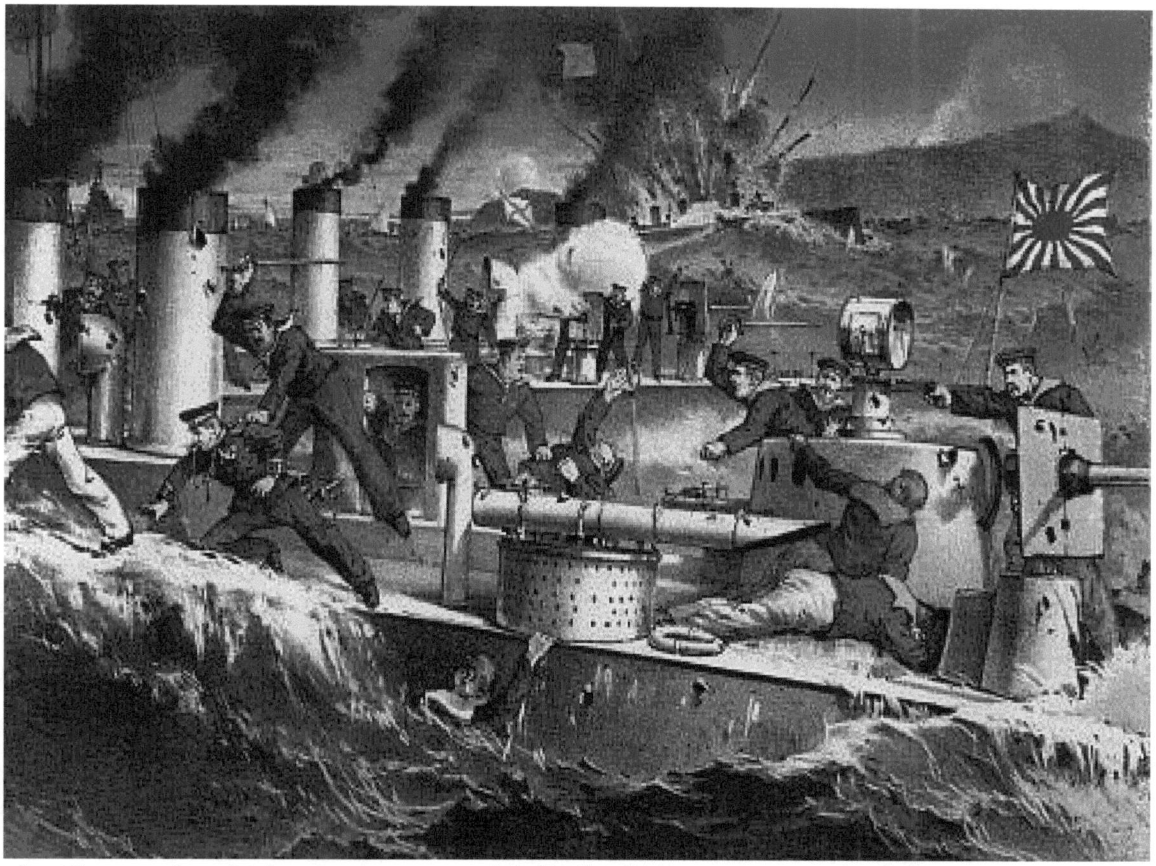

The battle was fought in stormy seas with little chance to rescue survivors. Above picture depicts a Japanese destroyer sinking a Russia destroyer with torpedoes. Japan surprised the Russians with their gunnery skills and highly advanced self-propelled torpedoes, as they surprised the Allies thirty-six years later with the "long Lance" torpedo in the Second World War. The long-lance torpedoes were especially deadly in the waters off Guadalcanal in 1942 where they devastated Allied warships early in the war. Artist Ryozo Tanaka National library of congress

In the 1930's from their land bases in Korea and Manchuria taken from Russia, Japan invaded China, claiming it was a peaceful occupation (the Rape of Nanking). Following World War I, Japan as an allied combatant took former German islands, included the Bismarck Archipelago, named for the 19th century German Prime Minister who had created Germany with "Iron and Blood", the Solomon Islands (King Solomon of the Old Testament) including Guadalcanal and Bougainville, the Marshalls (Majuro, Eniwetok), Carolinas (Truk) and Marianas (Guam, Saipan, and Tinian) islands. Between the World Wars Japan illegally converted these islands into a chain of fortified bases requiring thousands of American causalities to occupy. Currently China, North Korea and Japan are contesting tiny islands in the waters of Tsushima Straits, while China is building artificial islands in the waters of other Pacific nations.

Perhaps for the first time is history, it was possible that a fleet admiral could not only lose a battle, but a war in the space of few hours. This belief was so feared during the Great War 1914-1918, only one fleet action took place at Jutland where British and German fleets clashed for the only time in four years of war and the outcome determined ambiguous due to caution on both sides. The Battle of Midway in May 1942, while not ending World War II, destroyed Japan's offensive sea power in a single battle. At the Normandy Landings, the Allied admirals were so afraid of losing ships, they kept their floating gun platforms too far from the German shore batteries to inflict damages on the coastal forts. D-Day was the least effective naval gun fire and aviation bombing in the entire Second War.

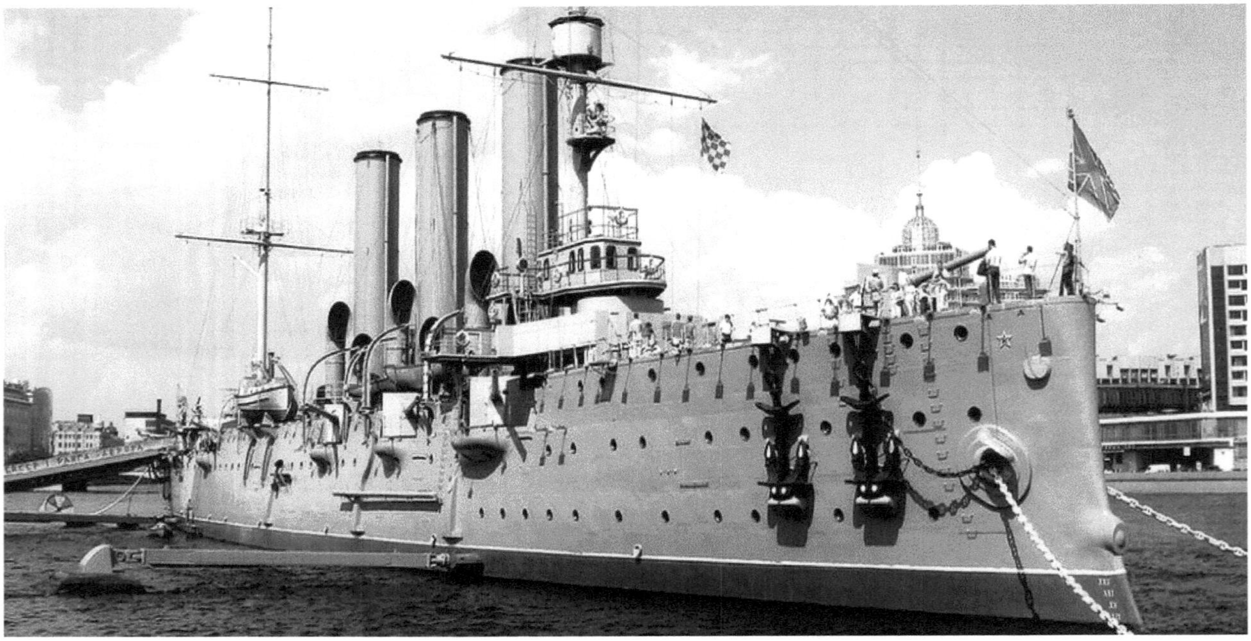

***Aurora*, One of few Russia survivors of the battle of Tsushima Straits, now a museum piece laying in Saint Petersburg harbor**

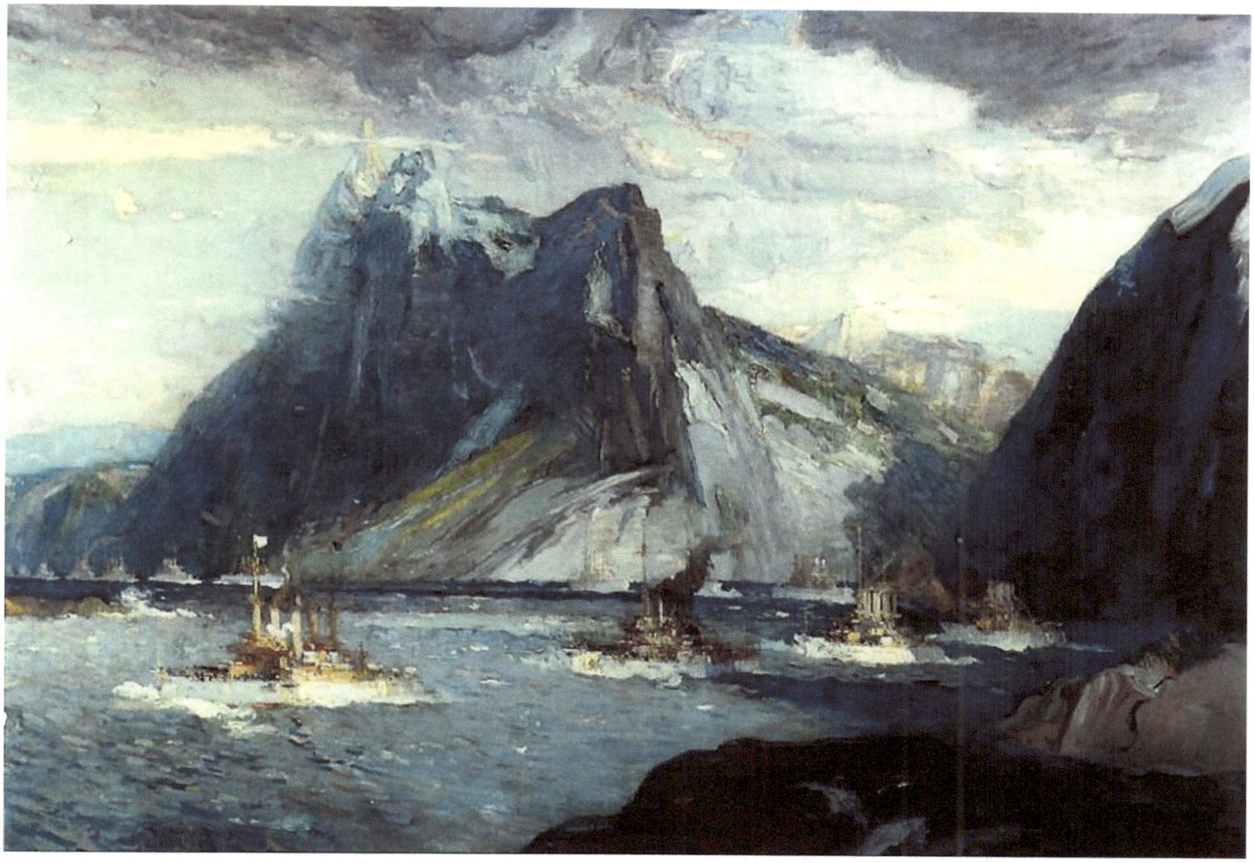

"The Great White Fleet" transiting Straits of Magellan by Harry Reuterdahl, America's first circumnavigation to show the American Flag.

Following the Russian-Japan War, in 1907 President Theodore Roosevelt sent the United States Navy's modern war fleet on a 43,000-mile circumnavigation of the world. All ships built since American Spanish War but by 1914, these coal-burning ships were obsolete after only twenty years of service. In addition to displaying America's naval, they provided humanitarian and field medical aid to the survivors of yet another earthquake on the sulfur island of Sicily and recovered the bodies of the American Consul Arthur S Cheney and his wife. In contrast to the early obsolescence of Roosevelt's ships, Admiral Nelson's flagship, the HMS Victory was over fifty years old at the Battle of Trafalgar. The 47-year-old one-armed sailor survived a serious upper extremity wound due to good wound care when wounds were often fatal and when not, left permanent disability. Nelson was one of several young naval officers that survived upper extremity injuries and went on to leave a mark in history. During the Battle of Tsushima Straits, a recent graduate of the Imperial Naval Academy serving as a junior gunnery officer on an Imperial Japanese cruiser lost two fingers on his left hand, had three fingers been lost, he would have been mustered from the navy as medically of unfit. With only eight fingers, he later graduated from the Japan's Naval Staff College, studied at Harvard, was allowed to attend the US Naval War College, at age forty became a naval aviator and became commanding officer of all naval forces. If his wounds had not been carefully examined, cleaned, repaired, dressed and cared for, the man that planned both the surprise attack on Pearl Harbor and the Battle of Midway, Admiral Yamamoto likely would not be in this book. While decoding the secret Japonese naval code, the Americans learned he was touring his Pacific bases by plane to promote

morale after loses at Midway and Guadalcanal. Knowing his flight plan, American P-38 fighters were sent over a long low altitude flight deep into enemy territory where Yamamoto's transport plane and escorts were shot down over the jungles of Bougainville Island. Some would despair the deliberate assignation of a foreign leader, while others might desire to preserve Yamamoto's leadership, since his attack on Pearl Harbor failed to destroy the repair docks or the extensive fuel tanks at Pearl Harbor, while sinking ships made obsolete with carrier warfare. Admiral Nagumo who commanded from the front at Pearl Harbor and Midway was strongly disliked by Yamamoto, yet the rigidity of the Japanese military hierarchy, dictates the most senior officer not the most competent, got command. Nagumo was too timid at Pearl Harbor. His fleet could have sent more waves of airplanes damaging the port severely, damage that would take a year to repair. The repair docks, cranes and especially the huge petroleum tanks were essentially untouched, high quality naval war assets left intact. Yamamoto's leadership from the rear was blunted by Nagumo caution, also a former gunnery officer and not an aviator. Much of Pearl Harbor was functional within weeks and all but three of the damaged ships in Yamamoto's attack were repaired and participated in Japan's defeat. Pearl Harbor was a huge strategic defeat for Japan and Yamamoto's' leadership. An example that leading from the rear is seldom as successful leading from the front. More aggressive leadership at Pearl Harbor could have allowed the entire Japanese fleet to sail into the nearly defenseless harbor and use their deck guns to wreak havoc, as the only US Navy warships available were trapped and sinking at their anchors. Admiral Halsey had taken Pearl Harbor's carriers and support ships days before from Pearl Harbor, delivering aircraft to Midway and were days away from the attack. Pearl Harbor, proclaimed by General Marshall to both houses of Congress in August 1941, "is the most powerful fortress in the world and is impregnable." It wasn't impregnable, it was vulnerable. After missing the American carriers at Pearl Harbor, in May of 1942, Yamamoto planned to lure the American Pacific carrier fleet into the open ocean and defeat it. The same plan the Confederacy deployed when General Lee entered Pennsylvania eighty years earlier. Both Lee and Yamamoto divided their forces with almost no intelligence of the enemy's strength or location, and both leaders were in the rear when the battles began. On the other hand, the Union at Gettysburg and US Navy at Midway had intelligence of the invader and aggressive leadership at the point of attack with their force concentrated. Japan had nine carriers available in May 1942, sending only four to attack Midway with its other forces widely scattered in the Pacific attacking Aleutians islands in a feint attack. Japan expected an American response to the Alaska invasion and were unaware that US Navy code breakers knew the real attack was at Midway. Yamamoto who planned the distracting attack with part of his forces awaited with huge armada of heavy warships under his personal command 400 miles away from Midway. And once again, the timid, rigid Nagumo was in command of a third force at the point of attack. There was a defect in Japanese military leadership by allowing Nagumo to lead another carrier fleet action and Nagumo's decisions and leadership at Midway were inadequate for the task. Had Yamamoto's warships appeared beside Nagumo's carrier fleet, this concentration of force would have overwhelmed the Americans with only three carriers and support ships. Men who knew Yamamoto at Harvard and as a Naval attaché' remarked on his aggressive poker play. Yamamoto did plan aggressive attacks, but his plans were placed in the hands of an inflexible field commander. Aggressive leadership by General Lee lost Gettysburg while

lack of aggressive leadership strategically lost Pearl Harbor and tactically lost at Midway. The enormous Japanese loss at Midway mimics the loss suffered by Ottoman Turkey at Lepanto. Cervantes, Yamamoto and Nelson had serious upper extremity injuries they survived due to good field medicine, and lived productive lives, becoming part of history.

Water-H2O

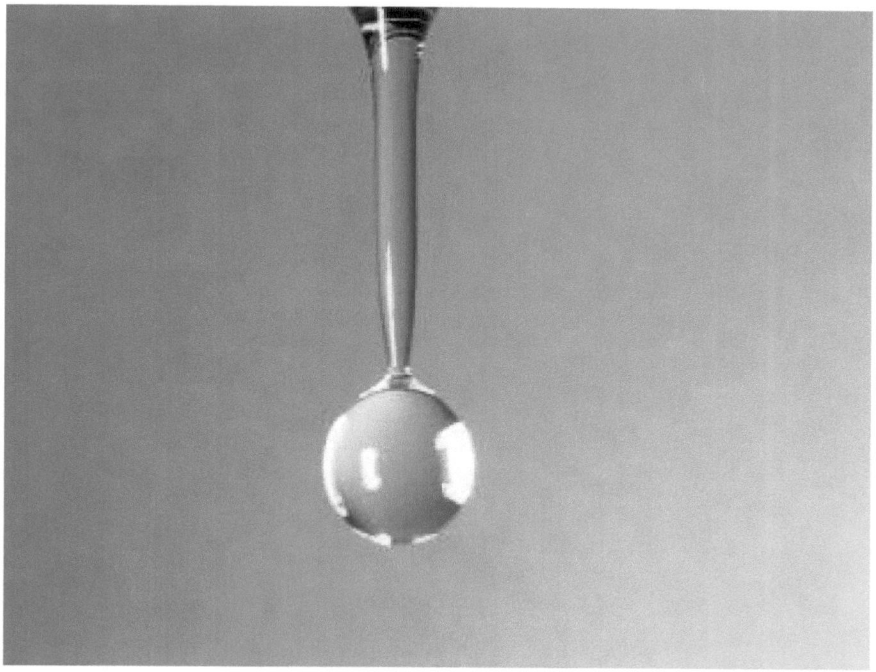

The unique properties of a drop of water are amazing and allow for much of biochemistry

If there is the ultimate chemical needed by all forms of known life, it is water. A simple, yet elegant molecule composed of two hydrogens bonded to a single oxygen atom, however, it is the complexities of these bonds that give water its highly unique behavior. H_2O owes much of its biochemistry to its ability to act as an acid or a base (+ positive and – negative charges), making water bipolar in a chemical sense. This bipolar behavior of water makes possible the important chemical reactions of life due to its ability to attract both + and – molecules. Water is the only molecule found in all three states on earth, i.e., liquid, gas and solid. It is the only chemical that freezes or becomes solid as it first expands and then floats! If water sank when it frozen, life would be much different if it existed at all on earth. Water molecules linked by positive and negative bonds create a special high surface tension, giving it both adhesive and cohesive characteristics. Adhesion allows a heavy drop of water to be suspended by a thin thread of water molecules, while its cohesive property allows water molecules to line up and "stick" to each other forming tension on the surface of water (like the esprit de corps of the US Marine Corps). Water can even overcome gravity as it climbs hundreds of feet from the roots to treetops.

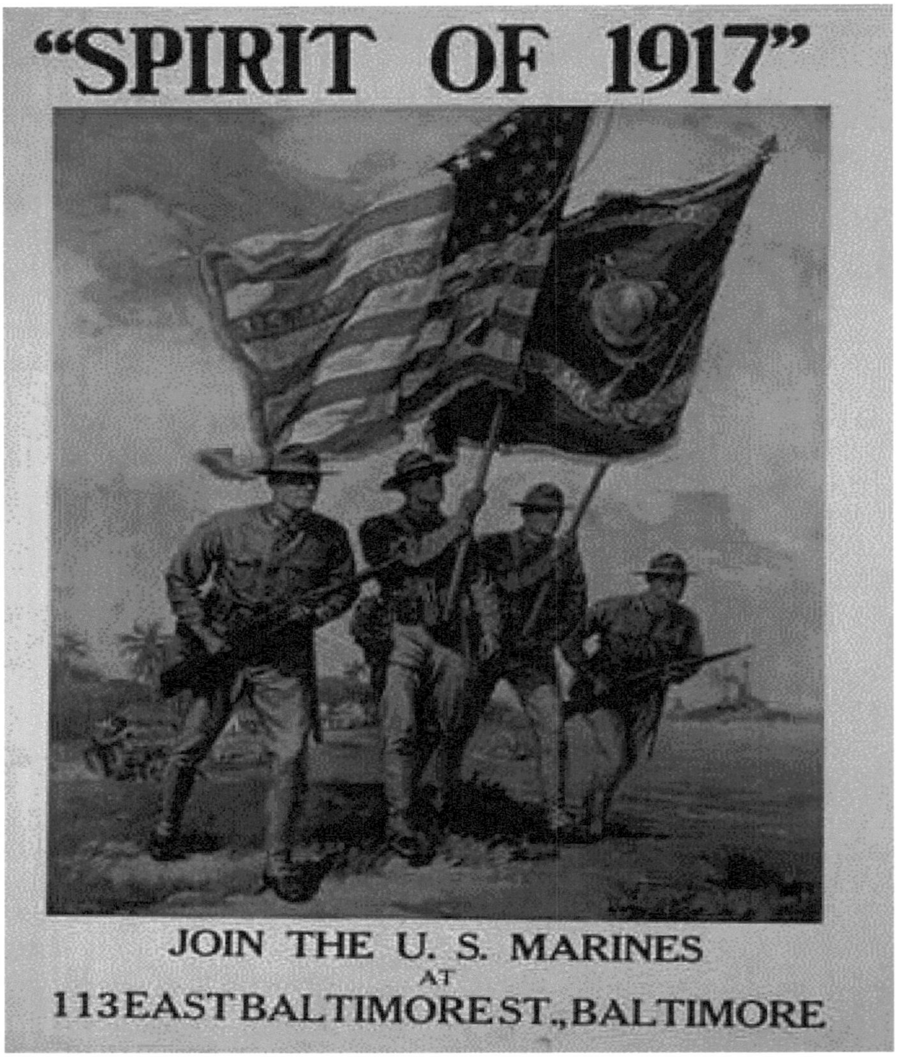
"SPIRIT OF 1917"
JOIN THE U. S. MARINES
AT
113 EAST BALTIMORE ST., BALTIMORE

United States Marines pride themselves on sticking together, National Archives

Water is such a powerful solvent; it has been called the "universal" solvent. It is amazingly effective as an insulator, since resisting temperature changes is vital in keeping the cell at near constant temperature. Just as being close to a large body of water insulates the land from extremes in temperature, as well as rapid changes. An example is the German Sixth Army deep in the Russian winter of 1942-43, thousands of kilometers from the sea. Germany does get cold; however, it borders the Baltic and North Seas which mediates its winters. At Stalingrad, the men, horses and equipment were thousands of kilometers from a large body of water and not prepared for temperatures of minus twenty to fifty degrees, and like Napoleon's army, were primarily defeated by the Russian winter described by historians as Generals January and February.

Everywhere there is liquid water there is life on earth. For many years it was believed that all life needed water and sunlight until life was found teaming in the ocean's dark deep depths where chemicals spewed from cracks in the earth and no solar radiation penetrated. This extremely hot chemical soup replaces sunlight as the energy needed for life since sunlight only breaches the shallow surface of the ocean.

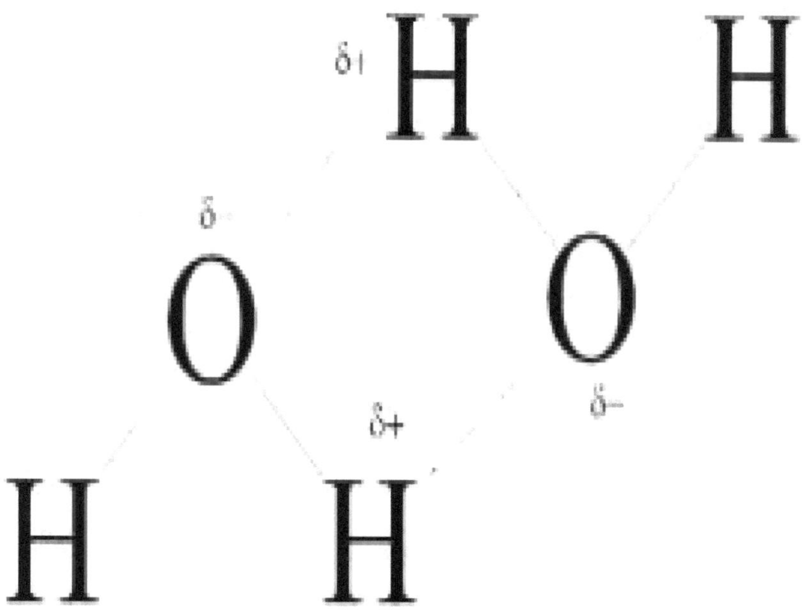

In theory, this represents one type of bonding between water molecules. Russian chemists have identified water molecules forming "clusters" when frozen that change with the water's reaction to sound. Frozen water crystals appear different when exposed to soothing symphonic music when compared to crystals exposed to discordant music. These clusters have been reported to have memory when thawed and refrozen. Wow! If this is true, what stories the Ocean could tell us as well as the water within our cells. They have also identified that rainwater water from high mountain tops is more reactive than water found in city water pipes.

Human activity requires lots of fresh water, without which war, a common human activity on land and sea would be impossible. Armies moved from water source to water source whereas at sea, water must be carried and stored. The weight of fresh water needed on a 19th century wooden combat sailing ship was more than the combined weight of cannons, gunpowder, cannon balls, food, sails, rigging material, anchors, crew and their supplies. A large sailing warship needed 2-4 tons of fresh water a day to stay at sea. Obtaining and maintaining water was a major part of seafaring as well as land-based activity. Fresh water was probably the most important item on warships during the Napoleonic Wars of the late 18th and early 19th century, where hundreds of ships were kept at sea for years. The *HMS Victory*, Admiral Nelson's flagship, with its 1000 souls of men, women and children needed a minimum of 6000 pounds of fresh water every day, primarily not for drinking but used to "steep" the salt from the preserved meat. Salted meats were poisonous until most of the salt was removed. Fresh water was certainly not used for bathing as the odor from unwashed humans, pigs, cows and chickens caused these ships to be so foul smelling that with the wind behind them, ship's odors preceded appearance. Fleets were sometimes smelled before they were sighted.

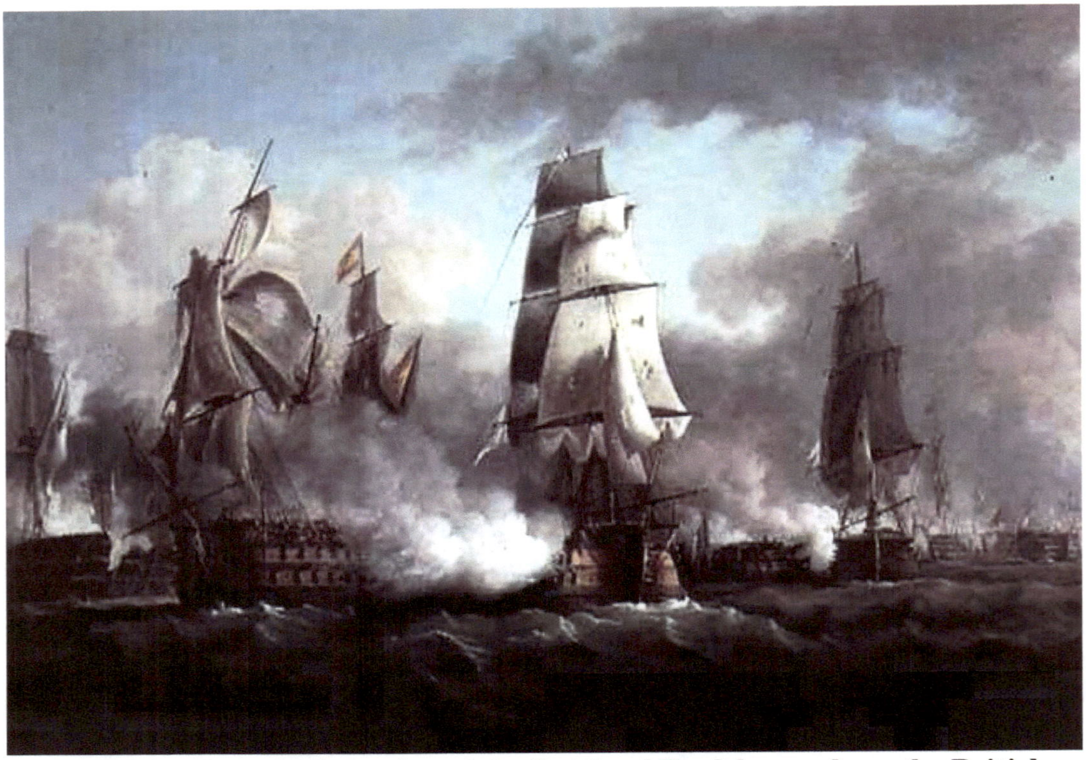

Painting by John Francis Sartorius of the Battle of Trafalgar, where the British under Admiral Horatio Nelson "crossed the T" and destroyed the combined fleets of France and Spain, one of the most important sea battles in European history. A storm following the battle destroyed even more ships and killed more sailors.

In addition to water, the major chemical components of life are carbohydrates (CHO), proteins, lipids and fats, usually combinations of the six most common elements (carbon, oxygen, hydrogen, nitrogen, calcium, phosphorus) found in every human cell. Human cells contain the machinery to combine or rearrange molecules to suit the cell's needs in the presence of water, which composes 50-70% of all cells. Water, like the earth has two poles, and this bipolar behavior makes water an excellent solvent especially with dissolving carbohydrates like alcohols. On the other hand, a characteristic of lipids is insolubility in water requiring cells to manufacture other organic solvents to break down fats.

Acid-base/oxidation-reduction chemical reactions

One of the most important chemical reactions in all forms of life, whether bacteria, plant or animal is the acid-base reaction or oxidation/reduction reaction. Although many would argue these are different, they are interchangeable in this text. In any case, energy and/or pieces of molecules are passed back and forth making life possible. An acid is a molecule that donates while the base is the acceptor. Acids tend to have hydrogen in front of the chemical, i.e., HCL vs bases which have an oxygen/hydrogen at the end of the chemical, i.e., NaOH. Acids give up a + charged proton while the base is the proton acceptor giving and accepting negative charged electrons. HCl (hydrochloric acid) in water is one of the most common chemical acid base reactions in the body whereby the chlorine molecule gives up a proton to water changing in from H_2O to H_3O (+) charge and HCl (-) charge. Charged particles are much more reactive than neutral particles and provide electrical energy to power the cells. Another common example of converting a neutrally charged chemical into charged one is dissolving a teaspoon of table salt in a glass of water. At the molecular level, sodium becomes (+) charged after accepting a proton while the chlorine molecule giving up a proton now has a (–) charge. Another method is by Na giving up negative electron and Cl accepting it. Na+ and Cl- now are polar or "ionic" charged particles and therefore more chemically active. Sodium and chloride found on the opposite sides of the Periodic Table, are two of nature's most reactive elements when alone yet combine to form one of nature's most stable chemicals. Until dissolved, table salt has no charge but when this molecule meets water, these charged particles serve as one of the cell's most basic functions. Cell function depends on the charged particles, as these charges are the micro-electrical energy that powers much of the cell (microscopic batteries). Although acid-base/oxidation-reduction chemistry is one of the fundamental reactions common to biochemistry and perhaps the most studied chemical reactions, much is still a mystery. How this happens at the cellular level is presently only theoretical and there are over ten different theories. One simple concept in oxidation, is it occurs when the radical and highly reactive single oxygen molecule inserts itself into a previously stable molecule. The radical influence of a solitary oxygen molecule desperate to fill its outer shell, disrupts the previously larger stable molecule, creating a more reactive new molecule. Many enzymes are oxidases that "speed up" chemical reactions within the cell. An example of this on a human scale occurs when peaceful protesters suddenly morph into mobs when a small element of violent individuals disrupts the stability the larger group.

Oxygen

Scientists in the 18th century proved there was some essential component of air that sustained animal life. The naming of oxygen and discovery in 1776, the year of the United States birth, is credited to the Frenchman, Antoine Lavoisier. Others with less credit made the similar discovery that air contained a vital element that was consumed by animals and replenished by plants. Lavoisier believed that oxygen was an acid, since he knew that oxygen "oxidizes" other chemicals, however oxygen is not an acid. Lavoisier named oxygen based on his belief, combining the Greek words *oxys*- "acid" with *geinomai* -"engender" meaning to beget or to birth. The transfer of energy with oxygen is the basis for human cells to consume and manufacture energy, i.e., the Krebs' Cycle. Oxygen in air is two oxygen molecules strongly bounded, O_2. Living cells in animals split the two oxygens into the single radical oxygen molecule. Oxygen in the air (21% of atmosphere) is colorless, tasteless, odorless, and even though it is not combustible, it enthusiastically supports combustion. In animal cells, this combustion is called aerobic metabolism. Oxygen readily combines with some metals, especially iron, making its transport possible in iron-containing red blood cells. Breathing atmospheric air under pressure as diving with scuba tanks increases oxygen pressure whereas going to high altitudes reduces oxygen pressure. Living at high altitude causes the bone marrow to produce more red blood cells.

Biochemistry vocabulary

Carbohydrates-(CHO) compounds made of carbon, oxygen and hydrogen are easily dissolved in water, found as chains and ring structures, examples are sugar, starch, alcohol

Isomer- two chemicals that are "mirror" images of each other, like the mirror image of the right hand to the left hand and isomers of each other and are referred to as right and left-handed molecules. Isomers allow the same chemical to exhibit different behavior, i.e., the right-hand and left-hand molecules behave differently because their structures differ as do the right and left hand in human activity.

Hydrocarbons-(CH) combinations of only carbon and hydrogens, classically called fossil fuels (although evidence is that coal, petroleum, natural gas are not exclusively formed from decayed plants and animals) gasoline, propane, butane are examples of hydrocarbons

Hydroxyl –an OH group when bound to a saturated carbon atom make an alcohol, the OH group gives the molecule its odor and polar (ionic) activity. Chemicals ending in "ol" are alcohols-ethanol, methanol (wood alcohol), cholesterol

Carboxyl group-a COOH addition makes chemicals an acid, i.e., proton donor activity-amino acids, nucleic acids, acetic acid (vinegar)

Ketone – organic molecule with carboxyl group, common product made by –OH (alcohol oxidation of protein waste). When cells are deprived of carbohydrates during fasting, shock or in diabetic disease states where carbohydrates are not available, the liver first converts some temporary stores of glucose stored as glycogen into energy. When this is exhausted, the liver turns to other energy sources and begins to dismantle, breakdown and convert protein and fats into energy for cells. Fasting at night often results in "morning breath", expelled air containing aromatic ketones. It can be a dangerous sign in a diabetic and is common in ethyl alcohol bingers. Confusion and heavily scented breath in diabetes has been confused with drunkenness by police officers, and diabetics have died in "drunk tanks". Breath like kerosene is a line from "Poncho and Willie", performed by Merle Haggard and Willie Nelson about a heavy drinker. His kerosene-scented breath from breakdown of fat and protein in the absence of food can fill the air.

Diabetes and biochemistry

There are two types of diabetes, Type I and Type II. Type I diabetes is due to a pancreatic defect of unknown cause resulting in an absence of insulin, whereas Type II is usually caused by excesses in lifestyle, i.e., overweight, inactivity, alcohol and excess fat intake. Central body fat is the hallmark of Type II. Type I requires insulin replacement, i.e., injections while Type II is managed with life changes (especially reducing body fat) sometimes augmented with oral medications and in difficult Type II patients, the added use of insulin injection. Insulin is the transporter enabling glucose to cross the cell membrane. Insulin is necessary for glucose to enter all cells except in central nervous cells, to protect them from glucose depravation. In the hyperglycemia of diabetes, glucose in the blood is not available to cells due to lack of insulin. Even though glucose levels are elevated, cells are deprived of their normal carbohydrate energy source, forcing cells to "burn" other chemicals for survival. Proteins and fats are more complicated and polluting to process when compared to the simple sugars, requiring more energy, and producing more waste. Ketones are one of these wastes and because it is aromatic and volatile, it passes out the lungs as gas in surrounding air. Fruity strong breath is a sign of ketoacidosis and is dangerous. Acid waste adversely affects cells resulting in lethargy, mental confusion, awkwardness and coma, not unlike alcohol intoxication. The body can only tolerate so much acid without damage to cells.

Ethyl-C_2H_5, a two-carbon molecule
Methyl-CH_3 only single carbon, less energy, in the past higher-octane fuel was called ethyl since it contained more carbon atoms
Propane 3 carbons (C_3H_8) butane 4 carbons (C_4H_{10})
Suffixes-endings of molecules names

- **"ide"** only 2 types of elements (sodium chloride-NaCl))
- **"ite"**-compound lower in oxygen (sodium nitrite-$NaNO_3$)
- **"ate"**-compound high in oxygen (potassium nitrate-KNO_4) explosive ingredient in gunpowder bringing its own oxygen to the explosion, needing no atmospheric O_2
- **"sis"**-to destroy, cleave or disable- (glycolysis-breaking glycogen into individual monosaccharide ie glucose)
- **"ase"**-enzyme enhances chemical reactions (protease-enzyme that inhibits AIDS virus by disabling proteins), lipase-breaks down lipids
- Metals-**"ic"** higher oxidation sate-stronger-sulfuric acid H_2SO_4)
- **"ous"** lower oxidation state
- Prefixes-beginning of word
- **"de"**-something has been removed (deoxyribonucleic acid-DNA)
- **"mono"**-single molecule (monosaccharide)
- **"di"**-two molecules connected (disaccharide sugars)
- **"tri"**-three molecules connected (trinitroglycerin-TNT)
- **"lyso"** prefix to destroy or degrade (lysomes)

Nucleic Acids- biopolymers, modified sugars (monosaccharide) combined with phosphate and purine (two ring structure) are essential to all forms of life for reproduction. These disparate molecules are connected by strong phosphate bonds, forming large spiral structures containing the blueprints for cellular biochemistry (reminds some of a spiral galaxy)
RNA (ribonucleic acid) five carbon sugar plus the nucleic acids of cytosine, guanine, adenine and uracil
DNA (deoxyribonucleic acid-one less oxygen molecule) five carbon sugar plus three of the same four nucleic acids found in RNA, cytosine, guanine, adenine while replacing uracil with thymine.

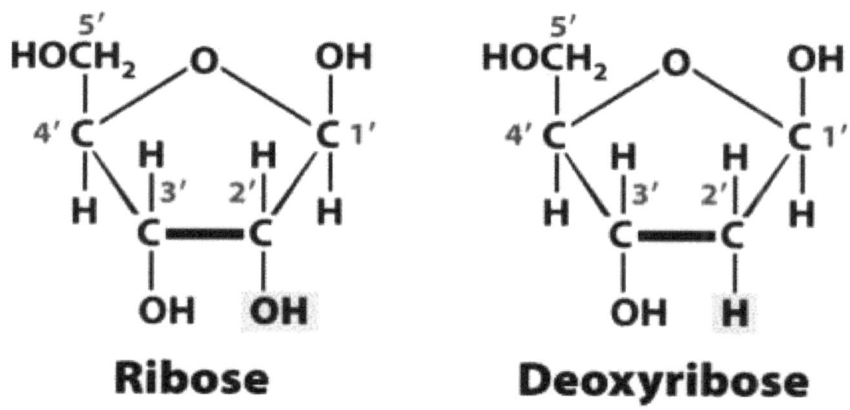

Note the missing oxygen atom on right molecule otherwise exact copies, yet vastly different actions-the numbers 1 thru 5 are the number of each carbon atom, numbered clockwise

Amino acids-compounds containing an amine group (NH) on one end and carboxyl group (COOH) on the other end, with a trunk of 2 carbons in the middle, chains of these form proteins like insulin, animal and plant structures

Fatty acids-not fats! Complex compounds of carbon, oxygen and hydrogen

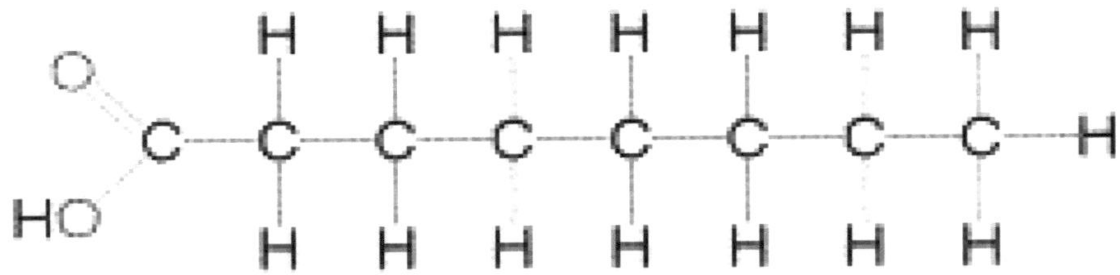

Saturated

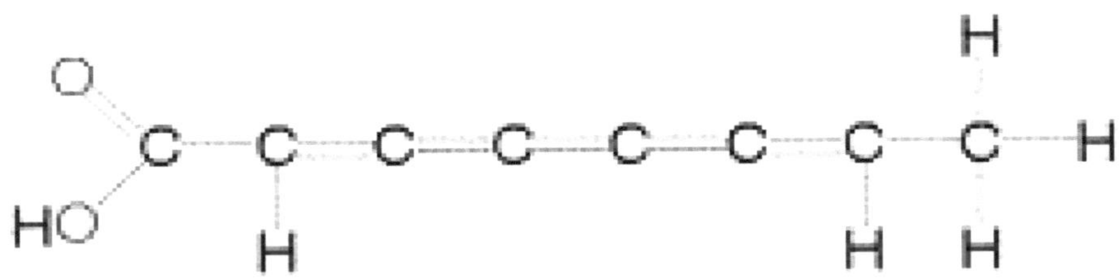

Unsaturated

The carbon atoms are much more exposed on the unsaturated chain, making these fats more reactive than the carbon atoms protected by hydrogen atoms on the saturated chain. The more reactive unsaturated fats are considered more corrosive to arteries. Triglycerides are formed when three of the above molecules combine

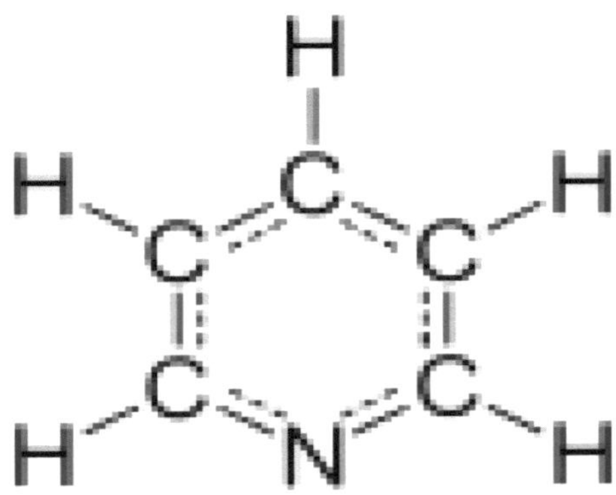

Pyridine - a five-carbon ring structure powerfully bonded, found in niacin (vitamin B3) and pyridoxin (B6) – the abbreviated lines on the interior side of the carbon atoms, reflects the uncertainty of what is happening at the molecular level

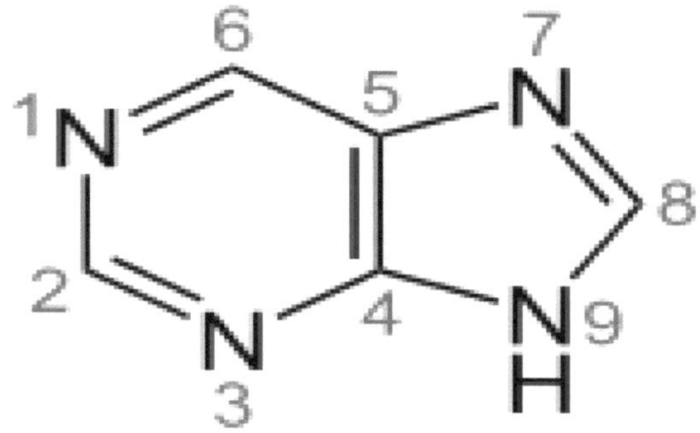

Purine - a two-ring structure difficult for human cells to break down, found in high concentration in rich foods such as meat and mammal organs (liver, kidney). Elevated purines lead to gout caused by elevated purine. A history changing chemical

Purines have been important to medicine and history and deserve a special place in the book. The basic two-ring structure of uric acid is common in nature and includes many of mankind's most notorious actors. Although all purines share the common structure of a five and six carbon ring securely bonded to each other, the chemicals attached to the rings, give purines widely different actions. The alkaloid plant purines of nicotine, caffeine, opiates, cocaine and most hallucinogens are of special interest to the biochemistry of the human cell.

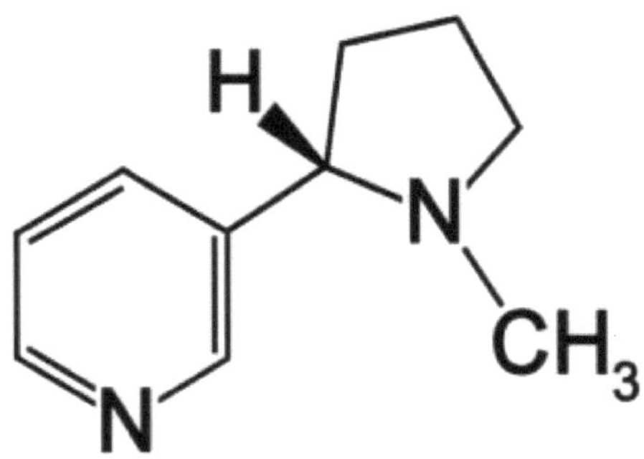

Nicotine is composed of carbon, nitrogen and hydrogen, containing two common rings, a five-sided carbon ring bonded to a six-sided carbon ring with alternating double bonds. It is believed that the plant produces nicotine as an insecticide discouraging bugs from eating it. Nicotine is considered too toxic by the USDA to be used as an insecticide.

Tobacco-the deadly plant alkaloid purine

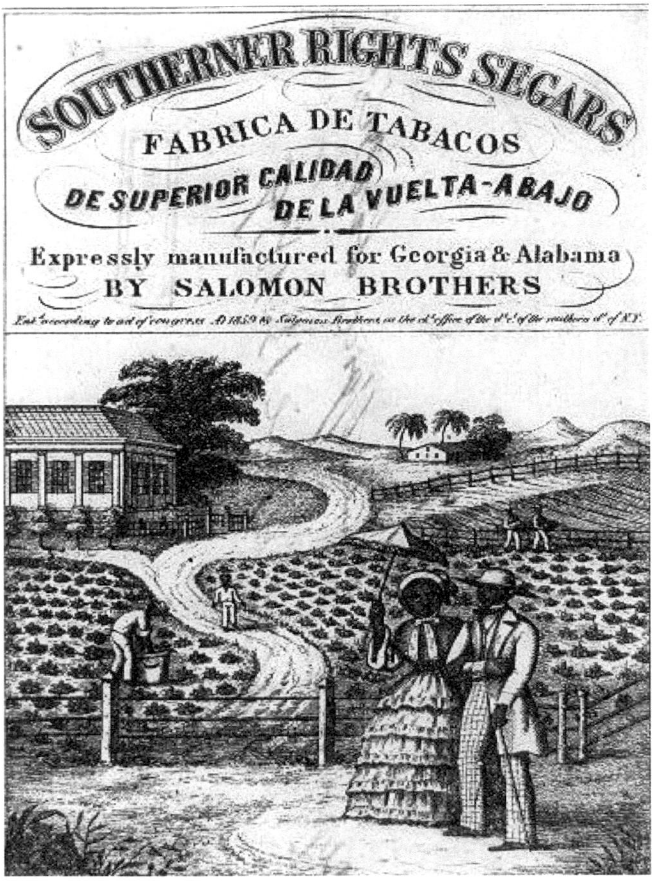

1859 ad for cigars by the Salomon Brothers of New York in a highly fictional image of tobacco farming in the south, in attempt to belay the true hardship of slavery-driven enterprise. Perhaps it would be more politically correct to smoke if one viewed tobacco cultivation in this picture. Cotton, sugar and tobacco were the main drivers of the Southern economy prior to the war and was due to slavery. Over 50% of the worth in the South was in human bondage on the eve of the American War Between the States. National library of Congress

In addition to nicotine, other important plant alkaloid purines of medical interest include cocaine, caffeine, theobromine (chocolate), dopamine, serotonin, theophylline and opiates. The most notorious of these plant purines in human history is nicotine. Nicotine is found in several plants, all in the nightshade family (which includes tomatoes, potatoes, peanuts, eggplant, digitalis and many others). Perhaps no other plant has caused as much human misery as tobacco. Since its introduction to Europe and ultimately to Asia following Columbus's return from America, its use and cultivation rapidly grew worldwide within a few generations. Tobacco quickly became a popular and deadly plant to humans and the land where cultivated. In addition to damaging the human cell in most of the body's systems, especially the respiratory tract, tobacco cultivation injures the land by leaching soil of nutrients. Successive crops require new land, leading to forest destruction and damaged watersheds. China suffered decades of famine, starving millions because of tobacco cultivation. Less than one hundred years after Columbus returned with tobacco, the demand in Asia was so high that previously uncultivated hillsides were planted. Tobacco unlike rice will grow on inclines and Chinese farmers denuded the hills above the rice fields to plant the cash crop. It was not long before major floods pounding down the now bare hills, poured their soil into the valleys, choking food crops. Tobacco continues to be consumed in large amounts around the world and remains a major health problem.

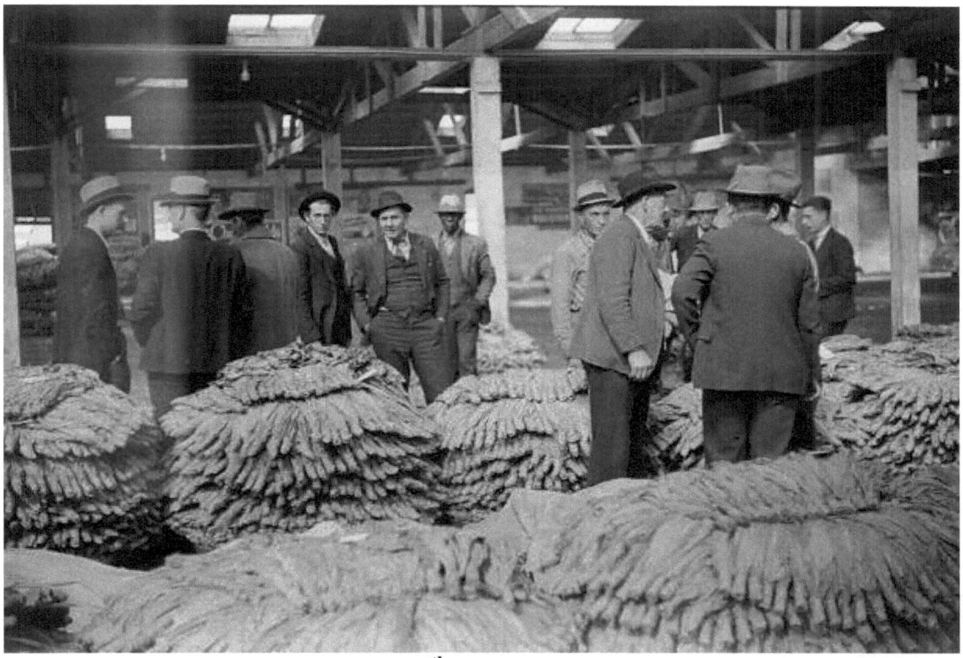

Tobacco merchants examining early 20th century bidding on the bales of "green gold". Cotton and tobacco, both highly dependent on slave field labor were primary forces behind the American economy in the 18th and 19th centuries. Both required slave labor. National Archives

Nicotine is a simple purine structure of only three different elements, not unlike many other purine molecules floating around in the body, however nicotine is no ordinary purine. To begin with, the human central nervous system appears to have nicotine receptors. Why would a plant produce a powerful alkaloid that directly stimulates a series of chemical reactions in the human brain? Is it by accident that nicotine, in addition to protecting the plant from insects, has a powerful effect on humans? Is it because tobacco is a special plant? The Native American tobacco Columbus bought back to the Court of Isabella and Ferdinand in Spain was special, containing psychogenic effects as well as nicotine. The immediate and prolonged central nervous effects of native tobacco were used primarily for spiritual activities and social interactions (smoking the peace pipe). Current commercial tobacco has removed the natural psychoactive chemicals, replacing them with pure highly concentrated nicotine. So powerful were its corrosive effects, some countries outlawed its use, punished by beatings, disfigurement and in 16th century Russia, was briefly a capital offense.

Nicotine has some limited medicinal uses such as a patch to reduce smoking and irritable bowel complaints. In the past, it has been used as insecticide, but its toxicity resulted in its banishment. In the human brain, nicotine enhances the release of acetylcholine, endorphin, dopamine, norepinephrine and serotonin, all powerful neurotransmitters effecting mentation, pleasure, appetite, and wakefulness. Withdrawal of these effects is why tobacco is habit forming.

The world-wide presence of human brain receptors for nicotine is hard to explain since at the time of Columbus, tobacco was only found on the American continent. Coincidence, or in the distant past did human ancestors have access to tobacco before the plant was isolated in America. Is it possible that nicotine has deliberately adapted human behavior to promote its own survival? If so, the same could be surmised for cannabis. There is evidence of tobacco in Egyptian mummies but no evidence of tobacco cultivation in Egypt.

Purine alkaloids- are a group of nitrogen containing compounds of plant origin (although can also be found in bacteria and fungi), generally bitter to taste (i.e., tea, coffee, chocolate, and cocaine), highly active in human central nervous system-caffeine, opiates, tobacco, atropine, strychnine, quinine, ephedrine, psilocin (magic mushrooms), mescaline, dopamine, serotonin. Cannabis has similar properties but does not contain nitrogen. One of the main biochemical effects of these chemicals within the human cell is the inhibition of the enzyme phosphodiesterase which increases the concentration of cyclic AMP. Phosphodiesterase inhibition is the mechanism by which Viagra works.

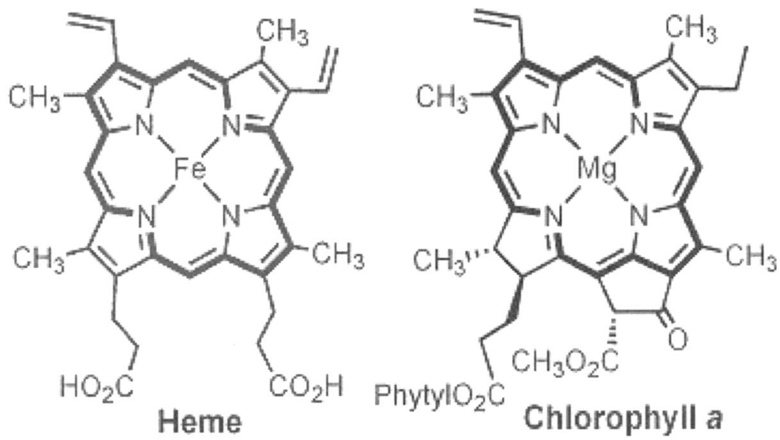

Porphyrins: complicated structures of multiple rings with an embedded metal: hemoglobin (iron), chlorophyll (manganese), vitamin B 12 (chromium). A genetic disease, porphyria, occurs when the liver is unable to breakdown accumulating porphyrins, poisoning the body.
The word root for porphyrin comes from the Greek word for purple derived from the Phoenicians for the deep purple dye extracted from purpura mollusks. Wearing of this purple was reserved for the royalty of the Byzantine Empire. The base word is also the name of a whale named Porphyrius, one of the author's favorite sea stories. During the forty-year reign of Justinian, a sperm whale appeared off Constantinople. It was very rare for sperm whales to enter the Mediterranean Sea and yet Porphyrius swam the entire length of the Mediterranean and entered the Black Sea. The whale arrived at Constantinople the same month that Theodora (who later became Empress) entered the city for the first time. The whale thrived in the waters, stationing himself at the narrow Bosphorus where the Black Sea meets the Mediterranean. Here, Porphyrius waited for schools of fish and even dolphins when he was not attacking boats.

Porphyrius terrorized shipping in and around Constantinople during the four decades that Empress Theodora ruthlessly ruled the Byzantine Empire with her husband Justinian who was weak, cowardly and duplicitous. Justinian let his wife, and her advisors govern while he spent time studying the minutia of Christianity and overseeing the codifying of Roman Law, some of which in use today. Justinian met his empress at a brothel, fell in love with her intellect, and after becoming Emperor, married her, disappointing families of senators and aristocrats. Antonina, from the same brothel, later married Belisarius, who became one of history's great field commanders. Antonina fought in combat with her husband as he reclaimed North Africa and Italy for the Eastern Roman Empire while her close friend and confidante Empress Theodora, governed the Empire. The author is unaware of any time when two women of common birth and lacking formal education, became the most powerful females in the Western World.

Not only did the whale and Empress arrived in Constantinople at the same time, but they also died decades later the same day. Porphyrius washed-up dead on the same day Empress Theodora died of aggressive breast cancer. Coincidence? Theodora, like Porphyrius, was feared and hated, becoming so unpopular that any negative comments about her were a capital offense. After their deaths, "the beast is dead" was spread throughout the Mediterranean empire and enthusiastically acclaimed, meaning the Empress, not the great whale.

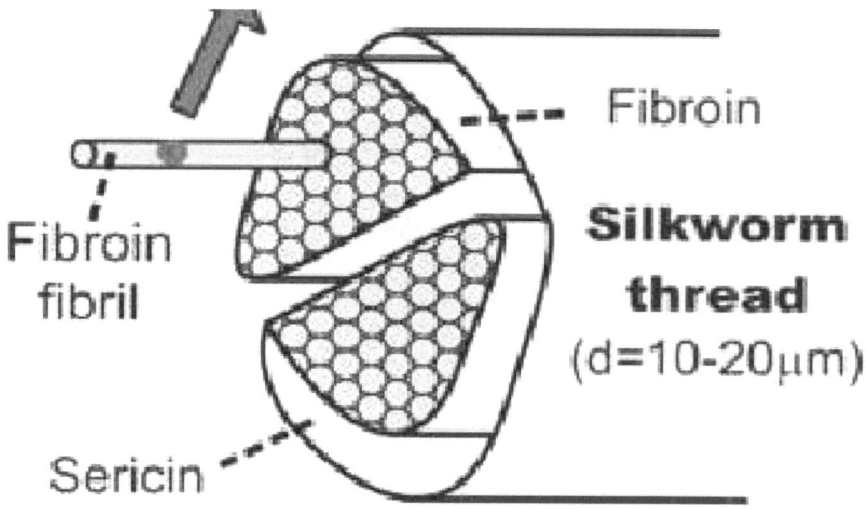

It is the microscopic structure of silk that made it so desirable for trade spanning thousands of miles and by weight as expensive as gold.

Justinian's empire relied heavy on silk from China accounting for 15% of Constantinople's revenue. Silk is hardly a simple structure, unique in nature composed of two protein chains mysteriously fused by heat into a single strand. A strand unwound from a single silk cocoon can be 500 meters long and legend tells a story of a princess accidently dropping a cocoon in a cup of hot tea. Silk in addition to its beauty, lightness and ease in manufacture of cloth had many practical uses including suturing wounds, ligating bleeding vessels and the Mongol soldiers wore silk shirts under their leather armor and if penetrated, the silk would envelop the arrowhead, enabling its removal. Silk garments and tapestries are so durable they can last a thousand years.

Carbohydrates (carbon + water)-CHO

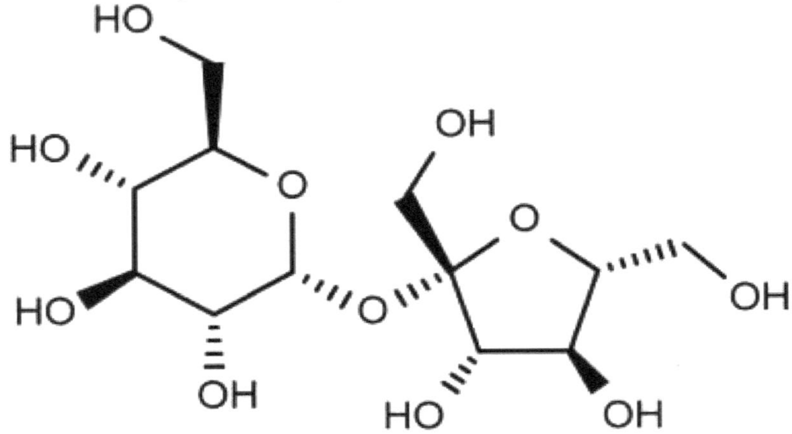

Disaccharide – two simple monosaccharide sugar molecules chemically connected

Carbohydrates have many forms and uses in the cell. Sugars and starches (polysaccharides) are primarily used for energy and when combined with proteins and fats become structures such as cellulose and chitin (exoskeletons in insects). Carbohydrates may come in two isomers, the mirror image of each other, left-handed (*sinister* in Latin) or right-handed (*dextra*). Imagine holding your hand in front of a mirror. The image is an exact copy but reversed, the thumbs appear on the same side in the mirror. Even though they look the same, each hand is different. The right hand in a right-handed person function much differently than the left hand (even though they have the same form). In chemistry, the dextro (dextrose) isomer of many chemicals often behave much different than its sinister twin. Animal cells are unable to burn left-handed glucose for fuel, however they can use it to manufacture other molecules.

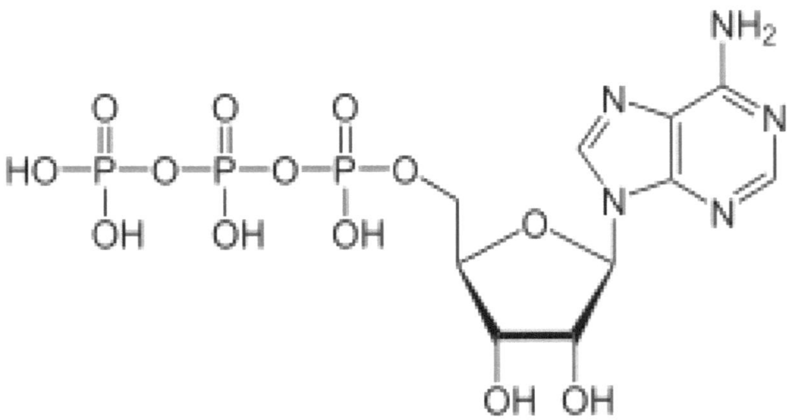

Adenosine triphosphate, ATP -the two rings on the right are a purine structure, connected to a five-carbon sugar ring with the chain of high energy phosphate bonds

Carbohydrates are a major food source for living things, animals, plants and fungi. The process of deriving energy from carbohydrates, as well as from lipids and proteins are the backbone of biochemistry. Two main processes are aerobic (with oxygen-O_2) and anaerobic (without oxygen-O_2). In both cases, sugars, fats and proteins are degraded inside the cell's energy producers, the mitochondria, to produce and store energy in adenosine triphosphate (ATP). ATP represents the primary stored energy source for the cell, like what wood, coal and petroleum products have been used for human activity. Imagine ATP molecules as intracellular "oil tankers" that are filled (loaded) with energy-containing bonds at one site and then travel to other areas in the cell where energy is needed. There is a great deal of energy in the chemical bonds that hold phosphate atoms to the adenine ring structure. The cell has chemicals that cleave off the phosphate atoms at one at a time, releasing stored energy. Energy is captured and used for needed chemical reactions elsewhere in the cell. With release of the first phosphate, the molecule has lost some of its stored energy, reducing it to adenosine diphosphate (ADP) and even though storage has been reduced, there is still energy remaining in the two remaining phosphate bonds. When the second phosphate is removed releasing its energy, adenosine monophosphate (AMP) is available to be refueled or used as a messenger molecule. Inside the cell, ATP, ADP and AMP are constantly recycled. The cell tries to use everything and now the near empty "tanker" molecule (AMP-adenine monophosphate) through a conversion whereby the chain structure folds on itself forming a ring structure, becoming one of the cells most useful recycled energy molecules, cyclic AMP (adenine monophosphate). Cyclic AMP is one of the mechanisms used by respiratory drugs to increase airway dilator in asthma and emphysema and a beautiful example of the cell's ability to recycle.

Metabolism

The breakdown and utilizing energy inside the cell, respiration or metabolism, occurs constantly even without the benefit of oxygen. Glycolysis describes sugar destruction and is the primary method of respiration in human cellular activity. Under normal conditions, human metabolism is aerobic (with oxygen), however in shock, O_2 is not delivered to cells, causing a diversion of metabolism into anaerobic or oxygen-deprived pathway. This anaerobic pathway uses much of the Krebs' Cycle, with the same electron transports system, however without oxygen to carry away the final electron. The electron acting like waste, is not removed, the system will slow and "back up" (imagine plugged toilet). The cell has a mechanism to bypass this "plugging", transferring to anaerobic respiration, which is less efficient than aerobic respiration, and produces more toxic waste. These toxic chemicals (especially lactic acid), when flushed from oxygen-deprived and stagnant tissues after CPR is successful, can be destructive to lung and kidney causing the delayed complications and sometimes death in successfully resuscitated victims of shock. The quicker the detection and management of shock, the better.

Lipid Metabolism

Lipids are composed of fatty acids connected by chemical bonds poorly soluble in water. Oil and water will not mix; however, they form a distinct layer separating the two disparate liquids, this "repugnancy" that oil has for water is the basis for membrane formation throughout the animal cell. Membrane formation is an example of life meeting chemicals within the cell and cell manufacturing structures from that interaction. Fats must be dissolved to be used, and since insoluble in water, the cell produces organic solvents. Lipid molecules can be saturated or unsaturated (see picture), they can be burned as energy, used as enzyme activators, stored as fat and because of the seemingly "repugnance" that fats and water have for each, they can be form into membranes! When lipids are metabolized, energy is released and stored if not needed at site.

Lipid molecules carry a high energy value, the bonds are more complicated and contain more energy than the simpler carbohydrates structures. It takes energy to break down these complex molecules, capturing some but not all in the phosphate bonds of the ATP structure. The Atkins diet of high protein and fat intake with no carbohydrates is built around this biochemical process.

The "excited" electron

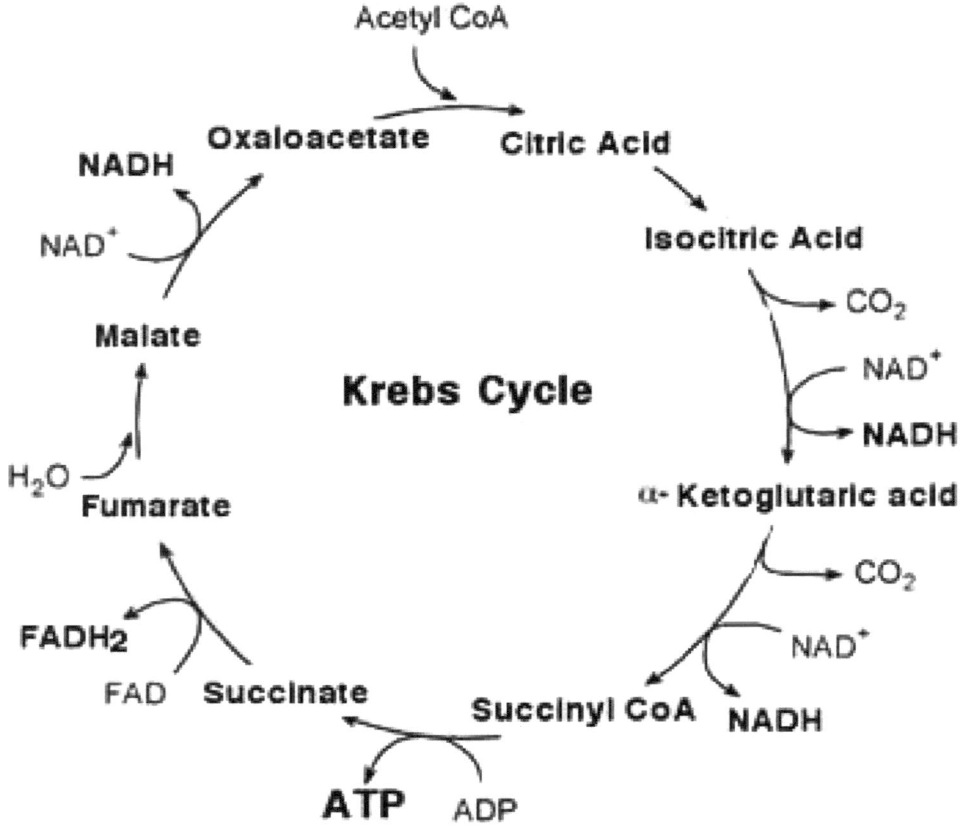

Simplified version of the Krebs' cycle beginning with the diaspora of an electron which jumps from its present location to another. Voluntary or forced migration?

At the molecular level, the energy captured in this cycle is one of the most important and most studied cascades of chemical reactions within the cell. An electron transport system known collectively as the Krebs' cycle or in the interest of purging men's names from science (courtesy of gender equality as Krebs was a male), the tricarboxylic cycle or citric acid cycle. This phospholipid-rich cycle is a series of eight reactions where an electron is passed from one molecule to the next, accounting for energy manufacture, storage and transport. In simple terms in this process, oxygen is burned and consumed (aerobic respiration) while discharging an electron, carbon dioxide and water as "wastes.

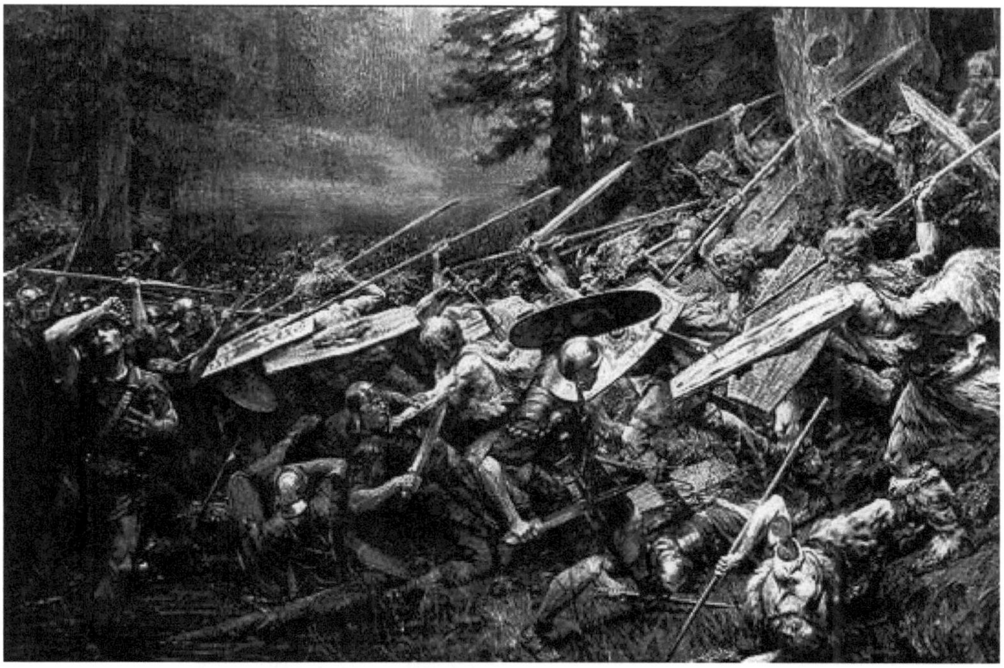

Picture of the Battle of Teutoburg Forest, September in the year 9 AD, where three Roman Legions, the 17th, 18th and 19th led by Publius Quinctilius Varus were destroyed by Germanic tribes beyond the Roman frontier. Varus a lawyer by training, married the grandniece of Augustus, where as a member of the royal family he became a rapacious governor of Syria and unfortunately later made governor of the lands beyond the Rhine. His Roman Army of 20,000 soldiers and perhaps 5,000 civilians (camp followers) were leaving the land beyond the Rhine for winter quarters after the Germanic tribes endured a summer of overly brutal Roman occupation under Varus. The army needed rest and better quarters as the medics (recently made officers by Julius Caesar) reported reduced fitness of poorly fed and ill-housed men. Varus placed his trust in Ariminis, son of a Germanic chief that been made a citizen and army officer of Rome, who encouraged a quicker route to the Rhine. Following advice from Ariminis and his German auxiliaries, Varus foolishly spread his army in a long 9-12-mile vulnerable army structure, easy to break apart. "Give me back my legions" Augustus shouted throughout the Roman capital after news of the total defeat. Not only did Augustus lose thousands of trained officers and men, huge amount weapons, armor, wagons and iron tools, making Ariminis and his chieftains the most powerful force in the Germanic tribes. Many historians point to this battle as a reason for two thousand years of warfare in Europe after the battle. Had Rome extended its control into central and Eastern Europe and civilized the discordant tribes and introduced Christianity, it is possible the European Union today could have been formed centuries earlier. Rome's inability to occupy and subdue the Germanic and other tribes, could explain the savagery of Germany in the Second World War. Had Augustus sent a better commander with his legions, history would have been much different. Since Roman legions normally marched and camped in stronger "ring" formations, they were much less likely to be overcome. In warfare and biochemistry, long chains are more vulnerable than compact ring structures. National Library of Congress

How does the Krebs' cycle happen? What starts the cycle? In theory, electron transport systems begin with the emergence of an "excited" electron (author's own word), one that is apparently unstable in its present state and seeks to change its current location (perhaps it is just curious and the same reason the bear went over the mountain). Could a curious electron be what started the "big bang" of the cosmos? For whatever reason or reasons, an excited electron feels the need to travel or is forced to travel, so it jumps or is pushed to the adjacent phospholipid molecule. Its arrival at a more stable lower energy position not only releases energy but displaces another, now excited homeless electron. That electron is ejected into the adjacent molecule and so on until the final system is reached. At the human level, this behavior compares to the pulses of migration out of central Asia pressing against the sprawling Roman Empire. Migration of particles when controlled is predictive, ordered and beneficial, however displacement of particles can disrupt large systems leading to mayhem. Strains on Rome's borders during the 6th century AD from people pouring through its former frontiers resulted in the city and the western part of the Roman Empire falling to "barbarians". The 6th century AD witnessed the fall of Rome, the Plague of Justinian (huge losses of human lives in a brief period), wars, famine, uncoupling of trade and communication. Rapid climate change was the primary reason for the chaos of the 6th century, chaos wrought by extraterrestrial impacts (Randal Carlson's lecture series) leading to centuries of stagnation known as the Dark Ages. Not unlike the chain reactions occurring in nuclear power plants and atomic bombs caused by impactions as well as the ovum (egg) enduring impactions from swarms of sperm. Comet and meteor impacts on earth have changed human history and to the author represent "excited electrons" on a large scale. In their search for stability, they enter human history.

Elements inside cells are seldom found alone. They are usually found in chains or ring structures. Chains are generally more easily disrupted and dismantled while ring structures are more durable, more resistant to change and contain more energy. Ring chemical structures, like forts are stronger, requiring more energy to construct and requiring more energy to disrupt. However, some rings are programed to open with just the slightest energy. Like a gate in a great fortress opened by a one person. A single photon of sunlight can open a ring structure in chlorophyll, vitamin D and vitamin B12. This is a unique function found in porphyrins and is responsible for almost all life on earth. Human skin color is part of this mechanism (imagine sunlight as a can opener).

For the systems of the Krebs' cycle to continue, there must be a final electron acceptor, and that final acceptor is the single negatively charged free oxygen radical. The unstable solitary oxygen molecule, in need of a free electron to fill its outer shell. Plucking that excited electron out of the system stabilizes oxygen with a paired oxygen molecule and allows the transfer of electrons to continue. The oxygen molecules in the atmosphere, like inhaled nitrogen, are inorganic molecules. Inhaled oxygen becomes "organic" at the molecular level, in an allegory, the author likens it to a "garbage collector" removing the now-unwanted electron, allowing the Krebs' cycle to continue. In the process of aerobic (with O_2) respiration, the animal cell gives off water and CO2. The animal cell's waste product, carbon dioxide is vital for plant's metabolism, and some believe it was the high concentration of oxygen on the land covered by oxygen-producing plants, that "lured" animals out of the low-oxygen sea. Animals "burn" carbohydrates, mostly made by plants, and in the presence of oxygen give off water and CO_2 as waste. Plants on the other hand make carbohydrates from water and CO_2 using the sun's energy, while giving off oxygen as waste. Solar energy drives plant life while animal life depends on consuming energy-releasing compounds from other living things. In both plants and animals, energy must come from outside sources. Animal cells produce other wastes in addition to CO_2, even in normal conditions, waste that must be removed. Waste products that allow them to accumulate, become harmful (as discussed in shock).

Oxygen and blood flow are the most important participants in waste management in human cells, providing energy while sweeping away the debris of energy production. In shock, stagnation deprives cells of oxygen, forcing them to adopt another form of metabolism without oxygen (anaerobic respiration), less effective and importantly, more polluting, as waste products such as lactic acid build up during the stagnation. When circulation is reestablished, these toxic waste products are flushed into circulating fluids causing adverse effects. This mechanism is discussed fully in the section on shock.

Proteins

To prevent protein starvation, only dietary proteins are acceptable. A diet rich in carbohydrates and fat will not produce cellular proteins and may result in malnutrition even in the face of continuous food intake lacking protein. Dietary proteins are large, complicated molecules that the cell is unable to use until broken into smaller pieces. This process begins in the gut and terminates inside the cell. Once through the gut, the now smaller pieces are carried to the organs of digestion, especially the liver for further processing. The cell is unable to utilize large foreign proteins from plants and other animals until converted to human proteins, primarily within the liver. The sudden appearance of large foreign proteins into circulation is dangerous as it does in snake envenomation.

Snake venom, when injected directly into circulation, has deleterious effects, sometimes fatal. If ingested through the gut with swallowing, it is broken down and utilized by the human cell. The exception would be an open sore in the mouth allowing snake venom to directly inter circulation. One the other hand injecting raw ordinary egg white protein could be dangerous as rattlesnake venom. Proteins after entering circulation are first degraded into smaller units of amino acids and later reassembled (mostly in liver) into proteins acceptable to the cell, a process requiring energy to process and later remove as waste.

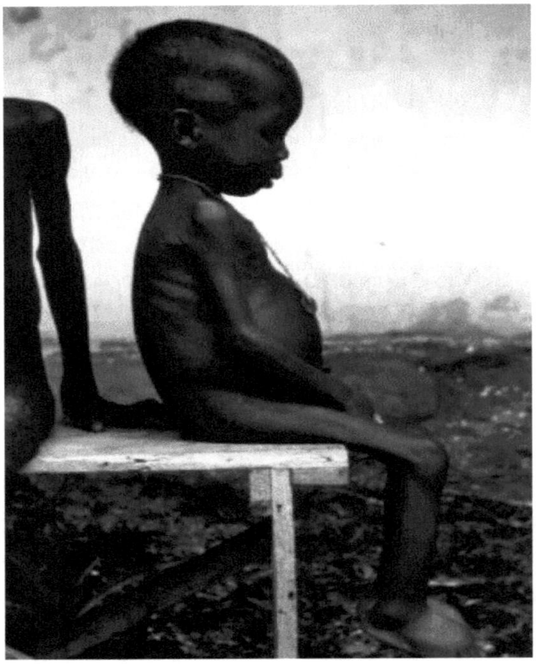

Kwashiorkor victim of the Nigeria-Biafran War 1960. Proteins have been stripped from muscle tissue and fluid has pooled in abdomen. National Archives

Urea-NH3

In animal cells, the major waste products of protein metabolism are excess water, carbon dioxide and the toxic ammonia-like substance, NH_3. Animals living in water find it easy to discharge NH3 into their surroundings, whereas land animals combine NH_3 and CO_2 to form the solid form, urea which is dissolved in urine. Even though it is a waste product, it still contains lots of energy, enabling Timothy McVay to use urea fertilizer as the primary explosive to destroy the federal building in Oklahoma City. Land animals that begin life in an egg are unable discharge the NH3 into their limited water reservoir but collect it as a solid in a separate sac. For the rest of their life, they will combine the urea with feces and discharge them together (thus bird droppings are high in urea and are generally more corrosive and useful in fertilizers and explosives). Placental animals discharge NH_3 through the maternal urinary tract via the placental exchange and later through their own kidneys. The exceptions to the above are amphibians like frogs, that live in water as tadpoles discharging NH_3 into water and yet emerge later as a land animal. Since all life needs organic nitrogen, where does the cell get it?

Act of God and the nitrogen cycle

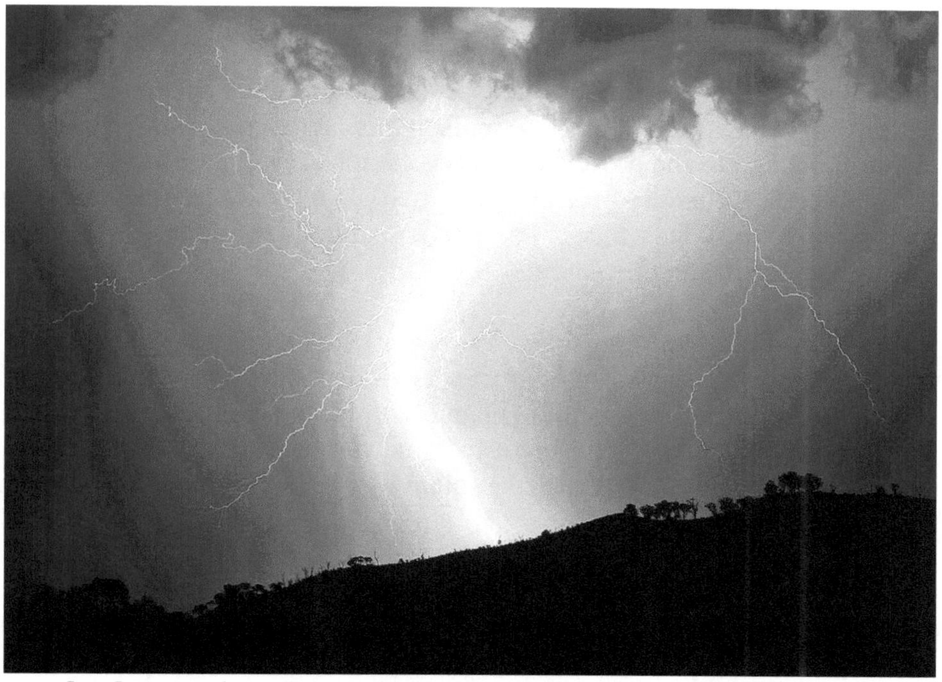

Lightening can be destructive, destroying forests with strikes, burning homes, frightening humans and all while playing a role in creating life on earth. National Library of Congress

Amino acids, nucleic acids, proteins, RNA, DNA, vitamins, purines, porphyrins and pyrimidines are all necessary for life requiring the presence of organic nitrogen. The nitrogen cycle was the sole source of all organic nitrogen needed for plants, fungi and animal cells until the Great War of 1914-18. Eighty percent of earth's atmosphere is nitrogen, acting as a vast storage vault. As an atmospheric gas, it is chemically inactive, passive, inorganic, and useless to living cells. Nitrogen gas is inert because its two nitrogen molecules are so tightly bound together (their joined outer shells are filled) that it takes a great deal of energy to separate them. Their separation allows the organic chemical to emerge. Some would say it takes an act of God to separate N_2, so powerful are their nitrogen bonds. Only two natural mechanisms are known whereby nitrogen is converted from inert or inorganic nitrogen into the organic nitrogen needed for plants and animals. Perhaps as much of twenty-five percent of nitrogen conversion is due to lightning strikes. Lightning strikes on the ground can be five miles long and as thin as the diameter of a 25-cent coin. For a moment in time, lightning is hotter than the sun (53,000 degrees F) and while this flash of energy, though lasting only a tiny part of a second, it is powerful enough to break both atmospheric N_2 and O_2 molecules apart, creating organic nitrous oxides which are readily used by plants. As exciting and violent as lightning is, most nitrogen conversion takes place in the dark silent underground home of plant's roots. Here, a symbiotic relationship between the roots, bacteria and fungi, "fix" inert nitrogen by combining Nitrogen with CO_2 and water. Plants merging sunlight with nutrients of the earth, along with its coconspirators, fungi and bacteria, forge the products necessary for the manufacture of amino acids, the building blocks of proteins.

In simple terms plants take in CO_2, organic nitrogen and water where using the power of sunlight manufacture organic compounds. In the process, plants exhale O_2 as an exhaust (like the exhaust pipe of a car expelling a waste product). Animals on the other hand, ingest compounds made by other lifeforms, burning these purloined chemicals as fuel, usually in the presence of oxygen, exhaling CO_2 as exhaust to be recycled by plants and so on in a constant cycle. What a wonderful symbiotic relationship between plants and animals. Once again, do plants attract animals out of the ocean and onto land due to the presence of oxygen-rich atmosphere compared to the oxygen-poor seawater? Oxygen levels were much higher when plants covered most of the world, as high as 24-26% compared to just less than 21% now. Animals were larger in the oxygen-rich atmosphere during the age of the dinosaurs.

Were plants aware they were being poisoned by their waste O2 and needed animals to consume it? Could plants have known their waste product was vital to animals? Since plants give animals, especially humans oxygen, food, medicines (plant alkaloids such as opiates, digitalis, vitamins), what do they get in return? Only CO2, which to us is waste and toxic? Many plants are highly valued by humans, giving rise to the theory that plants do get something in return, and may have deliberately altered human behavior.

One of the nature's most efficient plant converters of inorganic nitrogen into organic nitrogen is the lowly alder tree which in most cases is more of a flowering shrub than tree. Botanists consider the alder a pioneer plant, not unlike early human settlers in the American West that braved hostile natives, aggressive animals, storms and droughts provided an opening for further colonization. Like human pioneers, alders pave the way for other plants to come. As glaciers retreat in Alaska and Canada one of the first plant to appear is the alder, converting nitrogen and preparing the soil for other plants and later animals. The fields cultivated by the pueblo builders and cliff cites of the Anasazi (really a poor name choice for these people, as it is a Navajo word represented by the Zuni and Hopi, traditional enemies of Navajo and the probable real decedents of the pueblo builders) were surrounded with alders. Early Native American farmers realized the value of these plants in producing and maintaining fertile land. Alders grow along water courses, and like cottonwoods, reveal the presence of underground water. Alders contains drugs such as salicin, which Native Americans used for fever and pain, a plant chemical like aspirin. Two of the newer cancer drugs, botulin and lupeol are found in alders.

* 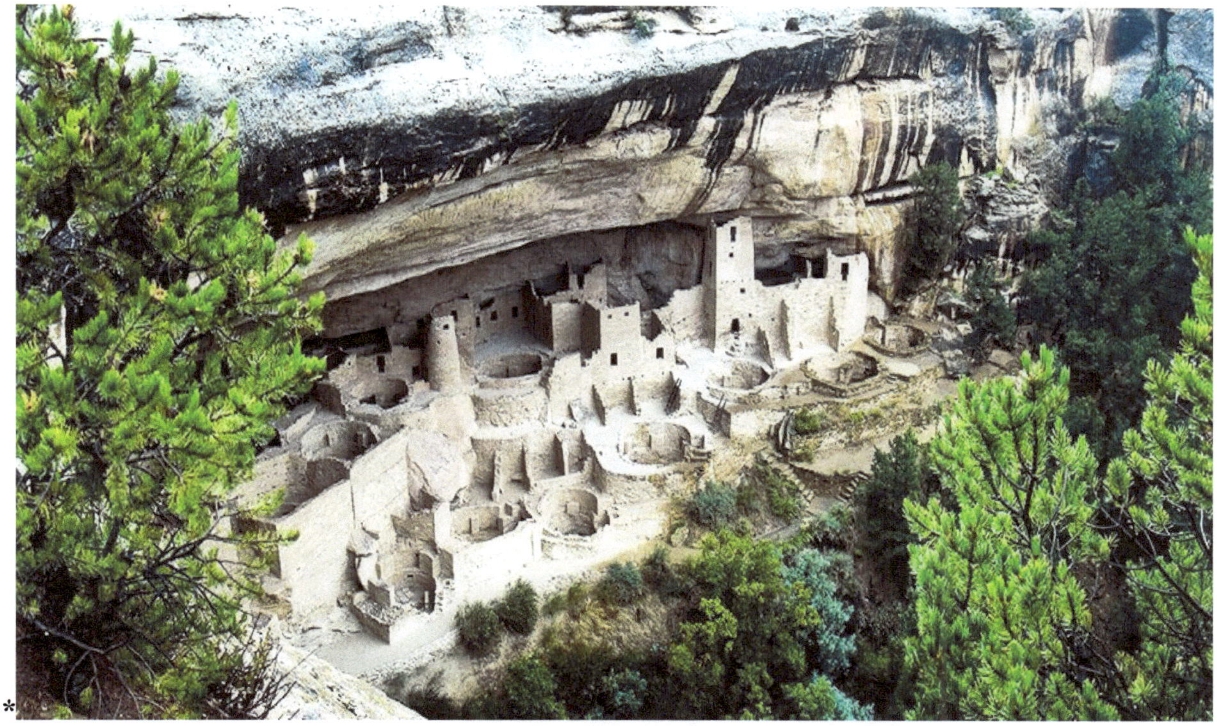

These people were afraid of something as they built their dwellings on almost vertical cliffs from natural shelves of rock. Their homes and storage bins were hundreds of feet above water and their fields of grain and maize. The Navaho have ancient verbal history of fighting giants". National Park Service

The brutal, powerful force of lightning and the slower, yet persistent conversion by plants roots and their symbiotic bacteria and fungi were the only known mechanism of N_2 conversion until late in the Great War 1914-1918. Germany was cut off by England's naval blockade from importing nitrogen-based chemicals from Chilean coastal islands of bird guano (solid waste rich in NH_3). Islands so valuable to the munition industry, armed conflicts were fought over in the "Guano Wars" between Chile and Peru. Without nitrogen-based fertilizer, central European crops diminished in amount and nutrition. People under German control were running short of food and Germany had to develop another source of organic nitrogen or starve. German chemists Haber and Bosch invented the process whereby atmospheric nitrogen under extreme heat and pressure with the addition of hydrogen and a metal catalyst produced NH3, the organic compound of Nitrogen, urea. ($N_2 + 3H_2$ converted to NH_3). NH_3 was also important ingredient of German explosives. There is a lot of energy in urea and is a powerful ingredient in munitions necessary for warfare.

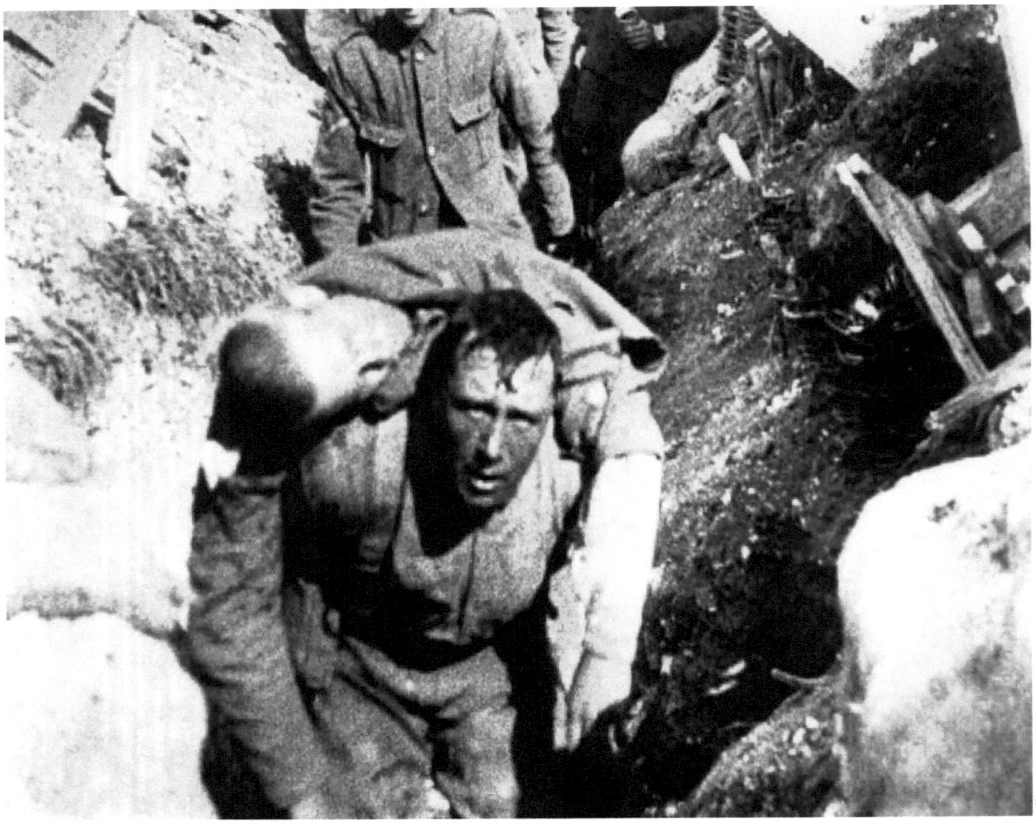

*

Still from moving film of wounded soldier at the Battle of the Somme, July 1916. Food for the soldiers and gunpowder for their guns came from urea-like chemicals. Many historians believe the British Empire died the morning of July 1 on the Somme River when over 100,000 of Great Britain's best men and her colonial soldiers "went over the top". Within two hours 57,000 were casualties. At Gettysburg, it took three days for the Americans to kill and maim that many. At the Somme River, the British attempted a frontal assault on the most powerful section of the 500-mile-long German lines. The Germans had 18 months to dig into the high ground overlooking the bare field of fire the British attack a force entrenched in tunnels and bunkers so deep, nothing short of an earthquake would damage. The first British waves became casualties within fifty meters, their graves marked in long lines just beyond their trenches. Medical officers serving close to the front at the Somme heard a "continuous nocturnal sounds" emanating from the wounded in No-Mans-Land following assaults, described as "enormous wet fingers screeching across an enormous pane of glass". Imagine working in a forward aid station by lantern light, awash in wounded, with such hopeless noises in the background. British commander, General Alexander Haig continued the attacks for months ending with occupying the same ground where the attacks started wasting tens of thousands more lives and continued the destruction of Pax Britannia. The battles of Caporetto, fought by Italy in the same Great War, made the Somne look like military genius. "Somme" by Lyn MacDonald is an excellent source. Imperial War Museum

Lipids/Fats-the best form of stored energy

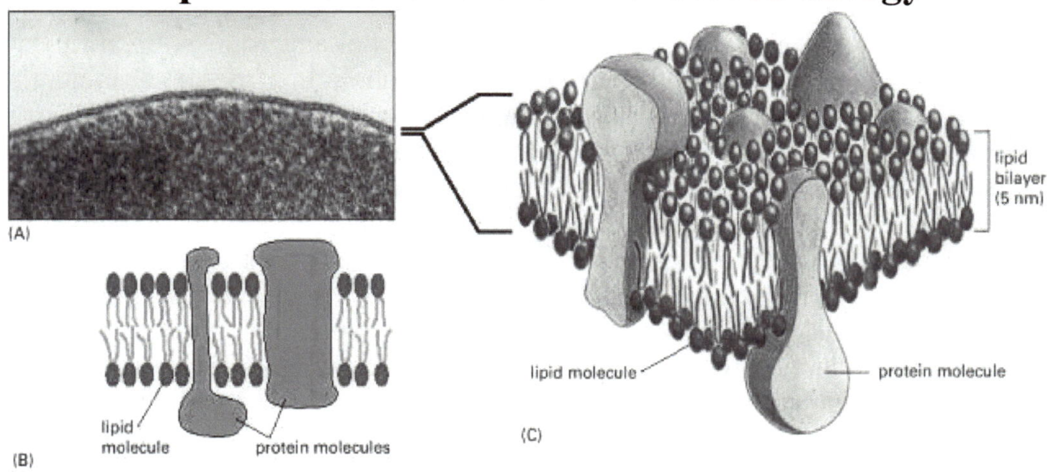

Electron microscopy of a cell membrane and an illustration of the results of water repulsion of lipid forming one on nature's most important interactions. National library of medicine

Fats are much more than just long-term energy storage molecules. Fat molecules serve as templates for vital compounds such as steroids, vitamins and enzymes. They require special tools to break down for cellular use (especially stored fats). The mechanisms whereby cells degrade fats were poorly understood until the discovery of the role played by the combination a cholesterol molecule and sulfur, creating the enzyme Co A (see Krebs' cycle). Coenzyme A is a complicated multi-ring structure that enables the Krebs' cycle to burn both carbohydrates and fats, turning fuel into energy.

Fermentation

A biochemical dance between yeast and sugar

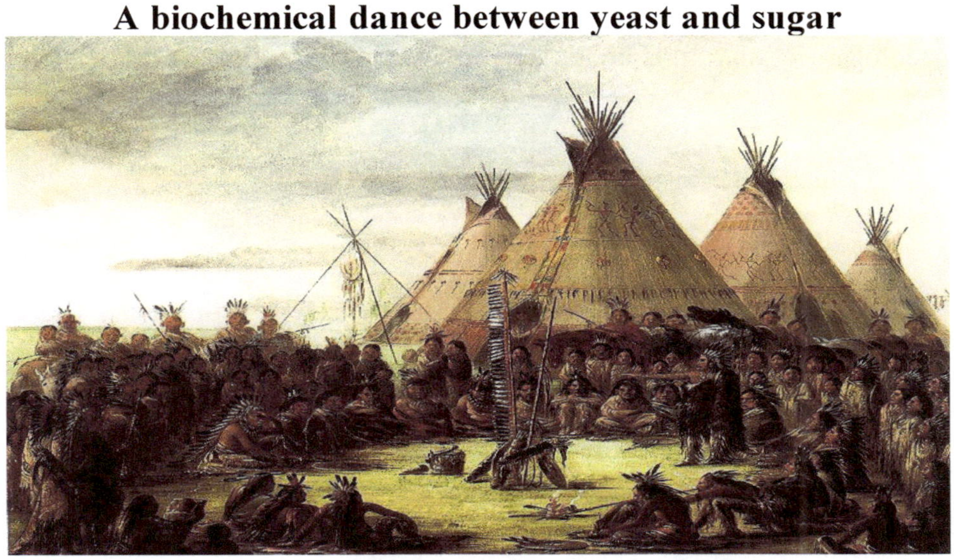

The Plains Indians were especially hard hit by the destructive effects of man-made interruption of fermentation, ethyl alcohol coupled with waves of infectious diseases. George Catlin, National Archives

Some cells only have metabolic pathways to produce energy occurs without oxygen, as O_2 is poison and deadly to these anaerobic organisms. One product of anaerobic respiration that is very destructive to human cells and human behavior is ethyl alcohol. In alcoholic fermentation, yeast convert sugar releasing CO_2 (bubbles in beer) transiently, producing ethyl alcohol, which then yeast can denature into acetic acid, vinegar. Since ethyl alcohol is a transient product, at some point in human history our ancestors discovered the right time to kill the yeast, thus retaining the ethyl alcohol. As previously stated, ethyl alcohol is toxic not just to yeast but to every human cell, especially brain cells. Converting grains and fruits to alcohol enabled calories to be stored prolonging shelf-life, enabling cultures to survive in the lean winter months. In some societies, beer and wine were a major part of survival diets. Human populations with access to alcoholic beverages slowly over generations acquired liver enzymes that denatured most of its toxic effects. However, when new populations were exposed to alcohol, the results were devastating. Native North Americans who had no previous experience with the products of yeast fermentation, were especially susceptible to drunkenness and aggressive liver destruction of ethyl alcohol, as were the Polynesian cultures. Later effects of ethyl alcohol toxicity include liver disease, diabetes, pancreatic dysfunction and mental destruction.

Ethyl alcohol is preserved by killing the yeast at the right time to stop fermentation. Sulfites added to wine and pasteurization of beer are used to kill yeast, while cold fermentation with near freezing temperature do the same. Before Pasteur, wine and cheese quality were not uniform and for unknown reasons some wine turned to vinegar, and some cheese spoiled. He discovered the role of yeast and how to control its role in the French wine and cheese industry. The process of fermentation occurs in the absence of O_2 and in fact, the presence of O_2 will destroy the chain of chemical reactions that produce ethyl alcohol. It is of interest that the pathway where energy and waste are produced in anaerobic metabolism is almost the exact pathway of energy production in aerobic metabolism, except for the last two chemical reactions. Energy production by cells is complicated and many things interfere with these reactions, spoiling both drink and food. Antibiotics are examples of chemicals that interfere with bacterial metabolism and are discussed in the pharmacology section of this book.

Vitamins

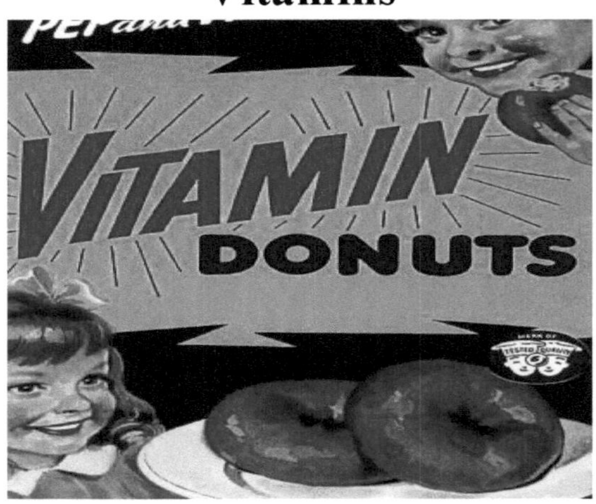

Not fake news, actual FDA poster as there are vitamins in donuts, its "science" like this that Robert F Kennedy Junior is going to change at the FDA

Vitamins are biochemical compounds (coenzymes) that enhance reactions and are required to maintain the cell's health. They come in many shapes and functions; some are manufactured in human cells while others must be supplied in the diet. An example is vitamin C, a vitamin most animals can synthesize, but not humans. The reader might enjoy the discussion of vitamins' role in health and disease as well as its place in history. Not all vitamins are discussed here and certainly there are other chemicals considered vitamins important in human health.

Vitamin A

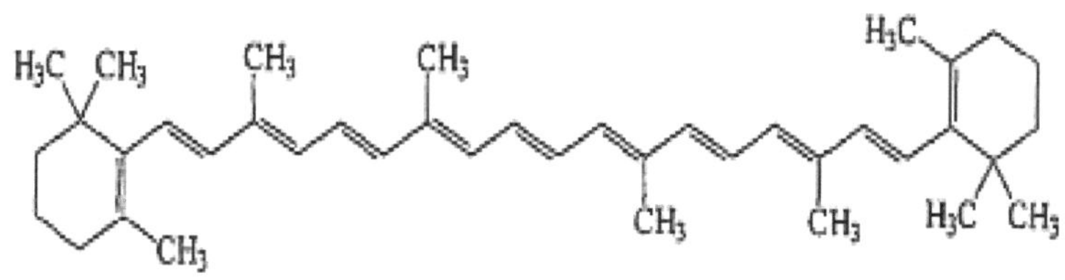

Beta Carotene

The light-changeable molecule is responsible for vision. This structure is like the hallucinogens found in the spices mace, cloves and nutmeg, *Myristica fragrans* which contain MDA which by adding a side chain chemical, becomes MMDA (ecstasy). Nutmeg was very expensive and desired as "narcotic fruit" used as snuff. Arab physicians used it for digestion problems and edema with kidney disease. Carotenes are molecules with carbon chains bookended by ring structures. Similar structures are repeated throughout nature in certain plants and animals. NIH

In the retina, a chain of chemical reactions begins when light strikes a carotene molecule coupled with opsin (visual protein), reconfiguring its structure to rhodopsin. Vitamin A has other uses in growth and repair of cells and is used to treat skin disorders as it is important in repair of DNA molecules. This repair of DNA is responsible for the "rejuvenation" of skin with topical Retin A.

Vitamin E

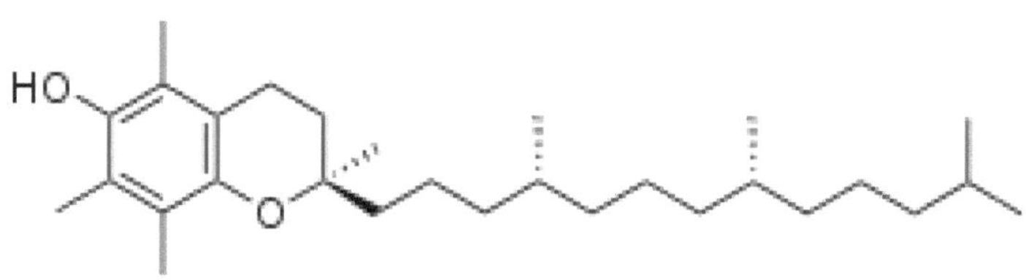

Alpha-tocopherol of vitamin E-fat soluble

Vitamin E is best known as an antioxidant, protecting other intracellular chemicals from oxidation. Anti-aging gurus believe the stiffening of young more flexible tissues become firmer with age, can be slowed by antioxidants (some authors believe antioxidants used to keep potato chips fresh, can help humans). It is found highest in many vegetable oils, especially beans, other seeds and olives.

Vitamin E has enjoyed intermittent success as a supplement, especially when used topically on wounds and scars. There is currently no proven use for supplementing diet with extra vitamin E.

Vitamin D

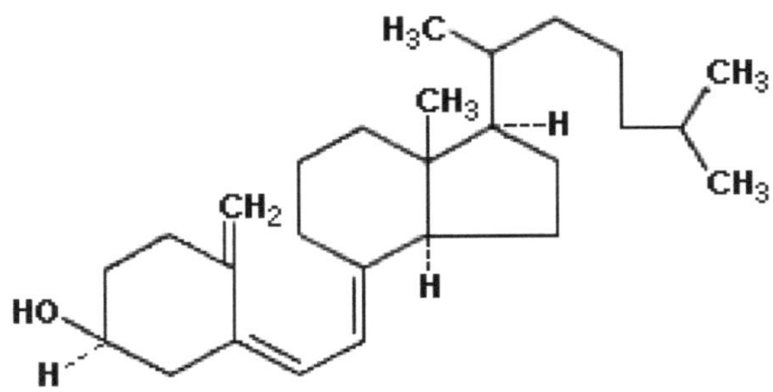

Vitamin D-cholecalciferol $C_{27}H_{44}O$ is composed of only three elements manufactured from a cholesterol molecule

Vitamin D is a group of fat-soluble steroid chemicals that allow the metals calcium, zinc, iron magnesium, phosphorous and potassium to be absorbed and combined into bone and other structures. Vitamin D deficiency causes Ricketts, formally a major nutritional skeletal defect. Because Ricketts was so common, the USDA required many prepared foods to be fortified with vitamin D beginning in the early 20th century. The active molecule of vitamin D is cholecalciferol (vitamin D_3). This cholesterol-derived chemical is part of a complicated and important chain of chemical reactions beginning with ingestion, followed by digestion and activation. This activation requires multiple organs and sunlight or artificial light in the 280-320 nm wavelength. It starts when the gut changes the shape of ingested vitamin D, enhancing its absorption as it passes through the walls of the gastrointestinal tract and into circulation. As it is carried through blood vessels, vitamin D passes under the transparent skin where penetrating sunlight or artificial UAB light "opens" a ring structure on the molecule exciting an electron (just as sunlight opens the ring of chlorophyll in plants). Light changes the structure of the molecule, preparing it for more modifications. The newly transformed vitamin D travels to the liver, now with an open ring in its structure, where a hydroxyl group (OH) is added on the number 25 carbon molecule. Now reconfigured it is carried by circulation to the kidney where a second hydroxyl (OH) is added at the #1 carbon, thus 1, 25 $(OH)_2$ cholecalciferol (an alcohol) becomes the metabolically active form. The final product can now build and maintain bones combined with metals imparting strength with flexibility to the hard tissues found in body.

Scandinavian governments provide lights producing the same wavelength as sunlight for use during the long dark nights of winter. It not only enhances bone growth but reduces the incidence of winter depression (Seasonal Affective Disorder). Light in the proper wavelength is the absolute ingredient needed to activate vitamin D, and therefore skin color has adapted in humans based on the amount of sunlight needed to change inactive ingested vitamin D_3 to its active vitamin D. People living along the equator became very dark as they experienced daily 12-hour doses of sunlight and added skin pigment prevented sun damage. Whereas people in the higher latitudes, being less pigmented, needed as much sunlight as possible during the short days of winter. This lighter skin, although helpful in high latitudes in bone formation does increase the risk of skin cancer when living in lower latitudes. Thus, Australia leads the world in skin cancer as it is now inhabited by Europeans from northern latitudes.

Vitamin K

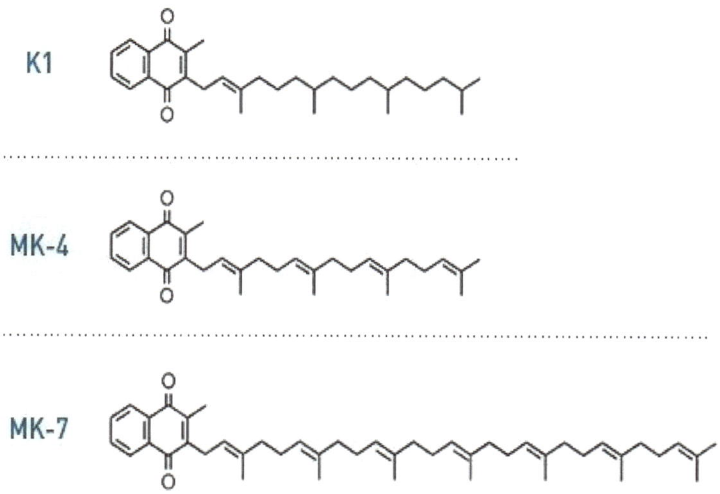

Vitamin K1, phylloquinone (phyllo-layered appearance, quinone-aromatic compound, highest concentration in rhubarb) three forms of vitamin K-K1 is dietary while K4 and K7 are transformed by microbes in colon

Vitamin K is found in plants and fungi (especially dark green leafy vegetables) and a large amount is transformed and manufactured into the human gut by anaerobic bacteria. This vitamin K is a necessary ingredient in blood clotting. The coagulation of blood is too complicated to even try to explain in this text, suffice it to say, "thanks to our gut bacteria for finding a way to help humans control bleeding". Vitamin K injections were given to infant boys prior to circumcision as their gut does not acquire bacteria until later (therefore in the Jewish ceremony, circumcision is delayed until the 8th day of life). Vitamin K is also needed for bone formation and repair as well as participating in other body functions.

Water soluble vitamins

Vitamin C

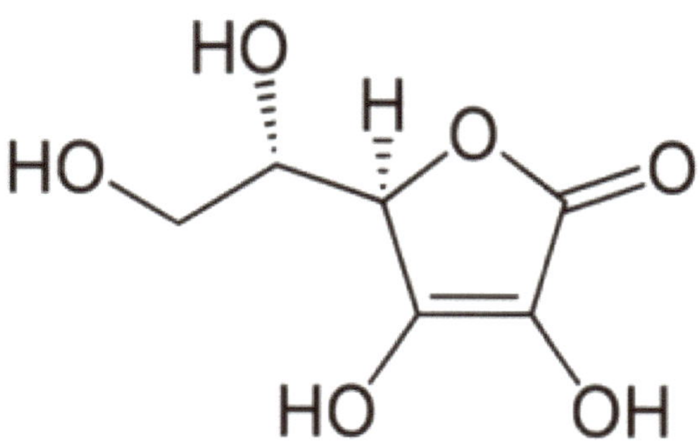

Ascorbic acid-C6H8O6 a simple yet eloquent water-soluble molecule

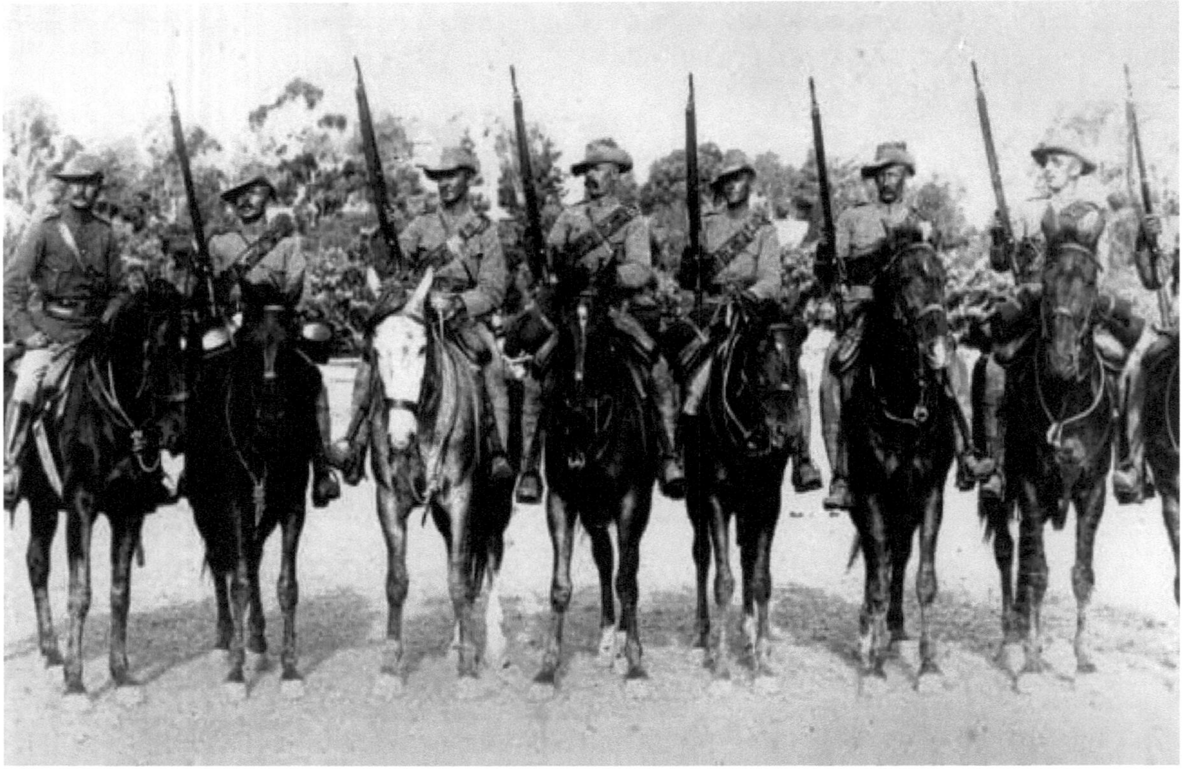

Scurvy, caused by dietary lack of vitamin C, decimated the women and children placed in concentration camps ordered by British General Kitchener during the Second Boer War, 1896. 60% of the children and 35% of the adult women perished in these camps, which modern Afrikaners believe reduced the white population in South Africa from a potential of 40% to less than 10% in the late 20th century. Pictured above are volunteer soldiers from Australia fighting with the English against the decedents of Dutch settlers, the 3rd from the left is Breaker Morant (his story is portrayed in the movie," Breaker Morant").

Vitamin C, ascorbic acid, is another necessary dietary nutrient. Vitamin C serves as a good reducing agent in oxidation-reduction reactions, where unlike most chemicals it can be reduced again after its first electron has been exchanged. This simple molecule is formed from left- handed sugar and is necessary for untold numbers of vital chemical reactions in cells, especially connective tissue formation and repair in wound healing. Chemically it functions as a weak acid (i.e. electron donor) and a strong antioxidant. Animals can manufacture their own vitamin C except bats, guinea pigs, primates including humans, and these creatures must be provided vitamin C on a regular supply. Because ascorbic acid is water soluble, it does not store well in the cell. The United States Navy medical officer turned Artic explorer; Dr. Elisha Kent Kane knew there was a plentiful supply of vitamin C on his ship trapped in Artic ice in the ship's rat population. With food-borne vitamin C stores gone, Dr. Kane encouraged his ice-bound crew to eat the rats in the ship to prevent scurvy. The crew that ate rats avoided scurvy, whereas those that found this rat-rich diet repulsive did not. In animals, vitamin C is found in high concentrations in adrenals, pituitary, thymus, ovary and retina.

B vitamins

All B vitamins contain at least one ring structure, except B5 (B2 and B12 have particularly complicated ring structures). B vitamins are found in most foods and like vitamin C, are water soluble vitamins requiring regular replacement in diet as they are also poorly stored.

Thiothiamine-B1

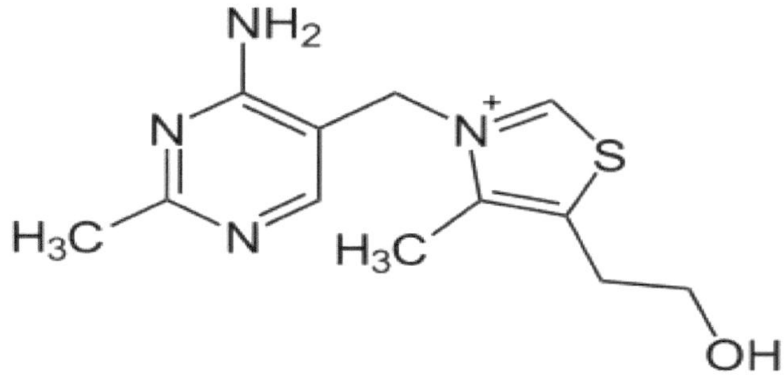

Note the sulfur molecule and the OH group making it water-soluble alcohol

B_1 or thiamine also known as thiothiamine (*thio* is Greek for Sulfur-containing) is necessary for living organisms to metabolize carbohydrates and amino acids. All microbes, fungi and plants make their own while on the other hand, animals require dietary thiamine. The first step of fungi fermentation of alcohol needs TPP (thiamine pyrophosphate) to produce one of man's favorite beverages, ethyl alcohol. One method of preserving foods is to block thiamine–driven reactions, thus adding sulfites (antibiotic to kill fungi) to wine stops fermentation, reducing risk of converting alcohol to vinegar. Thiamine deficiency (Beriberi) in milder forms affects peripheral nerves and later damages the central nervous system causing lethargy, coma and death. Beriberi not only affected the Japanese sailors in the Battle of Tsushima Straits but was rampant in the Imperial Japanese Army fighting Russia on the Asian mainland eating polished rice. Discovery of its cause has been credited to Patrick Manson who studied these symptoms in jails, mining camps and army concentrations mainly in India in late 19th and early 20th century. He called it a "tropical pathological puzzle" and initially thought it was a form of malaria. Beriberi continues today in famine-rich east Africa, where there are populations suffering from beriberi.

Riboflavin-B2

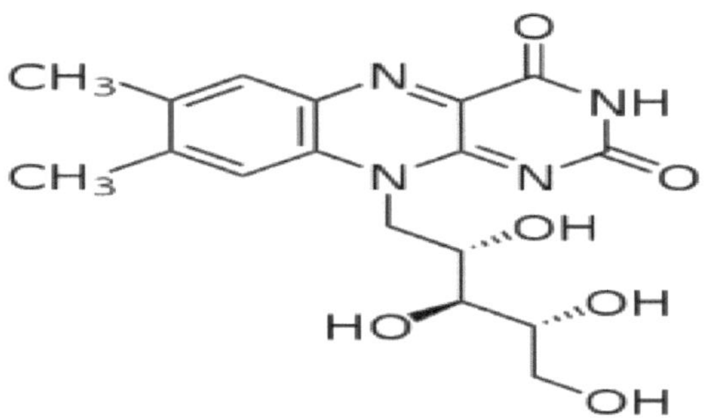

Note the OH group, allowing it to be water-soluble

B_2 is known as riboflavin, a yellow-orange color made from a simple sugar, ribose connected to ring structure. This important coenzyme is fortified by the USDA in many products such as wheat and cereals. Deficiency is rare except in poor diets (as in Japanese navy) Component of FAD and FMN in Krebs' cycle, considered vital parts.

Niacin-B3

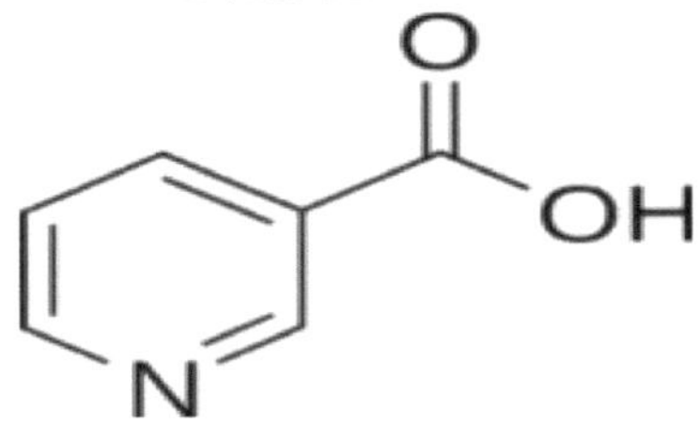

OH group, alcohol, water-soluble

B_3 also known as niacin $C_6H_5NO_2$, a simple compound found in high concentration in animal meat and organs, deficiency in diet leads to pellagra, a common illness in poorly fed populations. Less amounts found in fruits, fungi, whole grains and legumes (beans). Its structure is a simple pyridine (ring structure with 6 carbons) plus carboxyl group (COOH), component NAD in Krebs' cycle.

Pantothenic Acid-B5

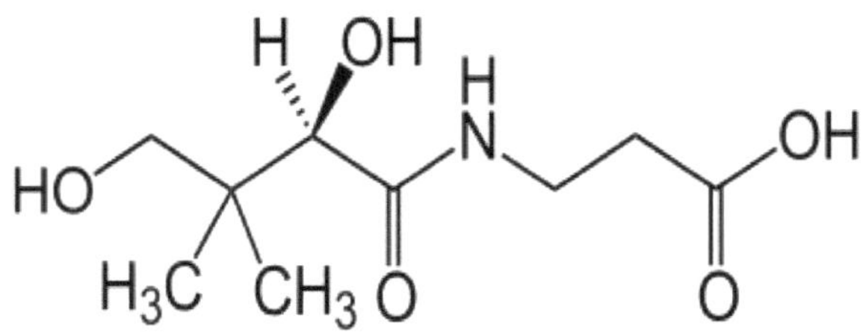

B5-C9H17NO5, known as pantothenic acid, precursor to CoA and steroid production, found in almost every food source, especially high in royal jelly of beehives. Royal jelly is secreted by nurse bees and used to nurture both developing larvae and the adult queen bees. It contains proteins, fatty acids and trace minerals. Although there is no scientific proof of value to humans it is widely acclaimed to have beneficial effects. It appears to have antibiotic effects within the hive.

Pridoxine-B6

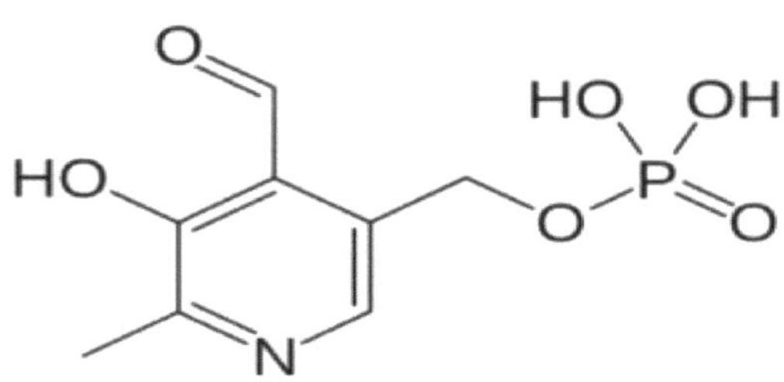

B6-pyridoxine note the pyridine ring structure –$C_8H_{11}NO_3$ needed for growth and repair, vital in the manufacture of nucleic acids and amino acids, glucose and lipid metabolism

Biotin-B7

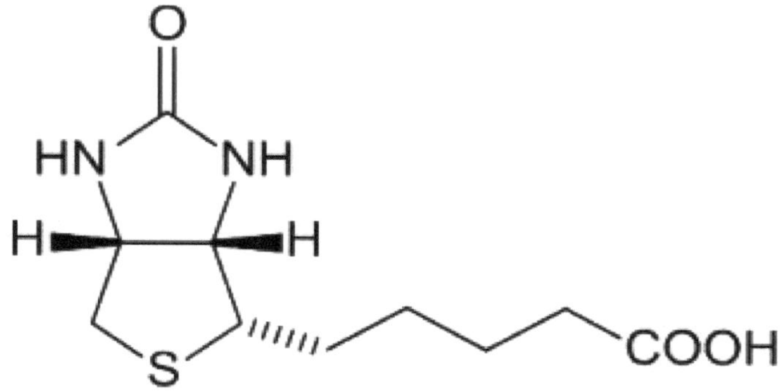

B7-biotin, a Sulfur containing B vitamin C10H16N2O3S, needed for cell growth and repair, fatty acid synthesis and gluconeogenesis (making new non-dietary glucose), deficiency is rare since B7 found in most foods and made by gut bacteria. Found in multiple commercial hair and nail products to fortify their strength? Note the sulfur molecule

Folic Acid-B9

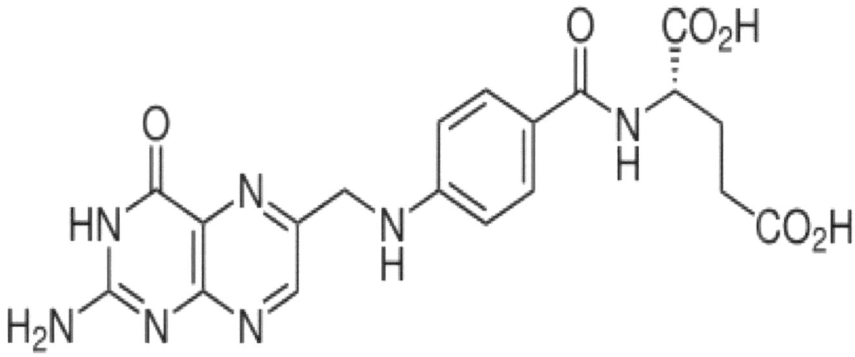

Anemias and spina bifida (birth defect) were greatly benefited by the discovery in 1931 by Lucy Wills that "brewer's yeast" was helpful and contained high amounts of folate. It was not isolated and delivered to medicine until the 1940s. Folic acid or folate is a vitally important coenzyme in pregnancy to prevent neural tube deformity birth defect, and its deficiency common in the elderly and alcoholics. It classically causes anemia with large red blood cells (macrocytic). Many countries require foods to be fortified with folate and recognized by World Health Organization as an Essential Medicine in basic health care. It is found in high concentration in liver and dark green vegetables. Folate deficiency, especially in alcoholics, requires prescription strength high dose.

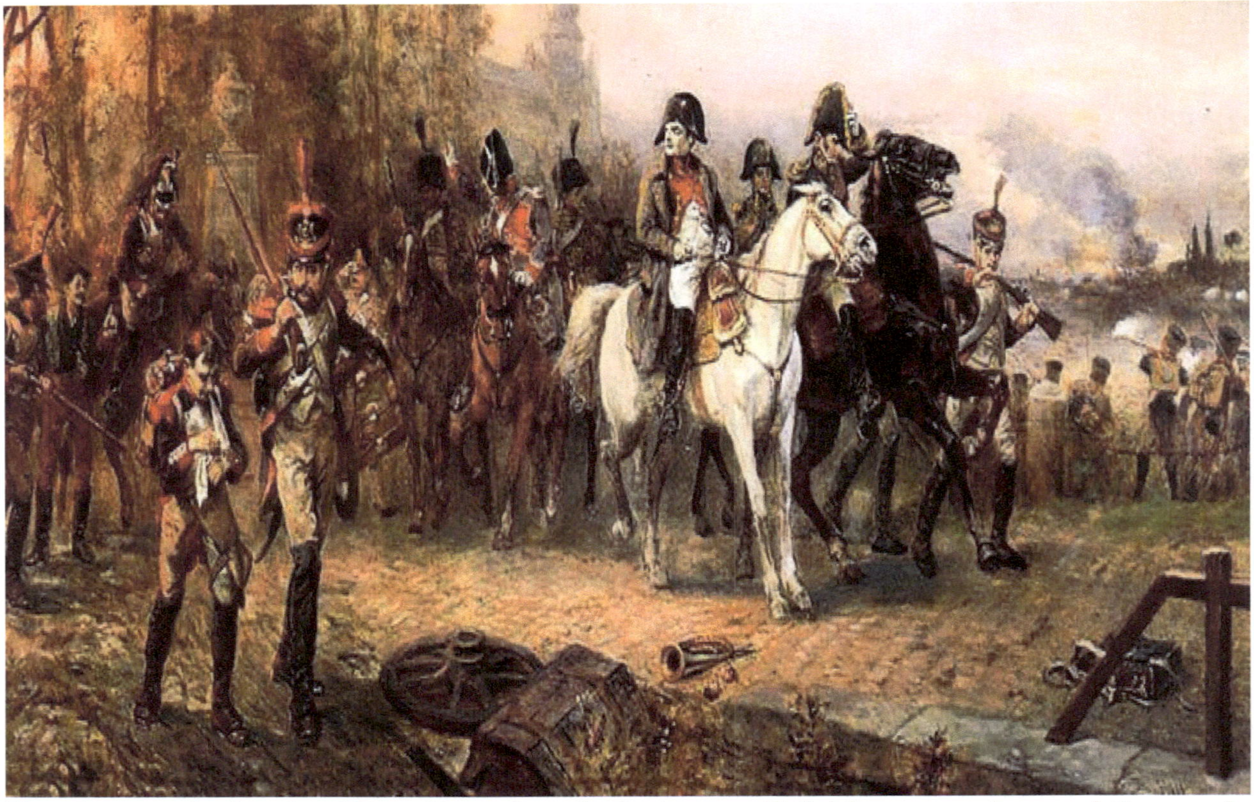

Napoleon at the battle of Borodino where he lost some 47 field commanders and thousands of frontline seasoned combat veterans, losses that fatally crippled his army in Russia and later. After the battle, his chief surgeon, Dominique Jean Larrey preformed over 200 amputations in 24 hours, including the first known successful complete amputation of a leg, where the hip joint was disarticulated, and the officer lived. A famous quote attributed to Napoleon but has never been documented was that "an army moves on its stomach", meaning the food and water needed for men and horses. An army really moves on biochemistry. Feeding a marching army has been a struggle throughout history and the best fed and least infected troops were generally more successful. Napoleon pushed the science community to provide "potable" rations for his army containing high concentration of iron-containing food protein products, later called "Iron Rations". Safe canned meats were not developed until late in the 19th century, but the can-opener was not invented until the 20th century. Current United States armed forces are provided with an 8,000 calorie daily ready-to-eat meals containing iron rations, vitamins and taste-enhancing condiments. Biochemistry and warfare are closely related. Painting by Alexander Hillingford, National Library of Congress

Cobalamin-B12

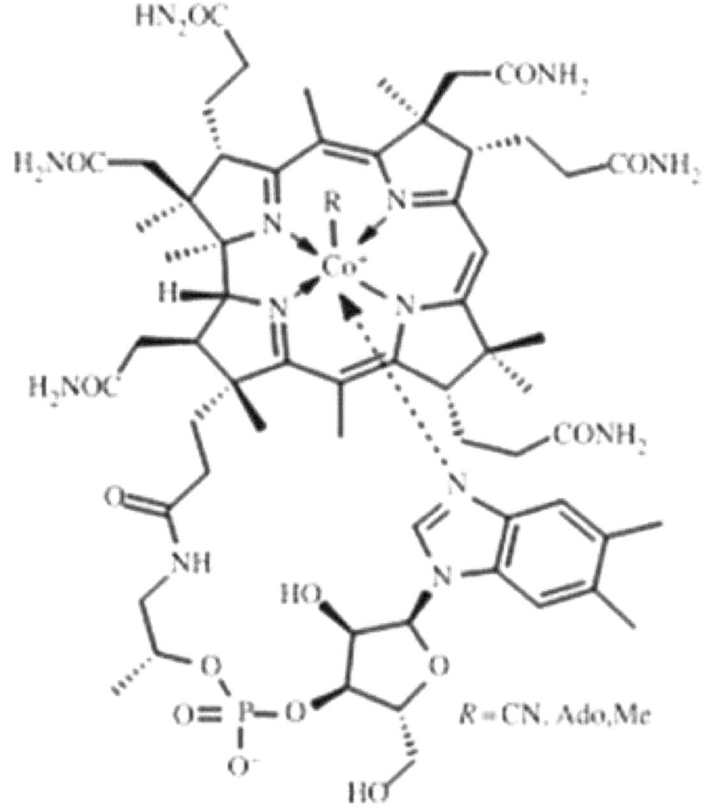

B12-$C_{63}H_{88}CoN_{14}O_4P$, cobalamin (contains molecule of the metal cobalt) is almost the same molecule as chlorophyll (manganese metal) and hemoglobin (iron metal). An elegant structure and life-saving vitamin, called the "ultra-trace element". Every cell requires its presence to make fatty acids, amino acids and DNA. The cobalt metal molecule surrounded by rings is by far the most complicated of B vitamins, and perhaps due to its complicated structure, there is no plant source for B12. Strict vegetarians often need supplements to prevent anemia. B12 anemias have long plagued mankind as meat was not always available but was not understood until the mid-20th century. It is found in almost all animal products, especially liver, however, without cooperation with stomach cells, it does not reach the bone marrow to be incorporated into cell manufacture. Cyanocobalamin is not absorbed without an intrinsic factor in the gut opening the gate to circulation. Injection or absorption under the tongue bypasses the intrinsic factor pathway delivering it directly to bone marrow. Mature physicians during the author's training spoke of making rounds on wards of patients dying with pernicious anemia. Until 1947 it was often fatal and the discovery that it was easily treated by simple B12 injections produced two Nobel Prizes in Medicine.

Example of chemistry in war and peace

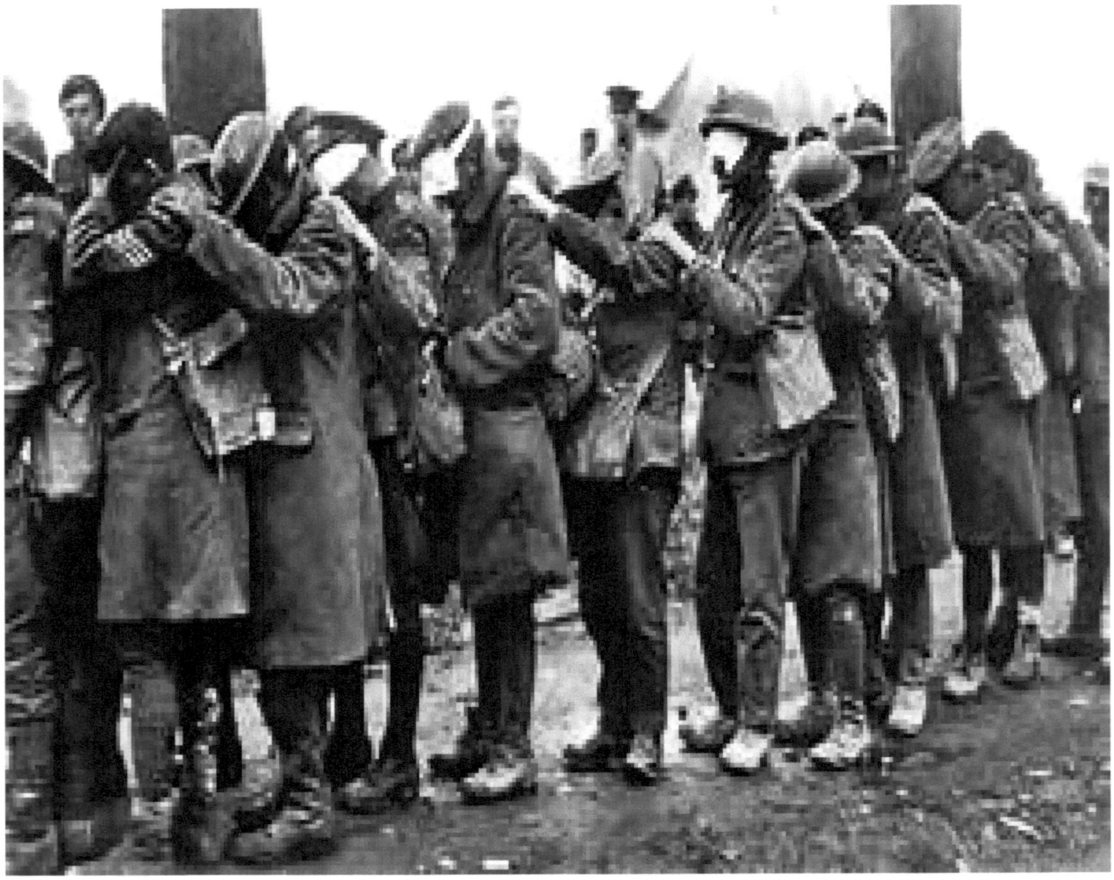

World War I victims of gas attack, probably chlorine. For the widespread use of battlefield chemical weapons, the Great War of 1914-18 has been called "the chemist war". In the last two years, both sides fired a tens of thousands of gas shells. Although no poison gas was used, chemical agents were just as important during World War II. Millions of Jews and other ethnics' peoples were killed with chemical gases by the German Nation, especially late in the Second World War. There is no evidence that Hitler authorized the use of poison gas in combat, perhaps because Hitler was "gassed" during the First World War. There is evidence he offered Franco, the Fascist leader of Spain, to gas those "British rats" out of the Rock of Gibraltar" if Franco would officially join his war efforts. Franco deferred and was the only Nazi to survive the war. The German army, especially later in the war was under the influence of DX-11 containing strong vitamins, methadone and amphetamine. Large doses of stimulants were distributed to German troop during the final months and the American army in Europe were also given amphetamines. Victor Hanson Davis, a favorite of the author reported his father needed months to wean of the stimulants he was given while flying combat missions. National Archives

Mustard Gas

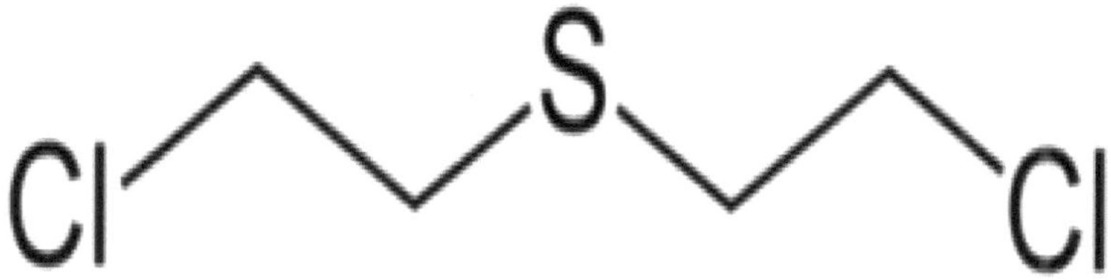

Mustard gas ($C_4H_8Cl_2S$) looks chemically benign, containing simple elements found in all cells, however the unique structure of these 15 atoms has profound effects on cells and tissues. Mustard gas was used later in the Great War, well after the introduction of chlorine gas and both affected survivors for decades. The prolonged effect of mustard gas on its suppression of the human immune system was noted and used to develop the first forms of chemotherapy for cancer. Almost every medical student is familiar with the pharmacology textbook by Goodman and Gilman. These two physicians discovered that survivors of mustard gas had chronically low white blood cells and perhaps in a "eureka" moment, surmised that since it killed normal white blood cells it would be effective in killing rapidly dividing cancer white blood cells. Thus, the first chemotherapy agent for leukemia was born of war.

The deleterious effects of mustard gas happen when a single chlorine atom is pulled off the molecule when it contacts human tissue and replaced by a nitrogen atom. This change in structure not only exposes tissue to the corrosive effects of chlorine but also exposes the sulfur molecule. The "freeing" of the sulfur molecule becomes a free radical which then forms a sulfur-hydrogen group. Acting now as a strong base (acid-base reaction), this changed molecule disrupts the alkylation (destruction) of proteins and nucleic acids, leading to massive blistering and tissue destruction on exposed skin, eyes and mucus membranes of nose, sinuses and lungs. This toxicity reduced its use in medicine until the offensive part of the molecule was removed by replacing a sulfur atom with nitrogen. It is called mustard gas because the color and odor on WWI battlefields resembled mustard and has nothing to do with the mustard plant.

Even though illegal after the First World War, there were massive stockpiles of mustard gas stored by both sides in World War II. However, there is no evidence that either side used poison gas in combat but there was a plan to use gas at Normandy if necessary (per Rick Atkinson). The *SS John Harvey*, an American Liberty cargo ship was secretly and illegally carrying mustard gas into the European war zone, and while awaiting to be unloaded in the Italian port of Bari, was attacked by German aircraft December 2, 1943. When the ship exploded and sank, a cloud of mustard gas settled over the port, maiming and killing hundreds of military and civilian personnel. The medical staff was unaware of the secret cargo and were at a loss on treatment since they did not suspect an illegal weapon was unleashed.

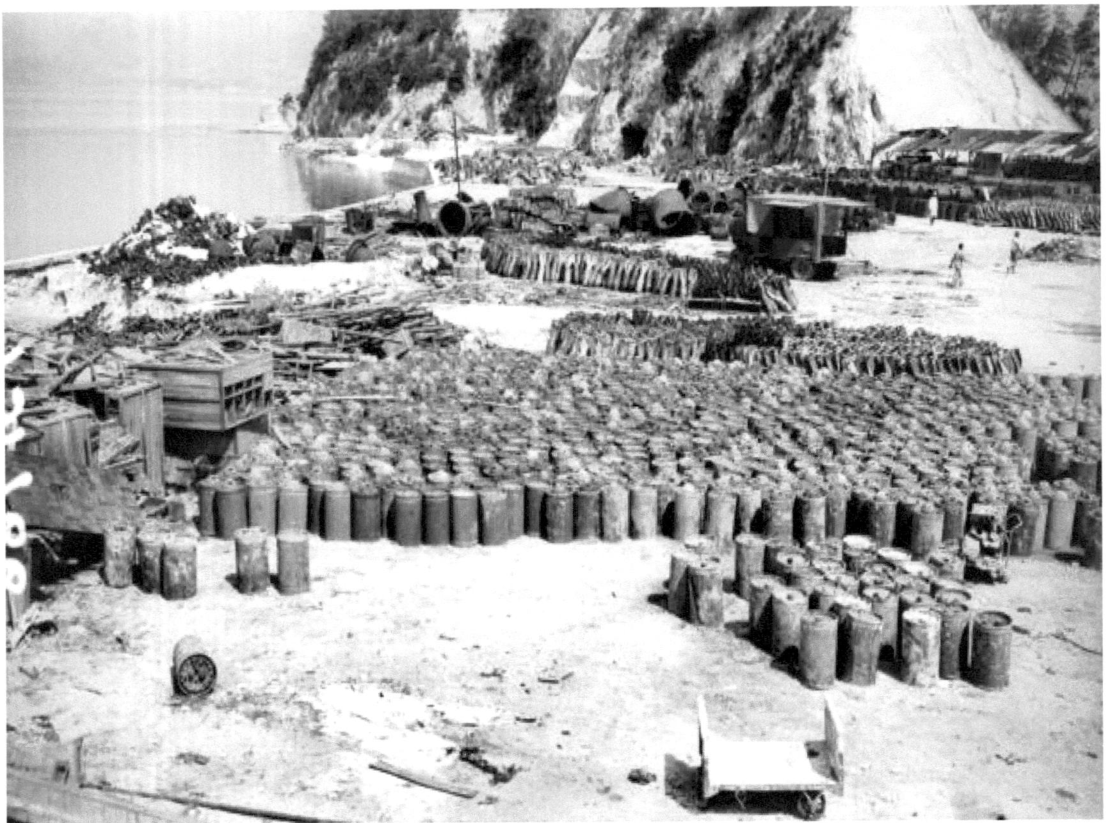

AUSTRALIAN WAR MEMORIAL 131766

One of many Japanese stores of poison gas found after World War II. No evidence that Japan used poison gas in combat but likely would have been used against invading Allied troops except for the atomic bombs. National Archives

One of the most exciting recent breakthroughs in treating cancer is another Sulfur-containing class of molecules, pembrolizumd (Keytruda) being the best-known drug of this class by author. It is composed of 5 of the 6 most common elements in the mammal cell, commercially manufactured in the ovary of Chinese hamsters producing a compound that blocks killer lymphocytes from being destroyed by the cancer cell's defense system. Keytruda is one of the results of Goodman and Gillman discovery of the beneficial effects of sulfur in cancer treatment. Its complete formula is $C_{6534} H_{10004} N_{1716} O_{2036} S_{46}$. The book "Blood and Money" by Thomas Thompson is an excellent read about the Keytruda story. By protecting the killer lymphocytes, Keytruda renders cancer cells more vulnerable to destruction by the host's immune system. It appears that cancer cells can trigger a "death switch" on killer T-cells and Keytruda prevents the activation of that death switch. One could say that Keytruda is the great grandson of mustard gas.

Antibiotics from sharks?

Sulfur is a fascinating molecule with double-edged biochemical activities within the cell. It is important in normal cellular chemistry but at the same time can be a powerful destructive agent in the same cells. Another exciting sulfur chemical is found in sharks, the chemical squalamine, a bile acid containing several amines (polyamine) and a sterol (alcohol OH group) with a sulfur molecule. It is believed to be the lightest oil in nature. Drugs made this molecule may be the next breakthrough in infection and cancer treatment.

Fishermen had long noted that sharks did not appear to have infections nor cancers, which eventually led to the discovery of a compound produced in sharks, Squlamine. This sulfur-containing chemical was first found in a primitive shark, the dog fish (*Squalus*–Latin for sea fish, *acanthias*-Greek for spine or thorn). Sharks have no segmented vertebrae yet like vertebrae (segmented backbone) animals; sharks use iron to carry oxygen, vs non-vertebrae animals that use copper and other metals. Another characteristic of iron-using animals is a complicated immune system. Sharks on the other hand, while using iron to carry oxygen have a simple immune system, a system much simpler than their segmented backbone fellow animals. It appears they rely on a sulfur-containing molecule to prevent disease. Sharks do not experience cancer even when exposed to known carcinogens, nor do their wounds get infected when also exposed to bacteria in repeated experiments. For these reasons, antibiotics and chemotherapy may someday resemble squalamine.

Squalamine

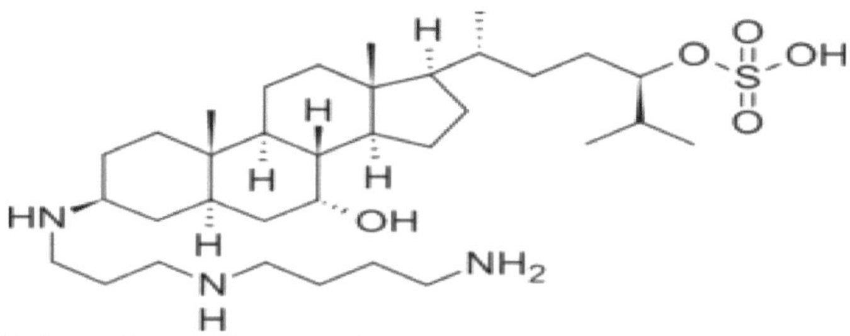

Note the alcohol (OH) hanging off an amine ring structure and the sulfur surrounded by 4 oxygens

Plucking antibiotics from nature is nothing new. The first antibiotics came from natural products, i.e., penicillin and streptomycin were grown from lowly mold fungi. American Indians used moldy spoiled food and lichens (which contain a fungi and algae) to pack into wounds. Before fungal-sourced antibiotics there were heavy metals, mercury, arsenic and lead. The first widely used antibiotic in the 20th century was sulfonamide, developed by the German pharmaceutical company, AG Farber in the 1930s. To discover the best method for administering sulfur as an antibiotic during World War II, the AG Farber company, with orders from their Nazi overlords, experimented on human subjects, especially Priests and Chaplains captured in Western Europe by the Gestapo. Although Germany was a Christian Nation, it became more barbaric as the Nazis continued in power. Using contrived wounds, gunshots, burns, amputations, topical sulfur was applied directly into wounds verses given by oral route. A common sulfur antibiotic in use today is sulfonamide combined with trimethoprim (Bactrim, Septra).

To continue the story of sulfur, there are "Sulfur-loving" bacteria, a key component of animals found surrounding hot vents deep in the ocean. Sulfur allows them to thrive without benefit of sunlight. These bacteria utilize sulfites for food in a world void of sunlight. Recently a shipworm bivalve species that bore into wooden ship's hulls, was found to use sulfides in wood for the creature's nutrition. This to the demise of wooded ships that left the safety of the worm-free

Mediterranean Sea. As European ships sailed into the Atlantic on long-haul voyages, their hulls literally fell apart from the effects of the "teredo" worms. These bivalves "rasped" their jaws into the hulls, using sulfur in the hull's wood as an energy source, to devour wooden ships. This was only remedied by using the antibiotic effects of heavy metals as ship's hulls were covered with thin sheaths of copper. Anti-fouling paint used on nuclear submarines contains high amounts of copper to prevent growths that reduce underwater performance and promote "silent running ".

There is still much to learn about biochemistry inside the cell as most discoveries that currently fill medical biochemistry texts have been in the recent past. Not until the mid-20th century was it known how the cell metabolized fatty acids. The 1964 Nobel Prize for medicine and physiology was awarded to Konrad Bloch and Feodor Lynen for discovering that a molecule manufactured by the cell combining cholesterol with sulfur, Coenzyme A (COA) enables the human cell to "burn" fat.

The author hopes these stories and concepts have been enjoyed by the reader, especially the author's fascination with sulfur, an element that is both necessary for the cell's health while at the same time dangerous. This concludes the discussion of medical biochemistry and though far from complete, hopefully it opened some doors in the reader's mind to further study. The world is full of biochemistry and there are many opportunities to learn and perhaps discover new explanations for how the cell interacts with chemistry. The author believes biochemistry in the cell is like a 3-D printer. The nucleus contains a blueprint in its DNA for every needed chemical and structure. Taking in raw materials, the cell builds, repairs and protects itself with manufactured products. The earth before life, contained all the raw materials, yet needed a force and a blueprint to assemble these into an organized pattern. The author believes life was that force and DNA the blueprint.

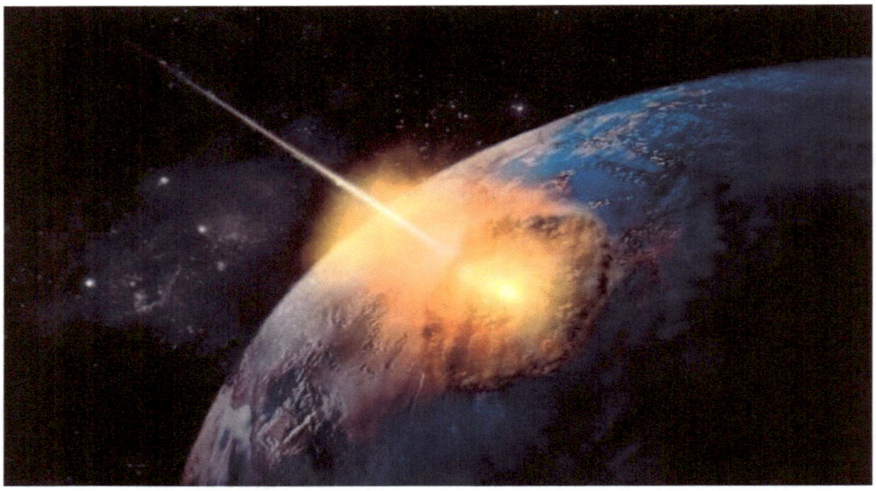

Comets containing blueprints (DNA) may have fertilized the egg of earth.

There are ancient stone records of such extraterrestrial events. One such record lies in east central Turkey, near the initial site of domestication of plants and animals in Western Civilization. Gobekli Tepe, "pot-bellied hill" in Turkish, is the site of a thirteen-thousand-year-old complex. The site is huge and carved into stone is the image of a comet-like object coming at earth. Eight thousand years ago, these structures were deliberately buried. For information, the author recommends Graham Hancock and Randall Carlson's presentations on YouTube.

Medical Microbiology

The study of life under magnification

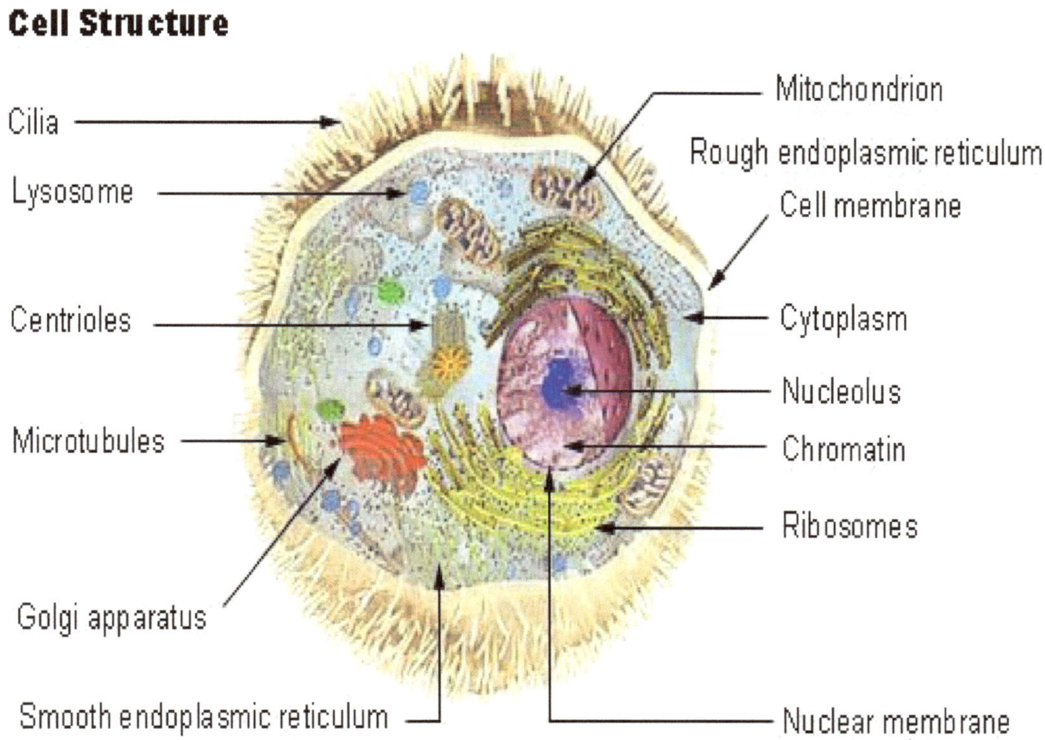

The cell is a natural work of art, as this beautiful illustration of the complexity and majesty of the animal cell portrays-NIH

The body is a complex entity containing trillions of its own cells living among trillions of alien organisms; bacteria, viruses, parasites, fungal colonies outnumbering human cells by a factor of at least ten. The native cells and their "guests" consume raw materials, manufacture chemicals, construct structures, generate waste, defend, attack, destroy and repair. The author's first medical microbiology lecture began with Professor explaining why study microbiology; "A cell can do everything an entire person can do and then some. It can make its own food, protect itself, communicates with its fellow cells, repairs damage, and reconfigure chemicals into new forms". It is within the cell, where chemistry meets life and controlled chemical behavior creates the evidence of life.

Microbiology is one of medicine's newest members, as the microscope has only been in widespread use for some 200 years. The microscope revealed an entire world to study, providing the foundations for the medical sciences of pathology and immunology. This chapter is primarily concerned with infections of cells and cellular tissues, describing structures, mechanisms of action and the mysteriousness of the human immune system.

Fever and microbes

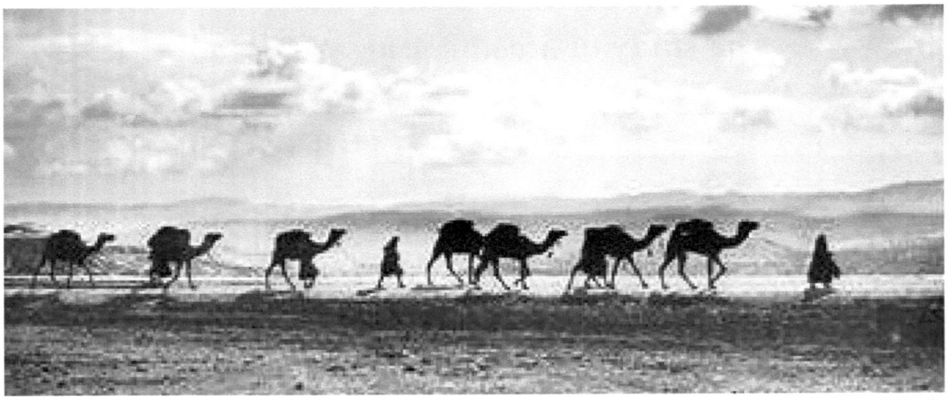

Some things are unchanged in Egypt as camels still transport materials and infections that plagued the ancient Egyptians and later the Greeks, Romans, British, still thrive in the Nile Delta. National Archives

Fever is a sign of infection in the field and at sea. There are other causes of fever, but they are not part of this discussion. This cardinal rule of fever as a cause of infection was driven home to me as a medical student in Cairo while studying medicine at the United States Naval Research Unit #3. I arrived in late 1981 as a newly minted US Navy Ensign just after the President of Egypt, Muhammed Anwar Sadat was assassinated. Egypt has known assassinations for thousands of years and the nation seemed to be soldiering on as the Nile flowed north. The Nile River had lured Ensign Hill to delve into the tropical medicine created by the river valley. The water from the interior of Africa and the delta the river creates in miles of sluggish flow provide environments for a host of human infections. One of my attending professors was a retired US Navy Captain and cardiologist, Captain Jack Dempsey. He became an important factor of my medical education.

Captain Dempsey was a well-travelled and well-read physician, historian and an interesting yet demanding mentor. His influence was one of the reasons histories is used as a conduit to teach medicine in this text. Our relationship started poorly on my part because of my misperception of fever. After listening to a case presentation of a 14-year-old male Egyptian farmer with a fever of unknown origin, Captain Dempsey was kind enough to ask my opinion. As the fever had lasted several weeks and the lab tests did not indicate an obvious infection, I felt the fever could be the result of an autoimmune disorder or perhaps some type of cancer. Captain Dempsey stopped me and in a scolding manner said, “This is the tropics young man and fever here and elsewhere is always presumed to be caused by an infection. Remember, the first 10 causes of fever are infections!”

Medical microbiology in this text concentrates on those infectious agents most likely to encounter or ones the author finds particularly interesting. Many infections encountered in Egypt and elsewhere were diagnosed with a microscope. Microscopes are rarely available in the field and the knowledge to use a microscope is even rarer. Pathogens and the conditions or diseases they cause can be usually identified by descriptions of the history and physical signs. Infectious agents include bacteria, viral, fungal and a bizarrely diverse group, parasites. In the Western World most infections are caused by bacteria and/or viruses, however in the tropical Third World, parasitic infections are as common. Malaria alone, an intracellular parasite, accounts for hundreds of millions new cases each year. Infectious agents has and will continue to change history.

Animal Cells

Just as humans look different than a tree or a mushroom, the cells of animals look different than the cells of plants and fungi. Human and other animal cells are unique, in that they are enclosed in a pliable cell membrane, whereas bacteria, fungi and plant cells have more rigid cell walls. The flexible membranes of animals have allowed them to move about in the natural world. Some have compared animal cell membrane to a soap bubble. If it is a soap bubble, it's a very complicated bubble, appearing more like the "Death Star" in Star Wars than one in a bubble bath. Membranes, being more flexible than walls, give the animal cell more mobility and allow the placement of mechanical devices. Human cell membranes are punctured with receptors, channels, dead end tunnels, sprouting antennae, projections containing protective mechanisms, both offensive and defensive. And there are still components yet to be discovered.

The membrane is so complicated, it is now considered a separate organelle of the cell. It is much more than just a flexible shell protecting the more fragile interior, as the more rigid cell wall does in bacteria, fungi and plants. The human cell membrane is semipermeable and selective, allowing entrance of fluids, nutrients, oxygen, chemical messengers while discharging waste and releasing its own messages to other cells. Admittance is strictly monitored, providing a secure border, serving as a barrier to unwanted visitors and chemicals. The membrane can and is breached by invaders such as bacteria, virus and in some cases intracellular parasites. Imagine a creature (protozoa) so small, dozens can live inside a human cell (malaria). The cell wall, a fixed fortress, strong but limited in motion, found in plants, bacteria and fungi, whereas a cell membrane, while providing less protection is more mobile. The tank was developed as a rigid protective wall that moves. Early tanks barely moved, but by World War II, tanks could fight and travel at 30-40 miles per hour. In the Great War of 1914-18, the fortresses of trench warfare became almost impregnable to infantry. To combat this obstacle, the tank was invented as a mobile fortress, a rigid wall that moved. Although early tanks travelled at 2-4 miles per hour while modern tanks travel at 60-70mph while accurately firing at targets miles away.

Cell membranes are composed of strands of proteins with amino acids and fatty acids form chains with fatty hydrophobic tails at one end and amino "heads" at the other creating a phospholipid bilayer membrane. Even though these structures are coupled, they have an aversion for parts of the other's chemical structure. The fatty acid tails are repelled by water (hydrophobic- "water-hating"), and the amino "head end" attracted to water (hydrophilic "water-loving"). Together they form the bilayer membrane molecule, thus creating a fluid, flexible membrane. It is the combination of proteins, fats and phosphates, all manufactured by the cell following the blueprints of DNA that gives the membrane of animal cells flexibility, passages and protective structures. Imagine the layer appearing when oil is added to water forming a layer of film at the point of contact where oil meets water.

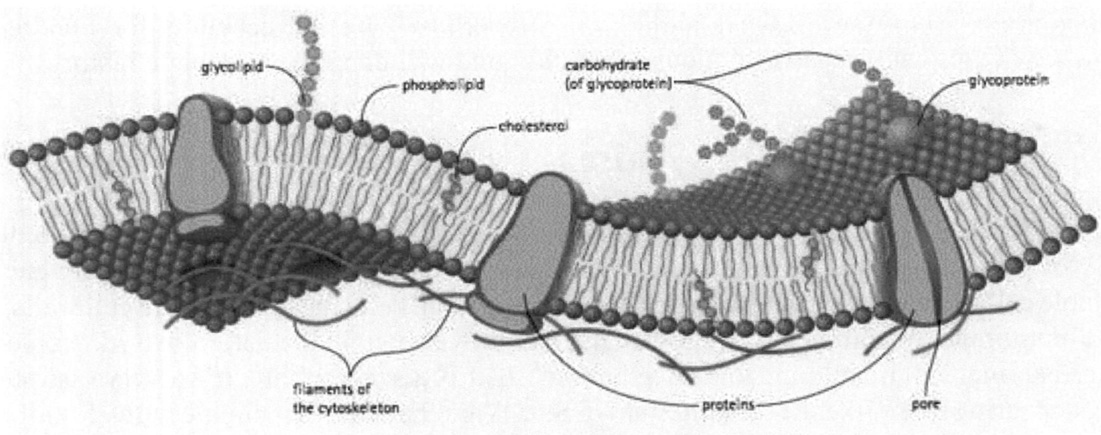

This bilayer plasma membrane of animal cells allows for both passive and active transport across the membrane, thus the protein channels. Glucose passively crosses central nervous cells but must be actively transported by insulin across all other cell membranes. NLM

Within the human cell are factory-like organelles, mitochondria, a Greek word meaning thread-like grain. In microbiology, similar cells working together normally would be recognized as tissue, except mitochondria are too small to rate as tissue (like Pluto is too small to be a planet). Mitochondria are the "power plants" of animal cells, where cellular respiration burns fuel in the presence of oxygen. Some of the energy is used on site in the mitochondria, while most is converted into portable energy stored in chemicals as high-energy bonds created when phosphate (oxygen-phosphorus) is strongly bound to a nucleic acid (adenosine) by being fused to the ring structure. When three phosphate molecules are bound, it is known as adenosine triphosphate (ATP). The manufacture and transfer energy in the form high-energy phosphate bonds within the microscopic mitochondria is not unlike oil refineries producing and loading petroleum products onto ships and trucks. Tankers, like ATP molecules, are under control of an organized distribution system of energy to designated areas of use. The energy needed to produce ATP resides in the furnaces and forges of mitochondria, where burning (oxidizing) carbohydrates in the presence of oxygen (aerobic respiration) process raw materials into chemicals and structures. And like human manufacturing plants, this process generates waste, especially excess heat and CO_2, exhausts the cell must expel. This is like a car's internal combustion engine burning hydrocarbons in the presence of oxygen and discharging the waste safely out the exhaust pipe, away from the occupants. Carbohydrates used in the cell contain oxygen, whereas hydrocarbons used by the internal combustion engine, only contain hydrogen and carbon.

Almost all human cells contain a nucleus (red blood cells do not) where the management and direction of the cell takes place. Animals, fungi and most plant cells have a nucleus (eukaryotic); however, bacteria and viruses do not (prokaryotic). Cells without nucleus can invade cells with nuclei and use the command center to make more copies of invaders. For these infectious agents, simpler is better. After all, we are perhaps the most complicated organism on earth and in some respects quite fragile, the result of too many systems. Infectious agents are designed to capture resources from the host's cells, organisms behaving as raiders, like the sea-borne Vikings that raided England and northern France. The Norsemen had little central control, and yet were able to terrorize and occupy more organized communities. Vikings spread their people and culture by taking from less aggressive and less protected people, like bacteria and viruses invading the host's vulnerable tissue. Bacterial infections include plague (Black Death), abscesses, pneumonia, TB, leprosy, syphilis, typhus, appendicitis. Tetanus, cholera, botulism and gangrene wreak their havoc with toxic wastes released by bacteria.

The human body contains trillions of cells; surprisingly, most are not our cells. For the most part, these organisms are happy partners, however some can become invasive. In some cases, normal inhabitants, always present within the host, can become a menace. These are the causes of "opportunistic" infections. The total number and species residing within and upon a human are currently unknown, as only some 3-5 % has been identified. Human bodies contain more foreign organisms than their own cells! The colon alone contains several pounds of bacteria. It has been known for decades that the upper respiratory tract, skin, oral cavity and colon are teaming with foreign life. Now it seems that areas formally thought of as sterile, harbor foreign creatures.

Even the tiny air sacks (alveoli) in the in the lungs long believed to be sterile, have resident creatures (*pneumocystis carinii*). This creature was discovered in the early 1900s but was ignored until it began to kill people in the AIDS outbreak. So new is this pathogen that microbiologists are undecided whether *pneumocystis carinii* are fungi or protozoa, but they are certainly not human. It is also known that this organism is found in the lungs of every mammal living on earth and was relatively unknown as a pathogen until it caused a deadly pneumonia in immune compromised humans. What could be the purpose of this organism living in our lungs?

In medicine, the human bite is considered the "dirtiest" wound due the large number of bacteria, followed by other primate and the bite of cats. The oral cavity of mammals, especially the human mouth, contains hundreds of millions, perhaps billions of bacteria, more than fish, fowl and reptile (with one exception) making these bites the most likely to get infected. Dog bites are considered less infectious than most pets, since for pathogens, the dog's mouth is much cleaner than a cat. Although hard to believe, the human mouth contains more bacteria than the rectum. Think about that with those deep wet kisses as the human mouth contains more organisms than there are stars in the Milky Way! Some studies reveal the clean kitchen sink contains more pathogens than the toilet.

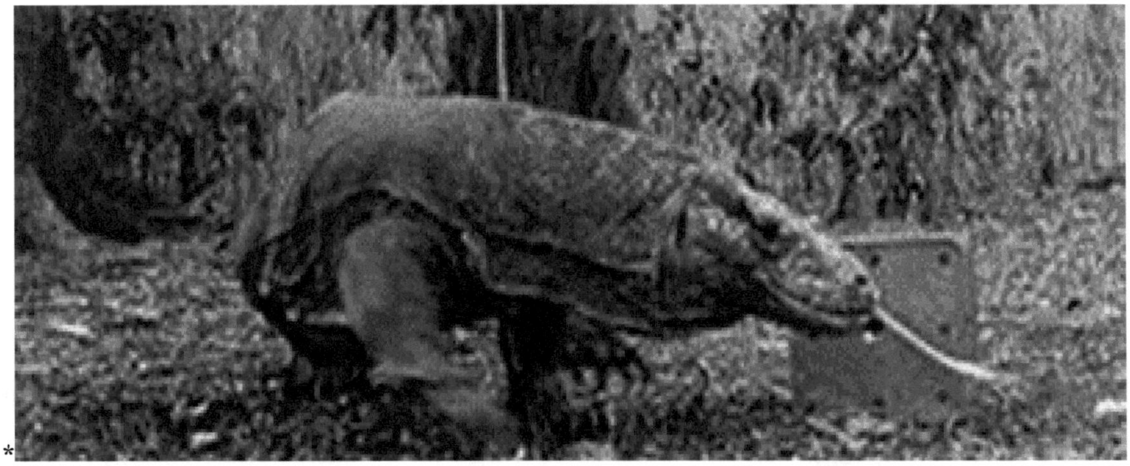

*

The Komodo dragon found only in Indonesia may have the "dirtiest bite" in nature but is fortunately found on just a few islands in the world, is slow moving and seldom encounters humans (excepting slower-moving tourists with cameras). In a world filled with millions of

bacteria, fungi, viruses and parasites, fortunately very few causes human diseases. National library of Congress

Infectious Diseases

Starting to medical school in the late 1970's, the author purchased the recently published textbook, "Infectious Diseases", 2nd Edition, in it, Hoeprich stated "Only some 50 infectious agents are of importance in Medicine." Currently there are many more, with new ones to be discovered. The list stands at 538 bacteria (includes rickettsia), 317 fungi, 287 helminths, 208 viruses, 57 protozoa and counting. Some "new" infections are coming from microbes residing permanently in the body's tissue, residents that have been living among humans from the beginning.

This is a good time to define infections that effect large populations. These are known as epidemics, pandemics and endemics. Epidemics are infections that begin with a common source and spread outward, such as the "Spanish Flu" of 1918, the plagues of Athens and Justinian. Pandemics are infections that seem to arise almost simultaneously from many sources infecting much of the world. Epidemics and pandemics arise and then fall, seeming to disappear. Some infections become endemic after infecting large numbers of people and remain infected for many generations. Smallpox became endemic after arriving in Europe, Asia and India in the Dark Ages and stayed for over 1000 years. It was not eradicated until the 20th century. Smallpox killed and maimed relentlessly, infecting much of the population in waves, killing 30-90% of infected. Many parasitic infections, especially malaria, have become endemic in many areas.

Bacterial Infections

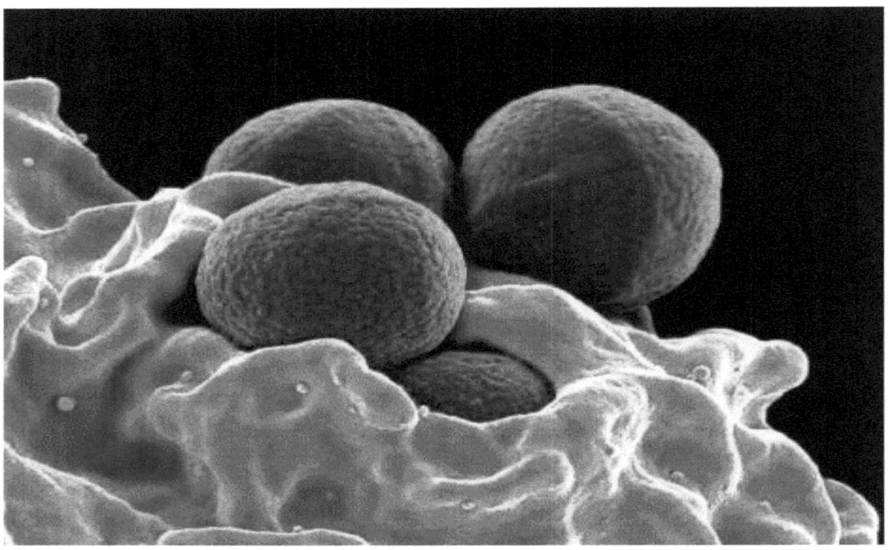

Electron microscopy of staphococcus (*staph*-Latin for grape cluster, *coccus* for round, streptococcus is round, bacteria found in chains as *strep* is Latin for chain). Bacterial disease varies widely, some like cholera can kill in hours, while syphilis takes decades. CDC

Bacterial infections are generally extracellular, meaning the infection is outside the cell in the surrounding tissue. In the skin, bacterial infections lead to swelling, redness, tenderness and heat. In the body cavities of lung, gut, reproductive and urinary systems it causes fever and pain. In response to bacterial infections, human cells and the immune system unleash a robust counteroffensive. Chemicals released by the violated cells and tissues attract "killer white blood cells", the immune system's bloodhounds, tracking down and attacking invasive cells. Chemicals released by other immune cells attach to invasive cells allowing them to be recognized, herded together and rendered disabled. As the body's immune system destroys bacteria there will always be collateral destruction of innocent human tissue, causing the cardinal signs of infection: redness, swelling, tenderness and heat. These four findings of bacterial infections have been chiseled into stone by the Egyptians and reconfirmed by following medical texts.

If not controlled, destruction expands in infection, providing more food for the bacteria. Bacteria are generally as large as human cells and in most cases do not attack individual cells but the tissue where similar cells reside. Bacterial infections are often non-selective as to type of tissue infected and many cases are opportunistic infections. Infections, caused by the body's normally present bacteria taking advantage of the opportunity provided by weakened immune activity or when the protective skin barrier is breached. Bacterial infections not contained and eliminated may lead to loss of extremity, organ failure or even death. The slow death of Rome can be perceived in a similar manner as tribes pushed around and into Roman territory, consuming resources previously consumed by Romans, which weakened the city-state. Finally, the invasive people broke into the walls of Rome itself after stripping the countryside and sacked the city. Rome fell because it could no longer protect itself. A weakened human immune system is vulnerable, increasing the risk of invasive organisms that live around and in the body. Not unlike the fall of Constantinople where the thousand-year-old walls of Theodosius finally yielded to gunpowder and the relentless of great numbers.

Bacterial infections generally occupy a single body system, i.e., sinus infection, pneumonia in lungs, abscesses in skin, bladder infections, and Helicobacter pylori in stomach ulcers. When multiple systems become involved in bacterial infections, it is a poor sign. Bacterial infections are best identified and treated as early as possible, while they still involve only a single site. An example is a skin infection that escapes the wound site and spreads through the lymphatic channels to distant sites. A red tender warm streak radiating from the wound site towards the central body means the infection has broken out and spreading. In the pre-antibiotic area, this sign often led to amputations above the streak to reduce the risk of spread and death. Fortunately, in most cases the immune system can "wall-off" and contain an infection, especially in skin wounds. An infection contained is easier to eradicate and will lead to a pocket of destruction containing pus and fluid that enlarges into an abscess. This is easily opened and drained thus removing the infection (described later). Wound infections resulting in spreading infection are known as cellulitis and discussed more fully in the skin section of this text. Proper wound care with clean hands, clean dressings, lots of clean water, removal of debris and dead tissue from wound (debridement) and prompt use of antibiotics greatly reduce the risk of wounds causing serious bacterial infections.

President Garfield was shot in the abdomen in an assassination attempt, and he might have survived except for the dozen physicians inserting unwashed fingers into the wound trying to locate the bullet. Of interest is that Garfield like every Republican president elected from Ulysses Grant in

1868 until William McKinley in 1897 was a former Union military officer. The lingering effects of the American Civil War not only produced soldier-presidents but kept some southern states occupied by Union troops for decades.

Antibiotics in most cases are effective in bacterial infections and not viral or fungal since they usually disable bacterial defenses or reproduction. The term antibiotic was coined by Louis Pasteur when he described "life against life" in the battles under his microscope. The earliest antibiotic in Western medicine was mercury, and it has been in use for thousands of years. It does kill bacteria but is highly toxic to the human cell. American Indians and other "primitive" cultures used combinations of "mold" (fungi) and lichens (an organisms contain both fungi and algae) both topically and orally for infections. These contain fungal produced antibiotics. Soon after the discovery of sulfa chemicals, the first safe and powerful antibiotic penicillin was derived from simple fungal mold, often found on old bread. The chemical isolated from the mold, penicillium ascomycetous is produced by the fungal colony to protect itself from bacteria. The "so called" broad spectrum antibiotics came after penicillin and are effective against several bacteria and multiple sites in the body. These are covered in detail in the section on antibiotics.

Viruses-Latin word for poisonous agent

Viruses are so small they require an electron microscope to be visualized. Early microbiologists suspected an agent capable of causing infection that crossed a filter that blocked other agents and was unable to be seen under magnification available. These were referred to as "unfiltered" agents. Compared to human cells, they appear not only much smaller but also much simpler. Probably only a tiny number of viruses have been identified and only a handful has caused important infections in world history include yellow fever, smallpox, influenza, measles, hepatitis, AIDS and COVID-19.

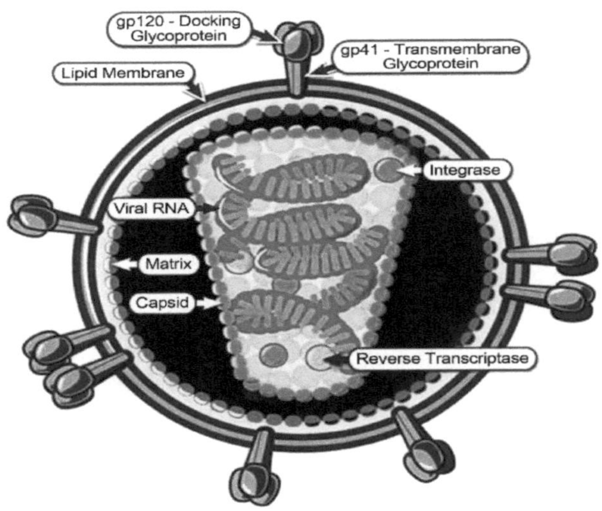

Illustration of HIV (AIDS) virus depicting its protective envelope with projections for attaching and penetrating host cell containing enzymes to cut and insert viral "software" into DNA or RNA redirecting the host cell activity. NIH

Viruses are intracellular infections, and it must gain access to the cell's interior to survive. Viruses generally attack only one type of cell, and the signs of viral infections are primarily due to the body's response to intracellular infection, i.e., rash of measles, chicken pox, yellow skin in hepatitis and yellow fever, bleeding under skin in hemorrhagic fevers. Some severe viral infection kills by triggering massive response from host immune system, causing body-wide bleeding from disseminated intravascular bleeding, DIC. Antibiotics in most cases are ineffective in killing viruses since they are safely inside the host's cells. Viruses appear to be only part of a cell, not a complete cell containing structures and internal organelles. They are tiny and simple when compared to a human, plant and bacteria cells as well as most parasites in that viruses are unable to reproduce without entering and "taking-over" a host cell. There is controversy as to their origin, whether a virus is "alive", did they appear before other cells or are they pieces of former cells, could they be aliens from space and do viruses have some form of primitive intelligence as well as other unknowns. They are everywhere, floating in the atmosphere and immersed in water. One investigator found that on every square meter of surface on the earth there are one billion viruses. Masks are hardly capable of preventing them from reaching the respiratory track as a chain link fence would block flies.

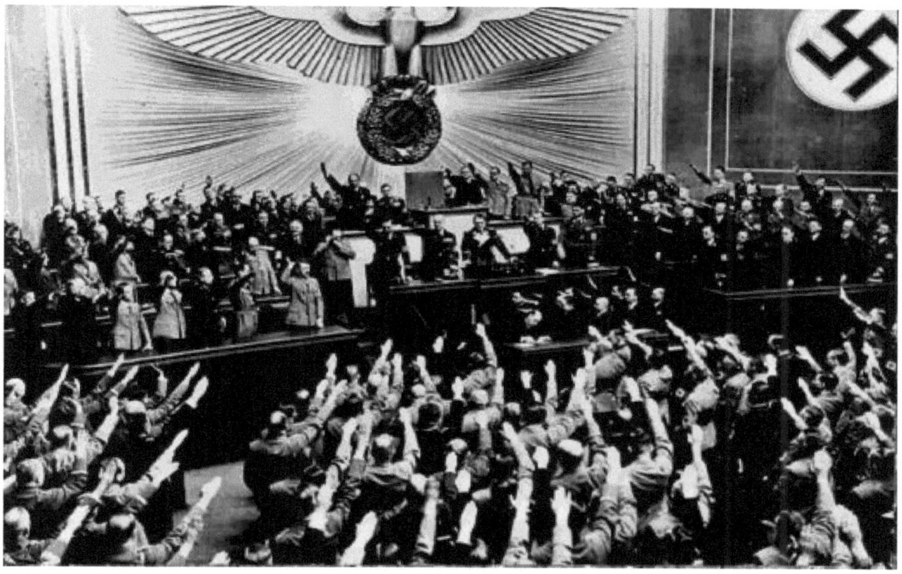

Hitler receiving adoration of the German people after "acquiring" Austria. National Archives

The actions of viruses is not unlike what happened in Germany in 1930's, where a tiny handful of National Socialists (NAZIs) took over first a single country, Germany and then most of Europe. Hepatitis, AIDs, influenza, measles, Ebola, smallpox, herpes and the common cold are examples of viral infections. Viral "organisms" appear much simpler than the cells they infect, being composed primarily of only three parts: a capsule protecting a small piece of DNA or RNA and two pairs of chemical scissors (enzymes that cut and paste changes to the invaded cell's blueprints). With the genetic code changed, the cell is forced to follow the "false information" to change normal cell function to a pathological pathway. Viruses can only reproduce by injecting themselves into a cell where it sabotages and takes over the cell's normal function, enslaving the cell to make copies of the viral components. Even though a virus is tiny compared to a cell, it is powerful enough to overcome the infected cell, where after a period of incubation, the cell is destroyed and releases copies of the invading organisms. These new viruses hungrily invade other cells.

Smallpox

"Envious and foul disease, could there not be one beauty in an age, free from thee." Ben Johnson

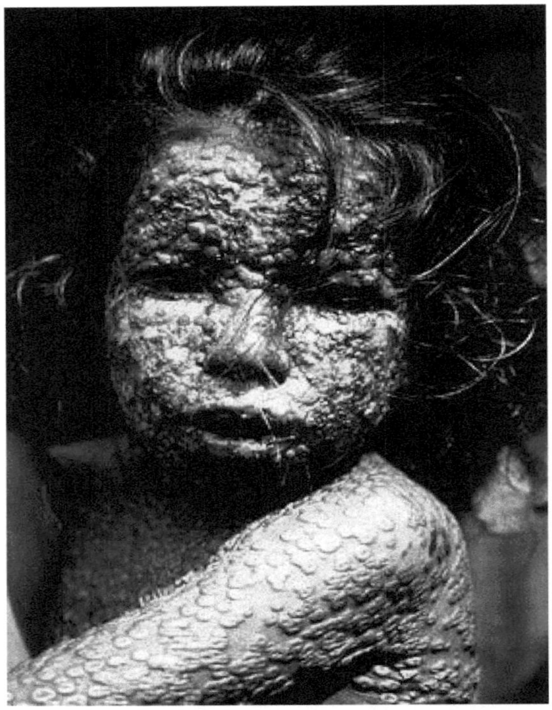

One of the last recorded cases of smallpox from Bangladesh 1977. There were rare cases in India and Somalia in the 1980's. This deadly virus continues to reside in a few virology labs and currently under tight security and is probably in biological warfare depots. NIH

Variola (smallpox) had all but disappeared from the study of medicine by the time the author (part the last generation of Americans to be mass vaccinated) entered medical training in the 1970's and what little was learned about this scourge was scant. The virologist at the author's school remarked "We really do not know how Variola killed". But kill it did and did so in great numbers in places the Europeans exploited. During the 17th and 18th centuries Age of Exploration, generations of Europeans lived and died, infecting perhaps half the world's population often killing one in two! Jared Diamond in his book "Guns, Germs and Steel" credits the domestication of animals where diseases were shared, and immunity obtained. This allowed Europeans to conquer much of the world where immunity to smallpox was unknown. Variola first appeared in Western Europe during the Dark Ages but increased dramatically at the end of the Crusades following on the heels of the Black Death. Both epidemics carried primarily by ships since land travel was too slow to allow spreading of the diseases. Centuries of strife in the Holy Lands had greatly changed the extent of Europe's contact with the outside world. Ships carrying men and goods had transformed the coastal shipping dominated by a few city-states on the Italian peninsula into large armed fleets containing infectious agents.

The Crusades stimulated military and commercial shipping for centuries after Europeans were expelled from the Middle East. And field medicine travelled with this traffic, carrying armies and pilgrims along with their supplies to the Holy Lands, returning with spices, silk (at times one pound of silk worth two-and one-half pounds of gold) and porcelain from the Far-East, purchased from Arab caravans. Trade kept education alive and two of history's best known field medical officers, Avicenna the Persian and Maimonides the Hebrew come from the Crusader period. Even though the European fought the Saracen, they kept open an active trade. Christian Venice with its large navy was often allied with the Ottoman Empire and France was treaty-bound with the Ottomans during the 16th-18th centuries when the rest of Christian Europe was fighting Islamic Turkey. Ships returning from the East, trading along the coasts of the Mediterranean, through the Pillars of Hercules (Gibraltar straits) and into the Atlantic carried smallpox as part of trade. When European cities grew, concentrating populations, smallpox became endemic, and medicine had no answer until vaccination (Latin for cow) centuries later.

Smallpox came to America with the Spanish and their slaves from Africa, decimating first the natives of Central America, later spreading north and south. Smallpox, unlike other infectious diseases, did not come in cycles, but remained in continuous contact with humans, killing in every generation. Until the advent of the smallpox vaccine, no mother could count her children until they had passed through the fire of smallpox. Ben Franklin lost a young son to smallpox, a loss he mourned all his life. Peter the Great's grandson, who revealed the same promise for leadership as his grandfather, unfortunately fell victim to smallpox and died before the age of 18. Those that survived death were often left with scars and broken health. It killed many soldiers both American and British in the American Revolutionary War while continued to kill and maim during the American Civil War.

Smallpox vaccination had been in use in India and Turkey for hundreds, perhaps a thousand years, by using scrapings from infected smallpox sores. Scraping causing milder symptoms but carried a high risk of pox scarred skin and even death. Though it was effective if the patient survived, it was not acceptable to most western physicians through the 18th century (although George Washington was vaccinated with smallpox as were many of his troops). Safer, effective vaccination was achieved by a general practitioner, Edward Jenner in rural England, who noted that milkmaids that contracted a mild form of pox known as cowpox, were immune from the more deadly smallpox. Edward Jenner in the 18th century with encouragement from his teacher, the great Scottish self-trained physician, John Hunter, inoculated several young patients, including his own son by scraping pus into their skin from a cowpox sore. His work was so successful that the medical community embraced this new technique within a few years. He was rewarded by Knighthood, numerous honors from European nations, even American Indian tribes. After Jenner's work, Spain introduced smallpox vaccine to the new world by sending a ship of orphan boys to its ports in Central and South America. Every week aboard this vessel, two new boys were inoculated from the still weeping sores of the previous two boys until they arrived in America. Two boys were inoculated, so that if one died, the other would carry the active virus forward as it was common for children to perish at sea, even without receiving experimental vaccines. From Cartagena, these boys spread the vaccine to America as fresh sores were passed on to other people.

Fungi
Latin word for mushroom

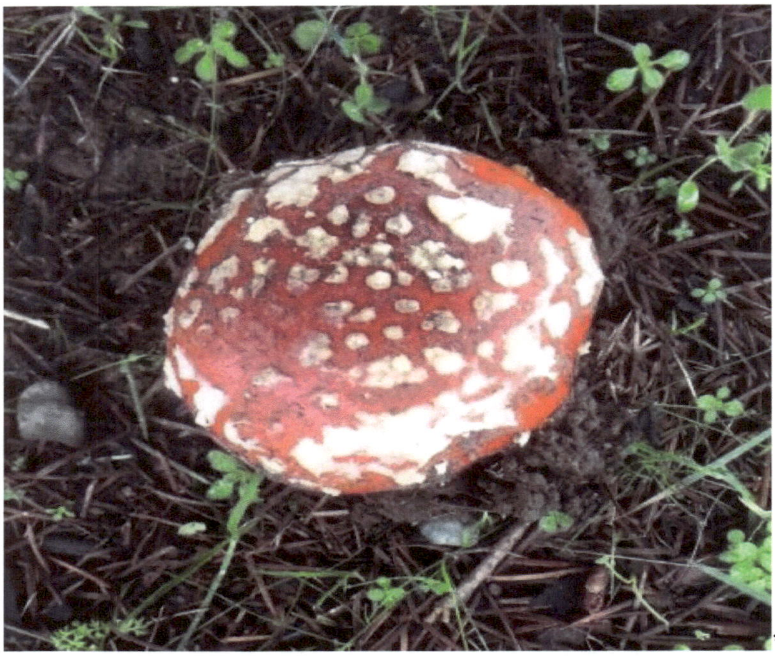

*

This mushroom, *amanita muscara*, considered toxic, is not deadly but will often cause nausea and vomiting. It does contain a powerful hullucigen and is the only hallucigen found above the Arctic Circle. Scandinavian Laplander legend have a myth that reindeer eat them, become intoxicated and "fly". This is likely the source of the legend of Santa Claus with his red hat with a white top and his flying reindeer. Mushrooms are the fruiting body of an underground fungus, just as apples are the fruiting body of the apple tree. Photo by author

Medical mycology (German word *myco* for fungus) is the study of pathological fungi. Neither plant nor animal, fungi occupy a separate Kingdom. They reproduce by releasing spores, tiny nearly microscopic "eggs", each capable of growing into a developed organism. Fungi are ubiquitous on land, where there is water and a food source, there are fungi. There would be no plants on earth without fungus, as fungi "invade" the roots of plants enlarging their surface area to enhance absorption of water, nutrients and enable plants to "fix" inorganic nitrogen. Organic nitrogen is "blessed" by a complicated synergistic process by which the plant, bacteria and fungi combine nitrogen and oxygen into nitric oxide, the organic usable chemical needed by all life. Fortunately, fungi cause few human diseases but has caused much human suffering. In destroying potatoes in the mid-19th century, both in the ground and in storage, the food supply for the Irish and other Europeans were starved by an explosion of phytophthora fungus. The potato blight converted tens of thousands Irish immigrants into factory workers and soldiers in North America just in time to help the Union win the Civil War. Fungi have served humans well in the 20th century since the first safe effective antibiotic was directly acquired from the mold fungus, penicillium. Pasteur's work with the wine and cheese industry in the 19th century greatly enhanced human enjoyment.

In humans, fungal infections are usually self-limiting, chronic, irritating and involve skin and nails, only rarely penetrating the interior of the body. Ringworm is one of the more common fungal infections has nothing to do with worms. It is a superficial fungal infection that forms a red ring that slowly expands leaving a clear center. It sometimes itches, is unsightly and generally resolved without treatment. Toenail fungus slowly forms thick yellow nails that continue to spread with aging. These fungal infections are usually cosmetic except in the diabetic foot, where it can expose the patient to deeper bacterial infections, resulting in cellulitis and amputations. Fungal dermatitis is common in dark damp areas such as the space between toes (athlete's foot), groin and genitalia (jock itch), vagina (yeast vaginitis), underarms and scalp. Keeping skin clean and dry is best prevention. As fungal rashes are itchy, red and scaly, diagnosis is generally obvious and treatment includes creams such as nystatin, clotrimazole (drugs ending in "ozole" are generally antifungal). To reduce the need to scratch a topical steroid or even petrolatum jelly is helpful.

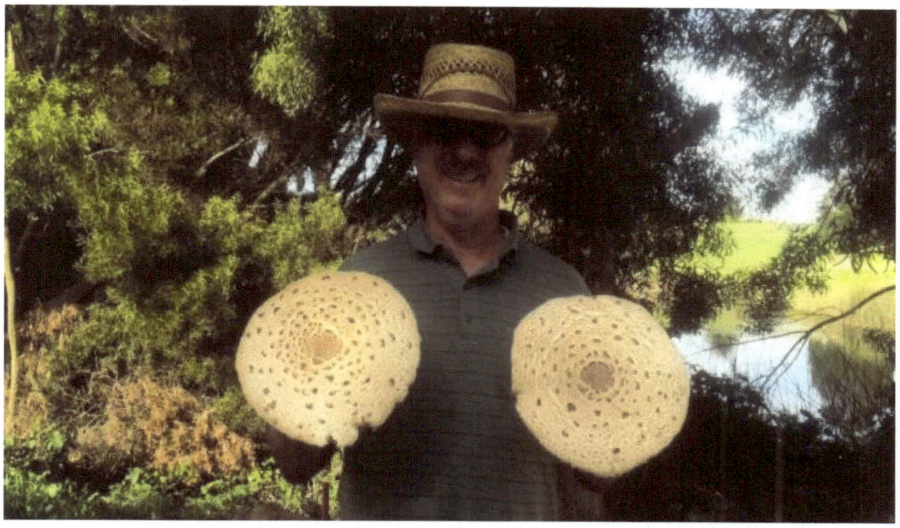

Tim Martin DO, interrupting his golf game to gather Shaggy Manes, *Corprinus comatus* growing in the same place year after year. They are easy to identify, excellent to eat and probably have immune enhancement properties.

Some believe the psychotropic effects of fungi have played large roles in human history. "The Food of the God's", "The Road to Eleusis", "The Sacred Mushroom and the Cross" and "The Immortality Key" are four books the author recommends to further explore the connection of fungi and the human mind, especially as it relates to Christianity.

There are safe oral medications for fungal infections, i.e. ketoconazole and terbinafine are well tolerated. However, it may require treatment for weeks or months due to the chronic nature of fungal infections. There are rare cases of systemic deep fungal infections that are not in the scope of this text to evaluate and treat. However, they do happen in the field. The author was involved with a Maritime legal case of a systemic fungal infection in a Merchant Marine steward with an extremely rare fatal form of fungal disease. After death he was found to have cerebral *cryptococcus neoformans*, the words mean: *cryto*-hidden, *coccus*-round, neoformans-new forming. This deep fungal infection involved his central nervous system causing confusion, central nerve dysfunction and ultimately death. This is a difficult diagnosis to make in the field. After he was removed from the ship and hospitalized in two different institutions, his diagnosis was only confirmed by the postmortem (after death) autopsy. There were many signs that this seaman had a compromised immune system. He was a poorly controlled diabetic, his lower extremities were covered with skin warts, he was pale, and reported to be often sweaty (fever). The captain of the vessel reported in his log that he felt the steward was too ill to go to sea when he boarded the vessel. The skipper's diagnosis was correct but was feared over-riding the fit-for-duty chit the steward presented. A chit later found to be fraudulent. In medicine, first impressions are often correct.

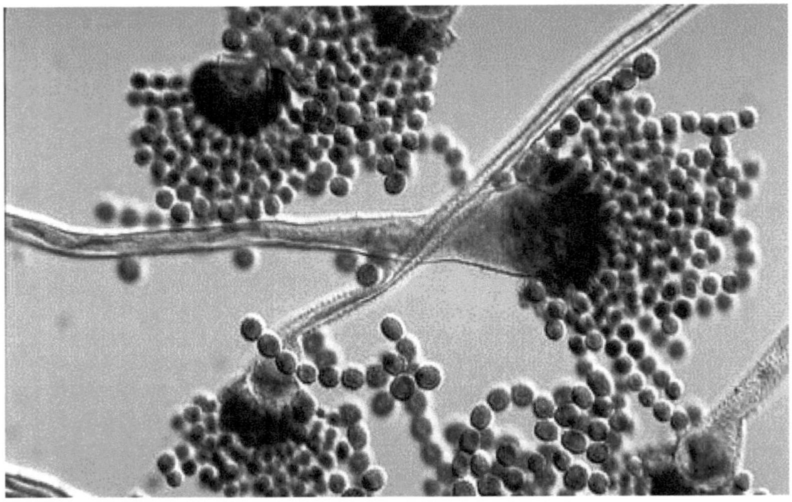

Microscopic view of "black mold" growing in wallpaper, an unscientific label that implies possible toxic effects if spores are inhaled and the resulting fungi grows in lung triggering respiratory complaints. Note the long strand of mycelium and the spores detaching. NIH

Parasites

Greek word *parasitos*-one who lives at another's expense, meaning guests

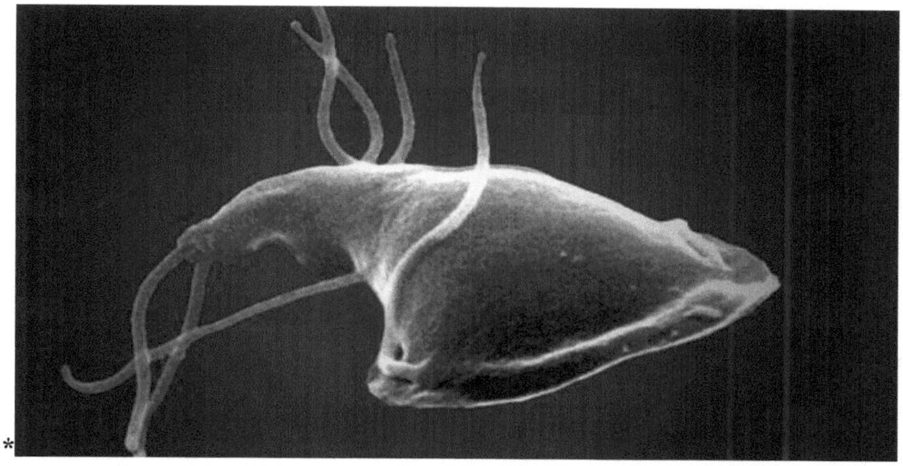

*

Giardia, a "simple" single cell parasite covered by a protective shell allowing it to live outside the host body for extended periods of time, surviving freezing and exposure to low-dose chlorine water treatment. The inventor of the microscope, Van Leeuwenhoek, discovered and illustrated this parasite in his own stools as well as lice found on his body. Looks dangerous! CDC

Protozoa are single-celled mobile animals causing common human afflictions of amoebas (liver abscesses) and flagellates (giardia, trichomonas). Other pathogens discussed, include trypanosomes (African sleeping sickness, an infection that saved Serengeti wildlife from human livestock), sporozoan (malaria), trematode (larger flukes, flatworms, Schistosoma (a gift of the Nile capable of penetrating intact skin), nematodes (hookworms, pinworms, trichinella). Trichinella, the result of poorly cooked pork and probably reason the pig is taboo in Hebrew and Islamic diet. These creatures all require different methods of destruction or eradication, while some cannot be killed and therefore require prevention or safe removal from the body.

Parasites are more widely varied creatures than the previously discussed pathogens. Many are multicellular creatures, some with extremely complicated life cycles, while some are large enough to be seen by the eye (worms) and others so tiny, require electron microscopy (leishmanial). Drugs, immunizations or physical factors (i.e., heat or cold) cannot kill or prevent all parasitic infections, although good hygiene greatly reduces risk. Many of the parasite drugs available in the Third World are effective but may be toxic. Once a parasite in the human body, it is difficult to harm (eradicate) the parasite without collateral damage on its host. Most parasitic diseases affecting humans and their animals are associated with fresh water in warmer climates and insects in the same geographic areas. There are places in the Third World where hygiene is suspected and carry a higher burden of parasitic diseases.

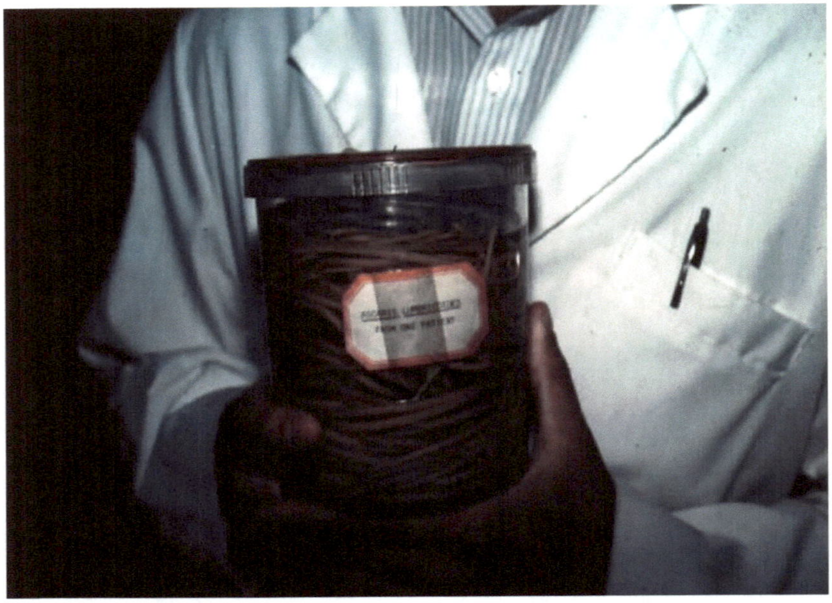

One of many specimens is contained at the Naval Medical Research unit #3 in Cairo, where the author spent three months of medical school. The above nematodes are not microscopic; however, most microbiology texts and medical courses include the larger parasites. The mass of worms in above image were removed from a bowel obstruction in an eight-year-old Egyptian girl. Parasites have plagued humans for thousands of years. Many of the world's capital cities were often built on malarial swamps and other well-watered ground, laden with human waste. Still today, hundreds of millions of people worldwide harbor pathological guests in densely populated coastal and river cities. A long way from classrooms in Oklahoma. Photo by author

Eradicating a parasitic disease is sometimes like fighting against guerrillas (Spanish for "little war") like the Vietnam War and the current wars in the Middle East. The enemy often occupy villages, schools and hospitals, making it difficult to kill the aggressors without harming the innocent. "Hiding in plain sight", a ploy of guerrillas, is common throughout history and in nature, as prey and predators use camouflage. Some parasites are experts at hiding as are cancers. The US Naval Medical Research Unit # 3 in Cairo, where the author studied tropical diseases in some depth, was especially focused on chronic parasitic infections. Since parasites evade the immune system as do some cancers, investigating the mechanisms whereby parasites elude the immune defense systems may explain how cancers also avoid detection. The human immune system is certainly powerful enough to eradicate parasites and cancer cells if it can recognize them.

When it comes to the study of parasitology, whenever possible, infections should be prevented! The most common dangerous parasitic infection is malaria, which even with survival, can lead to a lifetime illness. A chronic infection that shortens life and reduces quality of living. Avoiding pregnant mosquito bites especially at dusk and dawn (stay indoors under netting), insect repellent (DEET), anti-malarial drugs and sound common sense will go a long way in preventing malaria. It is helpful to avoid malaria if possible. Ivermectin is active against parasites, especially nematodes and appears to have effectiveness against viral infections such as COVID. Ivermectin is even therapeutic in some cancers.

Nematodes comprise a huge number of species (at least 25,000) and in individual numbers represent 80% of all animals on earth by weight! The vast majority living silently buried in the seabed, creatures living long lives are currently being studied for their mechanisms of their longevity. Fortunately, with these vast numbers, only a few nematodes cause disease in humans and our domesticated animals. Earthworms, important nematodes in American agriculture were nonexistent in the Americas until Europeans arrived with potted plants and within four centuries has spread throughout the American continents. Another beneficial invasive agricultural species in America is the honeybees brought by the same Europeans. Pathological nematodes species unlike common earthworms do not have segmented bodies and include pinworms, hook worms, round worms and trichinella. Hookworms are enjoying an increasing therapeutic role as they are deliberately given to patients suffering from asthma, inflammatory bowel disease, multiple sclerosis and other chronic afflictions with amazing outcomes for some.

Nematodes-round worms

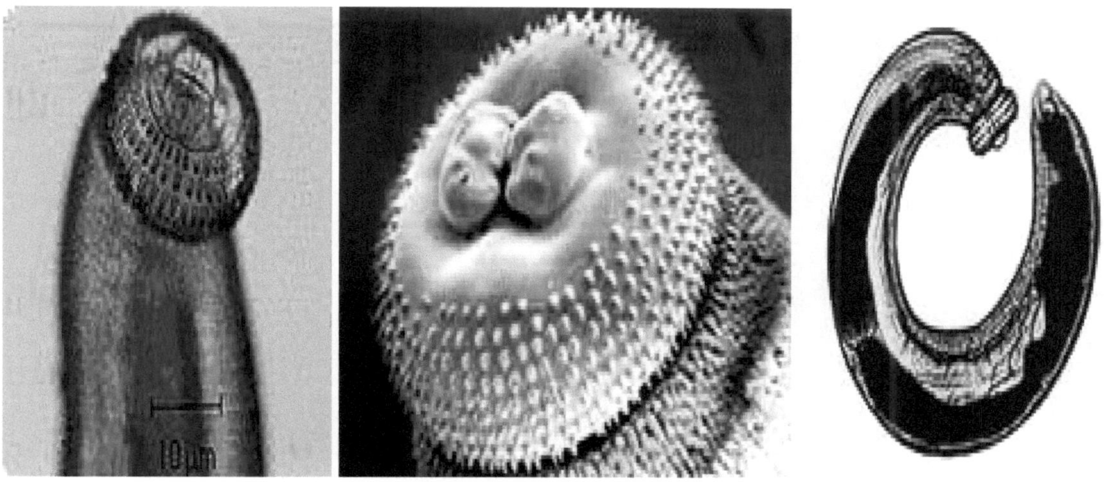

Nematode, *Gnathostoma spinige*, female, note the armored headpiece. NIH

And the pig, because it parts the hoof and is cloven-footed but does not chew the cud, is unclean to you". Leviticus 11:7. Leviticus is the book of laws in Old Testament and much of this law is public health. In the hot desert environment of the ancient Hebrews, meat spoiled quickly and there was probably a high incidence of contaminated pork by trichinella. It was good public health to avoid foods that caused disease. There have been recent outbreaks of trichinella, in Alaska with bear meat made into jerky, the nematode survived drying and smoking. In the South Pacific with the introduction of microwave ovens there are outbreaks of trichinella. The microwave cooks too briefly to kill the parasite. Pork must be cooked thoroughly if the flesh contains trichinella. Many meats can be eaten raw safely, pork products are not among them.

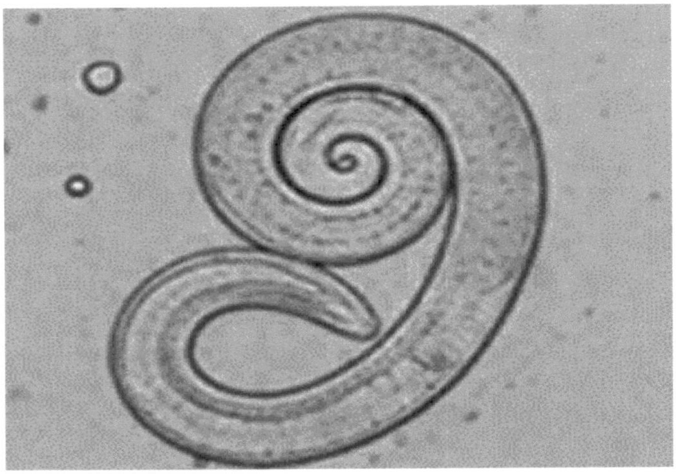

Trichinella spiralis **unlike other parasitic nematodes ingested are not content to stay in the gut. The females are larger than males, carry fertilized eggs in their uterus and juveniles in a separate sac. Upon her death, hundreds of her offspring eat their way through the bowel wall and enter blood vessels and lymphatic channels, allowing worms to travel and embed in muscles. These nematodes are found though much of the world and are a significant cause of disease worldwide. The parasite is found in bears, raccoons and pigs as well as humans. NIH**

Hookworms and pinworms

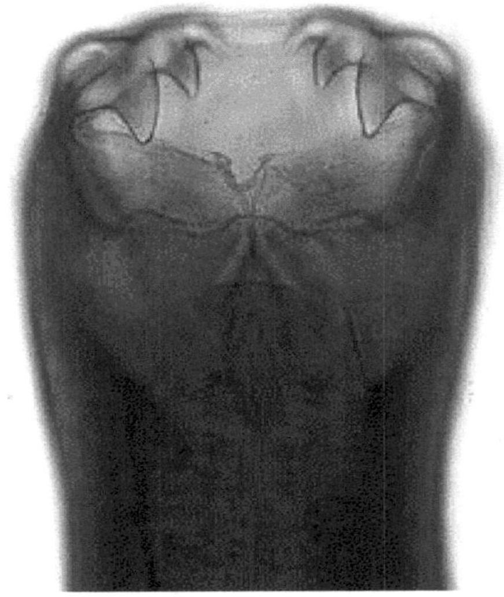

The mouth of hookworm that invades dogs, *Ancylostoma caninum*. These creatures have structures allowing for firm attachment. To "deworm" a dog or other infested animal, the worm must be rendered "asleep" causing it to lose its grip, fall into bowel and then flushed from gut. This requires 2 drugs, one to anesthetize the parasite and a laxative to flush the sleeping worms through the rectum. Imagine dozens or even hundreds of these suspended in the lower gut, their toothed mouths burrowed into the living bowel, stealing nutrients from their hosts. Worms are a major cause of anemia and malnutrition in human history. CDC

Hookworm and pinworm are common infections throughout the world, even in affluent communities. The diagnosis depends on finding parasites' eggs in feces. The worms are large enough to be seen, however the eggs are microscopic. Symptoms include pain, rectal irritation and bleeding. A simple way to diagnosis pinworms is to take advantage of their nocturnal behavior by placing a clear piece of tape over the rectum. If pinworms are present, they will migrate out the rectum at night where they become trapped on the tape in morning. Because medications do not kill the parasite but remove them from the gastrointestinal tract, the stool during treatment contains living worms and eggs which must be destroyed properly to prevent reinfection Mebendazole is the most common treatment for pinworms and is being touted for cancer. If nematode infestation is suspected while in the tropics, see local health care for the best care. Nematodes are living, feeding and reproducing in the guts of millions of people, stealing nutrients and blood causing a huge disability on populations in the tropics. Ivermectin is becoming the drug of choice to eradicate nematode and an older drug, Mebendazole is being used in some cancers.

Malaria

Latin word for bad air, modern name from the 17th century

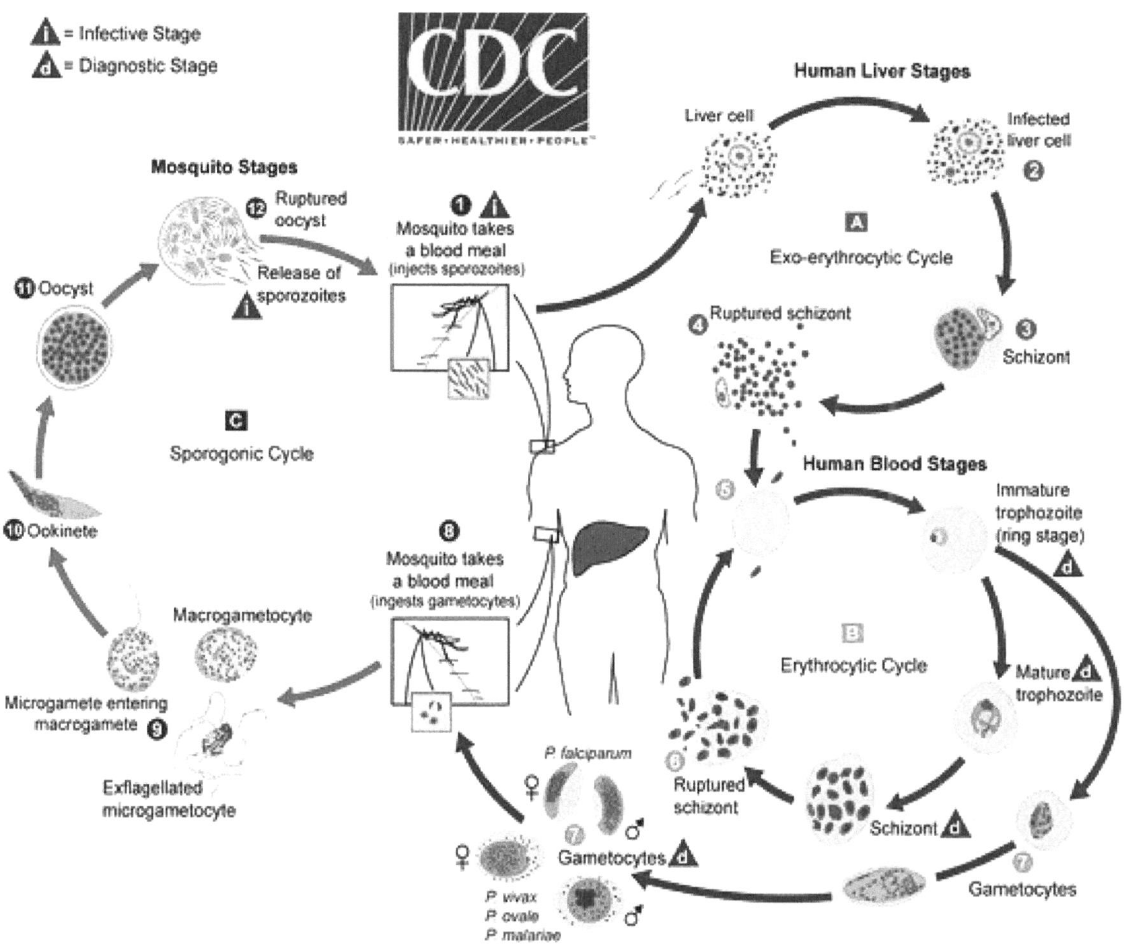

The complicated life or lives of malaria protozoa, 12 different lifeforms! CDC

Malaria currently afflicts over 200 million people worldwide and has been a threat since humans first started civilization, as all but a few great capitals were built on malarial swamps. Memphis in Egypt, Bagdad, Athens, Rome, London, Paris, the coastal great cities of India and China, even Washington DC were built around freshwater rivers and lagoons where water slows and pools. Since most cities were close to the coast if not on it, the slow-moving freshwater merging into the sea provided ideal mosquito breeding grounds. No effective immunization for malaria has been developed after decades of search and current antimalarial meds are losing their effects. There are primarily three species of malaria, *falciparum* being the most dangerous. *Falciparum* malaria can cause acute lethal disease, manifested with the occurrence of black urine, known to European explorers as "black water fever", a sign that was almost always fatal. Recurrent fever with hard shaking chills is diagnostic of malaria, lasting for decades in some. There are few diseases outside the tropics associated with hard shaking chills, kidney infection and pneumonia the most common.

It is far better to prevent malaria than treat, and prevention means avoiding mosquito bites at dusk and dawn as these are the periods when pregnant female *anopheles* mosquito feed by inserting her razor-sharp hollow proboscis through the skin, injects a prepared mixture of blood thinning anesthetics and siphons a blood meal. To keep the victim's blood from clotting and sealing off the bleeding, the mosquito's saliva contains a blood thinner which is frequently discharged into the wound. In the saliva there are thousands of sporozoites, looking like sperm in higher animals which enter the victim's blood stream and carried to the liver where they change into another life form. Most settle in the red blood cells where they consume and then destroy their host cells. Other sporozoites enter the liver cells and begin to reproduce, leading to enlarged livers. The stages of malaria symptoms correspond to the stages of its lifeforms and the fevers these stages cause. The intermittent fevers result from the cyclic death of host cells and the release of new malaria organisms. Quinine has been the treatment for centuries, but many organisms have developed resistance and for current information about risks and recommended medications please contact the Center for Disease Control (CDC), as they have the most thorough *and up to date management of malaria.

Quinine

-cinchona

The trees containing quinine were only found at high elevation along the east Andes among the headwaters of the Amazon and no place else in the world. In simple terms, they were unknown and almost inaccessible to Europeans. Natives of the western amazon jungle had used the tree bark for fevers and had no fear from malaria since it did not exist before the Europeans brought both the parasite and the mosquito. During the 17th century both Europe and the New World were experiencing "the scourge of malaria", depopulating wide swaths of land and devastating trade. There was no cure until the emergence of "Jesuit's bark". Jesuit priests armed with this alkaloid purine were able to penetrate and thrive in areas denied others, becoming the most powerful Catholic order since the Templers. And like the Templers, their power and wealth, brought jealousy and hatred. Without quinine, England, the Dutch and other European powers would have never penetrated and conquered their tropical empires. Pizarro and his captains, who conquered the Inca Empire were the first Europeans to encounter the antipyretic bark that was so effective in fevers, his ill soldiers quickly abandoned their own physicians for the local healers.

As effective as Jesuit quinine powder was, because of its connection to Jesuits, Catholicism and the Spanish Empire, it was castigated by Protestant nations. Not unlike the medical establishment disparaging hydroxychloroquine and ivermectin. Both effective and safe treatments for COVID-19, yet political physicians, especially Anthony Fauci and the CDC declared their use ineffective and dangerous. Quinine and its offspring continue to be one of the most important medical discoveries of the Age of Discoveries. The addition of the halogen chlorine and the hydroxy group has magnified its power, making it on the World Health Organization list of essential drugs. It is not coincidence, that countries where hydroxychloroquine and ivermectin are over-the-counter (Africa, SE Asia), COVID-19 is almost nonexistent. "The Fever Trail" by Mark Honigbaum is a good story for the search and development of quinine.

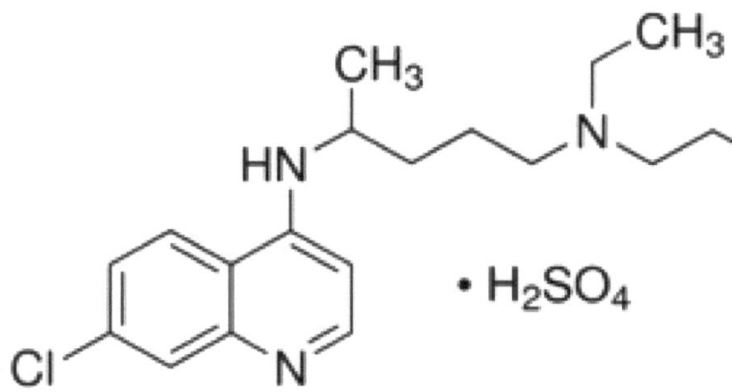

Quinine, an alkaloid purine-like chemical with a sulfate group attached

James Lind, a favorite naval medical officer of the author, was an early embracer of Jesuit's bark. Horatio Nelson and Captain James Cook were believers in Lind's entire shipboard medical care, including sanitation, citrus juice and cinchona bark. A Portuguese ships surgeon, Bernardino Antonio Gomez is credited with separating the active component, quinine by soaking bark powder in alcohol and potash. The name cinchona came from Contessa Cinchona who became famous for her cure from malaria by tree bark. After her miraculous recovery in Peru, she returned to Europe touting the cure. In truth, the Contessa died in Lima of fever, having never tasted the bitter alkaloid purine, yet her name has persisted, and the plant's scientific genus name is Cinchona. The author recommends CDC as a resource for current treatments for area of travel. Preventing bites at dusk and dawn is effective everywhere.

Trematodes – "flatworms"

Greek word meaning having holes, the Latin base means having suckers

Schistosomiasis, though appearing cylindrical is classified as a "flatworm", accounts for huge amount of human suffering, affecting over 700 million humans and untold animals. Like other trematodes, they have extremely complicated life cycles, reminiscent of the science fiction alien monster in the "Alien" movie series. There are depictions of this disease in Egyptian Hieroglyphics over 5000 ago describing abdominal bloating and bloody discharge from the penis. It was a major cause of disease and death in Egypt during the Greek and Roman times. English physicians in the 19th century mentioned "male menarche" when young adolescent men begin bleeding with urination. Bloody urine, a common finding in schistosomiasis infection (infestation) and years of chronic infections lead to permanent destruction of the urinary tract. Schistosomiasis is one of the few parasites that can penetrate intact skin, so swimming or wading in fresh water can result in disease. The eggs have a "sharpened" stake, a microscopic harpoon allowing them to attach and then bore through skin. After penetration, they flow through blood and lymph vessels, feeding along the way and like caterpillars' morph into butterflies, schistosomiasis morphed into a monster that feeds and reproduces within its host.

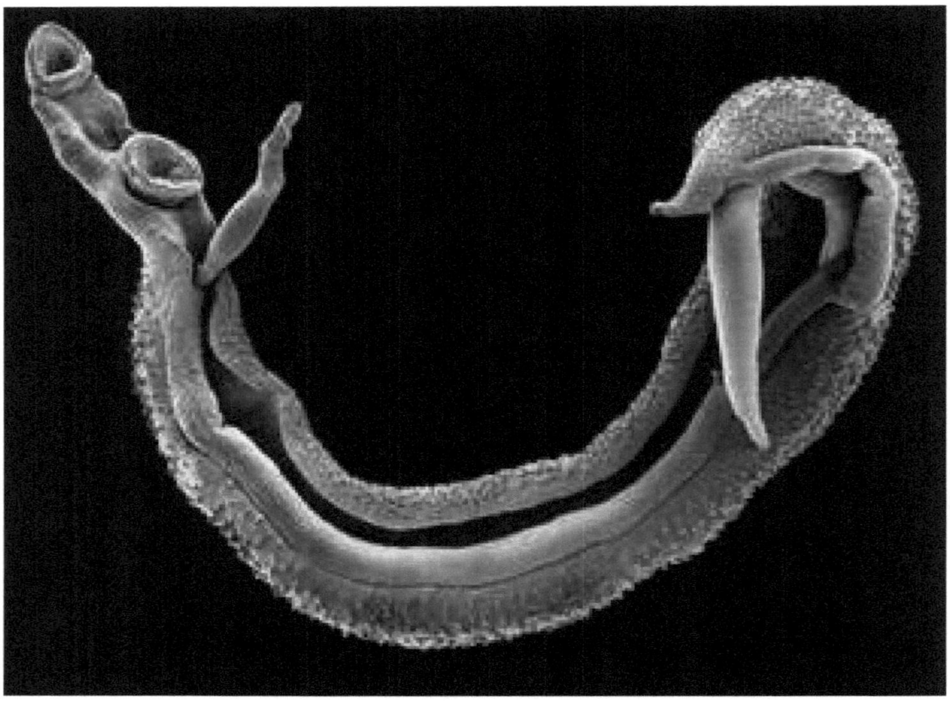

Schistosomiasis-note this creature is both male and female-CDC

There are two trypanosomes that cause significant human disease, *Trypanosome cruzi* and *Trypanosome gambiense*. The latter found in East Africa, home to the enormous herds of grazing wildlife of east Africa's Great Plains. Had it not been for this parasite, humans and their cattle would have moved centuries ago and settled in the fertile well-watered valleys and grasslands. *Trypanosome gambiense* is the reason the Serengeti Plain and its abundant wildlife is still in existence. African sleeping sickness, carried by the pregnant Tsetse fly, infects the mammal while taking a blood meal for her fertilized eggs. The cost to humans and their horses, cattle, sheep and goats to stay in the Serengeti, was too high a cost to pay.

Trypansome cruzi mode of infection is "crude" compared to previous parasites. The "kissing bug" is found primarily in Central America and South America with reports of cases in the Southern United States. Once again, a pregnant insect is carrying the infectious parasite, delivering the trypanosome during a blood meal. The bug comes down out of thatched roofs at night and is attracted to the moisture around the mouth in the sleeping victim bitten along the lip edge. To make room inside her enlarging pregnant body, she defecates, dispensing feces and parasites onto skin surface next to injection wound. After feeding, the bite site becomes inflamed and itches, prompting the victim to smear the bowel contents into the fresh wound with scratching. The resulting infection, Chagas Disease can be a major cause of death and disability in poor villages. When the trypanosome embeds in heart muscle, it is catastrophic.

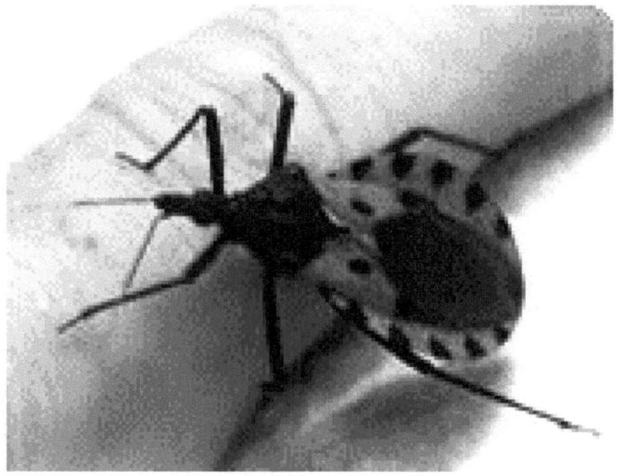

Reduviidae or for short, redivid bug harbors the trypanosome that causes Chagas disease. Infection rates are highest in poorer areas of southern North America and Central America. If you see a bug like this, sleep elsewhere! CDC

****There are many other parasitic infections, and this section only covers the ones most likely to encounter. For more information on parasites, the internet and the Center for Disease Control have a huge amount of highly specific and useful facts and recommendations for traveler.*

The Microbiota
-microscopic alien life within

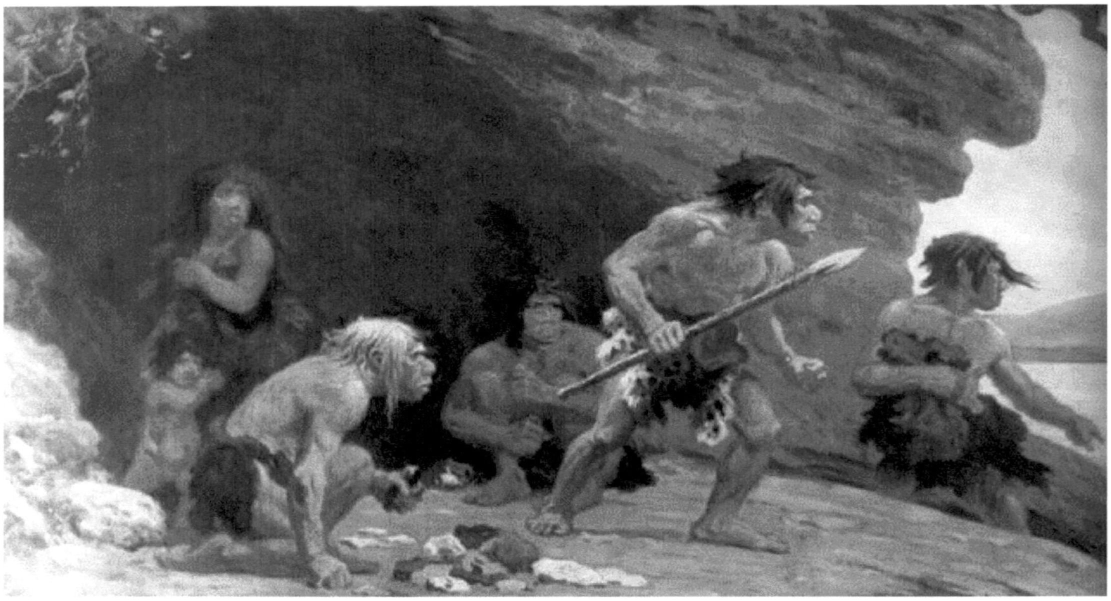

Primitive humans lived their lives with lice, witnessed by the early invention of nit combs. Lice, scabies and fleas were a part of human life until recently. These skin infestations pale when compared to the alien life within. zmescience.com

The organisms of microbiota studied by the author and others for decades were found primarily in the colon. Since it was believed the lower bowel, unlike the rest of the sterile internal body, contained only alien life. It has long been known of the great numbers and roles of colon bacteria in recovery of nutrients and manufacture of needed chemicals. The types and numbers of colonic bacteria now appear affect personality, behavior and even body shape! Fecal transplant, a new and promising treatment, is the transfer of feces from one person and depositing it deeply into in a recipient's colon. Legitimate positive results have been achieved in serious diseases such as ulcerative colitis and for weight loss. It appears that colonic bacteria can change overall health, body size and mitigate chronic diseases. Current belief is that foreign microbes occupy other spaces within the body, except for the central nervous system.

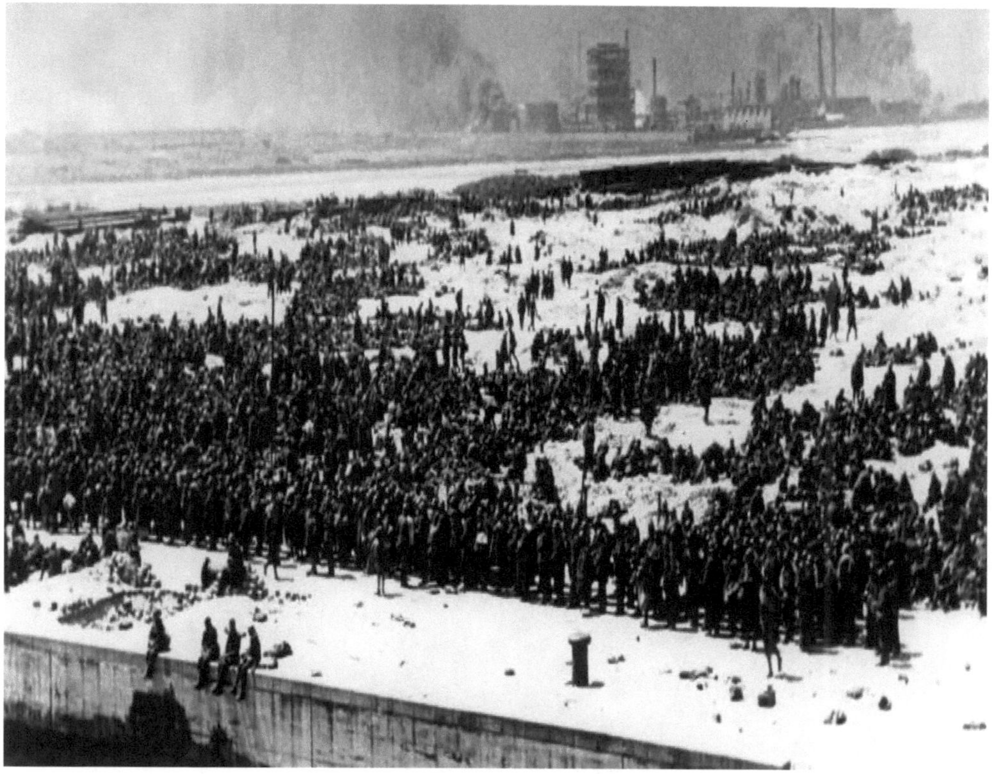

Over 330,000 British, Belgium and French soldiers removed from beaches after being flanked by German Army in six weeks of the summer of 1940. Many of the evacuated French officers and men later voted to return to Nazi occupied France. An act that greatly disappointed Winston Churchill. Imperial War Museum

There is a significant firewall separating the central nervous system from the rest of the body, especially the microbiota. This blood barrier is essential since the central nervous system is almost defenseless if breached. In May 1940, German forces flanked the barrier of the Maginot Line and pouring into the plains of central France almost unchecked, trapped the Allies on the beaches of Dunkirk and forced France to surrender. Throughout history, flanking the foe is a tried and proven maneuver to defeat and rout a foe. If the blood brain barrier is flanked, equally bad things happen. It was believed that the central nervous system is sterile as it has little defense beyond the barrier; however, some microbes, bacteria such as syphilis, the protozoan toxoplasmosis and a few viruses can penetrate. Rabies, West Nile Fever and rubella are examples of viruses that cause brain damage while herpes, chickenpox and polio are viruses that infect the outlying nervous system after penetrating a peripheral blood barrier. Meningitis, encephalitis and brain abscesses occur when the central nervous system is "flanked".

There are microbes known to cause pathological mental and personality disorders. The protozoan microbe toxoplasmosis found in cat litter can cause brain infections and birth defects in humans. Toxoplasmosis can cross the blood brain barrier and the placental barrier separating fetus from mother. Psychologists noted an increase in schizophrenia beginning the early 20th century when people begin keeping cats indoors as pets. Cats were traditionally outside pets, controlling rodents in barns and yards, in the last century brought in as house pets. There are many references concerning mental status changes and toxoplasmosis. An interesting article concerns the hunting of primates by big cats in the distant past. Hunting cats could identify primates and humans infected by toxoplasmosis by smelling urine, targeting them as easier prey. Another bad actor that flanks the central nervous is the brain-eating amoeba, *Naegleria fowleri*, lying dormant in warm stagnant water for decades, entering in human host when water enters the mouth or nose. Upon entry the spore sprouts dendrite-like tentacles and "claws" its way into the brain, where it slowly grows devouring brain tissue. The emergence of AIDs has led to the discovery of other microbes found in autopsies of AIDs victims. One study found all autopsied brains of AIDs victims contained bacteria and viruses not found in HIV negative brains. Perhaps the central nervous system also harbors microbes in "normal" brains?

The Human Immune System

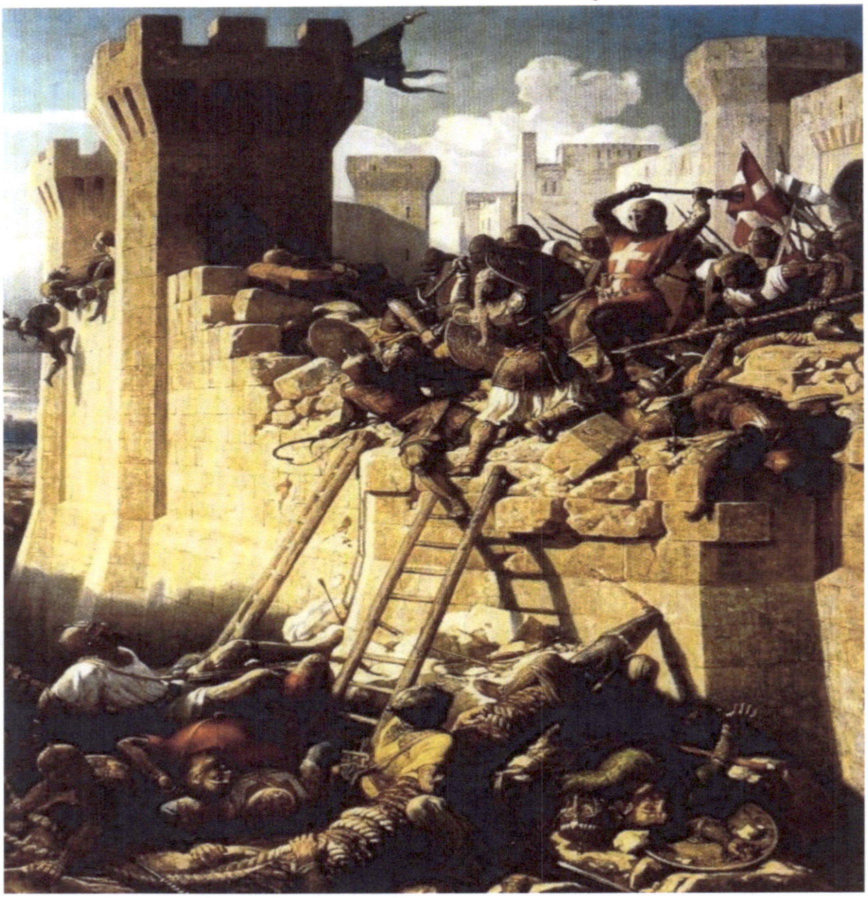

"The Siege of Acre" by Dominique Papety depicting Christianity's final enclave in the Holy Lands falling in 1291, two hundred years after the Crusaders took Jerusalem. The victorious Mamelukes, former slave-soldiers that overthrew their masters, conquered much of the Middle East, and drove the Europeans from the Holy Lands. By defeating the Mongrels at the Battle of Ain Jalut in 1260, the Mamelukes probably saved Islam. Acre had strong walls and behind the walls were hundreds of determined Teutonic Knights, Knights Templar and Knights Hospitallers (later becoming the Knights of Malta) with some 14,000 soldiers. The "Last Stand" of two centuries of conquest and retreat were concentrated at the Siege of Acre. Like the human immune system, the fortress at Acre represented strong walls and a strong defending force. However, the physical barrier of

the wall was undermined and breached, followed by overwhelming numbers of Mamelukes storming through the breach. The human immune system has strong determined internal components behind sturdy physical barriers of skin and mucus membranes, as the first line of defense. If the body's physical borders are breached, the invaders can sometimes overwhelm the body's interior defenses (white blood cells). Protecting the skin from injury along with cleaning and dressing these injuries, go a long way in containing invasion of the body's interior defenses. In Acre's fall, only seven of the eight hundred Hospitallers survived, and the city's 30,000 Christians were either murdered or sold into slavery.

The Mamelukes were slaves taken as young Christian and Turkic boys, converted to Islam, and trained into a soldier-class to protect the Empires in Mesopotamia and Egypt. Becoming more powerful and unified, they murdered their Egyptian masters and established a presence in the Middle East for 700 years. A Mameluke army defeated the Mongols in 1260 AD near Nazareth, inflicting the first significant loss on Genghis Khan's descendants. The victory may have saved much of Western Civilization's knowledge from destruction. Like the Mamelukes, some cancers and autoimmune diseases are examples of the immune system turning on its master. Autoimmune diseases can be caused by the immune system producing antibodies against its own human cells, as well as killer white cells attacking its own tissues. These diseases include rheumatoid arthritis, systemic lupus erythematous, rheumatic heart disease, Type I Diabetes, multiple sclerosis and others.

There were times in history that neither military power nor the human immune system is adequate for protection, like the fall of Acre's fortress. A similar story was about the 1918 influenza epidemic. No war, no famine, no plague has killed more humans in such a short period of time, along with hundreds of millions of pigs, chickens and other livestock. Pig deaths were strongly associated with *Hemophilus influenza* bacteria, implying most human deaths were likely from secondary bacterial-caused pneumonia and naming the disease, influenza. Some isolated villages in the northern latitudes of Europe and America, over 90% perished.

The story of the 1918 Flu Epidemic is an example of the human immune system, powerful and sometimes aloof, caught off-guard and overwhelmed in a moment of history. An avian (bird) RNA virus changed world history abruptly, killing directly and indirectly, perhaps 70 million people, while leaving tens of thousands of survivors mentally incapacitated ("Awakening", book and movie by Walter Sacks who is portrayed by Robin Williams). Influenza brought The Great War to a sudden collapse, initially called "The Spanish Flu" because large numbers of cases first appeared in Spain, however it may have begun in rural Kansas in 1917 and initially spread to a local army barracks. By 1918 it had changed, becoming more contagious and lethal, especially in the German Army and the civilians behind their lines dying in great numbers from starvation and influenza. The winter of 1918 was known in Europe as the "Turnip Winter", days short and rainy, nights long and cold. There was little food, and one of the few crops able to grow was turnips. The bulky tuber offers little nutrition, except in the green tops. Similar plagues including the Black Death in the mid-14th century, Plague of Justinian in mid-6th century, Plague of Athens in the 3rd century BC swept away much of the population, leaving a broken new world in its wake. All greatly changed the human world.

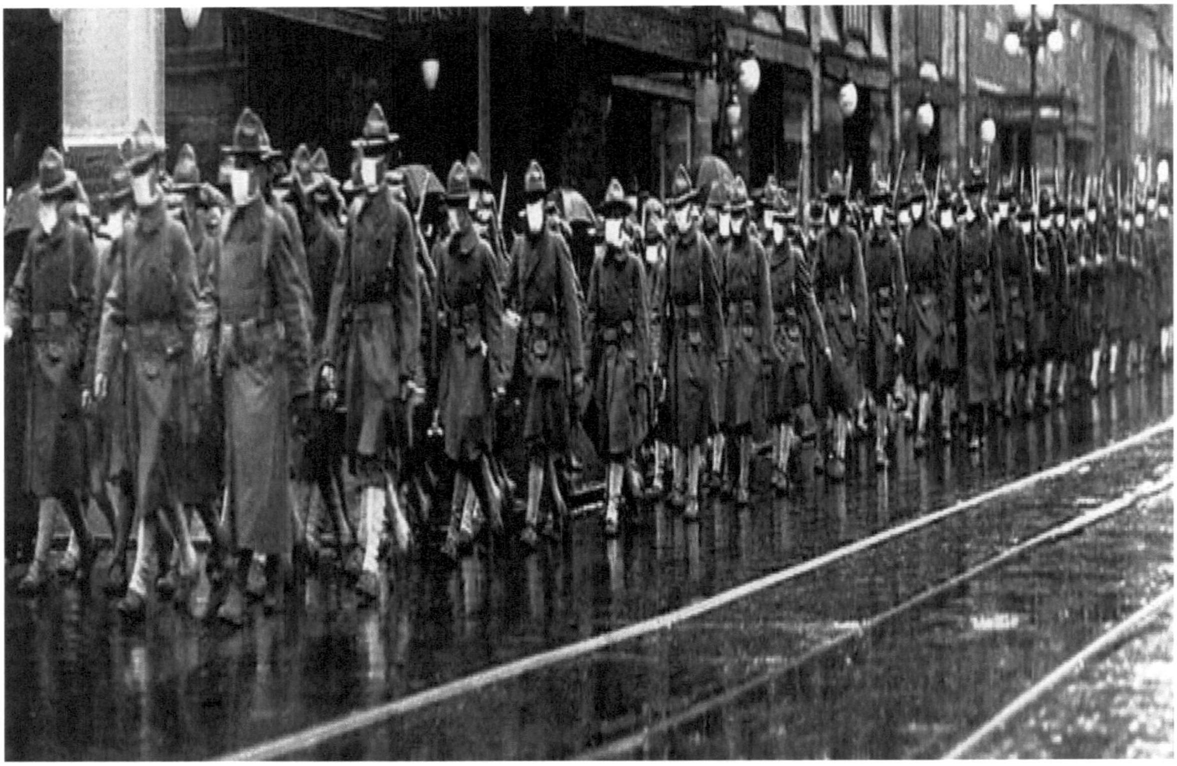

In an army stricken with flu in 1918, where cotton masks were an ineffective attempt to reduce spread. National Archives

The spring of 1917 saw the collapse of Imperial Russia and by summer, withdrew from the war, enabling Germany to move millions of soldiers to the Western Front. At the same time, American soldiers were pouring into France, however, one-third were either dead or too ill to fight from shipboard influenza. In 1918, 40% of American soldiers in Europe were hospitalized, the same as in the American Civil War sixty years earlier. German Generals Ludendorff and Hindenburg knew they must strike before the Americans were ready to fight, and before more of their dwindling number of German soldiers succumb to the flu. The French and English had arrogantly planned the use the incoming Americans as replacements spread among their depleted regiments. After Congress declared war, French and English officers came to the United States to help prepare the American forces for the Western Front. Initially, they demanded no American officer over the rank of major to be sent to Europe! Knowing this meant feeding American soldiers into the "meat-grinder" of the past four years, John "Blackjack" Pershing, commander of the American Expeditionary Army, demanded the Americans fight only after training and then to fight together and not spread among French and British units. 1918 was the year of the "pale horse, pale rider", a story by Katherine Porter surveying Paris's empty theatres and cafes, the streets filed with funerals. Some had falsely predicted the same with the corona virus of 2020.

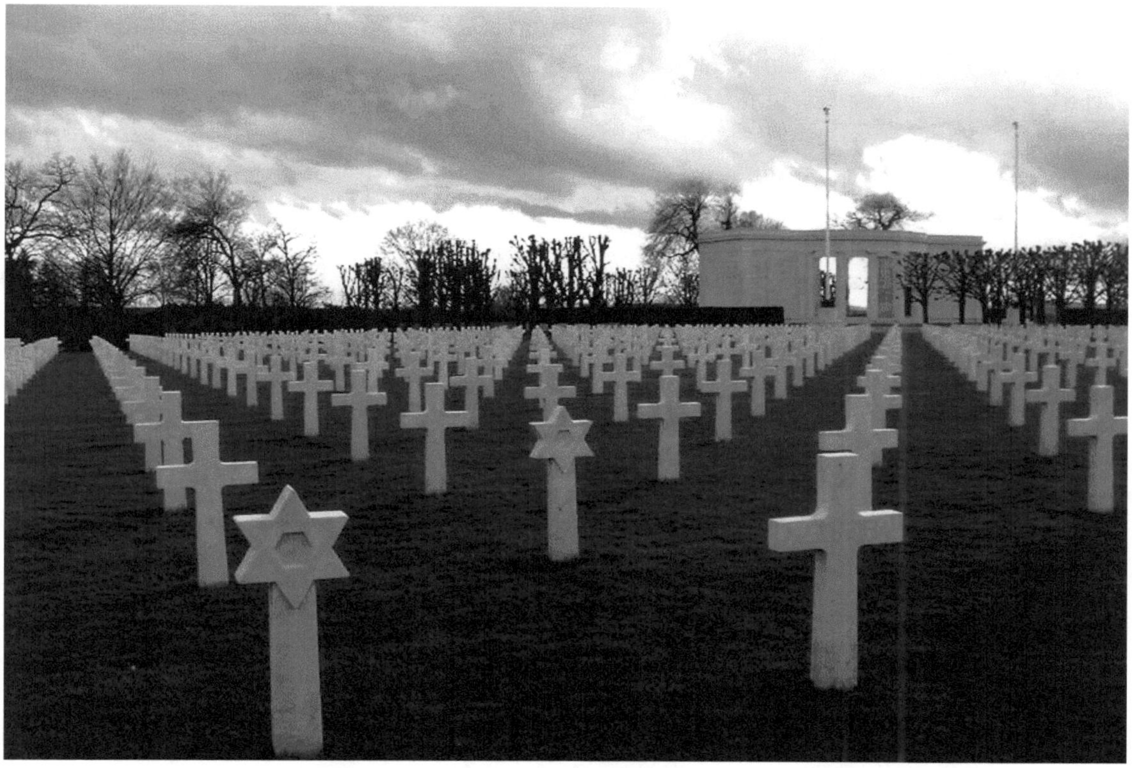

Final resting place in northeastern France for some of Black Jack's Pershing men. Note the Stars of David mixed with Christian Crosses. This land was occupied by Germany for four years during the Second World War and no Jewish graves were vandalized, even though Nazi Germany was rabidly anti-sematic! When the author questioned a veteran of World War II who had fought in this area, why the emblems of Judaism were left untouched, he replied, "the German soldiers I fought against were well disciplined and if their officers told them to leave the cemeteries alone, they obeyed". Note that no American flag is flying over our war dead. Photo by author

In 424 pages of Pershing's book on the American forces in the Great War, he only wrote one small paragraph on the flu. Influenza, the enemy he could neither defeat nor in any way control, killed and maimed many more of his men than did the Germans. Evidently influenza deserved little commentary in his memoirs.

Some infections seemingly unimpressed with the human immune system. One was Yellow Fever, which even killed its early investigators. The virus, a *Flavivirus* genus, cousin to the highly lethal viral West Nile Encephalitis are mosquito-borne RNA viruses that "slip" into the human cell due to a lipid chemical on their surfaces. Perhaps making them slippery? Yellow fever decimated Napoleon's army in Haiti and again later in the 19th century under de Lesseps, prevented the French from building the Panama Canal. Only a single animal, the pregnant female *Aedes aegypti* mosquito transmits Yellow Fever while siphoning a blood meal. The virus and mosquitos were endemic to central and West Africa, and slaves from this area were especially valuable in America, because of their immunity to yellow fever. So fearful was the disease, that ships flying the "Yellow Jack" flag prevented capture by pirates. Ships under the Yellow Jack flag were quarantined (a Venetian word for forty days), allowing no contact with land for six weeks. The Yellow Fever outbreak in the provisional capital of Philadelphia in 1793 was a major reason Philadelphia passed over as the site of the nation's capital. The book "Bring out your Dead" is a well-written account of that dark year in Pennsylvania, as the wealthier citizens, physicians and politicians who were at the time writing the Constitution, fled the city. The Constitution was written during this deadly epidemic and the Founding Fathers did not write that an infectious disease suspended either the rules of the government or the people's civil rights protected by the Constitution.

Native Americans and European immune systems did not fare well with this infection in the Americas. When the United States declared war on Spain and prepared to invade Cuba, the Army's Medical Department knew the island's jungles and rivers harbored Yellow Fever and the danger the disease presented to troops. The army sent to Cuba was 17,000 strong and 20% were descendants of slaves who were likely immune to yellow fever. The army's medical officers knew the biological value of combat soldiers resistant to fevers, as these diseases consistently killed many times more soldiers in history, than did combat. Another bad actor carried by mosquitos is West Nile Fever, which was endemic to the Nile River Valley when the author studied there in the early 1980's, has now spread to the western United States.

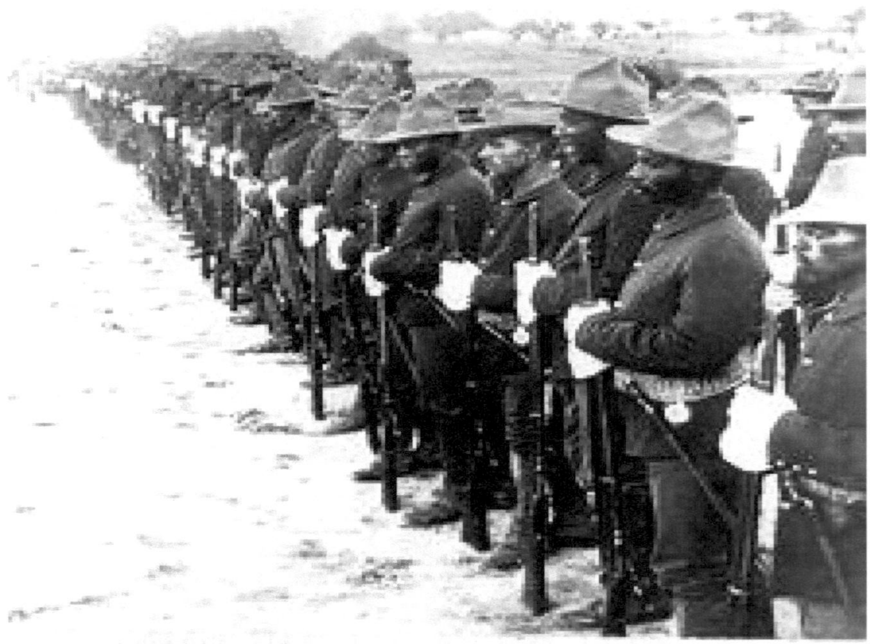

ACT (American Colored Troops) on their way to fight Spain in Cuba. "Blackjack" Pershing who led black troops in the West against Indians and in the Spanish American War, refused to allow black soldiers into combat in World War I, until forced by conditions on the ground. The orders against allowing blacks to fight alongside of whites came from directly from President Woodrow Wilson, an unrepented racist. He did not want the white and black races in close contact; however, the French had no such qualms. They had African troops in their army, and freely employed the unwanted American black soldiers, some transferred to French Army. The "Harlem Hellcats", a volunteer African American regiment became one of the war's most decorated units. The 369th Infantry regiment had no prisoners taken, lost no ground, were highly lauded by the French government and people, yet came home to segregation. The highest-ranking army general in 1917 when President Wilson declared war, was Leonard Wood MD, who after

graduating from Harvard medical school begin his army career as medical officer, where after winning the Medal of Honor, transferred to an army staff officer and rose to the senior officer in the United States Army. Most expected Wood to lead the American Expeditionary Forces in Europe as he had effectively led troops in Cuba and the Philippines while commanding black troops. However, because of his close association with Teddy Roosevelt and possibly his refusal to comply with Wilson's demand against using black troops in combat, the command was denied to General Wood. Museum of the United States

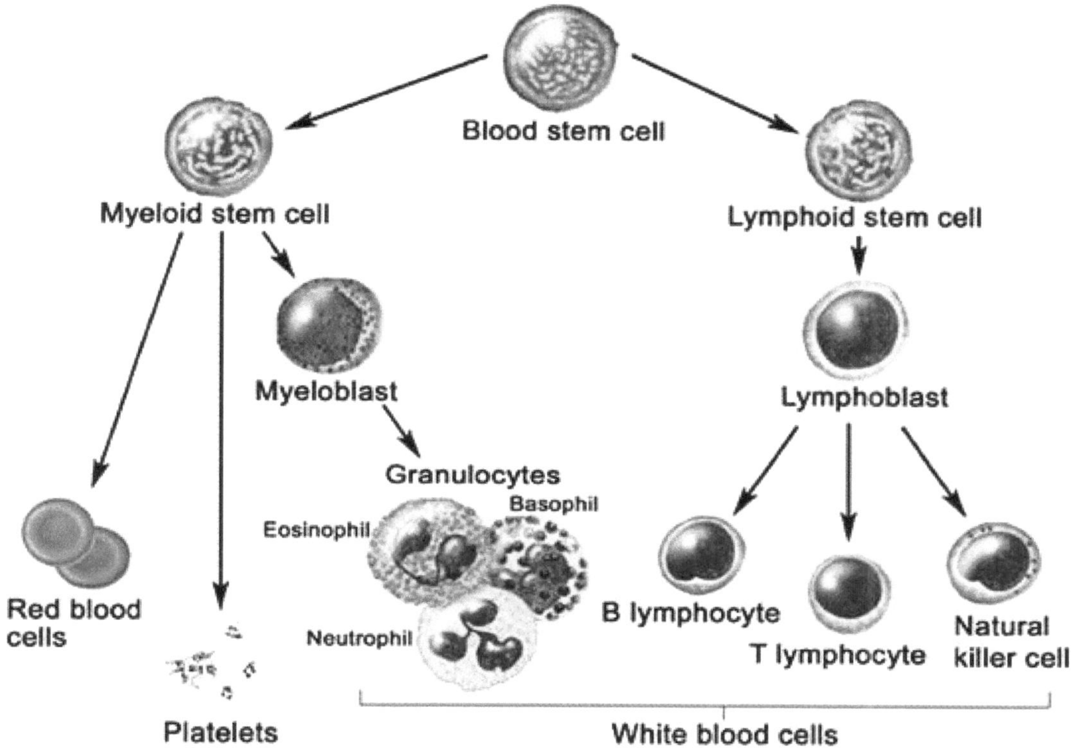

All immune cells produced by the bone marrow start life as a stem cell. Just as all soldiers and sailors start with basic training after recruitment, and later trained for specific purposes, the immune system recruits, and trains stem cells to become specialized defense cells. Many white blood cells live only a few moments in their defense of their host, dying in great numbers in the body's battles. National Institute of Cancer. Drawing by Terese Winlow

The human immune system is complicated, perhaps the most complicated in nature. Primitive lifeforms have primitive immune systems, probably because their enemies are primitive. Human enemies are not always simple, and even though they may appear to be primitive, some require a complicated network of defense systems to protect the human host. The immune system primarily functions on the microscopic level. On a larger scale, it controls body temperatures, directs blood flow and the manufacture of chemicals of destruction and the cells to deliver it. Immunology was an interesting field during the author's medical training in the 70s and 80s, however, little was of clinical use. AIDs supercharged the field of Immunology, making it a major part of medicine.

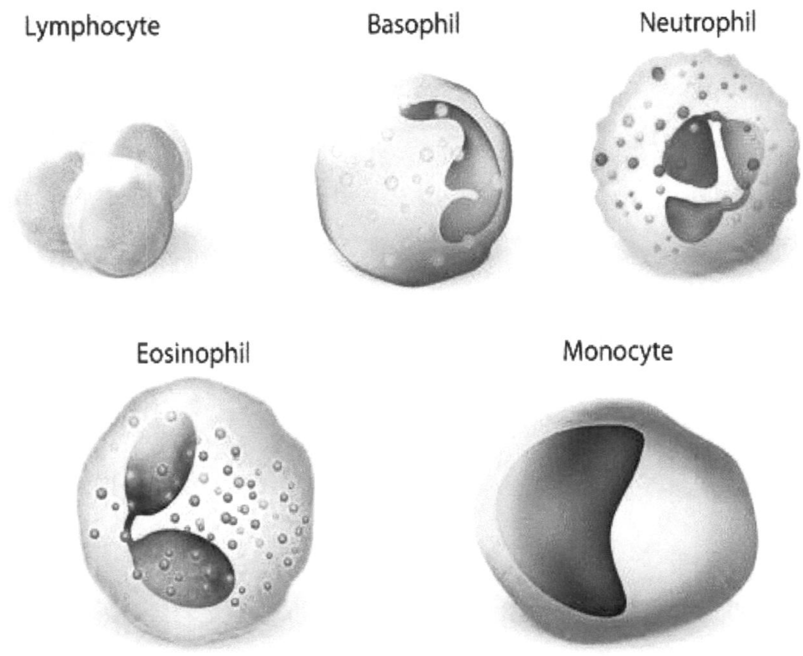

Five types of immune cells, each one "imprinted" with a purpose. NIH

White Blood Cells

Lymphocytes are the primary antibody factories, found in high numbers in lymph nodes producing Y-shaped proteins that attach to invasive agents at the three sites of the Y. Special lymphocytes "present antigen" to B cells, labelling antigen-containing cells to be destroyed.

Basophils are large white blood cells, few in numbers compared to other white blood cells, play a huge role in allergic reactions, including anaphylactic shock. These cells were discovered by Paul Ehrlich, German-Jewish physician who produced the first cure for syphilis since mercury, using a less toxic compound containing arsenic (Salvarsan). Dr. Ehrlich won the Nobel Prize in Medicine in 1908, dying in 1915 before his native Germany was overwhelmed with influenza. His treatment of syphilis with heavy metals was continued by Dr. Theo Morrel, treatment that affected decisions Hitler made in World War II.

Neutrophils are killers by design and nature, mechanically engulfing infections agents and digesting them as they digest themselves, not unlike suicide bombers. These are the "first responders", the author thinks of them as airborne troops quickly brought to fight. Larger macrophages of this type have been called "large eaters" as they consume and digest invaders.

Eosinophils are associated with allergic reactions along with basophils and mast cells. Parasitic infections greatly increase the circulating numbers of eosinophils, as does asthma.

Monocytes are generally the largest of white cells and are frequently associated with viral infections, especially mononucleosis. The author images these as artillery, releasing antibodies to aid the neutrophils

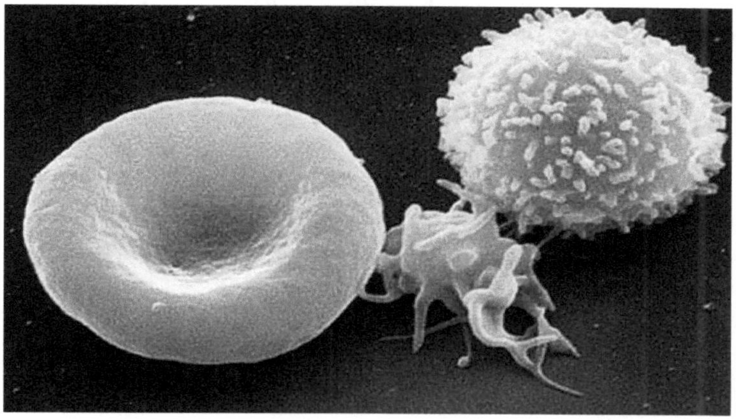

From left to right, red blood cell, platelet, white blood cell. All three started life as a stem cell. Keck School of Medicine, USC

All creatures have some form of an immune system. Fungal colonies manufacture antibiotics (penicillin) as a barrier to bacteria, and sharks manufacture squalamine as a defense against invasion and cancer. Humans deploy defense in depth with mechanical and chemical barriers as the first line of defense. Behind these physical barriers lies a body-wide defensive array of systems. Once an enemy penetrates the body, two major arms of the immune system are engaged. B cell function is primarily the production of antibodies designed to locate, attach and disable targeted cells. Invasive cells are marked as targets by the immune system of circulating immune cells in the blood and lymph vessels, and after being "labelled" are attacked by killer white blood cells.

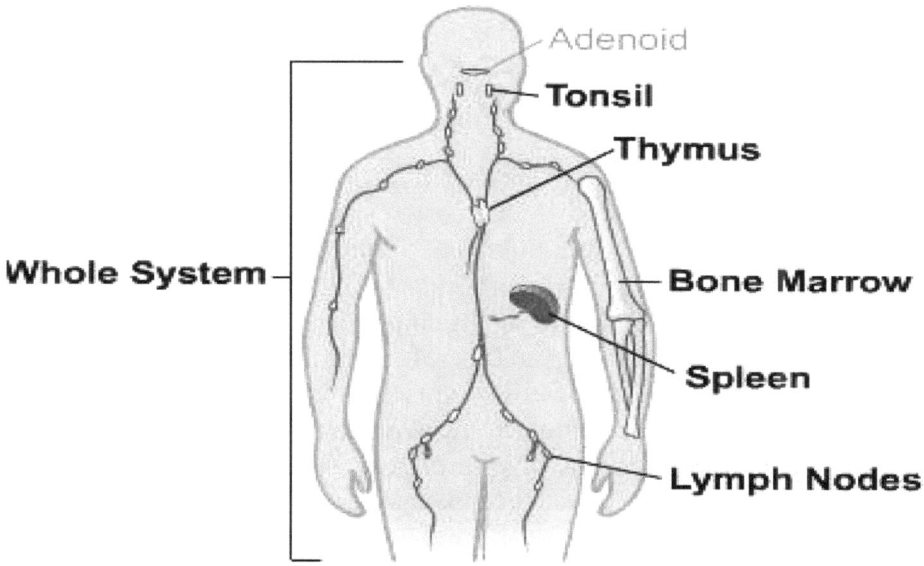

The immune is found body-wide and concentrated in the above areas. The thymus plays a major role in T-cell function while B-cells are "indoctrinated" in the small bowel, spleen, lymph nodes and elsewhere. NIH

Aggressive and effective defense cells, like the Knights that stood behind the walls of Acre and later at Malta, await agents that breach the body's walls. The "fighting monks" begin life like other humans are ordained into religious orders and trained to fight and kill. B and T cells, like all human cells begin life as untrained stem cells, but quickly ordained into one of the two orders of the human immune system. T cells are selected and trained by the thymus gland located in the upper neck around the larynx. A major medical mistake in the mid-20th century occurred when newborns, especially those in distress at birth, were found to have an enlarged thymus on X-ray. Called the "Sail Sign" because it looked like a boat's sail on X-ray. Unknown at that time was that the thymus normally enlarges in response to a stressful birth. In this case, the immune system was doing exactly what it was designed to do and was punished for it! Pediatricians at that time determined it was pathological and attacked it with ionizing radiation, which quickly shrank the gland and led to throat cancer later as adults. Medicine, like the human immune system, is often dangerous.

B Cell indoctrination occurs less centrally and is believed to take place in in the gut and lymph tissue. These white blood cells are primarily chemical factories, manufacturing antibodies engineered for only one purpose and one enemy. Antibodies, Y-shaped structures with three points of attachment to invaders greatly enhance the killing ability of the T-cells by attracting them with chemical scents, clumping invasive agents into herds and producing some antibodies that disables bacteria and viruses.

The lab test for white cells (part of a CBC-complete blood count) is based on the total number and the differential in types. Normal white cell count is 4-10,000 cells per cubic centimeter (cc). Two primary types of white blood cells are lymphocytes and neutrophils with a normal ratio of 60% neutrophils and 40% lymphocytes. In simple terms, the neutrophils are killers, dying in attack with help from lymphocyte's antibodies. Generally, in bacterial infections, the % of neutrophils increase, while in viral infections, the % of lymphocytes increase. In leukemia, the white cell count increases drastically, sometimes over 100,000 white blood cells per cc. Different infections illicit different responses from the immune system, causing other types of white bl ood cells to increase. Both arms of the immune system can turn on the host, as lymphoma, leukemia and ulcerative colitis attest.

Anti-inflammatory steroids based on hormone cortisol are the antidote for the immune system. Synthetic steroids and those derived from animal tissue are highly effective, and that effectiveness makes them potentially dangerous in suppressing the immune system. Chemotherapy and radiation are detrimental to the immune system since the rapidly reproducing cancer cells and normal immune cells are quickly dividing and therefore the most likely victims. Immune cells are fragile, many living fleeting lives sacrificing themselves in protection and in rare instances are deadly to their host. Good defense depends on sturdy walls of skin and mucus membranes, behind which stand resolute cells like soldiers, diligent in defense, not all injuries and invasions of the body can be mitigated even by an intact defense system. The difference between success and failure sometimes "hangs by a thread" with life and limb. The waxing and waning of the immune system mimics battles and wars both lost and won often by a single person or act. The following chapter is a story the author believes is an analogy to the human immune system when battling a potentially fatal invasion resulting from infection or injury. Strong walls, adequate fluid, nutrition, effective medical care and dedicated soldiers willing to fight to the death have won battles preserving their beliefs and culture.

The author served in the US Navy's submarine community and had exposure to the complexities and lethal capabilities of a nuclear-powered and nuclear-armed submarine. A single United States Navy ballistic-armed submarine has the destructive fire-power greater than the combined fleets of World War II. Almost every cell in the body has the complexity to produce this kind of power on a microscopic level. For defense to be effective, it must be powerful, and when the immune system defense is deployed, there will be destruction and some collateral damage to the innocent. The normally functional immune system is good at destroying invaders, but things can go wrong, and it can destroy the host it is protecting. Rheumatoid arthritis, Lupus, psoriasis and others are examples of slow attack of the immune system. In some infections, the immune system contributes to the damage initiated by the invaders and results in death. Many deaths of COVID were caused not by the virus, but the immune system unfortunate response.

The Siege of Malta

"Nothing is better known than the Siege of Malta" Voltaire

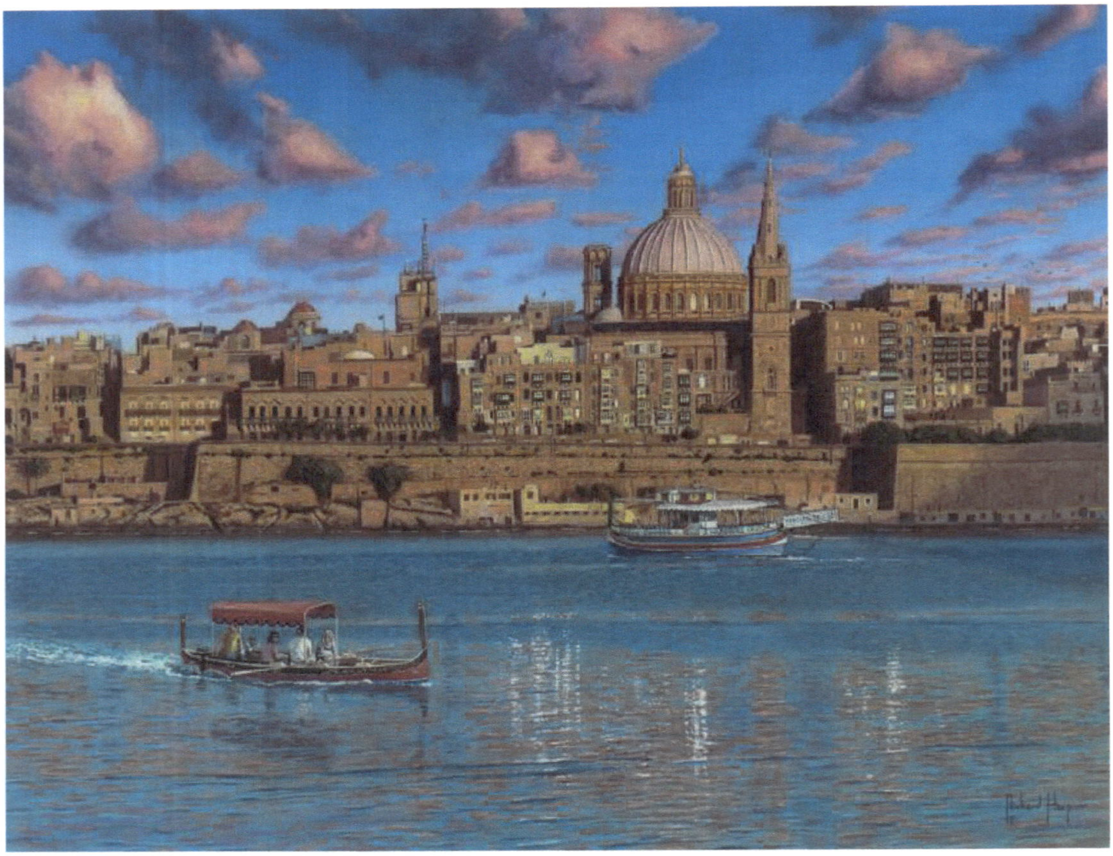

"Malta" by Richard Harpum

Malta is probably the most fought over piece of real estate in the world and the author uses Malta's fortifications and its defense in the summer of 1565 as a sea story to describe the human immune system.

Malta is a small archipelago of three islands and six rocks in the middle of the Mediterranean Sea, equal distance from Gibraltar to Istanbul. The islands are pieces of North Africa scattered towards Europe at the narrowest point in the Mediterranean Sea, fifty miles from Europe and one hundred and forty miles from Africa. The two major islands are Malta and Gozo, one hundred and twenty-two square miles of stony barren landscape greeted the former Hospitaller Knights on arrival in 1530. Wood so rare and valuable, it was sold by the pound, and yet Malta became a major sea power in the 16-18th Centuries. All east-west shipping in the Mediterranean Sea must pass by Malta's corrugated shores, containing some of the finest natural harbors in the world. Malta has been home to corsairs infesting these islands intermittently for thousands of years. The difference between piracy and nobility is subjective and depends on who documents the story. In recorded history, Malta has been occupied by Phoenicians, Greek, Carthage, Roman, Byzantine, Arabic, Norman, Spanish, French, and English invaders. There are ruins in Malta are believed to have been built by the ancient culture that built the Pyramids and the Sphinx over 10,000 thousand years ago. The first Christian church was founded on Malta, when Paul on his way to Rome, where he was to stand trial for his Christian beliefs was shipwrecked and bitten by a viper in the first century AD. The Great Siege of Malta in the summer of 1565 is considered by many historians to be the most important battle of the Western World.

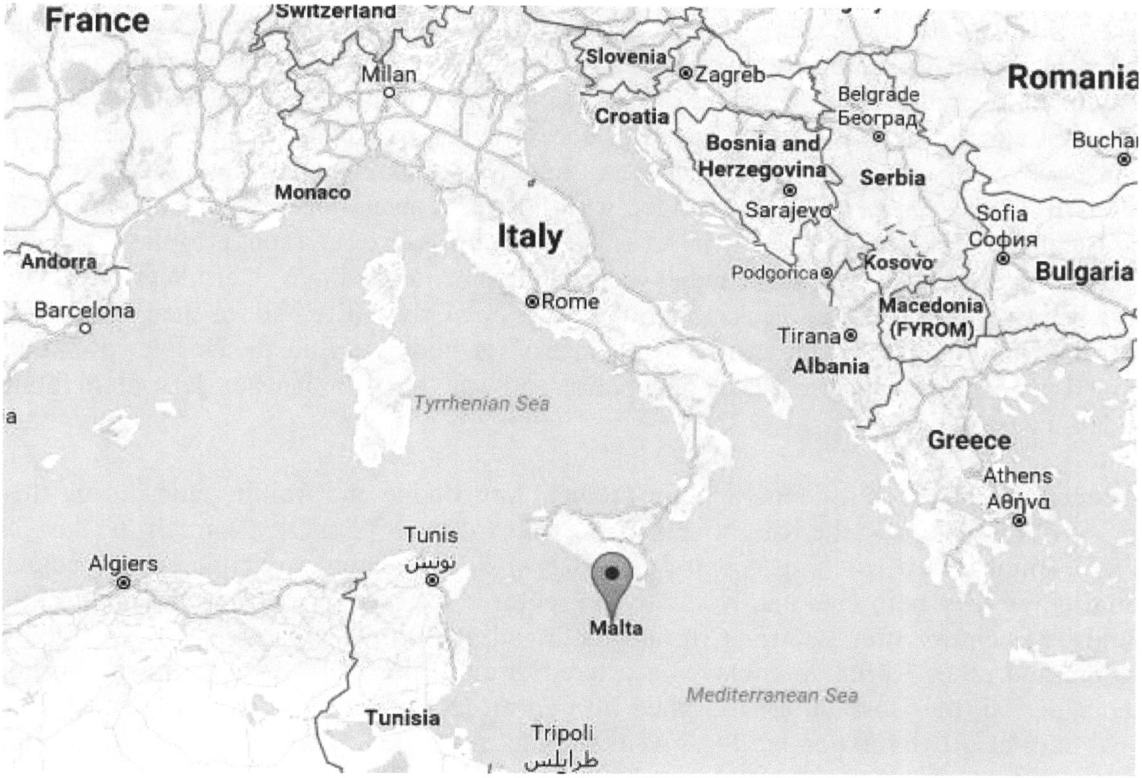

Malta is two islands, the smaller Gozo and the larger Malta. Gozo had been depopulated seven years before the siege by the pirate, Turgot. Turgot, the third leader of the Siege of Malta and 80 years of age, died leading from the front. In 1940, Malta was again besieged by the Germans and Italians during World War II. Their tenacious successful resistance played a huge role in winning another conflict against enemies of Christianity.

During the 16th century, the Ottoman Turks, under Suleiman the Magnificent had driven deep into Europe. Suleiman swept the Hungarians aside at the Battle Mohacs and his army was camped outside the gates of Vienna. Previously the Mamelukes had forced the Hospitallers off the Holy Lands in the 13th century and early in the 16th century, Suleiman drove them from the island of Rhodes, allowing them to surrender with their arms and unbroken spirit. An act of chivalry Suleiman would regret. The Hospitallers, also known as the Knights of Rhodes and the Knights of Saint John, were the final fighting Christian force of the Crusades. The Templars had been destroyed by the French King Phillip IV while the Teutonic Knights, first defeated by the Mongrels and later at the Battle of Tannenberg were destroyed and dispersed by the Poles and Lithuanians.

During the Crusades, the Hospitaller Knights maintained seven great fortresses in the Holy Lands along with dozens of fortified outposts protecting pilgrims that were built and garrisoned by the medical warriors in the Holy Lands. Each medical facility prepared to defend itself and surrounding lands with armed knights. These fortresses were captured over several generations until the Christian military orders were driven from the Middle East. Not until 1948 did a European nation return to the Middle East.

The Hospitallers that defended Malta, had their beginnings centuries before as a Catholic medical religious order, establishing hospitals and hospices to care for pilgrims traveling to and from the Holy Lands. In the beginning they were not a military fighting force, but trained medical officers, both male and female. Their hospital of Saint John in Jerusalem was staffed by teachers and students was functioning before the Crusades. Jerusalem under Islamic rule for hundreds of years was an open city where Christians, Hebrews and Moslems lived, worked, worshipped, and educated in relative harmony. This changed with the invasion and occupation of the Holy Lands by the Jihadist Seljuk Turks in 1070. In Jerusalem they massacred and sold into slavery thousands of citizens and destroyed Christian and Jewish temples demanded a Western World reaction. It was the behavior of the Seljuk Turks that prompted Pope Urban II to call for the First Crusade to liberate the Holy Lands from the infidels. Because of its medical value, the Hospice of Saint John continued to operate during the Seljuk occupation and was functioning when Jerusalem fell to the Crusaders in 1099.

Jerusalem had long been a depository for medical knowledge and training and during the two centuries of the Crusades, the Knights practiced "state of the art" medical care of the day. Saint John's Hospital was a teaching hospital training with lectures and practice. After education, Hospitaller recruits, both men and women were required to travel providing care and training in the field. The century after the First Crusade, the invading Europeans established the Kingdom of Jerusalem and other Christian enclaves scattered through the Holy Lands. It was during the Crusader period, the Hospitallers morphed into an armed force, fighting, dying and providing medical care at all the major battles. At the same time, they became a world-wide medical organization with thousands of knights and dozens of hospitals in Europe.

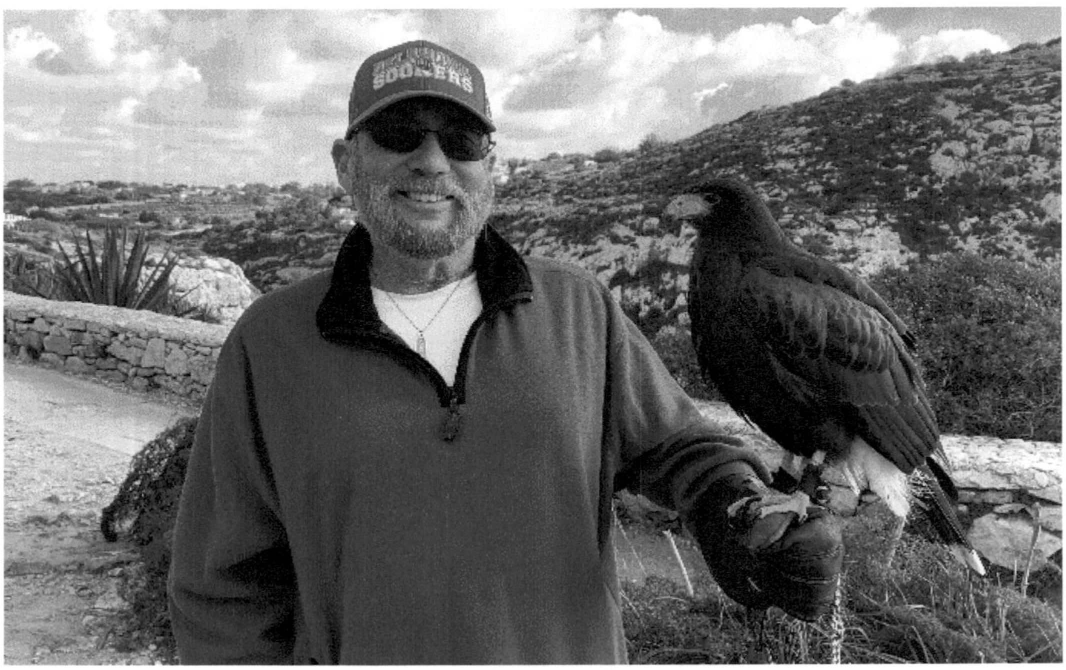

The author with a Maltese falcon

After the Knights Hospitallers were driven form Rhodes, "the garden of the Mediterranean", the new Pope, Clement VII, himself a former Hospitaller, convinced Charles V of Spain, to give Malta to the knights. Payment for this dry, nearly waterless rock, was a Maltese falcon, considered the premium hunting bird in Europe delivered to Sicily every year. After the lushness of their previous home Rhodes, Malta was a tiny desert. Almost all water was cistern-collected rain, as there are only a few small water sources on the island. The island had to import food as the rocky dry island did not produce enough. The Hospitallers becoming the Knights of Malta continued their seafaring occupation where both Turkish and some Christians considered them nothing but pirates. The Knights of Malta proved the difference between nobility and rouge is subjective and decided by the victors. They patrolled the sea in sleek fast narrow galleys of imported wood as there was no ship-building wood on Malta. Suleiman called them "sea-going scum" and described Malta as "a den of snakes"! When war was declared, Suleiman, who at seventy suffering from severe gout, was medically unfit to lead the expedition. In his place, an experienced general Mustafa Pasha led the army and Piyale Pasha while a youthful admiral married to his favorite wife's daughter led the fleet, sowing the seeds of defeat with a divided command. Turgot, the third leader, would further divide the Turkish command when he arrived from Tunisia after the siege had begun bringing more troops. As the more experienced soldier, Turgot was angered that the fleet was not in the Grand Harbor. Admiral Piyale feared losing the many Sultan's ships needed to force the gauntlet of Fort Elmo (a small fort protecting the Grand Harbor entrance). Turgot was further angered that the fortified central city of Medina left intact as Mustafa Pasha believed Medina insignificant. Had Turgot been there in the beginning, the fleet would have been in the Grand Harbor, Medina taken and Malta would have been lost.

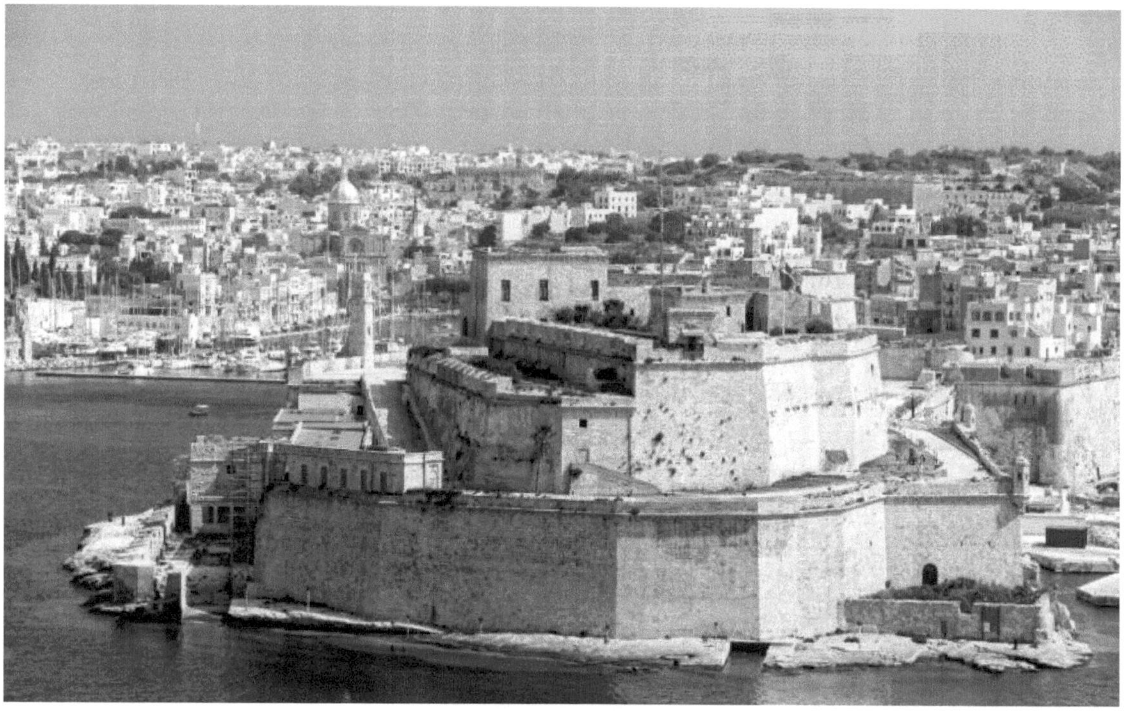

The fort of Saint Elmo guarded the entrance to Grand Harbor. A more aggressive admiral would have run his ships by the fort, accepting losses. Piyale was reluctant to risk his father-in-law's ships and choose to believe the Turkish engineers' estimate the small fort would fall in 3-4 days. The key to entering the Great Harbor held out 28 days consuming

the lives of hundreds of knights, soldiers and Maltese volunteers while inflicting much larger losses in Turkish soldiers, gunpowder, Turgot and resources that could not be replaced. At the final assault, medical officers strapped the wounded upright in chairs, dispersed weapons and fought to the death with their patients. The sacrifice saved Malta. Photo by author

In early summer of 1565, after the spring storms had dissipated, hundreds of ships discharged 40,000 soldiers, 10,000 slaves and horses, oxen, cattle, chickens onto an island with no water. The closest Turkish water was 140 miles south in Tunisia. What a nightmare for the Turkish army and naval medical officers to practice with extremely limited water. Ottoman field medicine was the best in the world with Arab, Christian, Hebrew, Armenian, Greek, Hungarian, Slavic, and Turkish medical officers trained in Istanbul. But it was summer, and the lack of potable water presented highly trained medical officers a huge obstacle for field medicine. The Ottoman military was known for clean camps and ships, experiencing a lower rate of dysentery and fevers than their Christian adversaries. On the other side, the medical monks of Malta had three hundred years of exposure to the same medical and surgical skills of the Islamic world. Skills were soon needed by both sides at the Siege of Malta. Good medical care is dependent upon several factors and one of the most important is safe drinking water. Adequate drinking water saved Malta.

The main Turkish army camp was placed in the only marshy area found on Malta, where men and animals concentrated around what they believed to be a water source. Proctomedicus (the senior medical officer on Malta) Camillo Russo predicting the Turks would encamp on the only water source had supervised the poisoning of the area after drilling deep wells throughout the marsh and placing hemp soaked in arsenic deep into ground water with large amount of feces and spoiled meat. Ottoman men and animals soon sickened from these waters, further adding to sanitation problems. Not long after landing the Turkish field hospitals were overwhelmed with wounded and ill with little chance of controlling sanitation. As water supplies dwindled, thirst drove Turkish soldiers, slaves and animals to drink from contaminated pools, even their own urine. The summer deepened, days became hotter and longer, fevers increased, Turkish medical facilities swamped, and except for initial wound care, Turkish field medicine, renowned for its effectiveness, like the army and navy, failed in its mission. Wounds, especially burns caused by fire grenades and fire hoops, exacerbated by the flowing robes worn by the soldiers, required frequent lavage with clean water. The author believes seawater, even though salty and stinging, would have sufficed; however, there is no record of its use. By the third month of the siege, dysentery was stalking the Turkish army and the autumn winds were stirring the sea. The siege was estimated to take a few weeks and neither the army nor the navy had prepared for the tenacity and dryness of Malta.

The Knights and soldiers of Malta, although outnumbered ten to one were behind their walls with extensive water storage and had accidently discovered a previously unknown well while mining for wall repair. A miracle was claimed by the church. Medical supplies, trained physicians and nurses, adequate food for nutrition and water to drink and to clean wounds, were available within the fortresses of Malta. The defender's access to drinking water, daily baked bread dipped in wine or vinegar and competent field medicine increased battle effectiveness and morale. Some days, 6,000 artillery rounds pummeled the fortifications, each shot (cannon balls rendered round by sculptors from granite) reduced the invaders' dwindling munitions. Imagine the Turkish logistics of getting hundreds of cannons, tens of thousands of cannon balls (all chipped from granite rocks mined in eastern Black Sea), tons of gunpowder, food, water, animal fodder and medical supplies to a tiny desert island in the middle of an ocean. After landing these stores without the benefit of docks, these materials were then transported miles to the walls of Malta in the summer with restricted drinking water and growing thirst.

Near the end of the siege, the Turks, personally led by Mustapha Pasha (his soldiers refused to make another assault without the commanding general leading) finally breached the walls of the main fortress, but at that moment of triumph, the rear of the invading force was attacked. Panic, the seed of defeat feared by commanders, spread through the attackers. Believing it to be the expected Spanish relief force, the nearly victorious Turks retreated from the walls they had entered at huge costs, in great disorder. In one of history's rare events, "defeat was snatched from the jaws of victory" when only one hundred horsemen sallied forth from the ancient fortress of Medina and destroyed the victory of ten thousand, by attacking their camp filled with wounded, foodstuffs and precious water supplies. After almost four months, the Spanish relief force arrived, and the Turks withdrew, its Empire greatly injured. Had the Ottoman Turks taken Malta, it would have opened the door into Italy and Europe. Just as the sacrifice of human immune cells protect the body, the sacrifice of the Knights of Malta and the Maltese population saved Christian Europe from a likely Islamic invasion and possible conquest. Western texts could have been written in Turkish. The successful Siege of Malta directly led to the Christian victory at the Battle of Lepanto six years later. In both conflicts, field medicine played its part in the story.

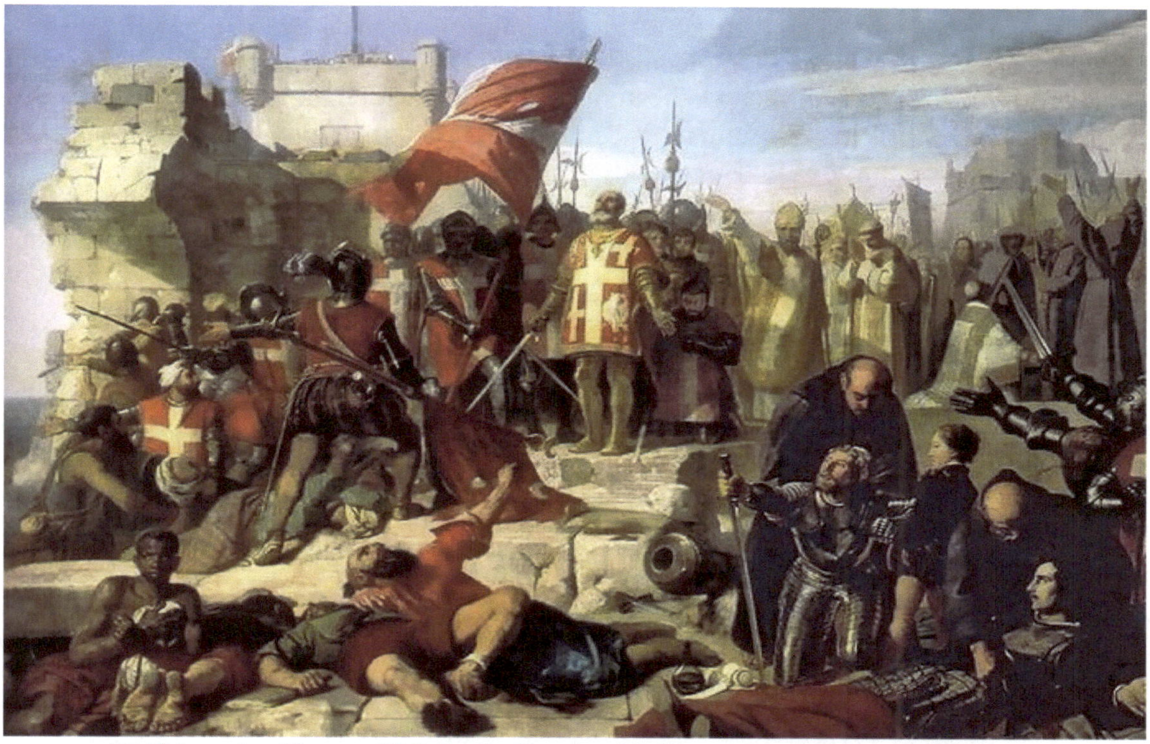

"Lifting the Siege of Malta" Charles-Philippe Lariviere (1798-1876)
Hall of the Crusaders, Palace of Versailles

The Grand Master, de Lavallette was seventy when the siege began many days, he donned over seventy pounds of armor and wielding sword and pike, fought hand-to-hand at the most perilous moments. As a younger man, de Lavallette was captured at sea and spent a year of slavery pulling an oar on a Turkish raiding galley. That year of slavery hardened de Lavallette who remained physically active and celibate. Celibacy was a powerful and respected mantle worn by the Knights and it protected them from the ravages of syphilis that was sweeping Europe during the 16th century, depriving men of strength and long life. Suleiman and some of his generals and admirals lived a life of luxury and multiple wives while de Lavallette and his knights primarily lived like monks eating simple foods and preforming daily labor. Suleiman at seventy was physically much older than his adversary, de Lavallette. Gout, congestive heart failure and lack of exercise were the result of years spent in Istanbul and Suleiman's mistakes in his planning and launching an amphibious invasion was likely affected by the Sultan's medical condition.

In 1566, one year after Malta, some 3,000 Christians held out against the aged and ill Suleiman, personally leading an army of 100,000 in Croatia at the Siege of Szigetvár. Near the end of the siege Suleiman with broken health and spirit died in is tent. To keep the news quiet, his physician was strangled with a silk scarf, as befitted an officer. These two sieges and the defeat of the Turks at Lepanto five years later, saw the maximum thrust of Islam into Europe until the Turks, under Kara Mustafa fought their way to the Gates of Vienna in 1683 with another huge army. History, like biochemical dynamics, can suddenly be changed by a small influence applied at the right time and location. In medicine, small things can affect a large change. This happened at the gates of Vienna in the late 17th century when a much smaller force of Polish cavalry under John Sobieski unexpectedly struck the flank of the Turkish army entrenched and stable, facing Vienna's walls. The charge suddenly changed both structure and orientation of the battle. In medicine, an enzyme has a similar effect on a much larger molecule. Free radicals such the single highly reactive oxygen molecules and enzymes such as phosphodiesterase are tiny compared to the molecules they disrupt. After the defeat, the Turkish commander Kara Mustafa (born from Christian parents), was strangled by a silk scarf, as befitted an officer.

Human skin like the walls of Malta is a powerful deterrent and can repair itself. Keeping the body's first line of defense intact requires skin and eye protection, good nutrition and when assistance is needed, good medical care. The body's internal immune system is aided by protecting the skin and eyes from sun, penetration by foreign bodies, hydration, caution when deploying hands, ingesting only safe fluids, frequently handwashing, avoiding motorcycles, obtaining immunizations for tetanus, diphtheria, pertussis, pneumonia, hepatitis, physical activity, staying hydrated and drinking apple cider vinegar.

During World War II, Hitler and his generals made a fatal mistake by taking the island of Crete at great cost when Malta was more important at a fraction of effort. Malta, unlike Crete controlled traffic from Europe to the Axis troops in North Africa. The unsinkable aircraft carrier, Malta, was the primary reason Germany failed in North Africa. As long as Malta held out, the Italian army and Germany's Africa Corps of men and equipment was doomed. The men and armor siphoned away from the invasion of Russia in a failed attempt in North Africa enhanced Germany's failure in Russia as well as in the Mediterranean. The second failed siege of Malta helped Russia, protected the oilfields, gave the allies control of the Mediterranean and played a large role in winning the Second World War.

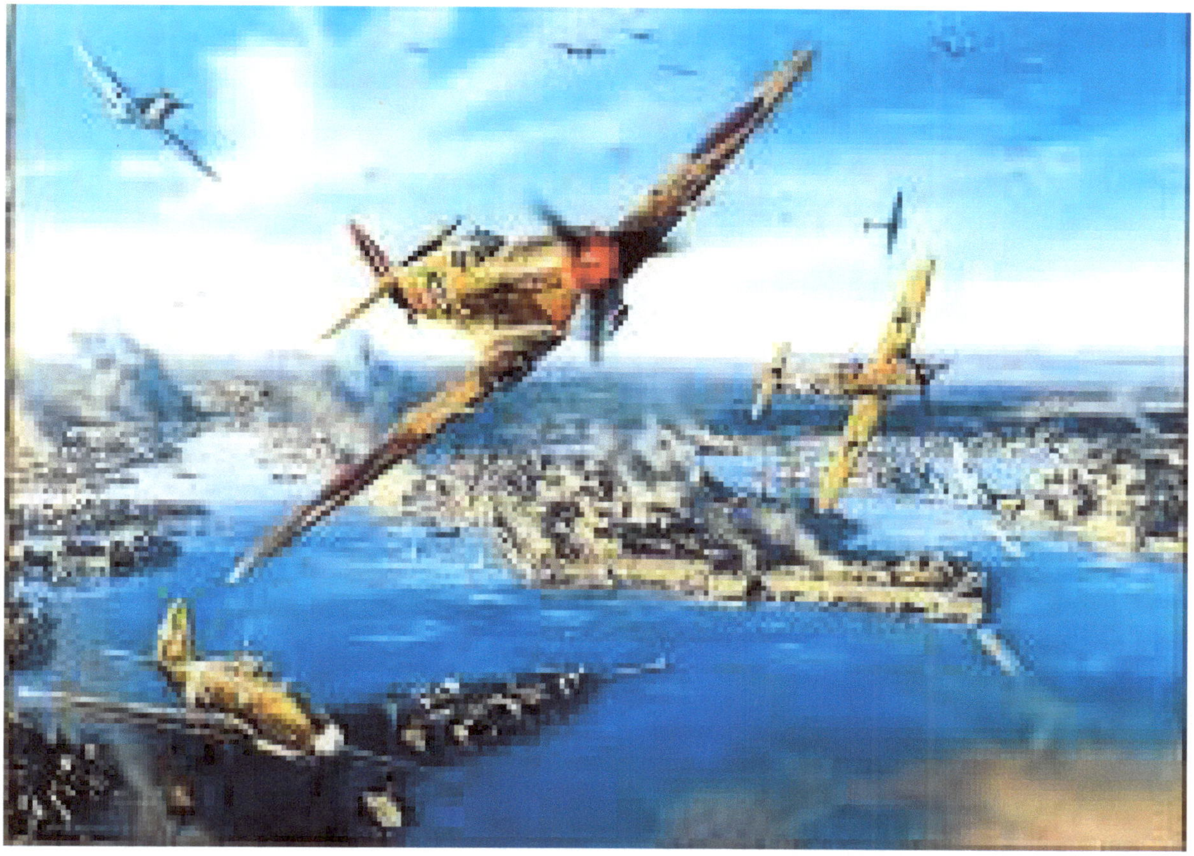

Malta was under siege again in the Second World War from German and Italian forces. Hitler, echoing Suleiman's words, called Malta "a den of scorpions". England's retention of Malta greatly inhibited the supply of men and materials needed by Hitler's Africa Corps. More bombs were dropped on Malta during World War II than the entirety of England. The island was partially saved when FDR in defiance of Hitler sent the USS Wasp steaming close enough to launch 47 British Spitfire fighters off her flight deck before America entered the war with Germany. Malta was later saved by the *SS Ohio* an American oil tanker when it barely floated into the Great Harbor at one knot, destroyers on port and starboard sides keeping it afloat. Getting the *Ohio* to Malta in late summer, 1942 cost England an aircraft carrier, two cruisers, several destroyers and fourteen merchant ships. The date of the arrival is still celebrated every year in Malta. In World War I, Malta served as a giant hospital and rehabilitation center, thus continuing the role Hospitallers have performed for over one thousand years. Image from Malta's Air Museum

Pharmacology
the study of drugs

Vitamin C, Scurvy and Mutiny on the Bounty

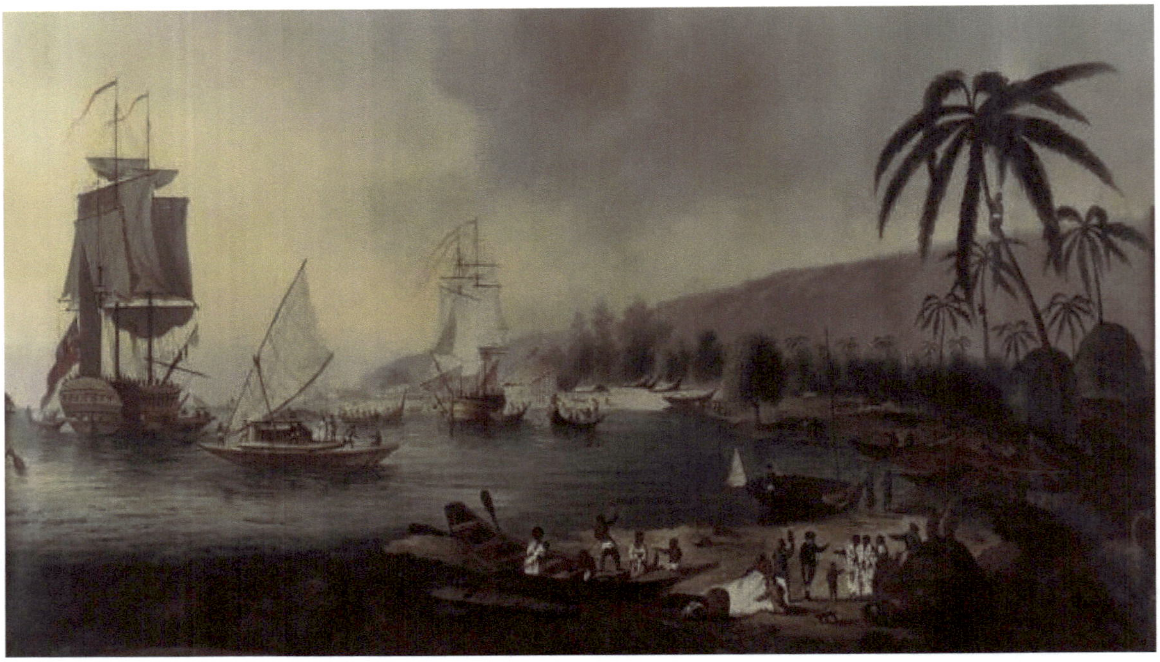

HMS *Discovery* and *Resolution* in Tahiti by John Cleveley the Younger (1747-1786)

There are important medications to carry at sea and in the field, a list that has changed significantly over the years, especially since World War II. The two of the most important class of medications per the author are antibiotics and heart drugs since these can play a huge role in saving lives. All ships venturing upon the ocean today should carry the most modern drugs available, since they are generally safe and easy to use. This was not always the case, as ships left port with few if any effective drugs. If there was a single most important drug to the history of world shipping, it could be vitamin C (ascorbic acid). The story of this simple vitamin supplement has played in history is long and tragic, as its absence killed many sailors, soldiers and civilians until the last century. Tragic, because using vitamin C to treat and prevent scurvy was known two hundred years earlier and likely even earlier. The story of Tahiti, Captain Bligh, the HMS *Bounty* and vitamin C is a tragic story explaining a role of medicine and history.

John Hawkins was a 16th century English sailor, knighted by Queen Elizabeth for his capture of foreign shipping and helping protect England from the Spanish Armada. He was a hero to Elizabeth while to the Spanish, Portuguese and Dutch considered him a pirate, who along with Sir Francis Drake were referred to as "sea dogs" and both carried large bounties on their capture or death from several nations. Sir Hawkins stated that he personally knew of 10,000 deaths from scurvy during his years at sea. So many lives wasted over hundreds of years for a disease that was easy to treat.

Long ocean voyages, besieged cities, marauding armies, concentration camps and where humans were deprived of fresh fruits and vegetables, brought on the symptoms of scurvy. It is caused by lack of ascorbic acid or Vitamin C in the diet, a substance vital for normal human physiology. Vitamin C is necessary for repair and restoration of tissues as they age or are injured. Animals such as the ship rat (*rattus rattus*) can manufacture Vitamin C, whereas humans must obtain it from food sources on a regular basis and historically, humans consuming rats in time of need prevented scurvy. Ascorbic acid, a water-soluble vitamin is poorly stored and must be consumed regularly. Symptoms of scurvy could appear as early as a few weeks, and without a source of Vitamin C, is fatal within two to three months in most victims. A deadly painful and disfiguring disease sorely limited sea travel.

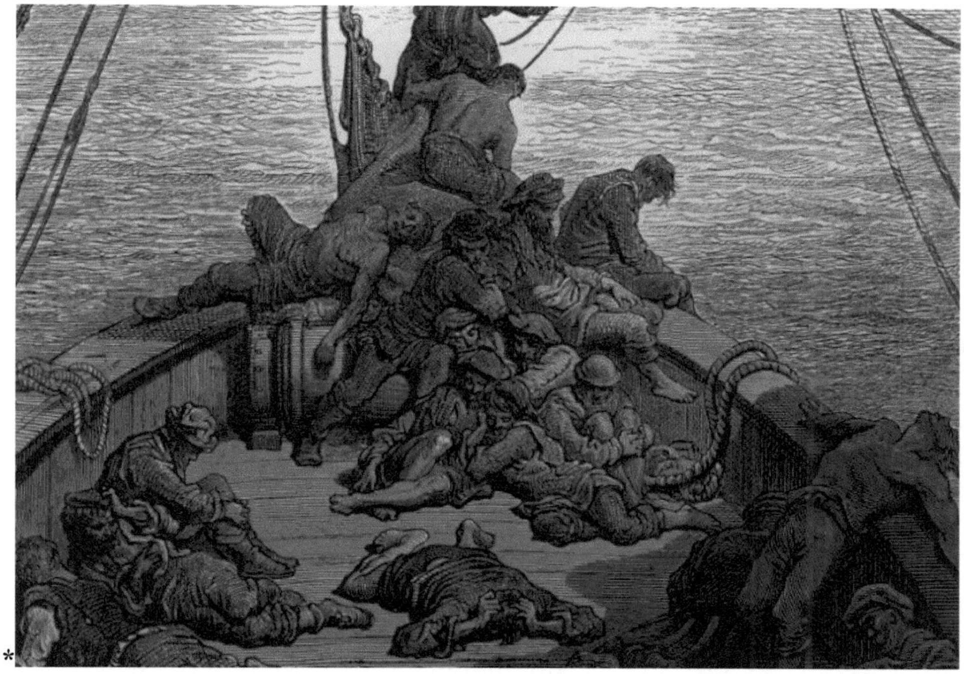

*

Image by Gustave Dore from book-length version of "The Rime of the Ancient Mariner". A rabble of crew can be converted into a fighting force with vitamin C.

Scurvy is easy to recognize, as its symptoms are well defined and occur only when people are deprived of fresh foods. But, since it was seen so often with diseases such as typhus, typhoid fever and jaundice, it was thought not to be a nutritional deficiency, but another infection. Ships surgeons and their captains proved that scurvy could be treated and prevented with fruit juice in the 18th century, knowledge largely ignored by generations of seafarers and unfortunately physicians. Vitamin C is a weak acid and a powerful reducing agent in the cell (because it readily gives up two hydrogen ions, thus reducing itself). It is easily rendered ineffective with heat and therefore prolonged cooking greatly decreases the amount of vitamin C in vegetables. Without vitamin C, the cement that holds the connective tissue of the body together, begins to fail.

Scurvy played a prominent devastating role in medical military history, spanning from the 12th century Crusades to the American Civil War. Representing seven hundred years of ignorance and mistreatment for a disease successfully controlled by ships surgeons and captains well before 19th century conflicts. Scurvy begins with fatigue and listlessness, followed by bleeding sores over the gums, which become spongy, allowing teeth to loosen and fall from the mouth. Few of the Age of Discovery sailors had a full set of teeth. Skin and underlying tissue darken as the flesh begins to decompose while still on the victim. The breath becomes foul, especially in the airless confines of a wooden ship's sickbay, located deep in the ship's bowels, devoid of light and ventilation. A place dreaded by sailors since few emerged alive. These foul quarters claimed men sometimes women and children, spending days and weeks in theirs and others filth, adding to the misery of a scurvy death.

Armies and besieged cities because of static position often suffered more from scurvy than the more mobile ships. An account recorded by John of Joinville, a member of Louis IX's ill-fated crusade of 1248 in his chronicles "The Life of St. Louis", the only complete record of St. Louis's Crusade. After a successful landing in Egypt, the Christian army was trapped in the Nile delta, cut off from its fleet's supply of fresh vegetables. Within weeks the disease spread, and men's flesh blackened and began to rot. "a great cry went up from camp like women in labor" as the barber-surgeons went about their grim tasks of cutting away dead flesh from living men. A painful and futile attempt to control scurvy. There are many sea stories about scurvy, the author's favorite is the story about the *HMS Bounty* and its relationship to scurvy and history. The portrayal by Hollywood of a cruel and inhumane Captain Bligh is far from reality. No surprise that Hollywood would distort history. By the time William Bligh was born in 1754, the Royal British Navy had recognized the rate of Ships Surgeon and Surgeon's Mate, an apprentice medical officer. The medical department of the British Admiralty had developed a standard apothecary (its contents dependent upon the integrity of the supplier) and every ship was supplied with a copy of "The Surgeons Mate". Unfortunately, many vessels carried medical officers that were almost illiterate or too much of a drunkard to do much reading in a text covering common diseases encountered at sea, care of surgical instruments and methods of amputations.

When the future Captain Bligh was fourteen years old, the first English textbook on tropical medicine was published by James Lind, the most remarkable ships surgeon of the 18th century. Lind, while a British Royal Navy Surgeon, studying literature and preforming his own research, proved the effectiveness of lime juice as both treatment and prevention of scurvy, publishing this information in 1747. Dr. Lind, a practical physician, was also responsible for the life-saving process of baking clothing and bedding to prevent the build-up of lice, which greatly reduced the incidence of typhus. Before Lind, typhus and scurvy killed more sailors than all other causes in the English navy and merchant marine. He stressed shipboard sanitation by fumigation with sulphur fogs (done thousands of years before by Greeks) and required crew personal cleanliness. James Lind left his government job for the lucrative and challenges of the Surgeon General of the British East India Company where in addition to training ships surgeons, he established the British Indian Medical Service. This medical education system in India, Burma and Malaysia has for over two hundred years supplied a greater number of English-speaking physicians than any other medical system in the world.

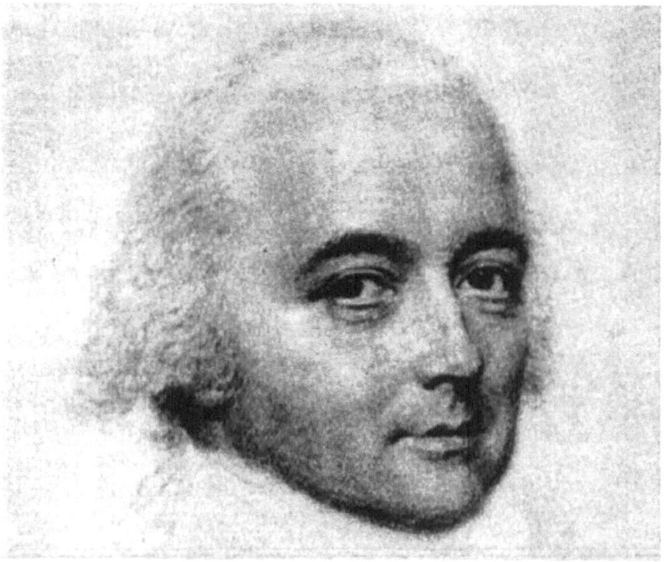

A young Captain Bligh, by J. Stuart

Lind's rediscovery that juices from certain fruits would prevent and treat scurvy, even when preserved for many months had likely been known and practiced by seafarers well before the time of Christ but like much ancient medical knowledge was lost. A tragedy that took centuries for Christian Europe to realize that scurvy was prevented by a substance found in fresh vegetables and in the flesh of tropical fruits found where there is sunlight all year and ample rainfall. Nations that had access to these fruits (Portuguese) were the most successful early European seafarers with fruits brought by the invading Moors from North Africa. Fruits that did well in the Iberian Peninsula. The Dutch had no access in the beginning to tropical fruits, although they could grow green vegetables. In their search for new markets, they pushed farther from Europe into tropical Africa and India (territory penetrated almost a century earlier by the Portuguese). Since military and merchant ships from the Netherlands had limited success using an anti-scurvy mixture of sauerkraut (partially cooked cabbage) and molasses preserved in vinegar (ascetic acid), were the first northern European power to follow the Portuguese into the tropics. This gruel-like mixture (vitriol) was a weak source of vitamin C, requiring large amounts of an unpleasant tasting medicine that was taken with little relish by the crew. Early Dutch captains and ships surgeons strictly dispensed this and other antiscorbics such as plain vinegar, often mixing it with the crew's evening ration of grog to further ensure its ingestion. So determined were so captains that no man should contract scurvy, flogging was used on men that contrived to miss their scurvy therapy.

Scurvy prevention was paramount in providing a nation with the ability for discovery and domination of far-off lands. After throwing off Catholic Spain, the Netherlands, a small country short in natural resources but rich in coastline and waterways, built and manned world-roving fleets. The Dutch were able to claim much of the early far eastern trade with the East Indies, returning ships laden with spices, tea and silk. Each ship is worth several fortunes for its owners and officers. By conquering scurvy as the Portuguese had previously done, the Dutch were able to compete with the maritime powers of the much larger nations of Spain, France and England.

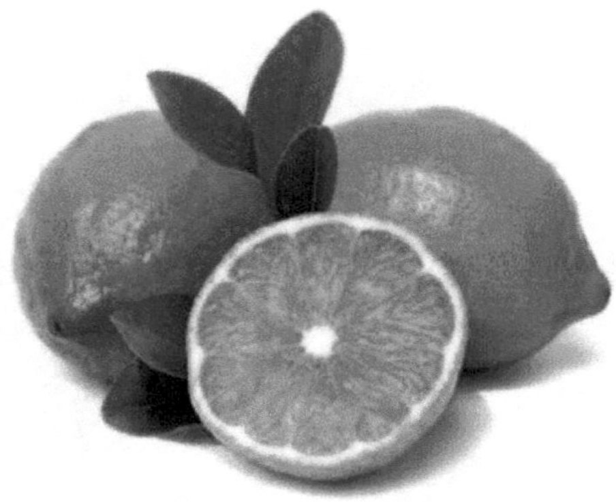

Lemons are a superior source of vitamin C, however for generations, the British choose limes and for centuries, British sailors were called limeys

By Bligh's time, sauerkraut and vinegar had been replaced with fresh fruits and vegetables, supplemented with a mixture of lime juice and diluted grog (making a far tastier totty than vinegar). Educated sailing officers knew the best source of vitamin C was found in tropical fruits, something the English did not have a steady supply of at the end of the 18th century. English shipping depended in a large part on the colonies of other powers for their antiscorbics. The Dutch operated a string of settlements from the Cape of Good Hope at the southern tip of Africa, along the coasts of India, and scattered among the islands of Malaysia and Indonesia. They supplied fruits and vegetables to passing ships of all nations for a price, sometimes even to ships flying the flag of the enemies of the Netherlands. Being rapacious entrepreneurs, the Dutch merchants sold vital medicine at inflated prices to adversary shipping. The British found the lack of their own citrus colonies a costly problem, one that was a high priority to solve. One of the purposes of Captain Cook's survey of the Pacific islands was a quest for a fruit high in ascorbic acid and one that was likely to be transplantable to a distant site. Plants found in Tahiti were believed to have the "right stuff" and Bligh, who had served under Cook was chosen for the task of harvesting these tropical plants and bringing them "healthy and hale" to British colonies in the Caribbean where these plants would be transplanted and thrive.

William Bligh first went to sea at the age of fifteen as an able-bodied seaman, spending time before the mast, and later being promoted to the officer ranks, as did Captain Cook before him. Bligh had spent six years as a junior officer when Captain James Cook chose him to be one of his Masters on the HMS *Resolution.* He must have been a promising young officer for Cook to pass him over more experienced officers when elevating Bligh for his third and final voyage to the Pacific. This was fortunate for Bligh, since James Cook was perhaps the most innovative commander of England's 18th century navy and a good mentor. Cook, already a captain in England's merchant marine chose to start all over as an able-bodied in the Royal Navy, spending twelve long years before making Lieutenant at the age of forty. As a commander, Cook had a remarkable record of sailing with fewer deaths and was an early follower of Lind's recommendation of fresh foods and citrus juices, personal cleanliness and baking the crew's clothing periodically. Captain Cook was elected to the Royal Society in 1776 for his improvements in medicine at sea and known as a merciful captain, sparingly flogging. All traits that Bligh embraced.

The English government, through the recommendation of several sea-going science officers had decided that the breadfruit plant of Tahiti could be transplanted to the West Indies. English planters with holdings in the Caribbean islands could then grow breadfruit, providing vitamin C for the navy and colonial army while furnishing a cheap source of food to feed the growing slave population. The *Bounty's* voyage was to be a botanical medical mission, carrying fifty-six souls on a ship built for thirty. The crew consisted of thirteen able bodied seaman, six midshipman, two cooks, an armorer, a gunner's mate, assorted carpenters, two gardeners and unfortunately for Bligh, a drunken incompetent ships surgeon. Bligh's mission was to sail southwest from England rounding Cape Horn, no small task in the southern winter and approach Tahiti from the east. After loading the *Bounty* with healthy breadfruit plants, he was to continue west, picking up additional types of fruit plants on the large island of Java. It was presumed that some of the breadfruit plants would expire, and these were to be replaced with mangosteens, durians, jackfruits, nancas, lanas and any other available tropical fruits in the gardens of the Dutch-held colonies. After crossing the length of the empty Indian Ocean and rounding the Cape of Good Hope, he was to continue to the Caribbean isles of St. Vincent and Jamaica, depositing one half of the surviving plants at each site. A circumnavigation of the entire globe in a time only a few ships had successfully completed. A command with no fellow officers, an overcrowded ship and a malignancy.

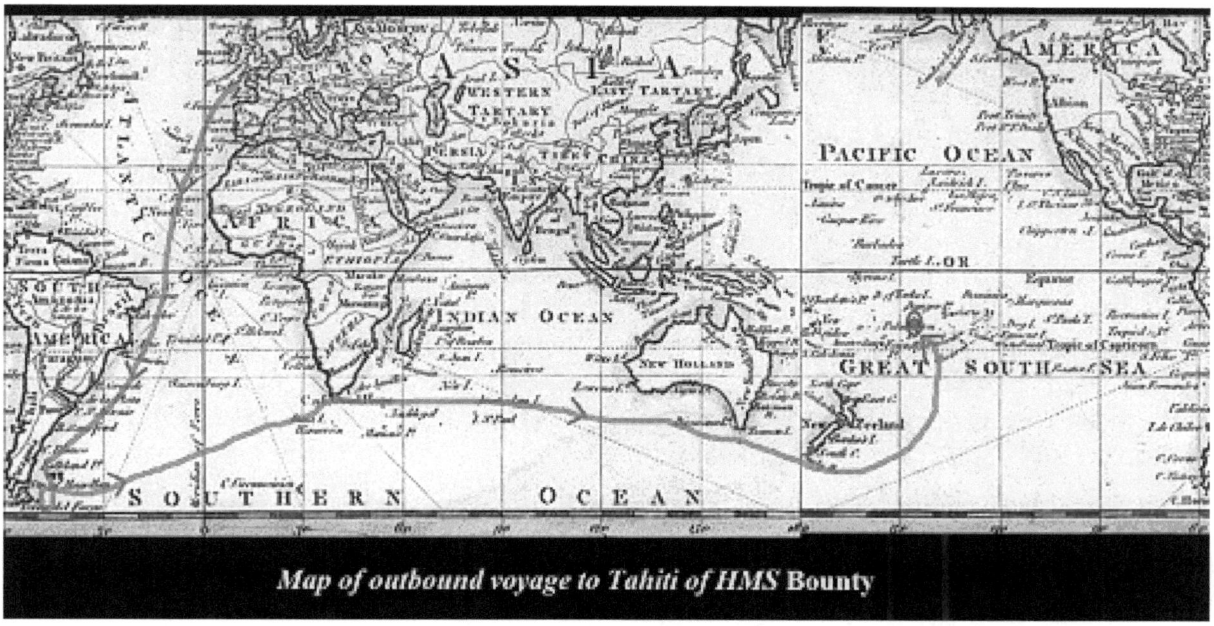

Map of outbound voyage to Tahiti of HMS **Bounty**

A very long voyage with a "cancer" on the ship in the form of the medical officer

This was perhaps the most ambitious attempt at nautical agriculture in history, and the Admiralty proposed to undertake this venture with a single ship overcrowded with men and not even a Lieutenant to serve as Captain Bligh's second in command. The Admiralty expected Bligh to train and promote one of the Able Bodied or midshipmen, which would have likely been Fletcher Christian. Christian, an experienced sailor, had served before as a third officer but had been "broken-back" to the enlisted rank of the forecastle for misconduct. Unlike most ordinary seamen, Christian was educated, literate, had seagoing experience as an officer, was born to a family with some connections and could get men to follow him. The story of the mutiny on the Bounty was primarily told by sources favoring the perspective of Christian Fletcher's well-connected family and surviving crew members spiteful of Bligh. No blame was placed on the Admiralty medical department that cursed the mission with criminally incompetent medicine at sea. Later, the British in the Crimean War were cursed with similar medical leadership.

Why the British Admiralty placed Thomas Huggan as ships surgeon on such a long and arduous mission, so important to British sea power in the Americas is a mystery. Perhaps someone in the medical leadership in the Admiralty wanted to get rid of Huggan and felt that medical care aboard the Bounty was a low priority. After meeting Huggan and deeming him unfit, Bligh was unsuccessful in having him removed, although he was granted a surgeon's mate. This fellow, Thomas Ledward, the last man to join the ship, had little medical training and was to learn the art of medicine at sea while underway, mentored by Huggan? It was the surgeon's behavior and incompetence that played the most important role in history's best-known mutiny. Early in the voyage, Bligh wrote in his personal Log of Thomas Huggan, "I now find my Doctor to be a Drunken Sot, he is constantly in liquor, having a private stock by him which I assured him shall be taken away if he does not desist from making himself such a Beast."

The Bounty reached the eastern gate of Cape Horn in late March (early winter on Southern Latitudes), where Bligh recorded the air suddenly became very sharp and some of the men were complaining of rheumatism. Bligh had not been to the southern tip of South America before and regarded the passage around it as "the most difficult and grandest part of our passage". Indeed, it proved so difficult that it was an impossible task as the Bounty was battered by continuous gales until late April. Green seas broke over the vessel as freezing rain and equally cold seawater poured through the leaking ship. There was no such thing as foul-weather gear, rubber boots nor winter clothes for the crew. Injuries and colds mounted as the men were battered as badly as the ship. By April 13th Bligh wrote, "I cannot expect my Men and Officers to bear it much longer, nor will the object of my Voyage allow me to persist in it." Rheumatism had struck down more men, the crew's cook had fallen and broke a rib, and the Surgeon fell while drunk and dislocated his shoulder. The weather became so bad towards the end and with fewer men to stand duty, Captain Bligh had himself lashed to the ship's mast as he stood watches day and night. Finally, on April 22, Bligh gave up and had the ship turned about and reached False Bay at the Cape of Good Hope one month later.

At the Dutch settlement, the entire ship had to be re-caulked, while the men rested and regained strength. While battling the Horn, Bligh had continued to serve his crew hot nutritious breakfasts and kept them as warm and dry as possible, even allowing the crew with the worst "colds" to sleep in his great cabin. While in the southern African Cape's port, a Dutch ship limped in with thirty men having been buried at sea and many others ill. A letter written at that time by the Bounty's new surgeon's mate Ledward, gave Captain Bligh high praise for the almost parental care he gave to his men. A quite different picture of the Bligh portrayed by Hollywood. On July 1st, the Bounty set sail for the empty continent of Australia, crossing some 6,000 miles of the Southern Ocean with no landfalls planned. Hot breakfasts, regular cleaning of clothing and bodies and daily ingestion of antiscorbics continued under Bligh's careful attention to the health of his crew. Thomas Huggan took little interest in these preventative medicine measures, he just continued to drink, often appearing drunk and disrespectful to Bligh in front of the crew.

After leaving the waters of New Zealand in early October, a medical tragedy occurred that shocked Bligh and his crew, sowing more seeds of unhappiness on the *Bounty*. Bligh had recently been furious at Huggan for placing men on the sick list for scurvy. Huggan knew that Bligh felt to have a single member of his crew "down" with scurvy was a disgrace. Bligh was with Captain Cook on a previous voyage and knew that it was preventable with daily doses of lime. By this time, Bligh and Huggan hated one another completely, and the surgeon seemed to draw his only delight in the bottle and aggravating the captain. Sometime during the night of October 8th, a popular young member of Bligh's crew expired under Huggan's care and not until the next day was Bligh informed, not by the surgeon, but through "scuttlebutt" from the disgruntled crew. The cause of able-bodied James Valentine's death was blatant medical malpractice by the ship's surgeon. He had repeatedly bled Valentine for some obscure reason and wounds became infected and continued care by Huggan only worsened the young sailor's condition. While young Valentine lay dying alone in sickbay on the evening of October 8th, Huggan was dining with Bligh, giving no indication that one of his charges was mortally ill.

Huggan continued to deteriorate after Valentine' death, becoming continuously drunk. Bligh in addition to his other duties became the ship's full time medical officer and as the crew's health improved, the surgeon had himself placed on the disabled list with a diagnosis of "paralytic affection". Bligh finally found the surgeon's hidden store of alcohol and destroyed it, so after 27,000 miles of sailing, his surgeon was sober for the arrival in the Tahiti Islands. Even sober he was incompetent. Captain Cook had always insisted that the entire crew was to be examined by the medical officer for signs of venereal diseases, primarily syphilis and gonorrhea. Any sailors found to have ulcers on the genitalia or any discharge from the penis was restricted to the ship. Captain Cook spent years in the Pacific visiting many islands without infecting the natives with syphilis. This changed with the *Bounty*, since Huggan cleared several men with the "Pox", even though they had sores or discharge. It is supposed that after such a long hard sail, Huggan thought it was asking too much for the diseased sailors to watch their crewmates enjoy the women of Tahiti. Or he was just evil. From this action, we can surmise that Thomas Huggan cared little for the misery and death that the introduction of syphilis would have on Paradise. This author is convinced that Thomas Huggan was never a true medical officer, but someone promoted up the ranks to pass a problem on. One of history's truly bad men.

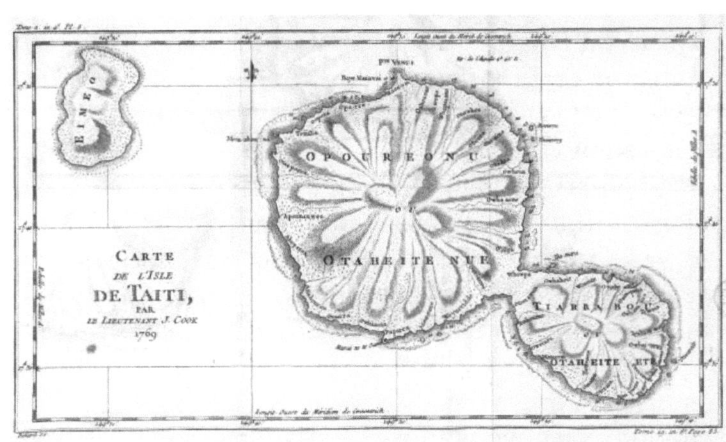

One of Captain Cook's survey charts. At the beginning of World War II, the American navy's only charts of many of the Pacific Islands were Cook's charts, drawn 150 years earlier.

Sometime after arriving in Tahiti, Huggan once again found a source of alcohol and drank himself into a drunken stupor, dying on the evening of December 10th, 1788. The surgeon's personal effects were held for auction but due to his lack of personal hygiene, his gear (clothing was generally valuable on ships at sea) went unsold. Thomas Ledward, a former regular sailor, was promoted to Acting Surgeon or the Bounty. In January, several men deserted, leading to floggings and further deterioration of the relationship between Bligh and the crew. Desertions and floggings later morphed into the mutiny occurring on April 28th, 1789, when Bligh and eighteen other men were cast off in twenty-three-foot open boat. Under Bligh's leadership, they traveled almost 4,000 miles of unchartered ocean with the loss of only one man. A nautical feat that places William Bligh as one of history's greatest sailors.

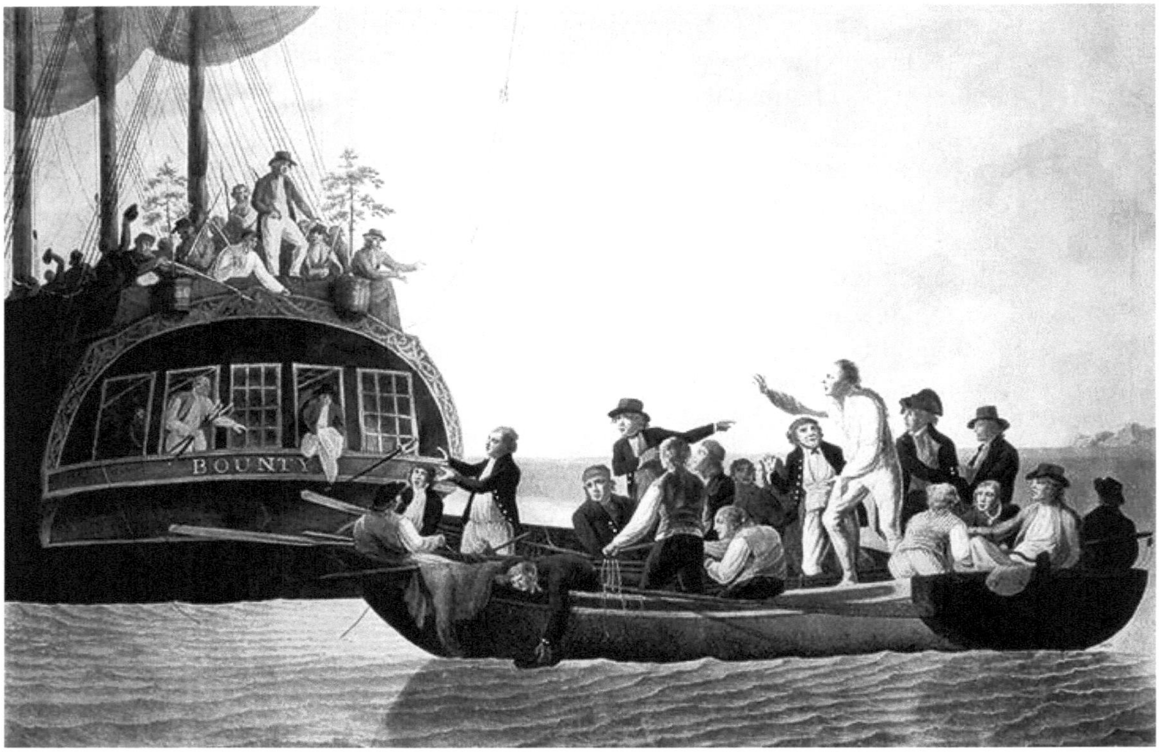

The mutineers are casting off Bligh and his companions for what Fletcher and the others thought was certain death. Engraving by Robert Dodd.

Bligh spent another twenty-eight years in his Majesty's Service and was at sea during the trial of the mutineers. Fletcher and others fled to the isolated atoll of Pitcairn Island where they avoided capture, and their decedents still live. Bligh fought valiantly with Admiral Nelson at the bloody battle of Copenhagen. It was this battle where history reports that Nelson put his telescope to his blind eye when he disregarded the admiral's order to disengage and Bligh, also disobeying the order to retreat led his ship in Nelson's wake and was instrumental in the victory. Nelson presented Bligh with his sword and thanked him for his support. Bligh, due to his outstanding record as a naval officer was appointed the Governor of New South Wales in Australia from 1806 to 1810 to reduce the rampant corruption by the British army's administration. Governor Bligh's clamp-down led to another mutiny against him in 1808 by corrupt army officers. Two of England's greatest sea officers, Captain James Cook and Admiral Horatio Nelson thought highly of William. He died at the age of 64 on December 7th, 1817, in his own bed in London. He should be remembered not as a tyrant, but as a sailor, explorer, exceptional Captain and medical officer.

Pain Medications-Analgesics

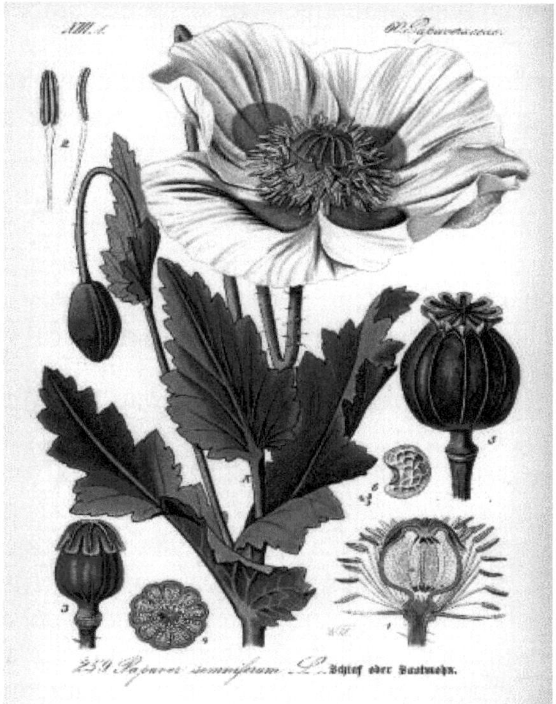

19th century drawing of the opium plant by unknown artist

Opium and its preparations are probably the longest and most used medicines are obtained from the unripe seed of the poppy, *Papaver somniferum*, after the milky juice is dried to a powder. Oil of the poopy likely originated in the Indian subcontinent and was brought to ancient Egypt where its use was widespread at least 5000 years ago. It was carried by Greek and later Roman shipping to all parts of their empire. Opium is a Greek word for the poppy juice made into an elixir. "Among the remedies which has pleased Almighty God to give man to relieve his sufferings, none so universal and so efficacious as opium" was written by Thomas Sydenham. Sydenham was a 17th century soldier turned physician after serving as one of Cromwell's captains in the English Civil War, entered medical training at the advanced age of thirty-three as did Albert Schweitzer. Combat experience had taught him the efficacy of opium and later medical officers would discover its dangers. The most common form of opium through the centuries has been a tincture where the drug dissolved in wine or other alcohols, known as laudanum. Some form of opium was found in most drug cabinets and medicine chests in the 18th and 19th centuries. All ships carried the drug, and it was readily available in any port-city apothecary. There were many opium addicts in the American West where isolation, boredom and frequent wounds made the drug an indispensable item. The tonics, cure-alls and theriacs sold by the traveling medicine wagons of the American western frontier was usually a mixture of opium, brandy and sometimes included actual snake parts. Although it seldom cured anything, it almost never failed to exert a positive mood change.

Opium use was ubiquitous in western medicine since the 18th century, driven by the British Empire trade in this commodity. Its value meant every ship, every medical officer and most people had some form of opium. It was carried in the covered wagons, on the backs of infantry and their mules. No army or navy took the field without it. There was no replacement for natural opium until Germany developed methadone eliminating reliance on imported opium. In the Second World War, Germany dispensed huge amounts of methadone combined with methamphetamine to its army. Methadone is a true synthetic opiate whereas the so called "synthetic" opiates, i.e. hydrocodone, oxycodone, hydromorphone begin life as opium and are manipulated in the lab to increase effects and minimize side effects. Morphine and codeine are the only natural opiates currently used, unchanged from the chemicals found in raw opium.

Raw opium contains over twenty alkaloids, one of which is morphine. The name is derived from the Greek god of dreams, Morpheus. Opiates are effective because they readily cross the blood-brain barrier where receptors on the brain are stimulated by these alkaloids, almost as if opiates were meant for mankind. Opiates are powerful analgesics in most cases, but this pain relief is sometimes accompanied by side effects of itching, nausea, vomiting, suppressed respiration, even respiratory arrest, urinary retention and constipation from bowel paralysis (this is useful when used in small amounts to control diarrhea). For these reasons and others, morphine is a drug that should be used carefully in the field. However, for pain relief, opiates are still the "King of analgesics". The author was taught by mentors in cardiology that reducing chest pain in a heart attack was the primary goal and opiates play a role. Relieving chest pain is paramount to saving heart muscle and life. Therefore, in a person with a history of heart attack or with a crew that has a high risk for heart attack, morphine could be a vital component of the offshore medicine chest. If used, the dose for morphine is 5-10 mgs every 2-4hours. Buprenorphine is a drug used to reverse fatal respiratory arrest in opiate overdose and at the same time is an excellent analgesic. It is safe, effective and easy to administer by dissolving in the mouth or by subcutaneous injections. In the field, **buprenorphine** is the drug of choice for pain relieve and should be part of the medicine chest.

A concern of possessing morphine is that it is tightly controlled in the United States. As a Class II controlled substance, it requires tight security when carried in an offshore medicine chest. Drugs in this classification are considered to have a high risk of abuse and therefore, must be kept under lock and key with careful recording of uses, dose administered, and disposal of out-of-date medicine. Class II drugs should be limited in the field medicine chest if possible. Controlled substances in the United States are rated from Class I to Class VI, depending on their level of control. Useful drugs such as diazepam (Valium) and buprenorphine in a medicine chest are Class IV. Class I drugs are considered so addictive or dangerous that they are not lawful to possess, even for research. Until recently this class includes LSD, psychotropic mushrooms and marijuana, even though individual states and the Veterans Administration have decriminalized them.

Synthetic morphine-like drugs have been developed to reduce the unwanted side effects while maintaining pain relief. For years, the author used and recommended sublingual buprenorphine for its pain relief without causing respiratory depression. In addition, it has a low risk of addiction when compared to Class II pain relievers. Unlike morphine and Demerol, buprenorphine causes little if any "euphoria" or the "high" associated with narcotics. Narcotic addicts seeking pain relief refuse buprenorphine as it may "uncover" opiates already onboard, as it is a traditional opiate blocker, can reverse respiratory depression with true opiates and usually just puts the patient to sleep while relieving pain.

When narcotic and narcotic-like drugs are given by injection they are often mixed with enhancers. Drugs such as promethazine (Phenergan) diphenhydramine (Benadryl) or hydroxyzine (Vistaril). Antihistamines may block any potential allergic reaction to an injected pain medicine and antihistamines reduce the incidence of nausea and vomiting so often associated with pain medicine injections. As previously mentioned, buprenorphine was developed to replace illegal opiate use and to reverse life-threatening opiate overdose and is effective as analgesic (pain reliever). It does relieve pain and does so safely. Fentanyl is a newer synthetic opiate thirty-three times more effective than morphine. It is highly effective in analgesia but has become a major killer in opiate overdoses in the United States. However, when used properly, it is an effective and safe form of pain control in the field. After fracturing four ribs in a motorcycle accident, the author found pain relief using fentanyl transdermal patch which delivered a low continuous dose for seventy-two hours. In fractures, burns and other painful conditions that last for days, the fentanyl patch would be the drug of choice. The patches come in 25mcg, 50mcg, 75mgc and 100 mcg. In the past the author supplied a sea-going medicine chest with the lower 25mcg dose.

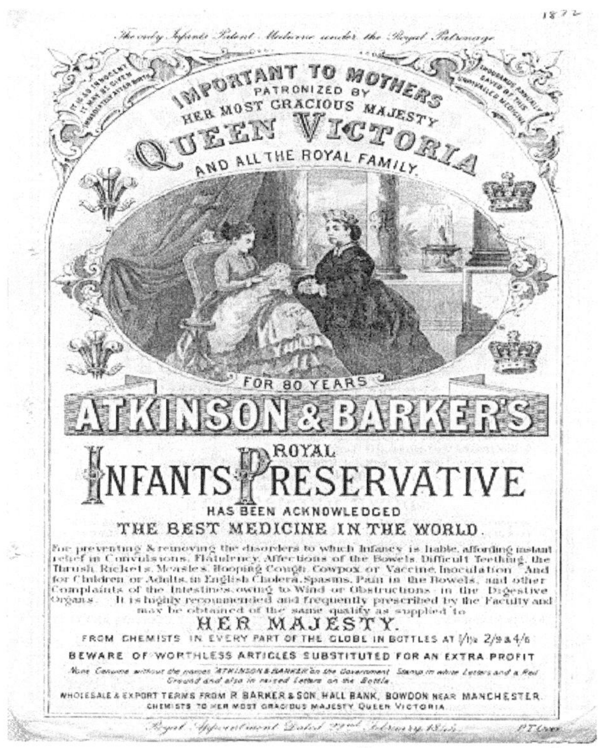

There were hundreds of opium products in the 19th and early 20th century, many brought to market by Victoria's British shipping empire. Opium, more than any other drug, always delivers effects, whether pain relief, anxiety, sleep or euphoria. There has been and will continue to be a market for opiates. Because of this, trade in opiates continues as a major component of criminal behavior. The current war with drug cartels using fentanyl on the Mexican-United States border in some respects, resemble Victoria's Opium Wars.

Aspirin

Aspirin-like drugs were first obtained from several plants. American Indians chewed willow bark for pain relief, fever and used it in poultices. The natural chemical salicin is the active ingredient in willow and other bark and in the mid-19th century chemist working for Bayer discovered a method to enhance its effect by adding an acetyl group. It soon became an important drug known as aspirin, its importance and use continue today. Aspirin has so many effects on the human cell that if it were developed and released today, it would not be an over-the-counter medication. Instead, be tightly controlled and probably cost $20 a dose. Aspirin reduces pain and fever, thins blood by poisoning platelets (this reduces the incidence of heart attacks and strokes), it inhibits parts of inflammation, making it useful in a host of medical problems. Aspirin in daily low dose may prevent heart attacks, strokes, colon cancer and perhaps delay symptoms of Alzheimer's disease. An effective cheap important component of any medicine chest.

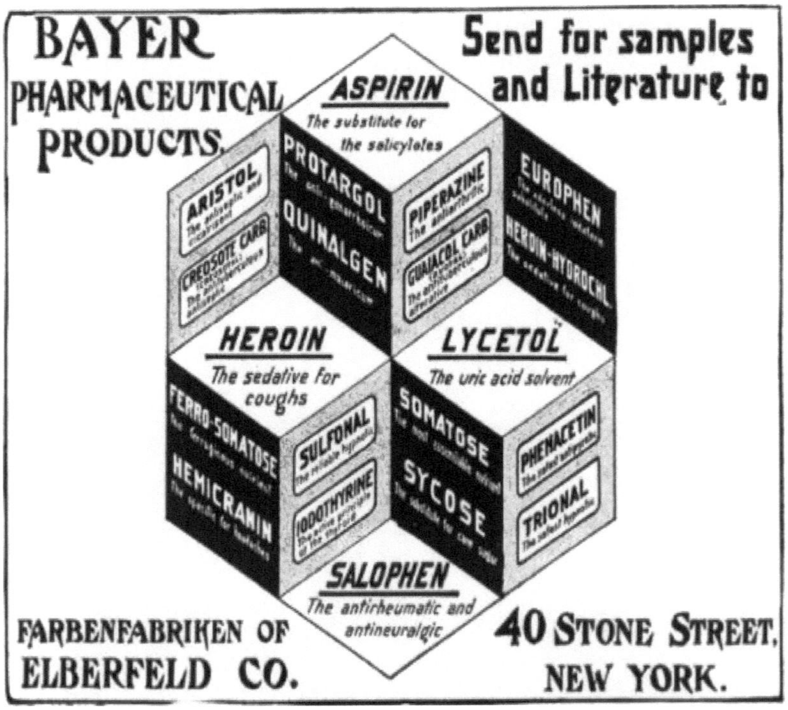

A group of pain relievers were available from Bayer one hundred years ago. In the 1920s, the Merck pharmaceutical company in Germany manufactured and sold 90% of the world's cocaine and heroin. It was legal and a huge source of cash flow for German industry. Phenacetin mixed with Tylenol (acetaminophen) was a common pain reliever until the 1950s. The author's students who served during WWII remembers huge jars of phenacetin and acetaminophen in the ships they served on and dispensed by the handful for headaches and hangovers. Phenacetin was later found to destroy kidneys after a certain dose achieved and no longer available.

One of the primary mechanisms of aspirin and the other anti-inflammatory drugs involves suppression of naturally produced compounds, prostaglandins. Although, this inhibition is beneficial in many painful problems, prostaglandin inhibition also can lead to ulcers in the stomach and small bowel. The corrosive effect of aspirin and other anti-inflammatory drugs is due to prostaglandin inhibition and usually occur in high doses (8-16 tablets a day for) several days, but some people may have stomach upset at lower doses. If indigestion is accompanied by blood in the stools, stop aspirin or other anti-inflammatory drugs and begin an acid blocker to reverse the damage. Prostaglandins come in many shapes and sizes and perform all kinds of services in the body. Kidney function, airway dilation, contractions of labor, fever and inflammation are mediated by prostaglandins. Therefore, many drugs taken for pain may interfere with other cellular activity.

The dose of aspirin required to relieve pain and inflammation is 1-2 tabs (325 mg) every 4-6 hours with food. This is the same dose for fevers over 102 degrees. **Aspirin should not be used in children and young adolescents for any febrile illness**. It is generally believed that aspirin is more useful in preventing heart attacks and strokes than its use for pain. The author had been taking aspirin for arthritic pain, perhaps two per day for four days when he experienced a vomiting episode resulting in a ruptured blood vessel in retina and subsequent eye bleeding. The ophthalmologist on exam reinforced the risk of aspirin effect of bleeding to the author when he stated rather sternly, “you should have known better!”

Low dose aspirin has been proven to lower the risk of stroke and heart attack by reducing the risk of blood clots forming in the blood vessels supplying heart muscle and brain tissue. This dose can be as small as a baby aspirin (81 mg) every other day. Aspirin will increase bleeding in trauma such as head injuries, fractures and lacerations. Surgeons strongly oppose aspirin use just before surgery. It should be used very carefully in people with a history of ulcers. If the author could only have four drugs in a medicine chest, one would be aspirin.

The Non-Steroidal Anti-Inflammatory Drugs (NSAIDS)

This class of drugs is a large one with over twenty members and growing with prostaglandin inhibition as their primary mechanism for pain relief. They are the most prescribed drugs in the world and ones with the most side effects. The first of this class (excluding aspirin) phenylbutazone (Butazolidin) was introduced in 1949 for the treatment of rheumatoid arthritis. It was effective for pain relief but accompanied with serious gastrointestinal bleeding, bone marrow depression, hepatitis and in some cases, death. Newer drugs in this class have proven effective with fewer serious side effects. NASIDs can cause gut bleeding in addition to cardiovascular problems. They should be used for as brief a period as possible with close attention to stomach upset and the possibility of blood in the stool. Use the stool guaiac test for occult (hidden) blood in the stool when using NSAIDS or when symptoms appear such as indigestion or abdominal pain. It is recommended to monitor blood pressure when using NSAIDs as they are known to increase blood pressure and increase cardiovascular risks.

Some cases of arthritis, gout, chronic headaches and other long-term pain, may require these drugs on an almost daily basis. Daily use of NSAIDs requires monitoring blood pressure, making patient aware that dark stools may indicate bleeding and periodically testing stool with the stool guaiac lab test. The presence of blood in the stool should either discourage continued use or the addition of an acid blocker to protect the stomach lining. The following is a list of most drugs available in this class of pain-relieving medications. These following NSAIDs will reduce pain and fever, however, have no effects on platelets and therefore have no heart attack or stroke protection. In fact, their use increases the risk of hypertension, heart disease and strokes!

A partial list includes: Indomethacin (Indocin), meclofenamate (Meclomen) tolmetin (Tolectin) propionic Acid (Daypro) ibuprofen (Motrin, Nuprin, Advil), naproxen (Naprosyn, Anaprox, Alieve) fenoprofen (Nalfon) flurbiprofen (Ansaid) piroxicam (Feldene) diclofenac (Voltaren) nabumetone (Relafen) ketuprofen (Orudus) etodulac (Lodine)

Antibiotics

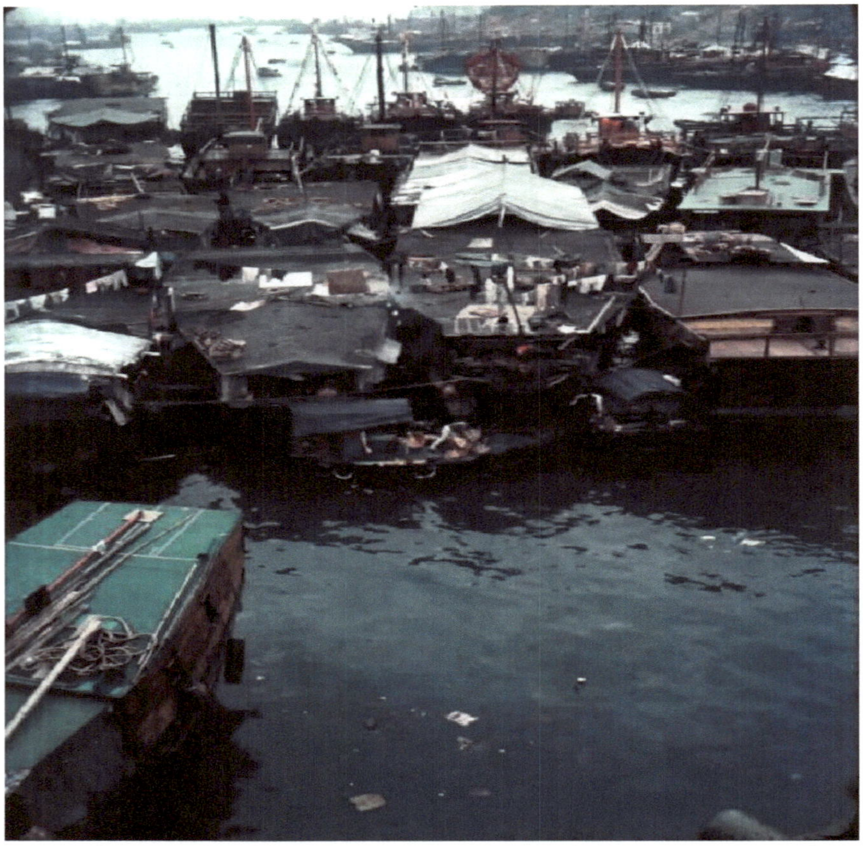

There are plenty of germs in this harbor as there are in many ports and crowded cities around the world. Water contaminated by human waste contains agents capable of causing disease and some are not responsive to antibiotics (like hepatitis). If one were unfortunate to fall into polluted water in the above image, take a long hot bath in medicated soap with brush scrubs, and consider taking a broad-spectrum antibiotic (cephalosporin) for 2-3 doses. Shaking hands with people living in this environment is potentially hazardous. One does not know where that offered hand has been. Photo Gail Hill

Although "germs" had been suspected as causing diseases for centuries, it was not until 1877 that Pasteur recognized that bacteria when placed into animals, multiplied and caused disease. Pasteur's study with anthrax bacteria led to an explosion of research for substances to kill bacteria.

Even though many experiments followed, and several substances were found that killed or limited the growth of bacteria, they could not be used because they were too toxic. Mercury, known to be very toxic, had been in use as an antibiotic drug for centuries. Paul Erlich's Salvarsan, a derivative of another heavy metal, arsenic was a great improvement in treating syphilis over the more toxic mercury, however it was still toxic.

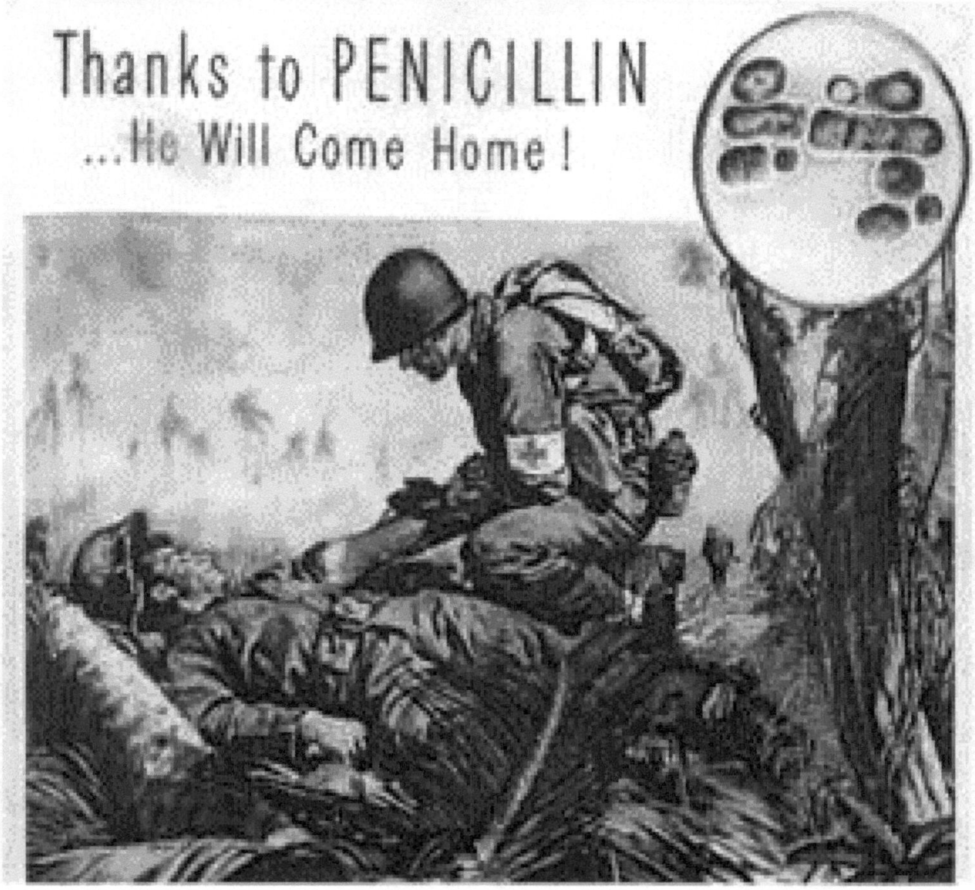

Penicillin was a huge morale booster for Allied soldiers, who knew there was a "wonder drug" available for their wounds. Given in the field and in the operating room, it saved lives and limbs. National Archives

In 1936 sulfa compounds were developed in Nazi Germany that the "age of antibiotics" began. The Germans went on to test sulfa compounds in experiments in large numbers on political prisoners and often Catholic priests that the Gestapo imported from Belgium, Denmark and Holland (where the Germans had difficulty in cowering the Catholics). Early in the war, the Allies used Dr. Fleming's ten-year-old research and mass-produced the first true antibiotic, penicillin. Penicillin was kept secret throughout the war, even though Germany had shared the benefits of sulfa compounds with the world. Before penicillin, wound care had taken a huge leap forward when John Lister proved that washing hands in an antiseptic, carbolic acid greatly reduced infections. However, his recommendation of washing wounds in carbolic acid and other caustic antiseptics caused more harm than good.

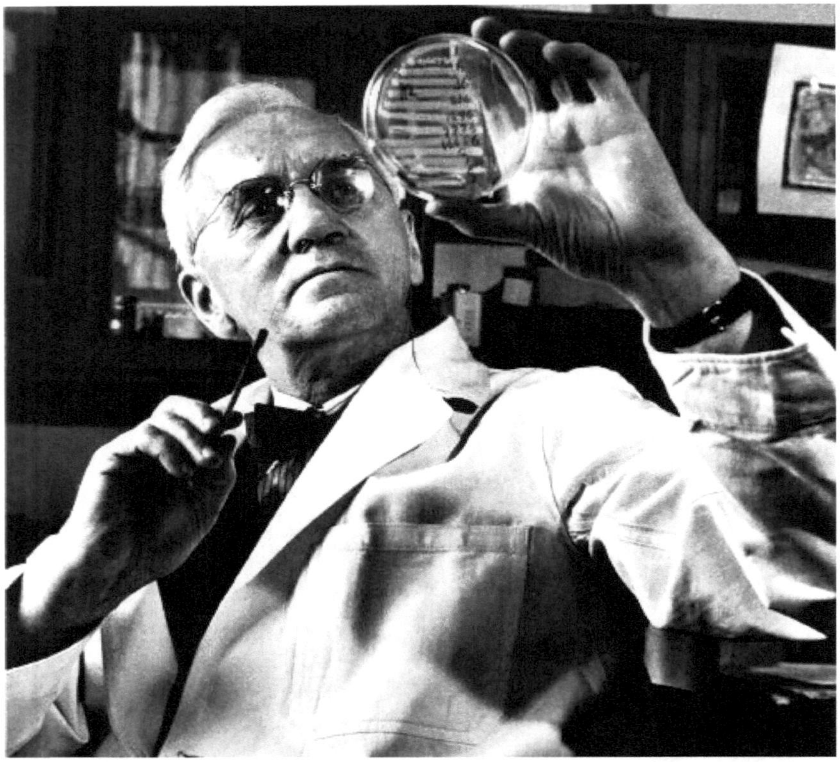

"One sometimes finds what one is not looking for" Alexander Fleming. Prior to service as a medical officer during The Great War, Fleming was captain of his rifle team in college and medical school. Throughout much of World War I, he served close to the front, coming under fire several times and his actions led to his mention in dispatches, something rare for medical officers. During the war, Fleming realized the corrosive antiseptic, carbolic acid Lister recommended on wounds were causing more harm than good, even though most of his fellow medical officers continued to employ them. Not unlike Ambrose Pare, who against common use, gave up the hot iron for soothing dressing in 16th century wounds. National Archives

Penicillin was a drug that was supposedly "accidentally" discovered. The story goes that Fleming, an English bacteria researcher in 1929 noted some cultures of bacteria had become contaminated by fungal colonies. Before discarding these cultures, he noticed a clear area around each colony of fungus. This could only mean that the fungus (penicillium) was producing a substance that either killed bacteria or inhibited its growth. Fleming discovered that fungus had solved a problem human had wrestled with from the beginning of medicine. The concept was first put forth by Pasteur, who noted that life destroys life among the lower species more than among higher animals and plants. This "life against life" defined antibiotics. Hand washing and cleanliness were just as important in managing infections as the discovery of antibiotics. However, its discovery and application has a tragic story. The following story proves what F Scott Fitzgerald said, "Show me a hero and I will write a tragedy.

If you do not like the message, kill the messenger

"Genius can be cruel, and those possessed of it, can be utterly helpless" Henry James

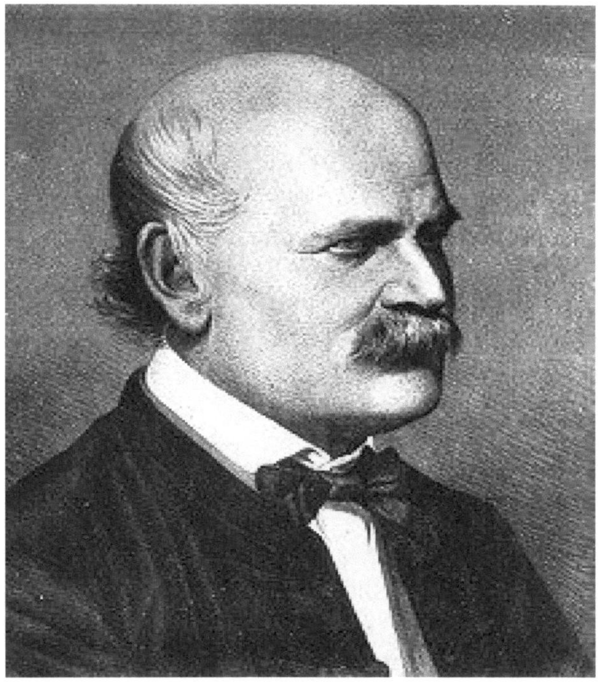

Ignaz Semmelweis, 1818-1865, woodcut by Jeno Doby. A Hungarian of German descent, who proved many things Joseph Lister, knighted by Queen Victoria was credited for later. After completing medical school in Vienna, where he was treated with some contempt by professors and fellow students for his accented German, he desired further training as opposed to primary care in Hungary. The only postgraduate program available to him was the obstetrical department, the least desirable training in Vienna. As a good medical officer, he paid attention and observed that infections following midwife deliveries were much lower than those performed by physicians. Semmelweis "rediscovered" field medicine techniques written thousands of years before in the proverb "cleanliness is next to godliness" about personal hygiene in the Book of Leviticus. Semmelweis recognized physicians coming from the wards and autopsy rooms to the obstetrics hospital where they thrust their unwashed hands into women and handled newborns, were carrying some form of infection. Semmelweis proved the existence of microscopic infections well before Pasteur. In addition to improving cleanliness, he added washing hands in an antiseptic, calcium hypochlorite (Lister used carbolic acid with hand washing and to lavage wounds). Semmelweis reduced mortality from fevers 90% is one study! His important discovery that would have revolutionized medicine was ignored by the medical establishment, further inflaming his belief in personal discrimination. With increasing bitterness in the rebuttal of his work, Semmelweis begins to blame physicians for deaths bordering on accusation of murder! The germ theory was not accepted by the Vienna medical establishment at this time and being called murderers by Semmelweis, did not encourage supporters. Because of his threat to the medical establishment and his increasing angry behavior, he was admitted

to an insane asylum by a colleague, where he was beaten so severely by guards, Dr. Semmelweis died of an infection from these wounds.

The discussion of antibiotics will be divided into four categories. These categories are the invention of the author and mean little outside this discussion. Perhaps one of the most difficult concepts for sea-going personnel has been the deployment of antibiotics and this discussion was developed to ease the confusion. Level I antibiotics are drugs that are used in the oral form and are more effective if the correct drug is matched for the system infected. Level II antibiotics are more powerful and offer a broader range of antibiotic activity in most systems. Level III antibiotics are the most powerful oral form, often as effective as injectable antibiotics and should be reserved for more severe infections. Level IV injectable antibiotics should be also reserved for serious infections when the patient is already ill or unable to take oral medicine. Since diabetics are more likely to develop serious infections quickly, they may receive more aggressive antibiotic therapy. Level III and Level IV antibiotics should be used in pneumonia, meningitis, peritonitis, kidney infection, or when the patient is deteriorating oral antibiotics. Deterioration manifested by rising fever, decreased alertness, increased respiration and heart rate. If the first antibiotic chosen does not improve conditions, then add a second antibiotic, probably an injectable, while continuing the first.

If the person worsens, it is not always necessary to stop the first antibiotic unless the patient has an allergic reaction, such as an itching rash, hives or gastrointestinal upset (erythromycin often causes mild gastrointestinal discomfort). Begin a second antibiotic and continue the first or consider an antibiotic by injection. The most powerful combination of antibiotics would be level III and the injectable level IV together in severe infections. This combination should be used in life-threatening infections mentioned above such as pneumonia, kidney infection, cellulitis, meningitis and abdominal rebound, especially when these are accompanied with high fever.

Level I Antibiotics

Penicillin, the first true "life against life" antibiotic, is still useful in many forms, ampicillin, amoxicillin, ticarcillin, Augmentin (methicillin and cloxacillin are powerful non-level I antibiotics) and others. As a rule, any drug ending with "illin" is a penicillin, even though other forms of penicillin, especially brand names, may not contain that suffix. Penicillin is the only antibiotic that will last ten days with a single injection. However, injectable penicillin is potentially dangerous, and may cause severe allergic reactions, even anaphylactic shock and death. In the oral form, penicillin allergy is unlikely to precipitate shock but may cause hives or itchy rash. If a penicillin reaction is suspected, immediately stop the medication, give Benadryl (diphenhydramine) 25-50 mgs and change to a different antibiotic. Injectable penicillin is too dangerous to administer in the field.

The author believes the best form of penicillin in the field is amoxicillin. It is well tolerated, only needs to be given every eight hours, as opposed to every six for plain penicillin, and is generally more potent in fighting infection than penicillin. Amoxicillin is effective in the upper respiratory tract, such as ears, sinuses, and dental. It works very well in the urinary tract, since the kidneys remove any penicillin as soon as the drug passes through the nephrons, concentrating it in the urine. This makes penicillin effective if the suspected infection is within the urinary tract.

Amoxicillin will work in the skin in treating and preventing wound infection, but other antibiotics (erythromycins) are likely more effective. The dose is 125 mgs three times a day in small children, 250 mgs for small adults and large children and 500mgs in most adults. Other Level I drugs are erythromycin (best in skin and lungs) and doxycycline (best in sexually transmitted infections as well as skin, respiratory tract and gut). Azithromax is a type of erythromycin that is especially useful in respiratory infections. It is the author's favorite antibiotic. Three doses, one each day, stays around for 10-14 days and is as powerful as Level II and III antibiotics.

Level II Antibiotics

Level II antibiotics are more powerful and may work in more systems (broader spectrum) than Level I antibiotics. They are used in more severe infections, where wounds more likely to become infected (burns, deep puncture wounds, bites, or in a diabetic) or when level I antibiotics have been less effective in previous infections. The major group of drugs in Level II are the cephalosporin drugs. These antibiotics include cephalexin, ceftriaxone, cefixime and others, usually beginning with "cef". These drugs are safe, well tolerated with few side effects and are useful in children. They are effective in the skin (wounds), respiratory tract (pneumonia), gastrointestinal tract (appendicitis) or for a fever of unknown origin. The dose is 125 mgs twice daily for children, 250 mgs. twice daily for small adults (under 125lbs.) and 500 mg twice daily in average sized adults. Since these are stronger antibiotics, try to limit use to five to seven days, sooner if the patient's symptoms are resolved. Sulfa combination antibiotics are Level II because they are effective in many infections and are somewhat more powerful than amoxicillin and erythromycin. Sulfa drugs do have high side effects and should be reserved for more serious infections or when the infection is in the urinary tract. As they are the drug of choice in bladder infections.

Level III Antibiotics

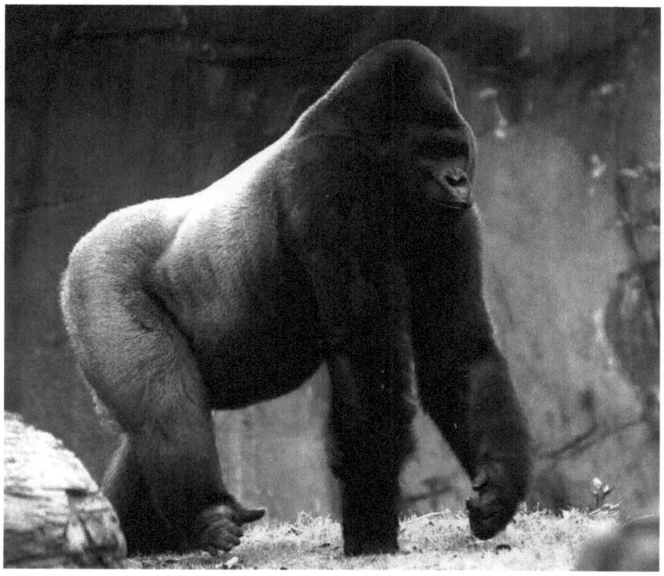

Five-hundred-pound male gorilla in Mexico City who later died of a heart attack when sedated for breeding (sex can be dangerous). In the field, Level III antibiotics are powerful

oral antibiotics effective for dysentery, wound infection and serious other infections. These powerful antibiotics have been labelled by the author "as the gorillas of oral antibiotics". Photo credit, Henry Romero/Reuters

These drugs are powerful oral antibiotics and should be reserved for severe infections such as pneumonia, cellulitis, deep infections or when patient has underlying medical problems. The major class of drugs in this level is the quinolones, which include ciprofloxin (Cipro), ofloxacin (Floxin), lomefloxacin (Maxaquin), levofloxacin (Levaquin). These antibiotics are well absorbed from the gut and because they penetrate tissue well, can be used for shorter treatment courses, 2-5 days. Quinolones work at the DNA level, interfering with the ability of the bacteria to replicate. These drugs should not be used in children or in adolescents, as they may damage still-forming joints. Quinones, especially cipro have been implicated in serious side effects and should be used when their power is necessity. The dose is 250-500 mg every 12 hours. The author prefers levofloxacin for use in the field.

Level IV Antibiotics

With the introduction of injectable penicillin in the 1940s, the course of serious infections was changed forever. No longer would wound infections, pneumonia and a host of other diseases so easily claim victims. However, it soon became apparent that there were many infections where penicillin was only partially effective or totally ineffective. In addition, bacteria quickly adapted to the mechanism of penicillin's action, requiring new, stronger antibiotics. Penicillin is still a valuable drug in its oral form, but has little if any use, as an injectable in the field. Not only are penicillin injections less effective than other antibiotics, but they are also more dangerous. Probably more people have died from penicillin injections (because of severe allergic reaction) than any other antibiotic in the past. If penicillin is injected, the patient must remain under direct observation for at least 20 minutes, and a syringe of epinephrine should be close at hand.

The class of antibiotics known as cephalosporins is the preferred class of injectable antibiotics to use in the field. They are powerful and at the same time safe for use in adults as well as children in the face of severe infections, even when the source or site of infection is not known. Cephalosporins have broad coverage, killing bacteria in skin and soft tissue (cellulitis), respiratory tract (especially pneumonias), urinary tract, nervous system (meningitis) and where the patient is worsening on a lesser antibiotic. These drugs are effective in preventing infections in burns, penetrating wounds and lacerations.

Cephalosporins have gone through generations of development and there are several injectable forms. It is in the second and third generation of these drugs, where the recommended injectable antibiotics reside. Two of these, cefuroxime (Zinacef) and cefotaxime (Claforan) will be discussed. These injectable antibiotics are carried as a powder, only mixed just prior to use. They have long shelf lives, are two of the most powerful antibiotics available and are safe. Cefotaxime is a third-generation drug that has enhanced activity against some bacteria due to its unique metabolism or breakdown in the body. The metabolism of most antibiotics renders bacteria less active or ineffective as their structure is changed and they are more efficiently destroyed. In cefotaxime's case, after the drug is metabolized, it is converted to another active cephalosporin. Therefore, injecting cefotaxime is like giving two drugs, increasing the time the active drug remains in the body, killing bacteria.

Cardiovascular Drugs

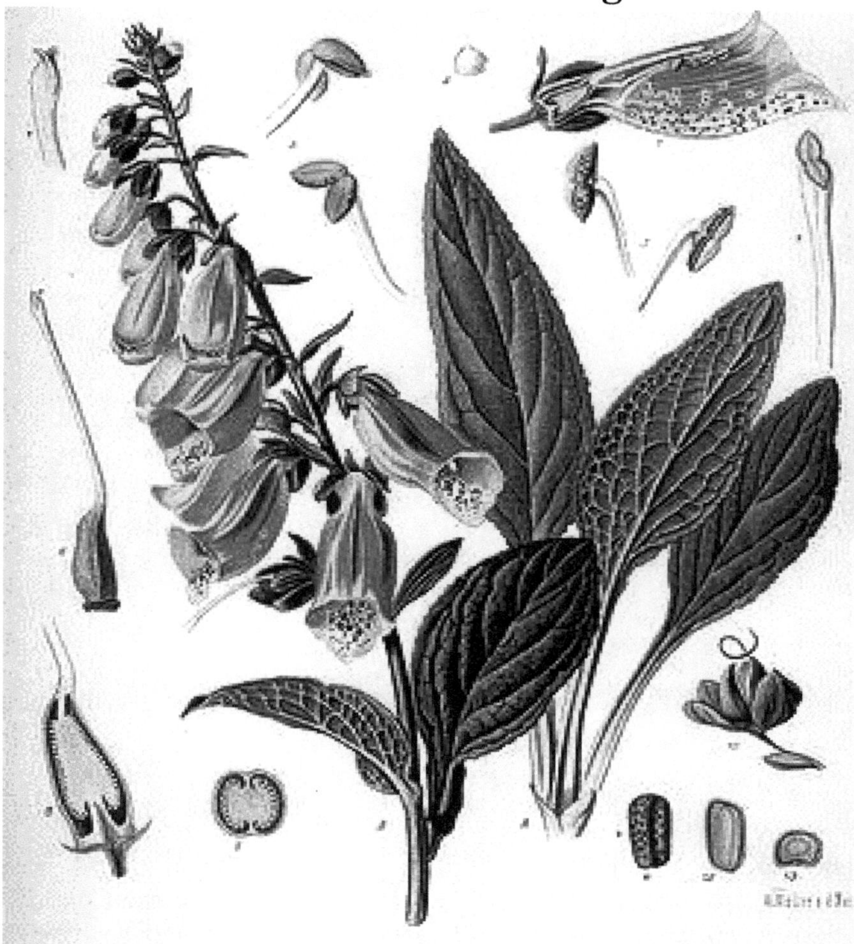

19th century drawing of digitalis, a member of the popular deadly nightshade family of plants. William Withering gets most of the credit for introducing digitalis as a treatment for dropsy, later called congestive heart failure. The Greeks and later Romans included this plant as herbal tonic and Hitler's physician was injecting him with it. Digitalis grows wild in most of the world and has been used as a poison in several cultures.

Many cardiovascular drugs are plant-based and the synthetic pharmaceuticals often mimic natural chemicals. Nitroglycerin, Beta blockers and Calcium channel blockers, ACE inhibitors and aspirin are common drugs acting directly, or indirectly on the heart and vessels. Drugs will be discussed by class, listing generic and brand name (Proprietary), uses and side effects. Doses are simple, in most cases one pill each 24-hour period unless otherwise noted. Cardiovascular drugs developed in the past generation has extended and saved lives. They should be part of any medicine chest.

Cardiac Glycosides – Digitalis

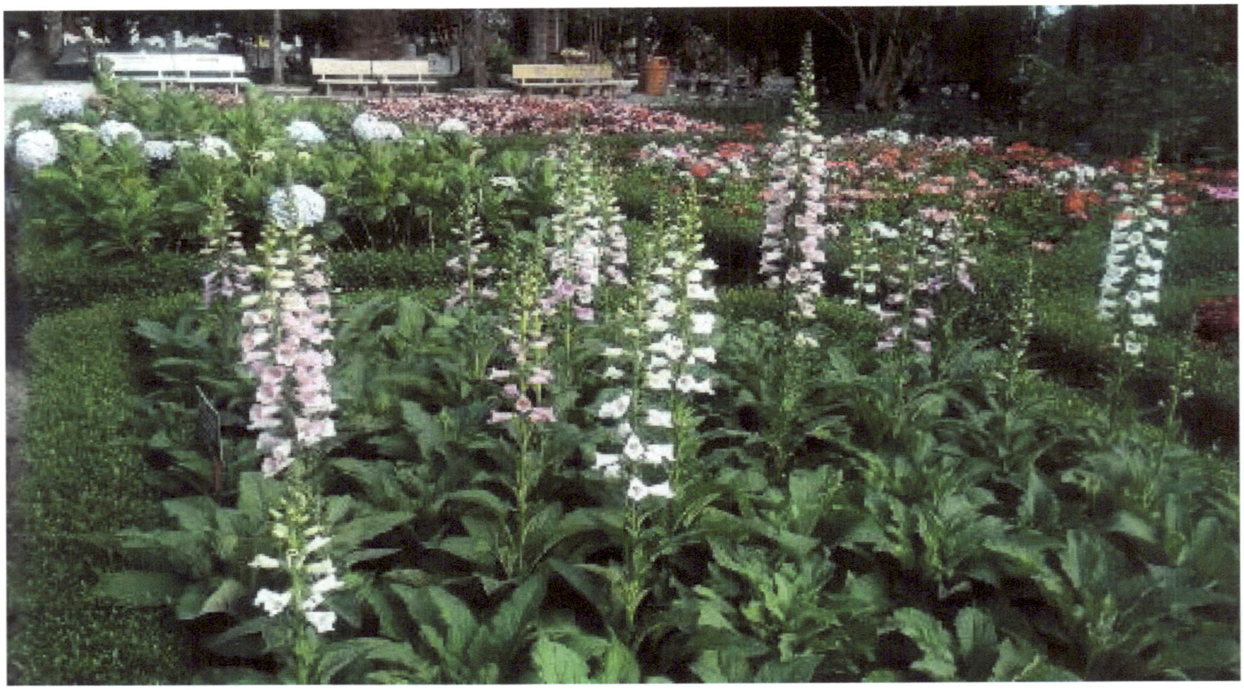

Digitalis growing in the central highlands of Viet Nam when the author visited on the 50th anniversary of the First Tet Offensive, January 31, 2018

The oldest currently used heart medication is digitalis (Lanoxin or Digoxin). This drug has been derived from several plants and venom of certain toads. Known to the Egyptians as squill and later used by Greek physicians as a diuretic, heart tonic, emetic and even a rat poison. In Medieval Europe, digitalis was used as human poison, as it was easy to administer and worked slowly, mimicking a gradual demise of the victim. Dried common toad skin was used by the Chinese for centuries. In the later 18th century, William Withering, an English physician, published his famous book showing the beneficial effect of digitalis on dropsy (congestive heart failure). During much of the author's practice, digitalis was the primary treatment of congestive heart disease and many pulse irregularities (arrythmias). Although digitalis in the form of Lanoxin (digoxin) is still used, its use is declining. In congestive heart failure and arrythmias, digitalis is being replaced by safer, more effective drugs such as ACE inhibitors and ARB blockers. It may be encountered in the hands of patients but has no place in a medicine chest. A side about the above photo: the author was in the southern central highlands of Viet Nam on January 31, 2018, on the 50th anniversary of the 1968 Tet offensive. As a senior in high school in 1968, the Tet Offensive was a big deal for young males as the need for combat soldiers escalated. Not a single Vietnamese that the author met knew the significance of that offensive. For them it was celebration of flowers including digitalis and not a battle that changed America in 1968 with unrest riots against the Viet Nam War.

Nitroglycerin

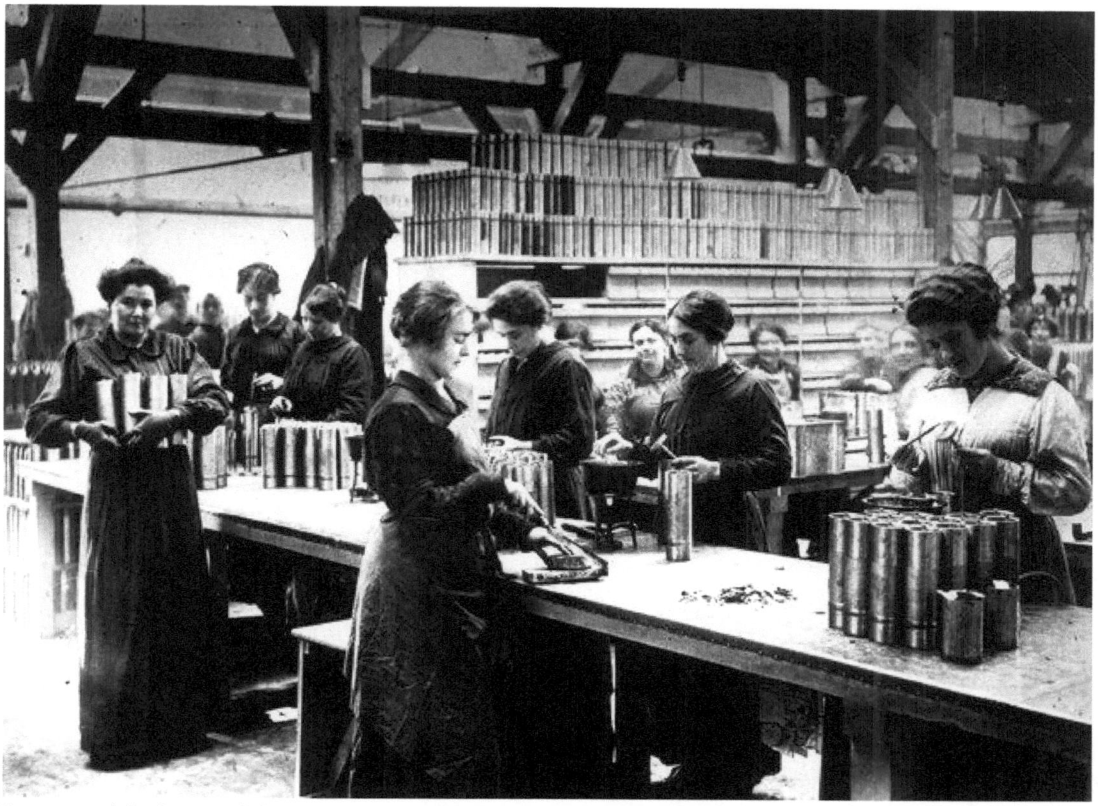

Females provided munitions workers in Paris during World War I as most of the men were in uniform. Many of these women developed short term headaches from nitroglycerin and life-long illness associated with the phosphorus and sulfur associated with making explosives. French National Archives

Nitroglycerin has been in continuous use for 100 years in management of chest pain. It was known as a vessel dilator, causing headaches in munition workers lasting all week and receding on non-working weekends. It was believed that the mechanism of action of nitroglycerin in relieving the chest pain of angina was due to its ability to widen the heart's arteries, improving blood to heart muscle. Although nitroglycerin causes vessel dilation, it does not reduce angina primarily by dilating the coronary arteries, since these vessels are stiff and blocked by hard cholesterol-filled scar tissue, more resembling an iron pipe as opposed to a flexible hose. Nitroglycerin reduces the heart's oxygen consumption by dilating large blood storage veins in the abdomen, thus reducing blood return to the heart. Less blood to pump, means a decreased workload on the heart, reducing the tension in the wall of heart muscle. These mechanisms reduce the amount of oxygen needed by the heart and is important in protecting heart muscle. By reducing workload, nitroglycerin relieves the discomfort of heart laboring under the pain of angina or heart attack. Chest pain of non-cardiac cause will not be affected by nitroglycerin and is safe to administer in the field in chest pain. The worst thing that could happen is a headache.

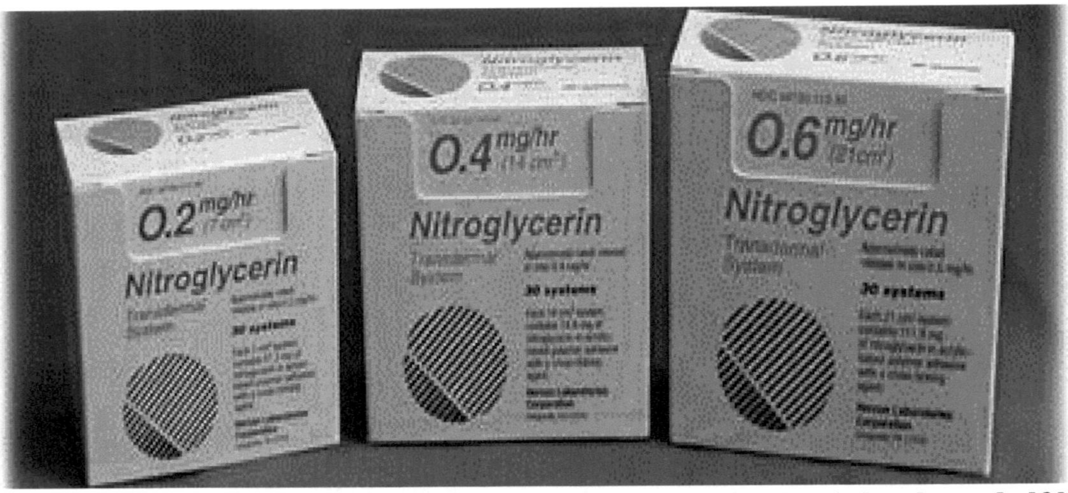

The transdermal patch of nitroglycerin is excellent in the field as it has long shelf life, is easy to apply and gives a steady continuous dose of drug for 24 hours

Nitroglycerin is effective in many forms, pills dissolving under tongue, ointments smeared over the chest wall, rapid-acting mouth sprays and in a long-acting nitroglycerin patch. The preferred method in the field is probably a patch placed over the heart which gives effective nitroglycerin levels within minutes, lasting for 24 hours. It comes in three strengths, .2 mg/hour for small adults under 150 lbs. and in .4 mg/hour for larger patients and .6mg/hour for large patients or with those needing a higher dose to relieve angina. Nitroglycerin used continuously for more than three days quickly becomes less effective unless the patient has a drug-free interval. The patch is usually worn during waking hours and removed for sleep, especially with headaches. By withdrawing nitroglycerin for a few hours or a day, it becomes more effective than when used continuously. Nitroglycerin in pill form is less effective, if at all for angina.

Beta Blockers

Beta blockers are a large class of medications used for angina, arrythmias, heart attack, hypertension, migraine headaches, glaucoma and mild tremors. They have been proven to decrease both death and disability in heart disease, especially sudden death. The mechanism of action of this group of drugs is blockage of a naturally released hormone, adrenalin or epinephrine. Propranolol (Inderal) was one of the first Beta blocker and had a major effect on preventing death after heart attack. Side effects include possible fatigue, decreased size and frequency of erections in males, worsening of asthma and emphysema, while may cause mild depression. Serious side effects are rare unless given with already low blood pressure and low heart rate. Monitor blood pressure and pulse when administering beta blocker.

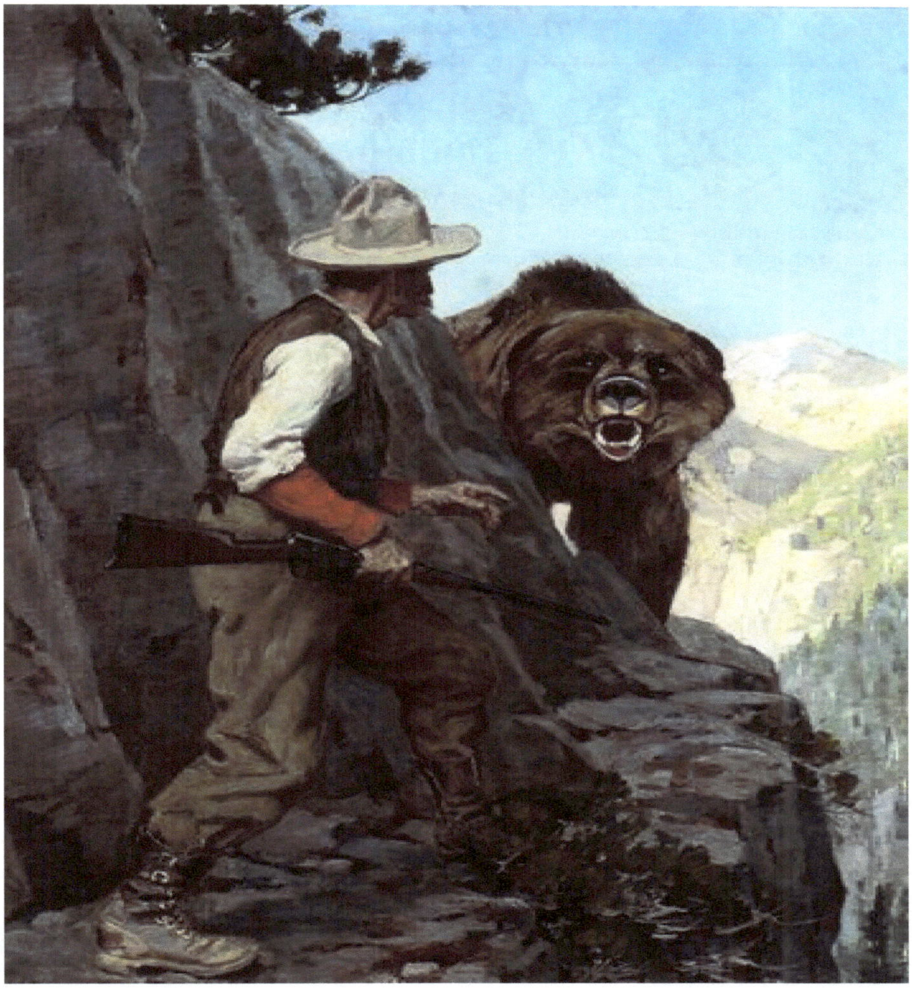

“Right of Way” by Philip Goodwin depicting a moment when both mammals would be releasing large amounts of catecholamines (adrenalin) in preparation to “fight or flight”. During and after a heart attack, these catecholamines can kill, by overstimulating an already struggling heart.

These are useful, perhaps lifesaving chest pain caused by angina or heart attack. By blocking the adrenalin released in pain and anxiety of the chest pain, beta blockers give the heart protection from its own defense. In acute stressful situations, the release of adrenalin and its sudden response is there for survival. In chest pain caused by heart disease, it can be a killer. If chest pain and elevated blood pressure persist, double doses of beta blockers may be necessary. It is important to prevent chest pain from returning when heart disease is suspected, since even intermittent episodes of chest pain can cause heart muscle damage. Atenolol or metoprolol are the beta blockers of choice in the field. There are other beta blockers available worldwide, most end with an “ol” indicating a well absorbed alcohol. These are safe drugs to administer in the field for chest pain, high blood pressure and rapid pulses. By slowing pulse and blunting the “fight or flight” response to stress, these drugs have found their way into athletics. In events of marksmanship (archery, rifle) where there is more time between heart beats to pull trigger or release an arrow, performance is enhanced. Finding beta blockers in urine testing will lead to disqualifying in these events. Professional golfers are using them to reduce the possible adrenalin surge with shots. **Do not use beta blockers in the presence of low blood pressure or pulse.**

ACE Inhibitors

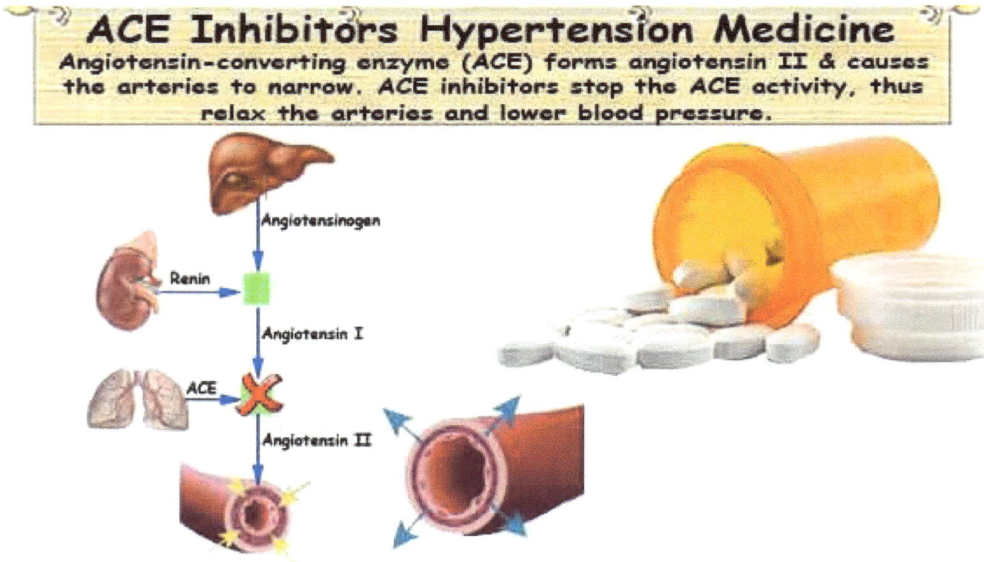

A commercial ad sketching the believed pathway and mechanisms of action of ACE blocking a naturally occurring chemical that can complicate high blood pressure.

This group of drugs, like the beta blockers are recent additions, becoming available in the 1980s. Angiotensin converting enzyme blockers have saved lives, extended lifespans, and improved the quality of life in many patients with heart disease. They are safe with few if any serious side effects. Common side effects include a dry persistent cough, rash and temporary loss of taste. The mechanism through which drugs such as quinapril, ramipril, lisinopril and others effect the cardiovascular by blocking an enzyme released by the kidney. A hormone, renin, was discovered in 1898 when this powerful "pressor" was extracted from a fresh kidney and injected into animals by researchers and is believed to be a major player in heart disease. Angiotensin I released by the kidneys is converted into a much more active compound, Angiotensin II by an enzyme. The Angiotensin Converting Enzyme (ACE) can be blocked by inhibiting drugs, thus ACE inhibitors. By reducing the pressure within arteries and the smaller more numerous arterioles, the vessels relax and dilate, increasing blood flow with less resistance. This in turn reduces workload on the heart while enhancing blood flow to vital organs. Most ACE inhibitors end in “pril”.

Studies show that ACE inhibitors protect heart muscle during the periods of reduced blood flow in angina and heart attack. Therefore, in suspected heart attack or angina, give an ACE inhibitor unless the blood pressure is lower than 100/60. Newer and improved angiotensin manipulating drugs are the angiotensin receptor blockers (ARBs), ending in “sartan” and include candesartan, azilsartan, valsartan, telmisartan and others. Doses vary and generally start with the lower dose and work higher to reduce blood pressure without side effects. These drugs are used in diabetes to slow and reduce kidney damage associated with diabetes. For the same reasons, using these drugs to control blood pressure, should help normal renal tissue live longer.

Calcium Channel Blockers

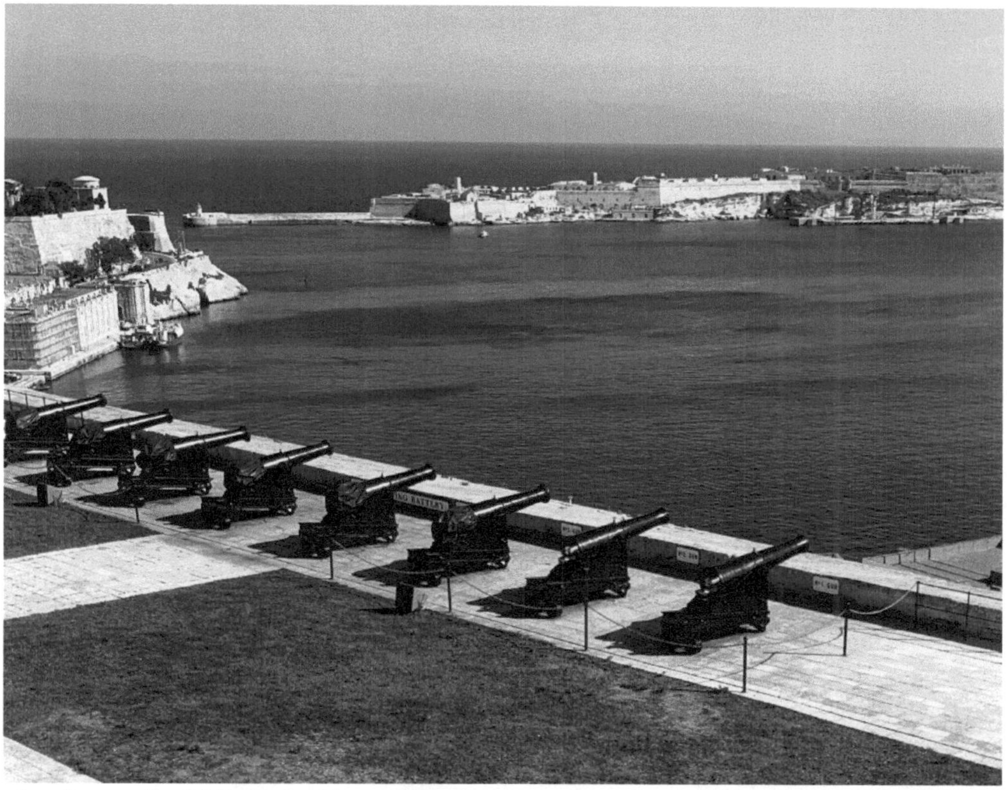

The main channel of Malta's Great Harbor was protected by cannon and blocked by a huge chain. Each two-foot link was forged in the arsenal in Venice at enormous expense. The Knights of Malta could not allow the Turkish fleet to occupy this harbor and blocking the channel into the Grand Harbor saved Malta in 1565 from the Turks. Photo by author

These drugs are used in hypertension, angina, arrhythmias and heart attack. They were studied along with another calcium channel blocker, the puffer fish poison, tetrodotoxin. By blocking calcium channels, blood vessels dilate, increasing blood flow to heart muscle. Decreased transport of calcium across membranes also reduces the irritability of the heart's electrical system, decreasing the likelihood of electrical disturbances such as arrhythmias. Perhaps most importantly, with less calcium crossing into heart muscle cells, the less the force of contraction and less risk of muscle damage. Calcium channel blockers have been proven useful in reducing the risk of a fatal heart attack and are also useful in controlling blood pressure. They should not be used if a person has low blood pressure, since the pressure could decrease further. Nifedipine, Verapamil, Diltiazem are three of the most used.

Lasix (furosemide) is a diuretic often used in heart disease by reducing circulating fluid and third space fluids that accumulate in the lungs and lower legs in heart failure. Remember to give potassium (K+) in the form of a pill (20-40 mgs.) or a glass of fruit juice with each dose of Lasix. Lasix should increase urine flow, improve breathing and decrease swelling in the legs. Lasix can be given several times a day since it has a short half-life.

Hytrin (Terazosin) is a drug that in addition to blood pressure lowering, has a useful side effect. While lowering blood pressure, it reduces the size of an enlarged prostate that may be blocking the outflow of urine as it transverses the core of the prostate. Decreased urination, "dribbling", urinary frequency, getting up several times each night and reduced urine stream are signs of a swollen prostate. Hytrin will lower blood pressure while relieving obstruction within the urinary tract.

Eye Drugs

Because the eye is composed of skin, respiratory tract tissue and very special nerve tissue several classes of drugs are used. Injury, infection and elevated pressure may cause eye problems requiring treatment in the field. Medicine chests should have a separate kit for eye care, containing equipment and drugs for treating complaints involving the eyes. Although a tiny part of the exposed body, the eye may account for a large amount of care in the field.

Topical eye antibiotics are necessary components of all medicine chests since eye infection and trauma are possible. A sensation of "something in the eye" is due to either a foreign body or a scratch over the eyeball. In superficial injuries to the eye, antibiotics should be placed early to prevent infection. Eye antibiotics are useful in conjunctivitis (pink eye) and post trauma. Sulfa or neomycin can cause irritation in many people; therefore, the author recommends gentamycin or erythromycin in an irritated eye. Ointments will stay in the eye longer, giving better antibiotic levels. Solutions, though easier to use, are quickly flushed out of the eye. Use ointments two to three times daily, apply solution three to five times a day.

Steroid eye drops are effective in reducing eye irritation; however, they may not be safe in the hands of non-physicians. If the eye irritation is caused by herpes, steroid use can lead to a scarred cornea. Steroids in the eye and steroid use in general, is discouraged in the field without good reason.

Eye irritation is common, made worse by wind and bright sunlight. Allergies also cause itching and irritation. Conditions helped with frequent cool wet compresses and gentle eye irrigation. Eye lubricants will usually decrease irritation and drying, while eye decongestants will reduce redness. Antihistamine drops will relieve itching, watering and some redness. These are unlikely to be effective in infections and should eye discharge become thick and creamy, use antibiotics.

Anesthesia are so effective that two drops are usually adequate to completely render the eye insensitive to pain and touch. It also ablates the protective blink reflex, and the eye that has been "put to sleep" must be protected with a patch. Eye anesthesia comes in preparations ending in "caine" (tetracaine). Early in the author's training cocaine was used extensively to examine eyes and vocal cords in the upper airway. These drugs give some twenty minutes of anesthesia, and if severe pain returns (as in a large corneal abrasion), the patch may be lifted, and a single drop placed in the injured eye but do not repeat more than three doses. Anesthesia may inhibit healing and should not be repeatedly instilled. Eye drops containing homatropine give safer long-lasting pain relief. If pain persists after injury, use two drops of homatropine to dilate and relax the pupil. Oral narcotics may also be needed for the deep pain of an eye injury.

Acute Glaucoma

This is a rare condition where the pressure within the anterior chamber of the eyeball increases over a short period of time, causing pain, redness and decreased vision or any vision change. Sudden stagnation and increasing pressure in the tiny, closed space of the eye is acute glaucoma. This serious medical problem is an eye emergency and if untreated, acute glaucoma will blind the eye with pressure destroying the optic nerve. Fortunately, it may be possible to be diagnosed and managed in the field. Acute glaucoma begins with a single painful red eye, pain that increases while the vision worsens. The eyeball becomes hard when compared with the normal eyeball's softness. Eyeball firmness can be measured by gently pressing the finger pad of the index finger over the closed eyelids of both the normal eye and the one suspected of glaucoma. When this diagnosis has been confirmed, the eye pressure can be reduced by instilling two drops of pilocarpine every six to eight hours. Pilocarpine will reduce intraocular pressure within minutes after treatment. Pilocarpine is a natural alkaloid found in shrubs (*pilocarpus*) of South America and a similar compound is in the betel nut, which is consumed as a euphoretic in the East Indies. If acute glaucoma is not recognized and treated properly, the eye will be lost. The more common chronic glaucoma is treated with beta blocker eye drops.

Eye Drugs

The eye is composed of skin, respiratory tract tissue and very special nerve tissue. Injury, infection and elevated pressure may cause eye problems requiring treatment in the field. Medicine chests should have a separate kit for eye care, containing equipment and drugs for treating complaints involving the eyes. Although a tiny part of the total exposed body, the eye may account for a large amount of care in the field.

Topical eye antibiotics are necessary components of all medicine chests since eye infection and trauma are possible. A sensation of "something in the eye" is due to either a foreign body or a scratch over the eyeball. In superficial injuries to the eye, antibiotics should be placed early to prevent infection. Eye antibiotics are useful in conjunctivitis (pink eye) and post trauma. Sulfa or neomycin can cause irritation in many people; therefore, the author recommends gentamycin or erythromycin in an irritated eye. Ointments will stay in the eye longer, giving better antibiotic levels. Solutions, though easier to use, are quickly flushed out of the eye. Use ointments two to three times daily, apply solution three to five times a day.

Steroid eye drops are effective in reducing eye irritation; however, they may not be safe in the hands of non-physicians. If the eye irritation is caused by herpes, steroid use can lead to a scarred cornea. Steroids in the eye and steroid use in general, is discouraged in the field without good reason.

Eye irritation is common, made worse by wind and bright sunlight. Allergies also cause itching and irritation. Conditions helped with frequent cool wet compresses and gentle eye irrigation. Eye lubricants will usually decrease irritation and drying, while eye decongestants will reduce redness. Antihistamine drops will relieve itching, watering and some redness. These are unlikely to be effective in infections and should eye discharge become thick and creamy, use antibiotics.

Anesthesia works very well in the eye. Two drops are usually adequate to completely render the eye insensitive to pain and touch. It also ablates the protective blink reflex, and the eye that has been "put to sleep" must be protected with a patch. Eye anesthesia comes in preparations ending in "caine" (tetracaine). Cocaine was used extensively in the past in the eye and the upper airway. These drugs give some twenty minutes of anesthesia, and if severe pain returns (as in a large corneal abrasion), the patch may be lifted, and a single drop placed in the injured eye. Anesthesia may inhibit healing and should not be repeatedly instilled. Eye drops containing homatropine gives safer long-lasting pain relief. If pain persist after injury, use two drops of homatropine to dilate and relax the pupil. Oral narcotics may also be needed for the deep pain of an eye injury.

Acute Glaucoma

This is a rare condition where the pressure within the anterior chamber of the eyeball increases over a short period of time, causing pain, redness and decreased vision or any vision change. Sudden stagnation and increasing pressure in the tiny, closed space of the eye is acute glaucoma. This serious medical problem is an eye emergency and if untreated, acute glaucoma will blind the eye with pressure destroying the optic nerve. Fortunately, it may be possible to be diagnosed and managed in the field. Acute glaucoma begins with a single painful red eye, pain that increases while the vision worsens. The eyeball becomes hard when compared with the normal eyeball's softness. Eyeball firmness can be measured by gently pressing the finger pad of the index finger over the closed eyelids of both the normal eye and the one suspected of glaucoma. When this diagnosis has been confirmed, the eye pressure can be reduced by instilling two drops of pilocarpine every six to eight hours. Pilocarpine will reduce intraocular pressure within a few minutes after treatment. Pilocarpine is a natural alkaloid found in shrubs (*pilocarpus*) of South America and a similar compound is in the betel nut, which is consumed as a euphoretic in the East Indies. If a*cute glaucoma is not recognized and treated properly, the eye will be lost. The more common chronic glaucoma is treated with beta blocker eye drops.

Gastrointestinal Drugs

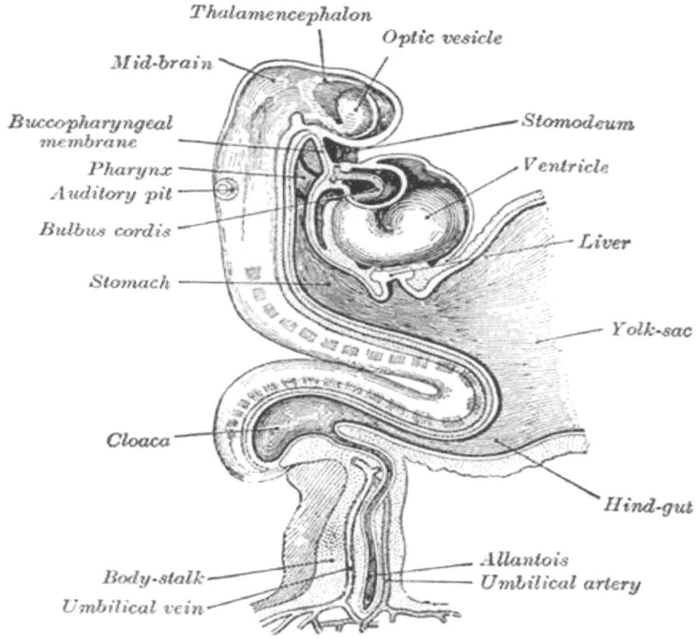

The 15-day old human embryo and the person's early gastrointestinal tract. Henry Vandyke Carter, Grey's Anatomy, 1918

The gut is a large organ, with many side passages and supporting organs. Most drugs use the gut to gain access to the body, since most medications are given orally. There are many drugs that affect the gut, and only a few will be covered in this section. These medications primarily reduce or neutralize stomach acid, reduce or enhance bowel motility (constipation, diarrhea), and antibiotics directed at gut infections.

Stomach acid is present for an important function of digestion and part of the body's barrier to invasion. However, it can cause medical problems such as heartburn (reflux), bleeding and ulcers. Under normal conditions, the stomach is protected from its own acid by secreting a thick coat of mucus. This mucus barrier separates the sensitive stomach lining (mucosa) from the corrosive acid. When this mucus barrier is breached, hydrochloric acid may devour stomach lining, leading to ulcers. Drugs and agents can disturb the delicate balance between stomach acid and its mucus barrier. Stress, alcohol and nicotine will damage the mucus barrier, leading to ulcer formation. Most ulcers do not occur in the stomach however, but in the first part of the small intestine, the duodenum.

Antacids

Most over-the-counter drugs for gastrointestinal problems are in this class of drugs including salts of calcium (Tums), aluminum (Maalox), and magnesium (Milk of Mag). These metal-based drugs work by neutralizing stomach acid, not blocking it. They are effective but must be used frequently, perhaps every hour to be effective in neutralizing acid that is produced constantly by the stomach. In mild heartburn, indigestion, belching acid and in abdominal pain caused by excess stomach acid, they can be used with few side effects. It should be remembered that by neutralizing stomach acid, there may be an increased risk of gut acquired infections. Stomach acid is an effective barrier to germs that enter the body through the mouth and lowering this barrier may enhance the survival of bacteria, viruses, and parasites that are ingested unknowingly with meals. Good practice not to use antacids if not needed, especially when traveling and eating in the Third World.

Acid Blockers

Heartburn and belching have been a common complaint of humans even before bad cooking. Few other human complaints have been more common. Some people belched acid burning breath constantly, much to their distress, as well as those around them. Samuel James Tilden, the Democratic candidate in 1876 won the popular vote following Grant's eight-year Presidency, only to have the electoral college vote go to the Republican, Rutherford Hays. Tilden was not pleasant to be around, constantly belching, complaining abdominal pain and was reported to have foul breath and flatus that would fill a room. He and those around him could have benefited from acid blockers. Another suffering from constant foul breath and frequent bowel gas releases was Adolph Hitler. In attempt to control his gastrointestinal complaints, Hitler ate a bland diet consisting primarily of lentil soup and handfuls of herbal supplements supplied by his drug dealer, Dr. Morrel. His generals in later life wrote about how distressing the constant bowel gas expulsions and the foulness of Hitler's breath in small spaces were difficult to bear. None dared to mention his gastrointestinal problems in Hitler's presence.

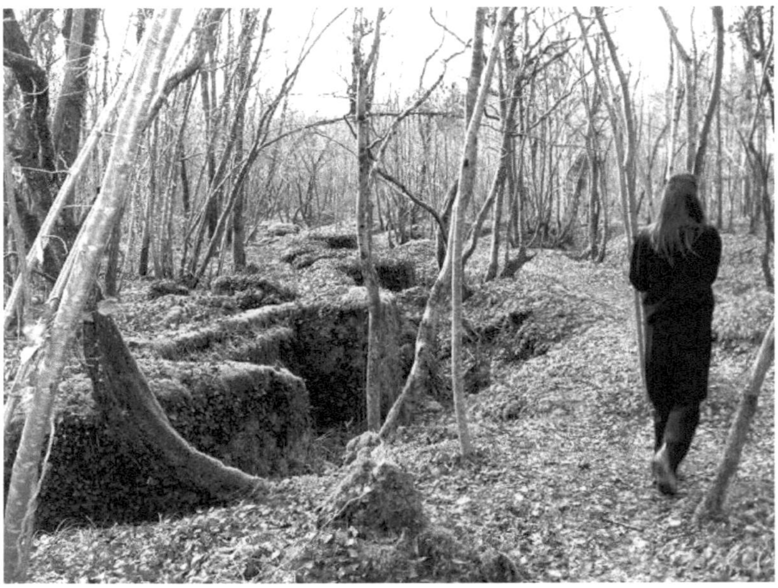

German trenches on the Western Front effectively blocked infantry attacks. Fixed barriers like the above, extended from the Swiss border to the North Sea, 500 miles of trenches opposing each other. These fortifications were three deep facing the enemy providing defense in depth. Just as trenches block attacks, acid blockers are effective in relieving as much human suffering as any class of drugs. Gastric acid is a normal and important component of a healthy gut, breaking down food and presents a hostile environment designed to destroy invaders. When there is too much acid or when the fragile stomach

lining is compromised, acid may become corrosive and in some cases prey upon its own tissue doing so in many patients. Prior to the development of acid blockers, surgery resecting (removing) part or all the stomach and proximal part of the small intestine, were being performed at thousands of hospitals every day. Surgeries are now rarely performed since acid injury to the stomach is reduced with medications. Photo by author

These drugs are particularly important medications to have in a medicine chest representing one of the most effective and safest class of drugs available. Few classes of drugs have relieved as much suffering in the past 100 years. Tagamet (cimetidine) was the first drug of this class and continues to be the used worldwide. The name Tagamet is the same in every country regardless of spoken language, making it easily recognized. Nizatidine, ranitidine, famotidine, omeprazole and a similar compound, Carafate (sucralfate) have all enjoyed success. Carafate is a not true drug as it effects through a mechanical mechanism and its effectiveness, unlike the others is not reduced in cigarette smokers. The newest and most effective acid blockers are the proton pump inhibitors, PPIs. The drugs in this class end in "prazole" and include esomeprazole, dexlansopraole, omeprazole, pantoprazole. These are once daily, usually 30 minutes before meals. The author recommends the PPI medications above others for control of acid complaints. Chronic reflux has been implicated in esophageal cancer, a very bad actor and probably preventable. Three of students in the author's first Medicine at Sea seminar in 1983 were three men who used antacid tabs regularly and all three died of esophageal cancer.

Drugs that affect Bowel Motility

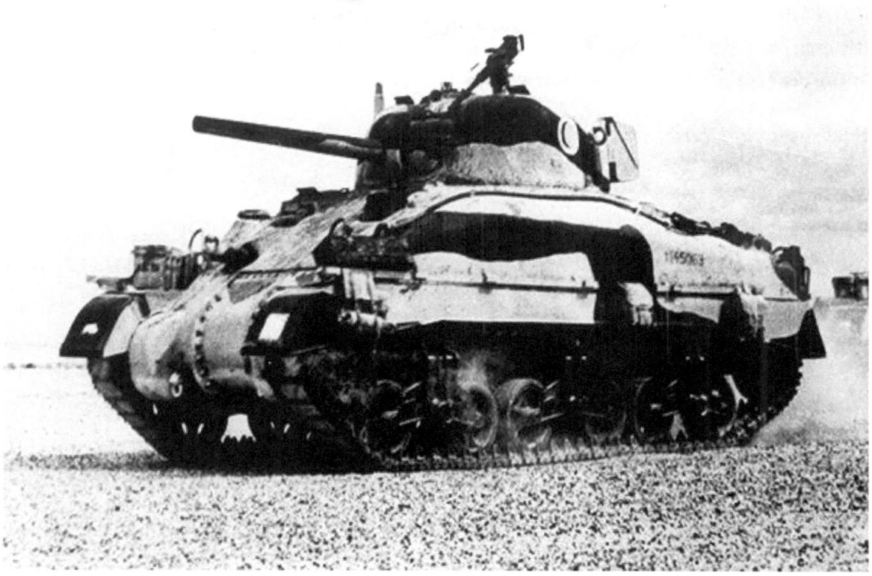

The American built medium M4 tank, better known as the" Sherman" pictured fighting with British crew in North Africa. Even though the British invented the tank during the Great War, they experienced difficulty in fielding an effective tank in WWII. American tanks arrived in Egypt ready for combat whereas the British tanks were ill-prepared for

the ocean trip and required maintenance before deployed and less effective. The Sherman carried a 75mm (3 inch) rifled cannon, multiple .50 caliber machine guns, sloped armor, was faster than most enemy tanks in the Second World War and carried a turret that hydraulically rotated. Most World War II tank's turrets were manually rotated which were slower in combat while the M4 in addition to its quicker turning cannon had motility, power and made in great numbers, overwhelming the enemy. The human immune system also fields a force of mobile armored killers produced in great numbers. The Sherman tank's major drawback was its gasoline-powered engine, much more flammable than a diesel. The United States produced many more gasoline engines prior to the War, and they were cheaper to produce than the diesel. Like the T-killer white blood cells, American tanks were expendable. And like the tank, the gut is mobile and in normal conditions, its constant motion protects the body from stagnation. National Archives

For centuries there have been herbs and compounds used to remedy complaints such as cramping, constipation and diarrhea. Some of these are still in use. The opiates reduce bowel mobility and are useful in diarrhea but because of reducing bowel motion often cause constipation in the unprepared. Extracts from the belladonna plants have thousands of years of use in reducing abdominal discomfort (Donnatal). Laxatives or purgatives have been used to treat almost all maladies throughout history (fortunately today they are only used for constipation). Laxatives promote defecation or bowel movements by increasing bowel motility and are used to treat or prevent constipation. The definition of constipation varies but usually includes reduced frequency of stools, hard stools, reduced bowel sounds or bowel movements consisting of small firm "rabbit pellets". The most common cause of constipation is inadequate water intake, and the most common symptom of constipation is lower abdominal pain. Laxatives work by three main mechanisms. The first is by pulling water into the small bowel (osmotic laxatives) which soften, dilute and loosen the stools. Other laxatives block the reabsorption of water in the colon, therefore increasing the amount of water in the colon contents, thinning the stools. The last and most effective but uncomfortable, is by increasing gut motility by irritating the bowel. Powerful laxatives aim to push the contents through the lower bowel in a more rapid manner.

Fiber and bulk-forming laxatives are the most gentle and useful of the group, especially if used daily. It is not unusual for mild dehydration to occur at the beginning of going to sea. Sea sickness decreases fluid intake, along with diet change will all contribute to constipation. Using agents such as psyllium (Metamucil), malts (Maltsupex), cellulose (Citrucel) and plain bran reduces the risk of constipation and have been shown to also reduce cholesterol while lowering the incidence of colon cancer (the most common cancer in Americans). Use of bulk-forming laxatives requires increased fluids to work. Stronger laxatives are often necessary to treat when abdominal pain and straining at bowel movements becomes a problem. The more irritating agents include bisacodyl (Dulcolax), phenolphthalein (Modane), senna pods, cascara (bark of the buckthorn tree), docusate (Surfak, Colace), castor oil, and the most powerful over-the-counter laxative, lactulose (Chronulac).

Constipation is the most common cause of abdominal pain, is usually self-limiting but can lead to serious problems. A submarine medicine lecture involved an emergency appendectomy on a Soviet nuclear submarine. The ship's medical officer required surgery performed by an assistant under the medical officer's direct supervision. When ask why the vessel did not surface and obtain better medical attention. "It was not appropriate place for the ship to surface at that time and place".

Antidiarrheal agents are some of the oldest drugs used by Ships Surgeons, since diarrhea is a common and ancient malady. Tincture of opium was carried in medicine chest for centuries, only recently replaced by safer preparations. Paregoric is a modern tincture of opium used to control chronic diarrhea and colic in infants, while diphenoxylate (Lomotil) is the most common opiate used for the diarrhea encountered by travelers. Opiates must be used carefully in children as they can be absorbed into the blood stream and cause respiratory depression and bowel paralysis. A metal, bismuth subsalicylate (Pepto-Bismol) is effective but must be used in large doses and repeated frequently.

Drugs for Nausea and Vomiting

Nausea and vomiting have several causes and several treatments. Acupressure, wristbands, skin patches, pills, suppositories and injections may all be effective in the management of nausea. Although nausea and vomiting are usually self-limiting and pass even without treatment, it can be serious. Persistent nausea and vomiting can lead to dehydration causing kidney damage and possibly shock. It is sometimes difficult to determine if an ill person is keeping enough fluid down, and the best method of measuring the person's fluid balance is the amount and color of urine. In prolonged nausea and vomiting, monitor the color and components of urine which reflect the body's fluid supply. Adequate fluid intake results in urine that is clear to light yellow, flows freely with regularity and contains no abnormal chemicals. The presence of dark, strong-smelling urine in scanty, infrequent amounts, means dehydration.

Nausea and vomiting of seasickness, even in a mild form, causes moderate distress to most people. Distress that can decrease their effectiveness, making it worthwhile to treat. In preventing seasickness, the scopolamine (Transdermal Scop) patches are sometimes effective. These work best if applied eight to twelve hours before sailing or in the face of oncoming rough weather. Ephedrine, Reglan (metoclopramide) or the mixture of promethazine and pseudoephedrine are generally effective after seasickness has begun. Antihistamines such as Benadryl, Atarax and Dramamine are also effective for many sailors. Injectable drugs such as Phenergan (promethazine), Compazine (prochlorperazine), Tigan (trimethobenzamide) and Valium (diazepam) may be necessary when the person is unable to keep pills down. In the author's opinion, the very best injectable for nausea is ondansetron. It is safe, almost always effective and can be given with tiny needle just under skin (subcutaneous) injection.

Actigall is a new drug made from dried cow gall bladder contents that has become the mainstay in non-surgical treatment of gall stones. In addition to reducing the formation of gall stones and the dissolving of the stones present, bile acids in Actigall reduce the abdominal discomfort by reducing motility and perhaps by tranquilizing the gut. It will dissolve stones over 12-24 months while reducing abdominal discomfort within days. Ox gall has been in use since Egyptian times for the relief of abdominal pain and not normally a component of a field medicine chest.

December 7, 1941

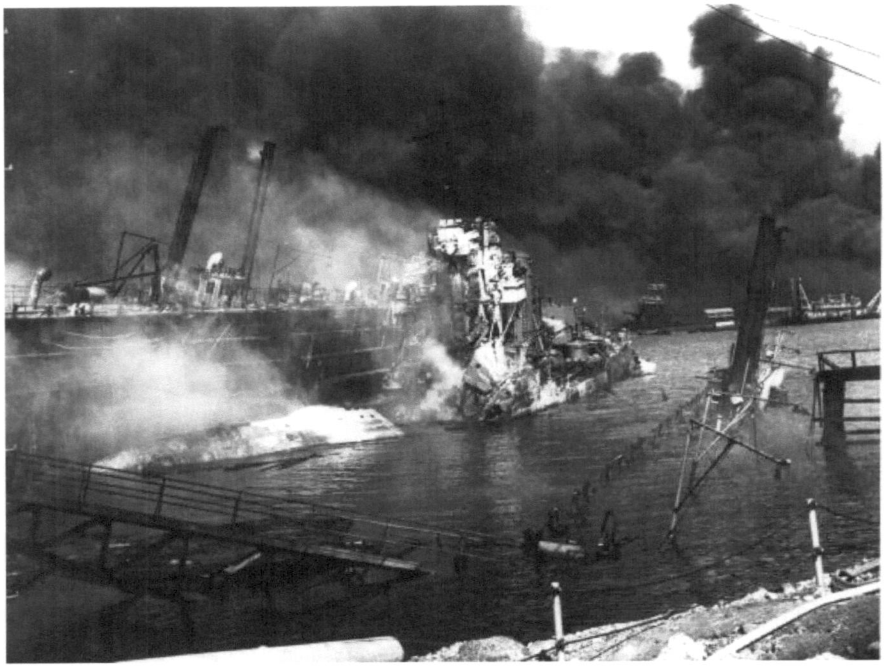

When Japan attacked Pearl Harbor and the United States entered World War II, America not only had a small army (17th largest in the world) but an inadequate number of medical services to cope with a world war. In 1941 there were no stores of penicillin or sulfa (the first effective antibiotics in human history), few surgeons trained in trauma, no effective treatment of shock without whole fresh blood, no system to pull medical personnel from their civilian duties into service and the machinery to increase training of new physicians and nurses as well as converting pharmaceuticals companies to produce wartime products. On the date above, the medical department of the US Navy, staffed by personnel long in years and short in combat experience consisted of 1,957 physicians and surgeons, 511 dentists, 10,187 corpsmen, 524 nurses worldwide. Three years later, October 1944 found an American fleet floating on Leyte Gulf invading the Philippines. The Battle of Leyte Gulf was not only the largest sea battle in the Second World, but it was also the largest sea battle in history. Field medicine's presence in the invasion was significant in its size and experience due to the high priority the military placed on medical care of the wounded. The fleet carried thousands of younger seasoned medical officers augmented by tens of thousands of trained and experienced medical, 200,000 tons of medical supplies all brought by sea. The investment in training and supply during the Second World War resulted in successfully treating 98% of the became ill and injured causalities. A vast improvement over the medical care of the First World War, primarily due to management of shock, discovery of medications, especially penicillin and IV plasma. National Archives

As stated before, the author begins the lecture series in field medicine with the concept if one could go back in time to the beginning of the Second World War, the student would be one of the world's premium field medical officers. This manuscript and a modern medicine chest would enable the field medical officer to diagnosis and treat problems in the field the mid-20th century medical officer would marvel at the knowledge and medicine chest. Management of heart attacks, trauma, shock, infections and many medical problems can now be successfully treated in the hands of non-professional individuals, as it has been done throughout history. If this text has been read, studied and comprehended, the author has reached the goal of writing this book. *Physician* is Greek word for "teacher" and hopefully "Medicine at Sea" has provided some teaching, some entertainment and stimulating the search for more medical knowledge.

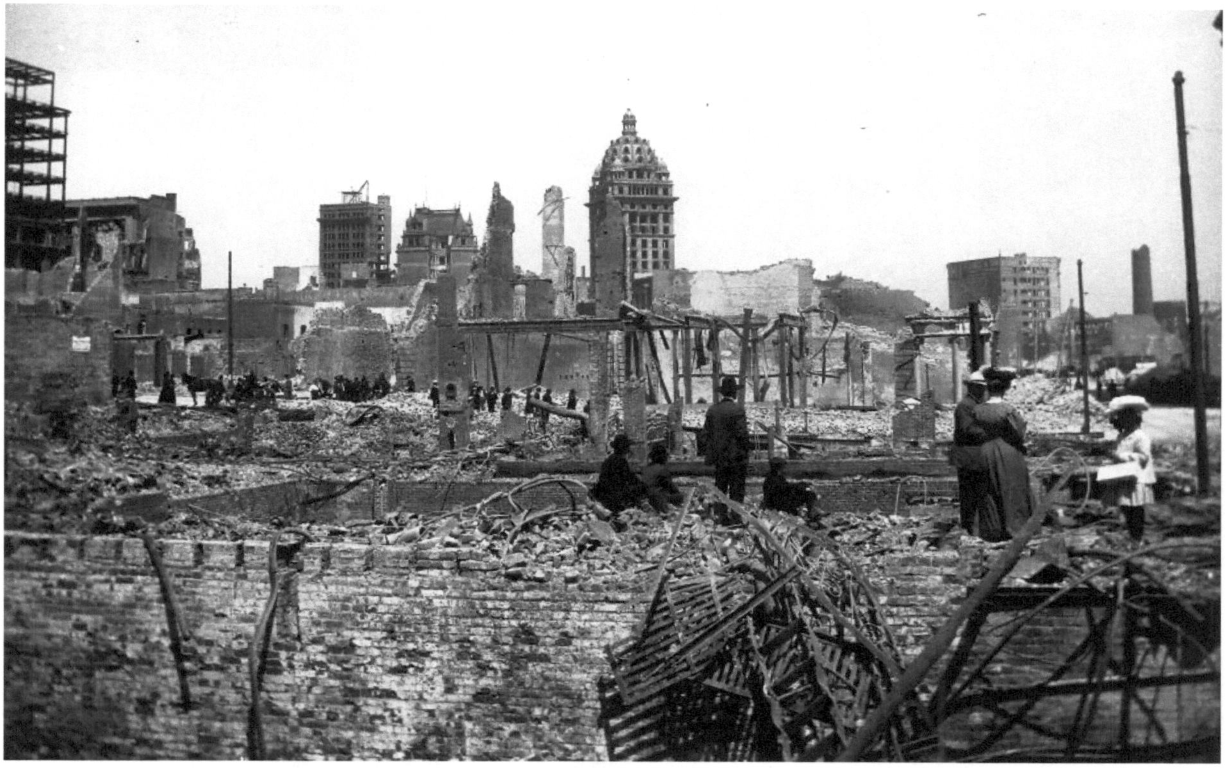

Earthquakes can remove medical services immediately, leaving victims to their own devices. The trauma to infrastructure and the fragile human body can be immense, with open fractures, penetrating objects and burns. Injuries resulting in tetanus and deep infections. The author recommends current Td immunization, and a pneumonia shot along with supply of antibiotics, wound dressings and the ability to recognize and manage shock. National Archives

The Medicine Chest

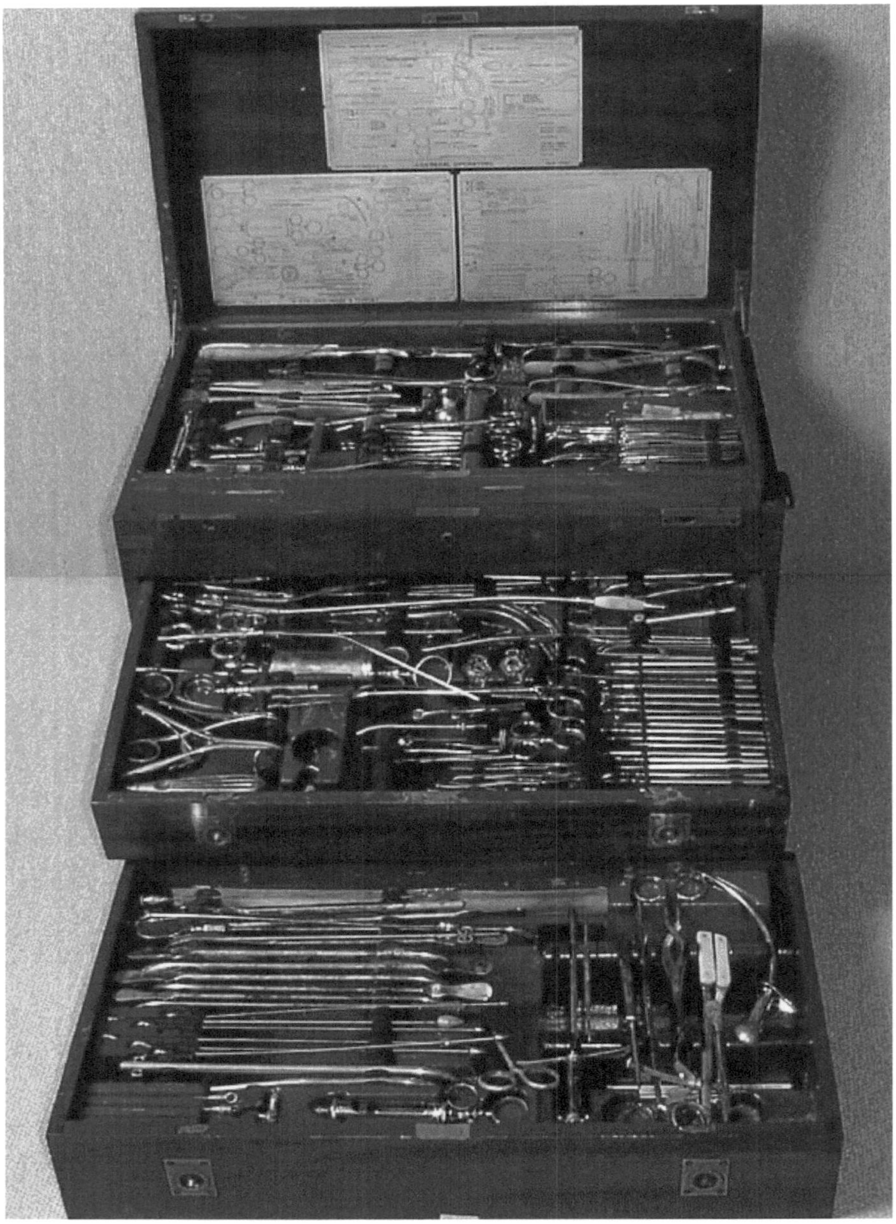

The late 19th century medicine chest above was primarily composed of hard and in many cases sharp cutting edges. Only a few instruments have found a place in the modern medicine chest instead containing soft plastic, soft pliable objects. The medicine chest has evolved greatly since the Second War, evolving into a small, effective and user-friendly unit. The chest above came off a late 19th United State Navy warship and would have changed little into the Great War 1914-1918.

Kits

Wound care
Silvadene, betadine, non-stick, sponges, tape, roll gauze

Trauma
Large blue pads, blanket, ace wraps,

Eye
Irrigation, lubrication, antibiotic sol and ointment, patches, tape

Wound closure
Steri-strips/glue, closure tape, surgical wound closure kit (includes material, needle drivers, local anesthetic)

Surgery
Suture kit, splinter removal, I&D kit, scalpel, anesthesia, injection of lidocaine

Burn
Silvadene, adaptic (non-stick dressing), sponges, roll gauze, compression wrap

Antibiotics
Amoxicillin, cephalexin, Zithromax, sulfa, doxycycline
Cephalexin class drug injection, injection kit (3cc syringe, 22 gauge needle)

Irrigation
Large syringe, irrigation fluid (any clean water), small flex tubing

Chest pain
Aspirin, beta blocker (metoprolol 50mg), nitroglycerin skin patch, angiotensin blocker, diuretic, calcium channel blocker

Fluid replacement
Powdered electrolytes or dilute saline solution-one teaspoon in liter of water

Diagnostic
Manuel blood pressure cuff, stethoscope, thermometer, flashlights (at least two), urine tests strips, consider ear scope or fiber-optic attachment for cell phone

Injection
Dexamethasone 4mg/cc 1-2 cc intramuscular every 4 hours as needed for shock, severe allergic reaction
bee sting/anaphylaxis kit (epinephrine, diphenhydramine)
Ondansetron (Zofran) 2mg/cc 1-2 cc subcutaneous (just under skin) for nausea/vomiting
IV solution-dextrose/normal saline-can be given rectally if an intravenous infusion not available

Miscellaneous medications
most are prescription in US, often over the counter in many countries
Diphenhydramine tablets 25mg 1-2 q 4-6 hours for allergies, sedation, nausea, itching

Respiratory
to reduce breathing complaints, helpful in bronchitis
Steroid/bronchodilator inhaler (Singular, Symbicort) for wheezing/asthma
Prednisone 5mg for severe asthma (use carefully)

Gastrointestinal
primarily for moving stool and for gastritis
Laxative for constipation-Metamucil, Miralax, Ducolax, Senokot
for more severe constipation use linaclotide (Linzess), extremely effective, always use increase fluid intake with constipation
Omeprazole 20mg 1 q day for heartburn, suspected gastritis, GI bleeding

Cardiac
blood pressure control, chest pain of heart disease
Beta blockers-metoprolol, atenolol, propranolol
ACE inhibitors-benazepril, captopril, enalapril, the best of this class include angiotensin receptor blockers-losartan, valsartan
Calcium channel blockers-nifedipine, diltiazem, Norvasc

Eye
primarily antibiotics, erythromycin, ciprofloxin-ointments more effective, however drops are easier to apply, treat both eyes

Skin
primarily antibiotics and steroid apply directly onto affected area
Antibiotics-silver/sulfa compound (Silvadene), bacitracin
Steriods-triamcinalone 1% ointment or cream, ointment more effective, hydrocortisone cream less effective than triamcinolone but can be used over longer periods, avoid stronger steroids such as those augmented with halogens such as fluorine such as fluocinolone especially on mucus membranes
Fungicides-clotrimazole, miconazole, ketoconazole, and terbinafine. Some are available in pill form for more difficult skin fungal infections such as toenail infections

Pain Relief
reducing pain in the field is important and has saved lives in trauma-induced shock since severe pain participates and may precipitate a falling blood pressure
Tylenol-500mg 1-2 q 6-8 hours, safe and effective
NSAIDs-ibuprofen, Naprosyn and many others are not always safe, used carefully at a low a dose as effective and for as short of time as possible
Opiates-considered the "gold standard" in pain management and like NSAIDs used at the lowest effective dose and for as short of time as possible. Codeine, morphine, hydrocodone, oxycodone and others are highly effective but have several side effects, the most serious is over- dosing, itching, nausea and constipation are the most common, recommended to add laxative if opiates used more than a few doses
Buprenorphine although not an opiate is highly effective and safe, long acting, effective quickly when absorbed in oral cavity, less effective if swallowed

Dressings-gauze in squares and in rolls, non-stick dressings (Adaptic)
ACE wraps-2 and 4" rolls, Q-tips, betadine on drumsticks, antibiotic soaps such as phisohex and all antideordorantnelson soap bars, with large wounds and burns, dressings must be changed daily requiring a large amount of soft absorbent dressings

Other medications may be needed for those with specific medical problems will require some not on the above lists.

The author recommends avoiding calling attention to the medicine chest containers painted bright red with white cross as it is valuable and often difficult to replace. Former students had chests taken after exposing and using the kit.

In conclusion, a modern medicine chest and the knowledge to use is it can be invaluable in situations where no other medical care is available. Medications alone are not effective unless combined with the patient's history and examination. There is no replacement for listening completely to the story about the complaint and a thorough examination using eyes, hands and diagnostic instruments. Do not make the mistake of sizing on the first diagnosis that "pops" into one's head. An example of focusing on something like appendicitis in abdominal pain. Appendicitis is more dramatic but unlikely to cause most abdominal pain. Take time, listen, touch, reassure, and consider all possibilities in managing medicine in the field. This text and the medicine chest is not meant for someone to be their own doctor when quality medical is accessible. The author's students report in travels, they were often better equipped than the local clinics to deal with their own difficulties. Good luck, hopefully keep the wind at your back, and approach medical problems with confidence and humility.

One of the secrets about medicine, it is mostly self-taught, one patient at a time.

www.ingramcontent.com/pod-product-compliance
Lightning Source LLC
LaVergne TN
LVHW070943210926
848482LV00002B/81
* 9 7 9 8 3 4 9 2 9 9 6 5 0 *